W9-CDC-448

Operative Laparoscopy
and Thoracoscopy

Operative Laparoscopy and Thoracoscopy

Editors

Bruce V. MacFadyen, Jr., M.D.
Professor
Department of Surgery
The University of Texas Medical School
Houston, Texas

Jeffrey L. Ponsky, M.D.
Professor and Vice Chairman
Department of Surgery
Case Western Reserve University School of Medicine
Cleveland, Ohio

With illustrations by Jan Ruvido

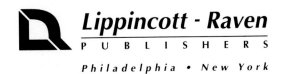

Lippincott - Raven
P U B L I S H E R S

Philadelphia • New York

Lippincott-Raven Publishers, 227 East Washington Square,
Philadelphia, Pennsylvania 19106-3780

Printed in Hong Kong

Library of Congress Cataloging-in-Publication Data

Operative laparoscopy and thoracoscopy / edited by Bruce V. MacFadyen,
    Jr., Jeffrey L. Ponsky.
        p.   cm.
    Includes bibliographical references and index.
    ISBN 0-7817-0279-8
    1. Abdomen—Endoscopic surgery.   2. Laparoscopy.   3. Chest—
Endoscopic surgery.   4. Thoracoscopy.   I. MacFadyen, Bruce V.,
1942–   . II. Ponsky, Jeffrey L.
    [DNLM: 1. Surgery, Laparoscopic—methods.   2. Laparoscopy.
3. Thoracoscopy.   WO 500 O6016 1996]
    RD540.O655   1996
    617.5′5059—dc20
    DNLM/DLC
    for Library of Congress   95-20399

The material contained in this volume was submitted as previously
unpublished material, except in the instances in which credit has been given to
the source from which some of the illustrative material was derived.

Great care has been taken to maintain the accuracy of the information
contained in the volume. However, neither Lippincott-Raven Publishers nor
the editors can be held responsible for errors or for any consequences arising
from the use of the information contained herein.

Materials appearing in this book prepared by individuals as part of their
official duties as U.S. Government employees are not covered by the above-
mentioned copyright.

9   8   7   6   5   4   3   2   1

To our wives, Rosemary and Jackie, and to our children.
We are greatly indebted for their help, patience, and understanding
during the many hours required to write this book.

Contents

Section VII. Retroperitoneum

Section VIII. Stomach

Section IX. Colon and Small Bowel

Section X. Hernia

Section XI. Thoracoscopy

Section XII. Future Technology

Contributing Authors

Mohan C. Airan, M.D.
Clinical Professor of Surgery
Finch University
Chicago Medical School
2340 Highland Avenue, Suite 250
Lombard, Illinois 60148-5396

Charles H. Andrus, M.D., F.A.C.S.
Associate Professor
Department of Surgery
St. Louis University
3635 Vista at Grand Boulevard
P.O. Box 15250
St. Louis, Missouri 63110

Maurice E. Arregui, M.D., F.A.C.S.
Director of Fellowship in Laparoscopy,
  Endoscopy, and Ultrasound
Department of Surgery
St. Vincent Hospital and Health Care
  Center
8402 Harcourt Road
Suite 811
Indianapolis, Indiana 46260

Robert W. Bailey, M.D., F.A.C.S.
Chief
Division of General Surgery
Greater Baltimore Medical Center
6569 North Charles Street
Suite 304
Baltimore, Maryland 21204

Robert W. Beart, M.D.
Professor
Department of Surgery
University of Southern California School
  of Medicine
1510 San Pablo, #514
Los Angeles, California 91103

George Berci, M.D., F.A.C.S, F.R.C.S.
Clinical Professor of Surgery
University of Southern California School
  of Medicine
EndoCare Center
Midway Hospital
5901 West Olympic Boulevard
Suite 405
Los Angeles, California 90036

Desmond H. Birkett, M.D.
Associate Professor of Surgery
Department of Surgery
Boston University School of Medicine
88 East Newton Street, D-507
Boston, Massachusetts 02118

Robert J. Burnett, M.D.
Senior Surgical Resident
Department of Surgery
University of Cincinnati College
  of Medicine
P.O. Box 670558
Cincinnati, Ohio 45267-0558

Stephen D. Carey, M.D.
Clinical Assistant Professor of Surgery
Department of Surgery
F. Edward Hibent School of Medicine
Bethesda, Maryland 20892

Ralph V. Clayman, M.D.
Professor of Urology and Radiology
Department of Surgery (Urology)
  and Radiology
Washington University/Barnes Hospital
#1 Barnes Hospital Plaza, Queeny Tower
Suite 5101
St. Louis, Missouri 63110

Thomas L. Dent, M.D.
Chairman
Department of Surgery
Abington Memorial Hospital
1200 Old York Road
Abington, Pennsylvania 19001

David W. Duppler, M.D.
Staff Physician
Department of Surgery
Appleton Medical Center
1818 North Meade Street
Appleton, Wisconsin 54911

David S. Edelman, M.D., F.A.C.S.
Director
The Gallbladder and Laparoscopic
  Surgery Center of Miami
8720 North Kendall Drive
Suite 204
Miami, Florida 33176

Douglas B. Evans, M.D.
Associate Professor of Surgery
Department of Surgical Oncology
University of Texas
M.D. Anderson Cancer Center
1515 Holocombe Boulevard
Houston, Texas 77030

Charles J. Filipi, M.D.
Associate Professor
Department of Surgery
Creighton University School of Medicine
601 North 30th Street
Omaha, Nebraska 68131

Aaron S. Fink, M.D.
Associate Professor
Department of Surgery
Emory University School of Medicine
1365 Clifton Road, N.E.
Atlanta, Georgia 30322; and
Chief, Surgical Service
Veteran Affairs Medical Center-Atlanta
1670 Clairmont Road
Decatur, Georgia 30033

Morris E. Franklin, Jr., M.D., F.A.C.S.,
  F.I.C.S.
Professor of Surgery
Director, Texas Endosurgery Institute
University of Texas Health Science
  Center
4242 East Southcross
San Antonio, Texas 78222

Eckart Frimberger, M.D.
Department of Gastroenterology
Medizinische Klinik
Ismaninger Strasse 22
8000 Munich 80
Germany

Nancy L. Furumoto, M.D.
Assistant Professor
Department of Surgery
University of Hawaii
321 North Kuakini Street, #305
Honolulu, Hawaii 96817

Michel Gagner, M.D., F.R.C.S.C.,
  F.A.C.S.
Associate Professor of Surgery
Department of General Surgery
The Cleveland Clinic Foundation
Cleveland, Ohio 44195

M. M. Gazayerli, M.D.
Laparoscopic Laser Surge-on Institute
1555 West Big Beaver Road
Building G, Suite E-18
Troy, Michigan 48084-3525

Peter M. Y. Goh, M.D., M.B.B.S.,
  F.R.C.S., F.A.M.S.
Associate Professor and Chief
Minimally Invasive Surgical Centre
National University Hospital
Lower Kent Ridge Road
Singapore 0511
Malaysia

John N. Graber, M.D., F.A.C.S.
Chairman, Institute for Minimally
  Invasive Therapy
Abbott Northwestern Hospital
Clinical Instructor of Surgery
Department of Surgery
University of Minnesota
2545 Chicago Avenue South
Minneapolis, Minnesota 55404

Richard Graves, M.D.
Assistant Professor
Department of Obstetrics and Gynecology
Division of Gynecology
University of California
Davis School of Medicine
1621 Alhambra Boulevard, Suite 2500
Sacramento, California 95818

Frederick L. Greene, M.D.
Professor of Surgery
Director of Surgical Oncology
  and Endoscopy
Department of Surgery
University of South Carolina School
  of Medicine
Columbia, South Carolina 29203

Mohamed Hakky, M.D., M.B.B.Ch., M.Sc.
Chairman
Department of General Surgery
  and Laparoscopy
Egypt Air Hospital
38 Gamet El Doul Al Arabia Street
12411 Imbaba
Cairo, Egypt

Makoto Hashizume, M.D., Ph.D.
Assistant Professor
Department of Surgery II
Faculty of Medicine
Kyushu University
3-1-1 Maidashi, Higashi-ku
Fukuoka 812-82
Japan

Stephen R. Hazelrigg, M.D.
Associate Professor and Chairman
Department of Cardiothoracic Surgery
Southern Illinois University
School of Medicine
800 N. Rutledge, Room D317
P.O. Box 19230
Springfield, Illinois 62794-9230

Hosam S. Helmy, M.D.
Lecturer, Department of Surgery
Cairo University
Cairo, Egypt

David F. Hickok, M.D.
Clinical Associate Professor
Department of Surgery
University of Minnesota Medical School
Abbot Northwestern Hospital
2545 Chicago Avenue South
Minneapolis, Minnesota 55405

Ronald A. Hinder, M.D., Ph.D., F.R.C.S., F.A.C.S.
Harry E. Stuckenhoff Chair of Surgery
Department of Surgery
Creighton University School of Medicine
601 North 30th Street
Omaha, Nebraska 68131

John G. Hunter, M.D., F.A.C.S.
Associate Professor
Department of Surgery
Emory University Hospital
1364 Clifton Road, N.E.
Atlanta, Georgia 30322

Daniel B. Jones, M.D.
Laparoscopy Fellow
Department of Surgery
Washington University
Barnes Hospital
One Barnes Hospital Plaza, Suite 6108
St. Louis, Missouri 63110

Robert K. Josloff, M.D.
Associate Professor
Temple University
Surgical Care Specialist, Inc.
1245 Highland Avenue
Suite 600
Abington, Pennsylvania 19001

Namir Katkhouda, M.D.
Associate Professor
Department of Surgery
University of Southern California
1510 San Pablo Street, Suite 514
Los Angeles, California 90033

Timothy King, PA-C
Coordinator of Physician Assistant
  Services
Department of Surgical Oncology
University of Texas
M.D. Anderson Cancer Center
1515 Holcombe Boulevard, Box 106
Houston, Texas 77030

Cheng K. Kum, M.B.B.S., F.R.C.S., F.A.M.S.
Senior Lecturer
Department of Surgery
National University Hospital
Lower Kent Ridge Road
Singapore 0511
Malaysia

Rodney J. Landreneau, M.D.
Associate Professor of Surgery
Department of Cardiothoracic Surgery
University of Pittsburgh
300 Kaufmann Building
3471 5th Avenue
Pittsburgh, Pennsylvania 15213

William S. Laycock, M.D.
Instructor in Surgery
Department of Surgery
Dartmouth-Hitchcock Medical Center
Lebanon, New Hampshire 03756

Tom Legge
Laparoscopic Laser Surge-on Institute
1555 West Big Beaver Road
Troy, Michigan 48084-3525

Jeffrey E. Lee, M.D.
Assistant Professor of Surgery
Department of Surgical Oncology
University of Texas
M.D. Anderson Cancer Center
1515 Holcombe Boulevard, Box 106
Houston, Texas 77030

E. Dwayne Lett, M.D.
Surgical Fellow
Department of Surgery
University of South Carolina School
*   of Medicine*
Columbia, South Carolina 29208

Demetrius E. M. Litwin, M.D.,
*   **F.R.C.S.(C)***
Assistant Professor
Department of Surgery
University of Toronto
Mount Sinai Hospital/The Toronto
*   Hospital*
600 University Avenue
Toronto, Ontario M5G 1X5
Canada

Bruce V. MacFadyen, Jr., M.D.
Professor
Department of Surgery
The University of Texas Medical School
6431 Fannin, #4292
Houston, Texas 77030

Michael J. Mack, M.D.
Clinical Assistant and Professor
Department of Thoracic Surgery
Southwestern Medical School
Medical City Dallas Hospital
7777 Forest Lane, A-323
Dallas, Texas 75230

Robert J. McKenna, Jr., M.D., F.A.C.S.
Assistant Clinical Professor
Department of Thoracic Surgery
University of Southern California
1245 Wilshire Boulevard
Suite 606
Los Angeles, California 90017

J. Barry McKernan, M.D., Ph.D.
Clinical Professor
Department of Surgery
Emory University School of Medicine
1364 Clifton Road, N.E.
Atlanta, Georgia 30322; and
Medical College of Georgia
1120 15th Street
Augusta, Georgia 30912-4000

John D. Mellinger, M.D., F.A.C.S.
Associate Professor
St. Mary's Health Services
Grand Rapids, Michigan 49503

Michael J. Miller, M.D.
Assistant Professor
Department of Plastic Surgery
The University of Texas
M.D. Anderson Cancer Center
1515 Holcombe Boulevard, Box 62
Houston, Texas 77030

Jean Mouiel, M.D., F.A.C.S.
Professor of Surgery
Chief, Department of Digestive Surgery,
*   Video Surgery, and Liver*
*   Transplantation*
University of Nice
St. Roch Hospital
5 Rue Pierre-Devolux
Nice 06006
France

Paul T. Morris, M.D.
Assistant Professor of Surgery
Department of General and Thoracic
*   Surgery*
John A. Burns School of Medicine
University of Hawaii
1960 East West Road
Honolulu, Hawaii 96822

Keith S. Naunheim, M.D.
Professor
Department of Surgery
St. Louis University
3635 Vista at Grand Boulevard
St. Louis, Missouri 63110

Douglas O. Olsen, M.D.
Assistant Clinical Professor of Surgery
Vanderbilt University
Baptist Hospital
2021 Church Street, Suite 502
Nashville, Tennessee 37203

Barry A. Salky, M.D.
Department of Surgery
Mount Sinai Medical Center
New York, New York 10029

Richard M. Satava, M.D., F.A.C.S.
Clinical Associate Professor of Surgery
Uniformed Services University of Health
   Sciences
Department of Surgery
Walter Reed Army Medical Center
Washington, D.C. 20307; and
Program Manager, Advanced Biomedical
   Technologies
Advanced Research Projects Agency
   (ARPA)
3701 North Fairfax Drive
Arlington, Virginia 22203

Bruce D. Schirmer, M.D.
Professor
Department of Surgery
University of Virginia Health Sciences
   Center
Box 181
Charlottesville, Virginia 22908

Leonard S. Schultz, M.D.
Clinical Assistant Professor of Surgery
University of Minnesota Hospitals
2545 Chicago Avenue South
Suite 611
Minneapolis, Minnesota 55404

Kurt K. S. Semm, M.D., F.R.C.O.G.
   (Ed), F.I.C.S. (hon)
Director of the Women's Clinic
Department of Obstetrics and Gynecology
Michaelis-School of Midwifery
Christian-Albrechts University
Michaelisstrasse 16
24105 Kiel
Germany

Robert W. Sewell, M.D.
350 Westpark Way
Suite 205
Euless, Texas 76034

Eric M. Smith, M.D.
Professor of Surgery
Chief Resident
Department of Urology
Case Western Reserve University
2074 Abington Road
Cleveland, Ohio 44106-5046

Lee E. Smith, M.D.
Professor
Department of Surgery
George Washington University
2150 Pennsylvania Avenue, N.W.
Washington, D.C. 20037

Roy T. Smoot, Jr., M.D.
Instructor
Department of Surgery
University of Maryland School
   of Medicine
22 South Greene Street
Baltimore, Maryland 21201; and
Chairman
Department of Surgery
Nanticoke Memorial Hospital
801 Middleford Road
Seaford, Delaware 19973

Nathaniel J. Soper, M.D.
Associate Professor
Department of Surgery
Washington University
Barnes Hospital
One Barnes Hospital Plaza
Suite 6108
St. Louis, Missouri 63110

Mary Lou Spitz, M.D.
Attending Surgeon
Department of General Surgery
St. Joseph Mercy Hospital
900 Woodward Avenue
Pontiac, Michigan 48341-2985

Charles A. Staley, M.D.
Assistant Professor of Surgery
Department of Surgical Oncology
Emory University School of Medicine
1365 Clifton Road NE
Atlanta, Georgia 30322

Thomas A. Stellato, M.D.
Professor of Surgery
Chief, Division of General Surgery
Case Western Reserve University
University Hospitals of Cleveland
11100 Euclid Avenue
Cleveland, Ohio 44106

Keizo Sugimachi, M.D., Ph.D., F.A.C.S.
Professor and Chairman
Department of Surgery II
Faculty of Medicine
Kyushu University
3-1-1 Maidashi
Fukuoka 812-82, Higashi-ku
Japan

David M. Ota, M.D.
Professor and Chief, Division of Surgical
  Oncology
Medical Director
Department of Surgery
University of Missouri
Ellis Fischel Cancer Center
115 Business Loop 70 West
Columbia, Missouri 65203

Margaret Paz-Partlow, M.F.A.
EndoCare Center
Midway Hospital
5901 West Olympic Boulevard
Suite 405
Los Angeles, California 90036

Margaret S. Pearle, M.D., Ph.D.
Assistant Professor of Urology
Department of Surgery
Division of Urology
The University of Texas Southwestern
  Medical School
5323 Harry Hines Boulevard
Dallas, Texas 75235-9110

Carlos A. Pellegrini, M.D.
Professor and Chairman
Department of Surgery
University of Washington Medical Center
1959 N.E. Pacific Avenue
Seattle, Washington 98195

Joseph B. Petelin, M.D., F.A.C.S.
Clinical Assistant Professor
Department of Surgery
University of Kansas School of Medicine
9119 West 74th Street
Suite 255
Shawnee Mission, Kansas 66204

Edward H. Phillips, M.D., F.A.C.S.
Director of Endoscopic Surgery
Department of Surgery
Cedars-Sinai Medical Center
8700 Beverly Boulevard
Los Angeles, California 90048; and
Clinical Associate Professor of Surgery
Department of Surgery
University of Southern California
Los Angeles County Medical Center
Los Angeles, California 90048

Jeffrey L. Ponsky, M.D.
Professor and Vice Chairman
Department of Surgery
Case Western Reserve University School
  of Medicine
University Circle
Cleveland, Ohio 44106

Joe B. Putnam, Jr., M.D.
Associate Professor of Surgery
Department of Thoracic and
  Cardiovascular Surgery
University of Texas
M.D. Anderson Cancer Center
1515 Holcombe Boulevard, Box 109
Houston, Texas 77030

Jose M. Ramos, M.B.B.Ch., F.C.S.(SA)
Consultant Surgeon
Department of Surgery
University of the Witwatersrand
7 York Road, Parktown 2193
Johannesburg
South Africa

Martin I. Resnick, M.D.
Professor and Chairman
Department of Urology
Case Western Reserve University
11100 Euclid Avenue
Cleveland, Ohio 44106-5046

Arlene E. Ricardo, M.D.
Resident
Department of Surgery
The University of Texas Medical School
6431 Fannin
Houston, Texas 77030

Mark W. Roberts, M.D.
Resident Surgeon
Department of Surgery
University of California
Davis Medical Center
2315 Stockton Boulevard
Sacramento, California 95817

Jonathan M. Sackier, M.D., F.R.C.S.
Associate Professor
Department of Surgery
George Washington University
2150 Pennsylvania Avenue, N.W.
#415
Washington, D.C. 20037

Lee L. Swanström, M.D.
Clinical Associate Professor of Surgery
Department of Minimally Invasive
  Surgery
Oregon Health Sciences University
501 North Graham Street
Suite 120
Portland, Oregon 97227

Kenji Takenaka, M.D., Ph.D.
Associate Professor
Department of Surgery II
Faculty of Medicine
Kyushu University
3-1-1 Maidashi
Fukuoka 812-82, Higashi-ku
Japan

Hugh R. Taylor, M.D.
Division of General Surgery
University of Toronto
Mount Sinai Hospital
600 University Avenue, Room 1225
Toronto M5G 1X5
Canada

Frederick K. Toy, M.D., F.A.C.S.,
  F.C.C.M.
Clinical Instructor
Department of Surgery
University of Maryland School of
  Medicine
22 South Greene Street
Baltimore, Maryland 21201; and
Nanticoke Memorial Hospital
801 Middleford Road
Seaford, Delaware 19973

Stephen W. Unger, M.D.
Director, Surgical Endoscopy
  and Laparoscopy
Department of Surgery
Mount Sinai Medical Center of Greater
  Miami
4302 Alton Road
Suite 820
Miami Beach, Florida 33140

Harold C. Urschel, Jr., M.D.
Professor of Thoracic and Cardiovascular
  Surgery
University of Texas Southwestern Medical
  School
Baylor University Medical Center
3600 Gaston Avenue
Suite 1201
Dallas, Texas 75246

Rosario Vecchio, M.D.
Clinica Chirurgic III
University Di Catania
% Aspedale Victtorio Emanuele
Via Plebiscito 628
Catania 95100, Italy

Garrett L. Walsh, M.D., M.Sc.,
  F.R.C.S.(C), F.A.C.S.
Assistant Professor of Surgery
Department of Thoracic and
  Cardiovascular Surgery
The University of Texas
M.D. Anderson Cancer Center
1515 Holcombe Boulevard
Houston, Texas 77030

Gerold J. Wetscher, M.D.
Research Fellow
Department of Surgery
Creighton University School of Medicine
601 North 30th Street
Omaha, Nebraska 68131

David J. Winchester, M.D.
Assistant Professor
Department of Surgery
Evanston Hospital
Northwestern University Medical School
2650 Ridge Avenue
Evanston, Illinois 60201

Catherine M. Wittgen, M.D.
Clinical Fellow
Department of Surgery
Division of Vascular Surgery
Massachusetts General Hospital
Harvard Medical School
15 Parkman Street
Boston, Massachusetts 02114

Bruce M. Wolfe, M.D.
Professor
Department of Surgery
University of California
Davis Medical Center
4301 X Street, Room 2310
Sacramento, California 95817

Karl A. Zucker, M.D.
Professor
Department of Surgery
University of New Mexico
718 Encino Place
Albuquerque, New Mexico 87131

Foreword

Good surgical practice entails more than competent execution of operative procedures, and this aspect of our profession has become more important in recent years with the advent of laparoscopic surgery and the reduction in the national health budget of various countries. However, unsavory as it may appear to physicians and surgeons, there is a limit, irrespective of the wealth of any nation, to the amount of the national income that can be allocated to the provision of private and public health services. In this respect, financial accountability and health economic considerations are here to stay and will dominate health budgets in the future.

Drs. MacFadyen and Ponsky must have had this message in mind when outlining the core essence of this excellent manual of operative laparoscopic surgical practice and, in my view, this aspect distinguishes this book from the many others that have preceded it. This book reflects the fact that the days of the surgical laparoscopic explosion or revolution are over and we are not at the mature phase of evaluation and critical appraisal of these new procedures. However, the book focuses on how these procedures are done safely and whether they really impart any benefit to the patient or health practice.

The book covers most of the surgical procedures on operative laparoscopy and thoracoscopy that have been introduced into clinical practice since the late eighties, and the editors have recruited a team of contributors that includes some of the pioneers and leading authorities in laparoscopic and thoracoscopic surgery. Each chapter provides background information on the current state on the subject together with a clear description of the operative steps of each procedure that are illustrated by excellent drawings and color photographs. Equally important is the emphasis throughout the book on both the advantages and the limitations of the various laparoscopic procedures. In this respect the various contributors have followed the directives of the two editors resulting in the cohesiveness of this operative manual. Furthermore, the morbidity of these various operations is emphasized, highlighting the importance of training in achieving surgical laparoscopic operative competence.

It is my view that this book will be well received as a useful and important addition to the established literature on the subject and by general surgeons who practice minimal access surgery. The two editors are to be congratulated for producing a volume that is both instructive and highly educational.

Alfred Cuschieri, M.D., Ch.M., F.R.C.S., F.R.C.P.S. (Hon), Fl.Biol.
Professor and Head, Department of Surgery
Centre for Surgical Skills, University of Dundee;
Honorary Consultant Surgeon
Ninewells Hospital Trust
Dundee, United Kingdom

Preface

With the introduction of video laparoscopy and new instrumentation and techniques over the past 5 to 10 years, the use of the laparoscope has developed greatly in general and thoracic surgery. When the first cholecystectomy was performed in 1987 by Mouret in France and later described and promoted by Perrisat, DuBois, Reddick, Olsen, and McKernan, general and thoracic surgeons saw the tremendous potential for the application of this new technique. This surgical revolution continues with 3-dimensional video laparoscopy and the emerging fields of robotics, tele-presence surgery, and virtual reality.

Several surgical textbooks have been written describing operative techniques and technology in this rapidly developing field. However, this book was written for the clinical surgeon to address the issues of not only *how* but *why* a procedure is performed. Each chapter illustrates pertinent anatomy and defines efficient and effective preoperative planning, and indications and contraindications so the surgeon is well prepared preoperatively. The pertinent steps to efficient intraoperative management is the primary feature of each chapter and includes potential complications. Surgical pearls are also provided to help the reader prevent or correct any potential problems.

Another important feature of this book is its inclusion of contributions from experts around the world. Authors were chosen not only because they were competent clinical surgeons but also for their vast experience. This aspect provides the reader with the decision-making process necessary for efficient and effective surgical care. It also gives the reader a more in-depth view of surgical treatment and the rationale for preoperative, intraoperative, and postoperative management. Each chapter contains Key Words to help the surgeon identify the important subjects. The diagrams, photographs, and illustrations clearly describe all aspects of patient management. The reader will find this book understandable, usable, and extremely applicable in clinical surgical practice.

Operative Laparoscopy and Thoracoscopy contains the latest clinical procedures and will aid the beginning laparoscopist in becoming more familiar with these techniques and will be useful as a refresher for the most experienced laparoscopist. There are several procedures that are particularly unique and have not been previously published in operative laparoscopy books. These include the laparoscopic management of the acute abdomen, trauma, pancreatic surgery, adrenalectomy, pancreatic pseudocyst management, spine surgery, liver resection, endoluminal rectal surgery, and esophageal surgery. Inclusion of all these techniques will bring the clinical surgeon up-to-date.

This book is particularly useful in the cost-conscious medical world. The chapter on the economic and environmental considerations in laparoscopic surgery explains the economic issues with regard to the physician, hospital administration, insurance company, and government. Attention to these issues will encourage the surgeon to be quality-oriented and cost-effective in conjunction with his/her management plan.

The unique formatting of chapters, the vast experience of the contributors, and the most applicable laparoscopic and thoracoscopic procedures in one source combine to help the surgeon become more skilled and efficient.

Acknowledgments

Many people were responsible for bringing this project to completion. We want to thank each contributing author for their effort, time, and expertise in preparing their chapters. In addition, we would like to thank Lippincott-Raven Publishers for their tremendous support. In particular, Joyce-Rachel John, Jodi Borgenicht, and Dennis Teston, without whose insights, persistence, and expertise the project would not have been completed in a timely manner. We also thank our secretaries, Mary Carson and Stephanie Larson, for their help in preparing and organizing the manuscripts for review and completion and Jan Ruvido and Cindy Eller for the great illustrations they created for the book.

SECTION I

GENERAL CONSIDERATIONS

The History of Laparoscopic Surgery

Thomas A. Stellato
Division of General Surgery
Case Western Reserve University
University Hospitals of Cleveland
Cleveland, Ohio 44106

Operative Laparoscopy and Thoracoscopy, edited by B. V. MacFadyen, Jr. and J. L. Ponsky. Lippincott-Raven Publishers, Philadelphia © 1996.

As we approach the twenty-first century, a reflection upon the advances in medicine will support the contention that the twentieth century is truly the "Age of Laparoscopy." This endoscopic technique began in 1901, and other milestones and advances subsequently occurred throughout this century (Fig. 1). In spite of a somewhat glacial acceptance initially and later improvement of this technology, laparoscopy during the last decade of the twentieth century has produced an unprecedented impact on medical care with enormous societal, legal, and economic ramifications. The personalities, the instruments, and the procedures, which together define the history of laparoscopy, provide a fuller appreciation for this powerful technology we now identify as videolaparoscopy. In attempting to portray this history from its inception to the present, in this chapter the chronology of laparoscopy is arbitrarily divided into four era: origin, early human experience, technological advances, and modern laparoscopic therapeutics.

ORIGIN

The credit for being the first to perform laparoscopy is shared—perhaps arguably—by two innovative physicians separated by land, culture, and medical discipline: Dimitri Oskarovich Ott and Georg Kelling. The resolution of this debate demands a definition of what laparoscopy encompasses, that is, what constitutes

1901 ⟶ 1911 ⟶ 1929 ⟶ 1937 ⟶

Kelling   Jacobaeus   Kalk   Ruddock
| | | |
Canine   Man   Dual   USA
                                 Trocars

1938 ⟶ 1960's ⟶ 1966 ⟶ 1986

Veress   Semm   Hopkins   Computer
| | | Chip
Needle   Automatic   Rod-Lens   TV
                 Insufflation   System   Camera

Figure 1. Milestones and personalities shaping laparoscopy from its origin to videolaparoscopy. Refer to the text for details. (From Stellato, ref. 6, with permission.)

a laparoscopy. Dimitri Ott, a Russian gynecologist, has been credited by some as the first to perform laparoscopy. He published his first description of this subject in 1901. The procedure described by Ott consisted of inspecting the abdominal cavity by creating a small incision in the anterior abdominal wall or vagina through which a speculum was inserted. Illumination was provided by light reflected from a head mirror. Ott called this procedure "ventroscopy." The term "laparoscopy" is one of many used to describe the use of an endoscope to view the abdominal cavity.

Georg Kelling, a surgeon from Dresden, Germany, demonstrated a procedure he termed "Koelioscopie" in the same year (1901) Ott launched his technique. Under local anesthesia, Kelling used a Fiedler puncture needle to introduce filtered air into the peritoneal cavity (pneumoperitoneum), inserted a trocar into the abdomen, and then used the trocar to introduce a Nitze cystoscope (laparoscope). This procedure was performed on a live canine during the Seventy-third Congress of German Naturalists and Physicians.

If a strict definition of "laparoscopy" is demanded, especially in terms of the procedure as it has been known through most of this century, then Georg Kelling's procedure fulfills the requirements essential to laparoscopy as we know it today, and credit as the originator of laparoscopy belongs to him. If a more liberal definition of "laparoscopy" is applied, that is, the use of an instrument (the speculum as a precursor to the endoscope) to aid in viewing the abdominal cavity, then Dimitri Ott should be credited with the first laparoscopy. However, the cystoscope—not the speculum—commonly served as the vehicle for viewing the abdominal cavity by subsequent investigators.

Early Human Experience

Although Georg Kelling later reported his experience with laparoscopy in a small number of humans, the first major clinical contribution is attributed to Hans Christian Jacobaeus. Jacobaeus achieved the distinction of rising to Professor of Medicine at the Caroline Institute in Stockholm, and in 1925 was Chairman of the Nobel Committee. His first publication on laparoscopy appeared in 1910. Like Kelling, Jacobaeus used the cystoscope, but unlike Kelling, he expanded the limits to include the thoracic cavity. Jacobaeus coined the term "laparothorakoskopie." His initial experience was restricted to patients with ascites. In 1911, he reported 115 examinations in 72 patients—45 of whom underwent laparoscopy and 27 thoracoscopy. He was able to identify syphilis, tuberculosis, cirrhosis, and malignancy at laparoscopy. Subsequently, Jacobaeus directed his attention mainly to thoracoscopy. He developed the technique and was the first to perform operative thoracoscopy to divide pulmonary adhesions with galvanocautery. This allowed complete pneumothorax, which was the major treatment for pulmonary tuberculosis at that time.

By 1911, laparoscopy arrived in the United States. In that year, Bertram M. Bernheim, a surgeon from the Johns Hopkins University, reported in the *Annals of Surgery* on a procedure he termed ''organoscopy'' and referenced Jacobaeus in the introduction of the publication. Rather than a cystoscope, Bernheim utilized an ordinary proctoscope. Illumination was provided by an electric headlight. No pneumoperitoneum is described in his technique. The procedure compares more to a minilaparotomy with the proctoscope (laparoscope) introduced through an incision in the epigastrium and the light directed from the headlamp to illuminate the peritoneal cavity through the same incision. In spite of what must have been a cumbersome and difficult technique, Bernheim described his experience with two patients, one of whom was a patient of William Halsted, with cancer of the pancreas and obstructive jaundice. Bernheim performed an organoscopy and ruled out metastasis. His findings were confirmed at laparotomy, which we can assume was performed by Halsted. In the second patient Bernheim identified chronic appendicitis. He also described a technique to inspect the gastric mucosa. During the organoscopy, the stomach could be identified and pulled out the wound. An incision was made in the anterior gastric wall and the proctoscope inserted directly into the gastric lumen. Bernheim's report, although meager in clinical experience, documents the entry of laparoscopy in the United States.

Following Bernheim's publication, additional sporadic reports emanated from the United States. In 1924, W. E. Stone, from Topeka, Kansas, summarized the work of Jacobaeus, Renon (importance of laparoscopy in inspecting the liver), Orndorff (first to devise a sharp pyramidal-point trocar), and Rocavilla (designed an instrument that permitted the source of light to remain outside the abdomen), and reported his own experience using a nasopharyngoscope to perform ''peritoneoscopy.'' He meticulously described the steps necessary to perform the procedure, yet his own experience was limited to canines. Despite his lack of clinical experience, Stone arrived at several important conclusions. He suggested that identification of pelvic organs during peritoneoscopy could be aided by vaginal and rectal palpation. He also concluded that the examination could be performed under local anesthesia with minimal discomfort to the patient, and that the peritoneoscope could afford a means of arriving at a more exact diagnosis in some cases of obscure intraabdominal pathology without resorting to laparotomy.

Although laparoscopy was slowly developing a foundation as an important medical technology, awareness of its existence was far from universal. In 1924, Otto Steiner, from Atlanta, Georgia, published two papers, one in English and one in German, both entitled ''Abdominoscopy'' (''Abdominoskopie'' in German). Steiner included no references to prior work and suggested that the technique of abdominoscopy was a new method that had never been performed on a living patient or human cadaver. Interestingly, the technique he described utilized a cystoscope, a trocar, and oxygen to insufflate the abdomen. To his credit, he carefully detailed several maneuvers, such as inflating the stomach during the abdominoscopy procedure to visualize a greater area of the gastric surface and the repositioning of the patient to bring the gallbladder into view.

The following year (1925) Nadeau and Kampmeier reported on their own experimental and clinical studies with laparoscopy, as well as a scholarly summary of the 24 prior years of work, beginning with Kelling. This important manuscript with 42 references was published in *Surgery, Gynecology and Obstetrics*, the same journal in which Steiner's paper was published the previous year, where he claimed to have no knowledge of prior references. Although their report was both scholarly and lengthy (12 pages) Nadeau and Kampmeier's clinical experience consisted of only three patients. Nonetheless, their attention to detail makes for

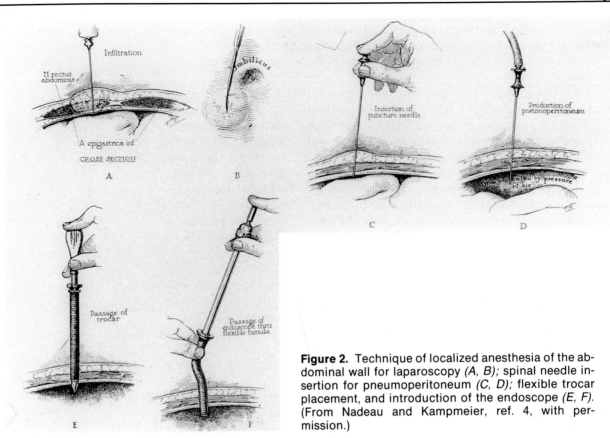

Figure 2. Technique of localized anesthesia of the abdominal wall for laparoscopy *(A, B);* spinal needle insertion for pneumoperitoneum *(C, D);* flexible trocar placement, and introduction of the endoscope *(E, F).* (From Nadeau and Kampmeier, ref. 4, with permission.)

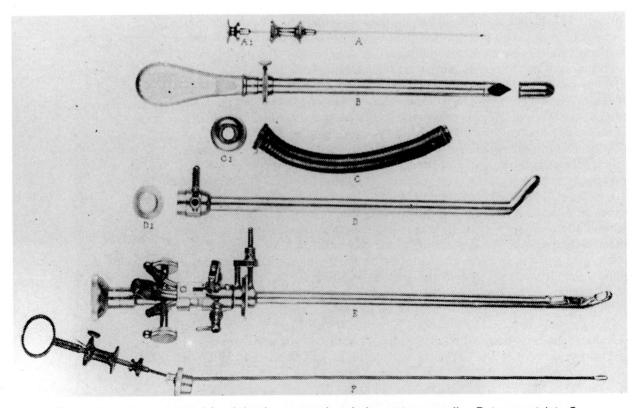

Figure 3. Instruments used in abdominoscopy: *A,* spiral puncture needle; *B,* trocar stylet; *C,* flexible trocar cannula; *D,* Braasch cystoscope (direct vision); *E,* Brown-Buerger cystoscope (indirect vision); *F,* operating forceps. (From Nadeau and Kampmeier, ref. 4, with permission.)

enjoyable reading. Figure 2 is taken from their paper, illustrating the method of local anesthesia, creation of a pneumoperitoneum, and the use of a flexible trocar, since the laparoscopes (cystoscopes) were angled. The angled cystoscopes and accessories used in laparoscopy during that era are shown in Fig. 3. Nadeau and Kampmeier recommended, as previously suggested by Orndorff, that advantage could be derived from inserting a second cystoscope into the bladder to allow transillumination of the bladder wall. They also reported that bimanual palpation of the pelvic organs during laparoscopy could improve inspection of that area. The importance of tilting the operating table was shown to improve the examination of the pelvis (Fig. 4) and the liver and diaphragm (Fig. 5).

The first report on laparoscopy from England was written in 1925 by a surgeon, A. Rendle Short, from the Bristol Royal Infirmary. Short concluded that coelioscopy (his term) had advantages over exploratory laparotomy, for example, "it can be done at the patient's own house." He also made the important observation that coelioscopy is "principally valuable for what is definitely seen and not for what is apparently absent."

TECHNOLOGICAL ADVANCES

Although there were numerous advocates of laparoscopy, in 1925 Nadeau and Kampmeier stated "the method is but little used." One explanation was the inade-

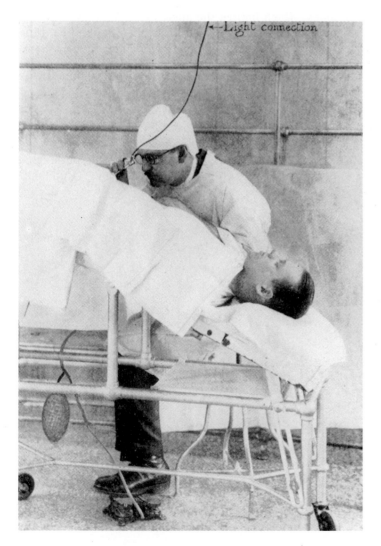

Figure 4. Tilting of the patient to permit an uninterrupted view of the pelvic interior. (From Nadeau and Kampmeier, ref. 4, with permission.)

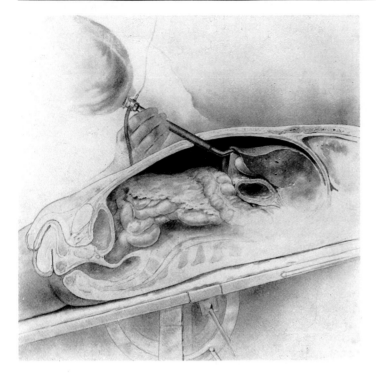

Figure 5. Tilting of the operative table to improve visualization of the liver and diaphragm. (From Nadeau and Kampmeier, ref. 4, with permission.)

quacy of the early cystoscopes, which limited the angle of vision to 90 degrees. In 1927, the German hepatologist, H. Kalk, devised a system of lenses that produced a forward viewing angle of 135 degrees. This modification, which greatly improved visualization during laparoscopy, remained essentially unchanged for three decades, and is credited with producing widespread adoption of the procedure. Kalk also introduced the dual trocar technique, which would later be a necessary component for therapeutic laparoscopy. In 1929, he reported his experience with 100 laparoscopic examinations, and 22 years later, in 1951, he reported his personal series of 2,000 laparoscopies without any deaths.

In 1933, C. Fervers reported his experience with peritoneoscopic burning of abdominal adhesions and peritoneal biopsy. Four years later, John C. Ruddock,

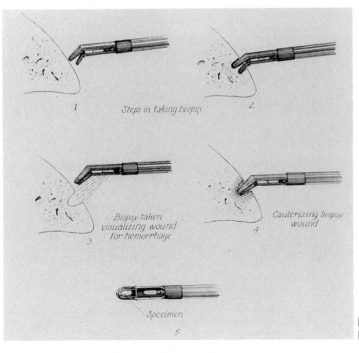

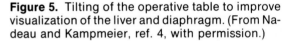

Figure 6. Technique of obtaining liver biopsy. (From Ruddock, ref. 5, with permission.)

an American physician, reported in *Surgery, Gynecology and Obstetrics* a personal series of 500 consecutive laparoscopies, including 39 biopsies, over a 4-year period—one of the earliest reports of a large series of biopsies (Fig. 6) and one of the first major clinical reports in the American medical literature. Ruddock recognized the importance of cytologic examination of ascitic fluid taken during laparoscopy and documented the usefulness of laparoscopy to evaluate a variety of malignancies (Figs. 7 and 8). Up to that time, instrumentation for laparoscopy could best be described as "makeshift." Ruddock perfected his own instruments and, more importantly, organized a complete set of laparoscopic instruments and accessories (Fig. 9), which subsequently became commercially available through ACMI.

In 1937, the same year as Ruddock's publication, E. T. Anderson, from Corpus Christi, Texas, published a report entitled "Peritoneoscopy," in the *American Journal of Surgery*. Anderson described a laparoscopic method for performing tubal ligation. In addition, he created an instrument he called a "gastrodiaphane," which would allow both insufflation and transillumination of the viscus into which it was inserted. He noted that the gastrodiaphane permitted dilation and illumination of the stomach or sigmoid colon during peritoneoscopy, and thus helped determine the operability of each of these organs.

As early as 1918, an automatic pneumoperitoneum needle was developed by O. Goetze. However, the spring-loaded needle developed by Janos Veress in 1938 remains almost unchanged to the present day. The Veress needle was initially created for use in the thorax as a means for safely creating pneumothorax in the treatment of tuberculosis. Today the Veress needle is used as a means to produce pneumoperitoneum in closed laparoscopy.

Although the safety of closed laparoscopy was greatly enhanced through the use of the spring-loaded Veress needle, injury to intraabdominal or retroperitoneal structures could still occur from either the needle itself or the first trocar, especially in the previously operated abdomen. Open laparoscopy reduces the likelihood of these complications. The difficulty of maintaining a pneumoperitoneum

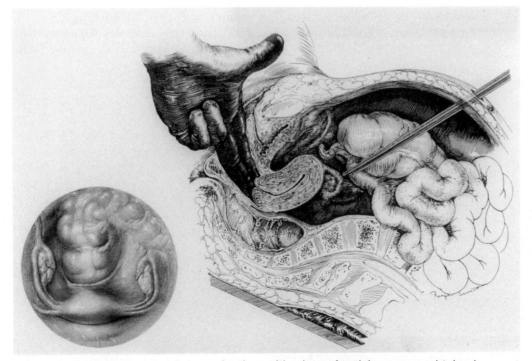

Figure 7. Technique of pelvic examination with view of pelvic organs obtained through a peritoneoscope after pneumoperitoneum is produced, and manipulation of pelvic organs through the vagina. (From Ruddock, ref. 5, with permission.)

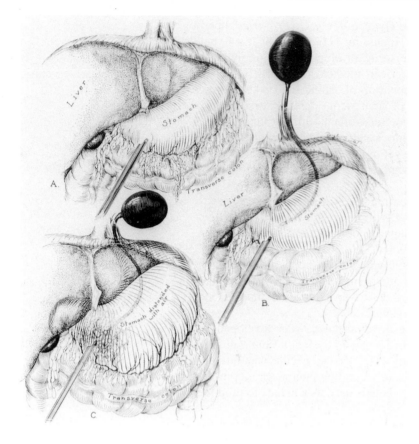

Figure 8. Operability of gastric malignancy. *A,* visualizing stomach, liver, and adjacent tissues and localizing malignancy; *B,* unfolding stomach under vision with air; *C,* transillumination of inflated stomach. (From Ruddock, ref. 5, with permission.)

during open laparoscopy was solved by H. M. Hasson, who developed a laparoscopic cannula fitted with a cone-shaped sleeve that is movable along the shaft of the cannula. The cannula itself is fitted with a blunt-tipped obturator. Hasson, an obstetrician-gynecologist, first reported this instrument and technique in 1971, and today the "Hasson technique" is equated with open laparoscopy.

Controlled, automatic insufflation for laparoscopy was developed by Kurt Semm in the 1960s. Before this time, pneumoperitoneum was a primitive affair,

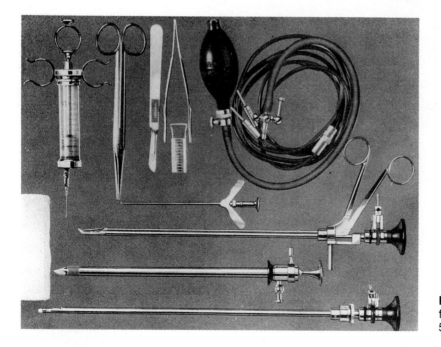

Figure 9. Instruments and accessories for peritoneoscopy. (From Ruddock, ref. 5, with permission.)

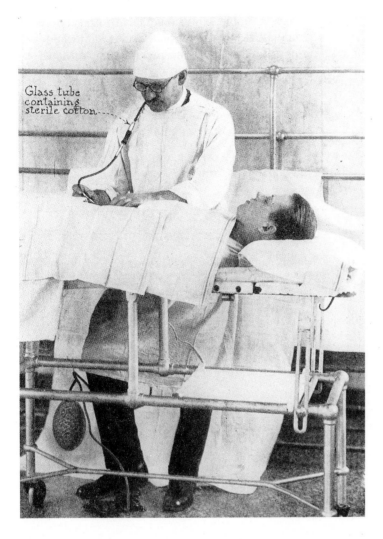

Glass tube containing sterile cotton....

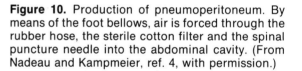

Figure 10. Production of pneumoperitoneum. By means of the foot bellows, air is forced through the rubber hose, the sterile cotton filter and the spinal puncture needle into the abdominal cavity. (From Nadeau and Kampmeier, ref. 4, with permission.)

created using either a hand-held bulb (Fig. 9) or a foot bellows (Fig. 10). Semm also developed a number of endoscopic instruments that would become necessary in performing therapeutic laparoscopy and endoscopic abdominal surgery.

Although these advances improved the procedure, further progress and acceptance of laparoscopy mandated improvement in optics. In 1952, Fourestier, Gladu, and Valmière used a quartz rod to transmit light through the laparoscope. This device produced cool illumination and eliminated the dangers of electrical hazard. In the late 1960s, the British physicist, Hopkins, arranged rod-shaped lenses as light transmitters with air lenses between the rod-shaped glass elements. This became known as the Hopkins rod lens system, which markedly improved resolution and contrast. While improvement in visualization was markedly better with the Hopkins rod lens system, it is not a coincidence that the development of laparoscopic cholecystectomy occurred shortly after the introduction of the computer chip TV camera.

MODERN LAPAROSCOPIC THERAPEUTICS

Although therapeutic laparoscopy (e.g., tubal ligation and appendectomy) occurred prior to laparoscopic cholecystectomy, the latter was solely responsible for mandating a role for laparoscopy in general surgery. The first reports of successful laparoscopic cholecystectomy in humans emanated from France. J. Perrisat and colleagues of Bordeaux and F. Dubois and colleagues of Paris, share the fame of this innovation. What followed was a veritable explosion of laparoscopy into general surgical practice. It can be said without exaggeration that almost any abdominal or retroperitoneal operation performed "open" has been attempted laparoscopically. The subsequent chapters of this text narrate the methods used in performing a number of laparoscopic abdominal surgical procedures.

ACKNOWLEDGMENTS

Special thanks to James M. Edmonson, Ph.D., Curator of the Dittrick Museum, Cleveland, Ohio, for his invaluable assistance.

RECOMMENDED READING

1. Braimbridge MV. The history of thoracoscopic surgery. *Ann Thorac Surg* 1993;56:610–614.
2. Edmonson JM. History of the instruments for gastrointestinal endoscopy. *Gastrointest Endosc* 1991;37(Suppl):S27–S56.
3. Gunning JE. The history of laparoscopy. *J Reprod Med* 1974;12:222–226.
4. Nadeau OE, Kampmeier OF. Endoscopy of the abdomen: abdominoscopy. [A preliminary study, including a summary of the literature and a description of the technique.] *Surg Gynecol Obstet* 1925;41:259–271.
5. Ruddock JC. Peritoneoscopy. *Surg Gynecol Obstet* 1937;65:623–639.
6. Stellato TA. History of laparoscopic surgery. *Surg Clin North Am* 1992;72:997–1002.

Anesthetic Considerations

Charles H. Andrus and Keith S. Naunheim
Department of Surgery
St. Louis University
St. Louis, Missouri 63110

Catherine M. Wittgen
Department of Surgery
Division of Vascular Surgery
Massachusetts General Hospital
Harvard Medical School
Boston, Massachusetts 02114

Operative Laparoscopy and Thoracoscopy, edited by B. V. MacFadyen, Jr. and J. L. Ponsky. Lippincott-Raven Publishers, Philadelphia © 1996.

Although laparoscopic and thoracoscopic techniques may be visually "minimally invasive" to the patient and nonendoscopic surgeon, significant physiologic changes are observed, some of which are unique to these procedures. While many of the anesthetic techniques employed are comparable to those used during standard laparotomies and thoracotomies, the unique physiologic changes produced during laparoscopy and thoracoscopy require diligent observation and possible alterations in "standardly" employed anesthetic techniques and monitoring methods.

LAPAROSCOPIC ANESTHESIA

To provide for better overall airway control, muscle relaxation, and adequate pneumoperitoneum, most laparoscopic procedures are performed under general anesthesia (1,2). Studies of laparoscopies performed under a general anesthesia have attempted to compare different types of inhalation or intravenous agents (3), tube versus mask anesthetic techniques (4), and neuromuscular blocking agents (5,6). Local anesthesia during laparoscopy is limited by the significant peritoneal irritation that occurs when carbon dioxide is used as the insufflating gas (7), the increased risk of viscus and solid tissue injury due to patient movement, and the very real potential of hypercapnia, hypoxia, and emesis with subsequent aspiration in the conscious, nonintubated patient.

GENERAL ANESTHESIA

Most laparoscopies are performed with endotracheal tube intubation and under a general anesthesia to ensure an adequate airway and ventilation and to prevent aspiration during the period of positive-pressure pneumoperitoneum (12–20 mmHg insufflation pressure) (1,8). Due to the increased pneumoperitoneum pressure, increases in mechanical ventilation pressures are utilized to ventilate a patient adequately (9). Positioning the patient in a Trendelenburg position may affect ventilatory pressures (10). In order to minimize reflux of gastric contents intraoperatively, a nasogastric or nasoduodenal tube should be employed. Transurethral urinary drainage catheters are also recommended in an effort to prevent inadvertent bladder injury during trocar placement.

Current recommendations for minimal routine patient monitoring include continuous electrocardiographic monitoring, intermittent noninvasive blood pressure monitoring, precordial or esophageal stethoscope monitoring, and pulse oximetry (10,11). If carbon dioxide is employed as the insufflating agent, capnography (measured exhaled end-tidal CO_2) should also be employed (11). Since CO_2 may still cause hypercapnia in the hyperventilated chronic obstructive pulmonary disease (COPD) patient, end-tidal CO_2 monitoring may severely underestimate serum CO_2 levels, and serial arterial blood gas analyses are often indicated to provide more accurate information (12).

Inhalation anesthetic agents used during laparoscopic procedures may vary, but halothane, isoflurane, and enflurane are most commonly administered with or without nitrous oxide (N_2O) (1,8). While the occurrence of N_2O-induced bowel distention during laparoscopy is debated as being neither absolute nor predictable, many laparoscopists routinely request the avoidance of this agent (8,13). Increased emesis after laparoscopic procedures are associated with N_2O anesthetic techniques, and this seems to indicate an N_2O effect on intestinal motility and distention (14).

Propofol, etomidate, and ketamine with midazolam are used as total intravenous anesthesia agents during laparoscopy (1,3,15). Considered by many most appropriate for outpatient laparoscopies, total intravenous anesthesia, especially when propofol (Diprivan, Zeneca Pharmaceuticals, Wilmington, DE) is employed, demonstrates a much more rapid recovery from anesthesia and diminished postoperative nausea and vomiting (1,3). Balanced general anesthesia techniques with fentanyl or butorphanol and N_2O have failed to demonstrate a similar advantage (16).

Adequate abdominal and diaphragmatic musculature relaxation is mandatory during most laparoscopies. An inadequate neuromuscular blockade will hamper abdominal distention and visualization and uncontrolled diaphragmatic movements can impede delicate laparoscopic maneuvers. Neuromuscular blocking agents such as atracurium, vecuronium, pancuronium, and alcuronium have demonstrated equivalent usefulness with some minor differences (1,17,18), and the reversal of all such agents is readily accomplished, making them all applicable to the same-day laparoscopic setting (19).

REGIONAL AND LOCAL ANESTHESIA

During laparoscopic procedures that take longer than an hour, general anesthesia provides better airway control, adequate ventilation so hypoventilation and hypercapnia are minimized, and effective abdominal and diaphragmatic muscular relaxation. For short laparoscopies, regional and local anesthesia have been used in the outpatient setting (1). Traditionally, during a laparoscopy with local anesthesia and conscious sedation, N_2O has been utilized for the pneumoperitoneum agent because of its diminished systemic absorption and minimal local irritation of the peritoneal cavity when compared to CO_2 (20). N_2O, while not inflammable, supports oxidation, and this precludes the recommendation of thermal or laser cauterization.

Bupivacaine epidural anesthesia has been used during pelvic laparoscopic procedures, but the assumed advantage of less physiologic stress has not been demonstrated (21). Comparable levels of circulating stress hormones can be measured when compared to general anesthesia. Even with the resultant increased intraabdominal pressure and concomitant increased gastric intraluminal pressure due to the pneumoperitoneum, no increase in gastroesophageal reflux has been documented during laparoscopies under local or epidural anesthesia. This may be explained partially by the concomitant increase in lower esophageal sphincter pressure, which also occurs with the pneumoperitoneum (22).

Successful completion of pelvic and limited abdominal diagnostic laparoscopic procedures can be accomplished under local anesthesia (23). There has been no definite physiologic advantage demonstrated for the use of local anesthesia during laparoscopy except in those cases where a genetic defect or previous adverse reaction preclude a general anesthetic or neuromuscular blocking agents.

POSTANESTHESIA RECOVERY

Although patient and physician perceptions of diminished postoperative pain, discomfort, length of hospital stay, and the early return to routine activities have made laparoscopic surgeries extremely popular, postanesthetic and postoperative morbidity, including incisional pain, nausea, vomiting, anorexia, constipation, and urinary retention are still very real after laparoscopic surgeries. Although these complications are less severe in intensity and duration when compared to standard laparotomy, postoperative analgesia and antiemetics are usually required. Using muscle relaxants during laparoscopy has demonstrated a decrease in the incidence of postoperative sore throats and abdominal muscle pain (24). Rectus sheath blockade with 0.25% bupivacaine at the termination of the laparoscopy diminishes the need for postoperative analgesia (25), but the use of preoperative analgesia to diminish postlaparoscopic analgesic requirements have not been successful (26).

In the immediate postlaparoscopic period a small supplementation of O_2 (2 L oxygen per minute per nasal prongs) will prevent transient hypoxemia (27). Nausea and emesis are common in the recovery room setting after laparoscopy (14). Nitrous oxide, etomidate, and fentanyl have all been implicated as potential causes (1,13,14), and droperidol seems to diminish nausea and emesis, while the efficacy of metaclopramide has been equivocal in comparative trials (28).

PHYSIOLOGY

Many of the variations in the physiologic responses observed during laparoscopy are secondary to patient positioning during the procedure and to the pneumoperitoneum, which can be the direct effect of abdominal distention or can be secondary to direct pharmacologic effects of the specific gas employed for insufflation (2,29). The physiologic changes observed during a pneumoperitoneum period can be classified as alterations in hemodynamics, pulmonary function, acid-base balance, and changes in hormonal secretion.

Hemodynamic Effects

With insufflation pressures used during most laparoscopic procedures ranging from 12 to 20 mmHg (average: 15 mmHg), the inferior vena caval and portal venous pressures have been observed to increase with concomitant decreases in flow in the superior mesenteric artery and portal vein (30). A measurable decrease in venous return to the heart may also occur. In a canine model, it has been demonstrated that these effects can be minimized with insufflation pressures of 8–12 mmHg (31). Central venous pressure has been recorded as unaffected or mildly elevated during the positive pressure pneumoperitoneum (2). Cardiac output and stroke volume are reported to decrease or remain unchanged during the pneumoperitoneum period, and heart rate is increased or unchanged, which have been attributed to the increased abdominal pressure impedance of venous return (32). These effects appear to be independent of the gas utilized, since they are reproducible with many different insufflation agents such as carbon dioxide, nitrous oxide, oxygen, helium, and argon. Two studies have reported an increase in cardiac output (33,34). In their original study, Smith and colleagues (33) suggest that the increase in cardiac output might be the true cardiac response to an increase in intraabdominal pressure and is observed only in the absence of myocardial depressant anesthetic agents such as halothane.

The CO_2 pneumoperitoneum produces additional hemodynamic changes—due to the unique acid-base properties and rapid systemic absorption of this gas—that are not observed with other gases; hypercapnia and acidemia may result, along with the initiation of pulmonary hypertension and systemic vasodilation (35). These cardiac effects are balanced by the hypercapnia, which also stimulates a sympathomimetic response of hyperventilation and systemic vasoconstriction (36). Demonstrated experimentally, these hemodynamic effects are clinically overshadowed by the pneumoperitoneal baroeffects and the myocardial depressant effects of the anesthetics.

Acid-Base and Pulmonary Effects

Regardless of the insufflating agent, the positive intraperitoneal pressure employed during laparoscopy causes a linear increase in peak airway pressure during artificial ventilation (37). This mechanical effect is the result of increased intraabdominal pressure from the pneumoperitoneum with an upward displacement and distention of the diaphragm, causing a decrease in thoracic cavity space. Due to the subsequent decreased tidal volume and in order to maintain an adequate minute ventilation, the intraoperative tidal volume or respiratory rate delivered must be increased to compensate. Despite these increased ventilatory requirements, hypoxia has not been a complication detected with the use of any of the insufflation agents studied.

While the need for increased minute ventilation has been observed during pneumoperitoneum, persistent respiratory acidosis is a complication unique to the utilization of CO_2 for insufflation. In laparoscopies without cauterization, research has demonstrated nitrous oxide to be superior as an insufflation agent due to the elimination of the potential development of hypercapnia and acidosis with CO_2 (38). For general surgery laparoscopies requiring cautery or laser, the most commonly used and frequently available gas is CO_2. With prolonged insufflation, the development of hypercapnia and subsequent acidosis has been documented in patients with underlying pulmonary pathology (12). More recent animal and human studies have repeatedly documented the consistent development of hypercapnia and acidosis during prolonged periods of CO_2 pneumoperitoneum (2). No increase in ventilatory dead space has been observed with any insufflation gas including CO_2, which eliminates the physical properties of the gas as a cause of the acidosis (39). The severity of the observed hypercapnia is a function of pulmonary excretory ability as seen in a COPD canine model (34).

To prevent hypercapnia and acidosis, inert gases such as helium have been studied in animal and human subjects (34,35). Although no adverse outcomes have been reported, the diminished solubility of helium versus carbon dioxide in the serum limits its use as the ideal alternate agent. Avoidance of CO_2 as the insufflation gas is impractical, and a more realistic approach to this problem of hypercapnia is to identify those individuals at risk to develop severe CO_2 retention, marked hypercapnia, and subsequent significant acidosis. Patients with abnormalities in preoperative pulmonary function testing, especially those demonstrating a decrease in the diffusing capacity of the lung for carbon monoxide ($D_{LCO} < 70\%$ predicted), and those with cardiac atherosclerosis, diabetes, and renal failure have been demonstrated to be at higher risk for the development of intraoperative hypercapnia and acidosis (40). For these patients, intermittent arterial blood gas monitoring during the procedure is recommended, since end-tidal carbon dioxide (ET_{CO_2}) may underestimate the severity of hypercapnia secondary to the defect in the diffusing capacity of the lung (12,41), and modifications in the choice of anesthetic (intravenous versus inhaled), better ventilatory support (increase in the minute ventilation), and lower insufflation pressure (8–12 vs. 15–20 mmHg) may help minimize the resultant hypercapnia.

Even with hypercapnia and intraoperative acidosis, most laparoscopic cholecystectomies have been completed without adverse outcomes (42). High-risk patients undergoing laparoscopic cholecystectomy demonstrate less perioperative morbidity and mortality than those undergoing open cholecystectomy (43). Despite the potential for intraoperative hypercapnia after laparoscopic cholecystectomy, postoperative pulmonary function testing values are decreased when compared to preoperative values, but these changes are significantly less severe than those observed after traditional open cholecystectomy (44).

Very significant pulmonary and acid-base changes can occur during laparoscopy performed with a CO_2 pneumoperitoneum. In those individuals at risk for the development of hypercapnia, it is advantageous to monitor the patient's acid-base status intraoperatively—with continuous end-tidal carbon dioxide monitoring methods as well as with intermittent arterial blood gas analysis (40).

Hormonal Effects

During laparoscopic procedures, changes in hormone release are the combined results of variable increases in abdominal pressures, pain and discomfort, and the manipulation of the abdominal contents; and there is not a straightforward predictable physiologic response during laparoscopic procedures. Studies of normal patients undergoing laparoscopy have demonstrated a rapid rise in serum arginine vasopressin (antidiuretic hormone [ADH]) levels upon insufflation (45,46). Severely cirrhotic patients with increased intraabdominal pressure from ascites demonstrate increased ADH release. The actual physiologic mechanism in cirrhotics that accounts for this increased secretion in response to elevated peritoneal pressure is unknown, but it has been postulated that increased abdominal pressure in these patients stimulates the ADH response; and the response to positive-pressure pneumoperitoneum may be by a similar mechanism.

Other serum metabolites and hormones increased during laparoscopy are those related to operative stress: glucose, cortisol, prolactin, β-endorphin, epinephrine, norepinephrine, dopamine, and interleukin-6 (IL-6) (21,47,48). In comparative trials of general (less painful) versus epidural anesthesia (21) and of laparoscopy (less painful) versus laparotomy (47), β-endorphin secretion is notably less. When laparoscopic colectomy was compared to traditional laparotomy, the rise in cortisol was similar for both operative procedures, while the rise in IL-6 was muted during the laparoscopic colectomy (48). The acute-phase immune response as measured by T-cell proliferation is less inhibited after laparoscopic cholecystectomy (49).

The generalization can be made that laparoscopy increases the release of stress-related factors, but the magnitude of the biologic response is generally decreased when compared to the open operative equivalent procedure. In terms of physiologic response, the body may indeed perceive laparoscopy as a less invasive procedure.

▲ COMPLICATIONS

Most of the complications unique to laparoscopy that influence anesthetic care are attributable to the pneumoperitoneum, and hypercapnia and subsequent acidosis are the most common physiologic changes observed when the insufflation gas is carbon dioxide (2,50). Subcutaneous emphysema, pneumothorax, pneumopericardium, pneumomediastinum, or gas embolism are complications dependent on the gaseous properties of any insufflation agent. Subcutaneous emphysema is a minor complication that is frequently seen in prolonged laparoscopies where the insufflation gas has dissected in the subcutaneous tissues, in obese patients where the gas can diffuse along the longer trochar tract, and where higher-than-normal pressures are used to fully distend the abdomen (51). Scrotal subcutaneous emphysema is frequently seen after laparoscopic varicocelectomy due to the retroperitoneal dissection. Once the gas dissects subcutaneously, it can spread extensively and has even been seen as periorbital subcutaneous emphysema. If CO_2 is the insufflation gas, the subcutaneous emphysema generally resolves over a 24-hour period; but if an inert, insoluble gas like helium is used, and subcutaneous emphysema develops, it may take many weeks to subside after the laparoscopy.

Although rare, pneumothorax, pneumomediastinum, and pneumopericardium have been reported as complications of the pneumoperitoneum (52,53). Where a defect may be found in the diaphragm or pericardium as in a laparoscopy for penetrating trauma, the positive pressure of the pneumoperitoneum can cause a potentially life-threatening pericardial tamponade or a tension pneumothorax. Immediate deflation of the pneumoperitoneum is indicated with additional corrective actions such as tube thoracostomy or pericardiocentesis if symptoms persist.

Venous gas embolism is the most dreaded of the laparoscopic complications directly attributable to the insufflation agent, with a reported incidence of 0.0016% to 0.013% (54,55). This potentially lethal complication can occur during any laparoscopy performed with positive-pressure pneumoperitoneum by entry of gas emboli through some major venous structure: uterine veins, hepatic veins, portal vein, or inferior vena cava (54–57). The initial clinical presentation is sudden cardiovascular collapse with loss of pulse and blood pressure, and precordial or transesophageal auscultation reveals a "mill wheel" murmur. To help alleviate the pulmonary outflow obstruction created by the gas embolus in the right ventricle, the patient should then be placed in a left lateral decubitus Trendelenburg position to help alleviate the pulmonary outflow obstruction created by the gas embolus in the right ventricle (55). The pulmonary outflow obstruction can be relieved by these maneuvers as CO_2 or N_2O are highly soluble in blood and the ventricular embolus will rapidly dissolve; but if a relatively insoluble gas like helium has been used as the insufflation agent, this dissolution process may require a considerable length of time.

Regardless of the insufflation agent utilized, there is a decrease in abdominal venous flow and a postulated diminished venous return to the heart due to the pressure of pneumoperitoneum (30,31). Duplex scanning and indwelling venous catheters have confirmed the loss of venous pulsation and diminution in venous blood velocities (58). With venous stasis during all positive-pressure pneumoperitonea, some form of deep venous prophylaxis like pneumatic compression hose is probably warranted.

As with any laparotomy, during laparoscopy the patient's core temperature will decrease with time due to patient exposure in a cool environment. In addition, there has been reported a 0.3°C decrease in core temperature per 50 L volume flow of carbon dioxide pneumoperitoneum could be avoided by warming the insufflation gas (59).

Cardiac arrhythmias, mainly ventricular ectopic beats, have a reported incidence of 13% during laparoscopy and occur more frequently during CO_2 pneumoperitoneum versus N_2O (17% vs 4.4%) (60). This increased incidence during CO_2 pneumoperitoneum has led to the assumption that the underlying acid-base disturbances are the etiology of the arrhythmias observed. Although arrhythmias are relatively common, cardiac arrest and cardiovascular collapse are extremely rare (0.04% incidence). The causes of these severe cardiac complications are most likely multifactorial in origin and may include increased ventricular irritability, decreased venous return, decreased cardiac output, hypoventilation, gas embolization, myocardial infarction, or profound vagal response due to peritoneal insufflation (61,62).

Although rare, venous gas embolism has a reported incidence of 0.0016% to 0.013% (54,55). The initial clinical presentation is sudden cardiovascular collapse with loss of pulse and blood pressure, and precordial or transesophageal auscultation reveals a "mill wheel" murmur. The patient should be placed in a left lateral decubitus Trendelenburg position to help alleviate the pulmonary outflow obstruction.

THORACOSCOPIC ANESTHESIA

Since most patients undergoing thoracoscopy have underlying pulmonary, cardiovascular, and/or pleural pathology, the choice of anesthesia, intraoperative monitoring, postoperative recovery, and complications are directly related to the patient's underlying pathology (2,63). Most thoracoscopic operations are performed as inpatient procedures under general anesthesia, which provides for better overall ventilation, differential airway control, and intrathoracic visualization. Administration of a general anesthesia during thoracoscopy involves choices in the method of ventilation, bronchus cannulation, and technique for achieving an intraoperative pneumothorax. Traditionally, local and regional anesthetic techniques have been limited to use during brief thoracoscopy for pleural effusion sampling, diagnostic evaluation, or pleural biopsy.

GENERAL ANESTHESIA

Adequate airway control is mandatory, so thoracoscopy is most often performed under controlled conditions with general anesthesia. Thoracoscopy that is quickly done and involves minimal intrathoracic manipulation can be performed with the patient spontaneously breathing, which enables the use of a light inhalation or intravenous general anesthesia without muscle relaxation (64). With the lateral decubitus position utilized for most thoracoscopy, selective ventilation of the unaffected, fully expanded, dependent lung is especially important. With routine single-lumen intubation, both lungs are fully ventilated, and to adequately visualize the operative field, mechanical retraction of the involved lung or compression is required. Compression can be accomplished with a controlled, low-pressure pneumothorax from insufflating CO_2 gas; however, visualization of the lung and pleural cavity remains somewhat limited (65). Double-lumen endobronchial tubes are frequently employed as they allow selective ventilation of the dependent lung with optimized visualization by passive atelectasis of the involved nondependent lung (66–68). Single-lung ventilation not only improves visualization of the operative field but also minimizes the ventilation-perfusion mismatch.

In pediatric patients too small for the use of double-lumen tubes, selective ventilation can also be achieved utilizing a standard single-lumen endotracheal tube in conjunction with an inflatable bronchial blocker, which is guided by bronchoscopy into the appropriate mainstem bronchus (69). Recently, commercial vendors have developed a special endotracheal tube with an integrated bronchial blocker (Univent), which can also be used to achieve one-lung ventilation.

Routine patient monitoring should include continuous electrocardiography, intraarterial blood pressure monitoring, precordial or esophageal stethoscope placement, pulse oximetry, and capnography (ETco_2). In the chronic obstructive pulmonary disease (COPD) patient, end-tidal CO_2 monitoring may underestimate serum CO_2 levels, and serial arterial blood gas analyses are often indicated to provide more accurate information (12). Frequently, pulmonary artery catheter placement with cardiac output monitoring is advisable because of the pulmonary shunting that occurs with patient positioning, pneumothorax development, and selective ventilation of the dependent lung.

The methods of inhalation anesthesia routinely employed during thoracoscopic procedures vary according to preference because there are no comparative studies analyzing different inhalation agents. In conjunction with nitrous oxide, halothane, isoflurane, and enflurane are commonly used.

REGIONAL AND LOCAL ANESTHESIA

Regional and local anesthesia have a role during the performance of minor thoracoscopic procedures that are quickly performed and involve minimal intrathoracic manipulation. Without endotracheal intubation, intravenous sedation during thoracoscopy can be administered, using such agents as ketamine, diazepam, or fentanyl with infiltration of thoracostomy sites with xylocaine prior to trocar placement (70,71). Regional anesthesia ("rib blocks") with 0.25% bupivacaine, xylocaine, or other local anesthetics involving the posterior infiltration of at least one intercostal nerve above and below the thoracic interspace chosen for trocar placement can provide adequate anesthesia (72,73). Stellate ganglion blockade upon entry into the thoracic cavity can be employed to obliterate the cough reflex caused by visceral pleural traction (74).

POSTANESTHESIA RECOVERY

After any thoracoscopy, parenchymal lung damage with a continuous air leak may result in a persistent pneumothorax, which may be identified before the procedure is completed by attaching the operating room mass spectrometer (SARA: system for anesthetic and respiratory analysis) to a thoracic trocar (75). Any amount of anesthetic gas identified during this maneuver implies lung parenchymal incompetency, which may require further treatment. If there is no identifiable air leak and the lung has not been injured, lung reexpansion and subsequent airtight closure of all incision sites can be attempted. At the conclusion of the thoracoscopy, positive-pressure ventilation is utilized to expand the nondependent lung, and pleural evacuation is performed by tube vacuum suction through one remaining open trocar site (72). With complete evacuation of the pleural cavity, the tube is removed with rapid occlusion of the remaining incision by a pursestring suture closure or incision site compression with an occlusive dressing of Vaseline-treated gauze and cotton pads.

If the thoracoscopy performed involved lung parenchymal biopsy, injury, or repair, it is more appropriate to place one or more indwelling tubes through the thoracostomy sites for continuous postoperative pleural evacuation under water-seal control with or without vacuum suction. When it can be radiologically demonstrated that the lung parenchyma is fully expanded and there is no air leak while under water-seal, the thoracostomy tubes can be removed in the usual manner.

The patient's and physician's perceptions of diminished postoperative pain have made thoracoscopic procedures extremely popular (76). As with any thoracotomy, the presence or absence of a persistent pneumothorax, ongoing air leak, and severity of the underlying thoracic disease are the limiting factors that determine the thoracoscopy patient's postoperative course. Postoperative analgesia requirements are significantly diminished when compared to thoracotomy, but in the immediate postoperative period most patients will require some form of analgesia (76). The frequently prolonged postoperative incisional pain due to muscle division and rib spreading experienced after thoracotomy is avoided.

When treated by thoracoscopy, the length of hospitalization for spontaneous pneumothorax is significantly shorter than after axillary thoracotomy (76). The overall postoperative morbidity and the length of stay after the thoracoscopy for other pulmonary diseases (especially malignant pleural effusions and severe emphysema), are probably more dependent on the underlying disorder than on the nature of the procedure itself.

PHYSIOLOGY

Most of the variations in the physiologic responses observed during thoracoscopy are secondary to patient positioning, the subsequent intraoperative pneumothorax and concomitant lung parenchymal compression, and the resulting changes in ventilation and perfusion.

Pulmonary Effects

As with a thoracotomy performed with single-lung ventilation in the lateral decubitus position, during thoracoscopy the Pao_2 has been observed to decrease (77–79), while the hemoglobin oxygen saturation (Sao_2) remains unchanged (80); these signs are indicative of an increased ventilation/perfusion mismatch (shunt) induced by one-lung ventilation. During thoracoscopy under local anesthesia, patients respond to this hypoxia with a concomitant increase in spontaneous respiratory frequency and develop hypocapnia due to the hyperventilation (77). Under general anesthesia, modifications in ventilatory techniques are frequently required to reverse the hypoxemia induced by one-lung ventilation. The recommended maneuvers include initiating continuous positive airway pressure of 5 cmH_2O pressure to the nondependent lung and, if this does not reverse the hypoxemia, then the addition of positive end-expiratory pressure of 5 cmH_2O pressure to the dependent lung (78,79). With the resumption of two-lung ventilation at the end of the thoracoscopy, the Pao_2 has been noted to return to insignificantly less than baseline levels and a mild hypocapnia has also been observed (77–79).

There have been no adverse long-term effects on pulmonary function attributable to thoracoscopy, and in those patients that have undergone thoracoscopies for recurrent pneumothorax disease and treatment of bullous emphysema, spirometric measurements have demonstrated long-term improvement in the majority of patients studied (81,82).

Hemodynamic Effects

As with the pulmonary effects of one-lung ventilation in a patient in the lateral decubitus position during thoracoscopy, significant hemodynamic changes are anticipated. During carbon dioxide insufflation to establish and maintain the pneumothorax in a porcine model, significant decreases in cardiac index, mean arterial pressure, stroke volume, and left ventricular stroke work index and significant increases in central venous pressure have been observed (83). In a recent human study, which did not directly evaluate any other cardiac parameters and was inconclusive as to the overall effect of thoracic CO_2 insufflation on cardiac output, significant central venous pressure elevation was observed but without changes in the mean arterial pressure or heart rate (80).

Without CO_2 insufflation but with dependent one-lung ventilation, hemodynamic variables have been noted to be quite stable (79). The mean cardiac index and mean arterial pressure have been noted to be unchanged during and after

PEARLS

Since the majority of patients undergoing thoracoscopy have underlying pulmonary, cardiovascular, and/or pleural pathology, the choice of anesthesia, intraoperative monitoring, postoperative recovery and complications are directly related to the patient's underlying pathology (2,63). Double-lumen endobronchial tubes are frequently employed, as they allow selective ventilation of the dependent lung with optimized visualization by passive atelectasis of the involved nondependent lung (66–68). Single-lung ventilation not only improves visualization of the operative field but also minimizes the ventilation-perfusion mismatch.

After any thoracoscopy, parenchymal lung damage with a continuous air leak may result in a persistent pneumothorax, which may be identified prior to the completion of the procedure by attaching the operating room mass spectrometer (SARA: system for anesthetic and respiratory analysis) to a thoracic trocar (75). Any amount of anesthetic gas identified during this maneuver implies lung parenchymal incompetency, which may require further treatment.

As with a thoracotomy performed with single-lung ventilation in the lateral decubitus position, during thoracoscopy the PaO_2 has been observed to decrease (77–79), while the hemoglobin oxygen saturation (SaO_2) has remained unchanged (80), which are indicative of an increased ventilation/perfusion mismatch (shunt) induced by one-lung ventilation. Under general anesthesia, modifications in ventilatory techniques are frequently required to reverse the hypoxemia induced by one-lung ventilation, which include initiating continuous positive airway pressure of 5 cmH_2O pressure to the nondependent lung and, if this does not reverse the hypoxemia, then the addition of positive end-expiratory pressure of 5 cmH_2O pressure to the dependent lung (78,79).

one-lung ventilation except in two individuals with poor cardiac reserve whose hypotension was improved by pulmonary artery catheter-directed preload volume expansion.

Thoracoscopic access for sympathetic chain ablation is gaining favor in the treatment of primary palmar and axillary hyperhidrosis and reflex sympathetic dystrophy (causalgia) (84). Although no consistent cardiac rate or rhythm disturbances due to the procedure have been identified, thoracoscopic stimulation or blockade on the stellate ganglion can produce profound cardiac effects. Previous experimental work has demonstrated that stimulation of the right stellate ganglion shortens the QT interval and suppresses tachydysrhythmias, while the opposite effect can be observed with blockade of the right ganglion or by stimulation of the left stellate ganglion. β-Adrenergic cardiac blockade can be obtained by sympathetic ablation bilaterally or of the left stellate ganglion alone, while the opposite effect has been observed in isolated right ganglion ablation.

▲ COMPLICATIONS

Most complications during thoracoscopy that will influence anesthetic care are attributable to underlying lung pathology and parenchymal injury. Although the reported postthoracoscopy 30-day mortality ranges from 0 to 19%, none of these deaths are attributable to the procedure itself; these statistics point to the severity of underlying disease found in patients undergoing thoracoscopic procedures (67,71,85).

Morbidity attributable to thoracoscopy includes persistent air leak and pneumothorax, atelectasis, pneumonia, subcutaneous emphysema, air embolism, and metastatic implantation along trocar tracts (86,87). A persistent air leak and pneumothorax is the most common significant morbidity observed posthoracoscopy (3–15%) (67,71). The most significant potential intraoperative complication is air embolism, which with the dependent lung selectively intubated and the nondependent lung collapsed, it is postulated the initial placement of a Veress needle below the third intercostal space may insufflate air into the lung or major vascular structures (69). Aspiration of the needle prior to insufflation for creation of the pneumothorax is advised to avoid instilling the gas into a vascular structure. With collapse of the nondependent lung, elevation of the ipsilateral hemidiaphragm occurs making the subdiaphragmatic organs subject to inadvertent puncture during Veress needle placement and aspiration prior to insufflation may identify potential intraabdominal injury.

REFERENCES

1. Smith I, White PF. Anesthetic considerations for laparoscopic surgery. *Semin Laparosc Surg* 1994;1:198–206.
2. Andrus CH, Wittgen CM, Naunheim KS. Anesthetic and physiologic changes during laparoscopy and thoracoscopy: the surgeon's view. *Semin Laparosc Surg* 1994;1:228–240.
3. DeGrood PMRM, Harbers JBM, Egmond J, Crul JF. Anaesthesia for laparoscopy: a comparison of five techniques including propofol, etomidate, thiopentone, and isoflurane. *Anesthesia* 1987; 42:815–823.
4. Kenefick JP, Leader A, Maltby JR, Taylor PJ. Laparoscopy: blood-gas values and minor sequelae associated with three techniques based on isoflurane. *Br J Anaesth* 1987;59:189–194.
5. Dodgson MS, Heier T, Steen PA. Atracurium compared with suxamethonium for outpatient laparoscopy. *Br J Anaesth* 1986;58:40S–43S.
6. Sengupta P, Skagel M, Plantevin OM. Postoperative morbidity associated with the use of atracurium and vecuronium in day-case laparoscopy. *Eur J Anaesth* 1987;4:93–99.
7. Gomar C, Fernandez C, Villalonga A, Nalda MA. Carbon dioxide embolism during laparoscopy and hysteroscopy. *Ann Fr Anesth Reanim* 1985;4:380–382.
8. Monk TG, Weldon BC, Anesthetic considerations for laparoscopic surgery. In: Clayman RV, McDougal EM, eds. *Laparoscopic urology.* St. Louis: Quality Medical Publishing; 1993:19–27.

9. Alexander GD, Noe FE, Brown EM. Anesthesia for pelvic laparoscopy. *Anesth Analg* 1969;48: 14–18.
10. Marco AP, Yeo CJ, Rock P. Anesthesia for a patient undergoing laparoscopic cholecystectomy. *Anesthesiology* 1990;73:1268–1270.
11. Webb TD. Monitoring for laparoscopic surgery. *Semin Laparosc Surg* 1994;1:223–227.
12. Wittgen CM, Andrus CH, Fitzgerald SD, Baudendistel LJ, Dahms TE, Kaminski DL. Analysis of the hemodynamic and ventilatory effects of laparoscopic cholecystectomy. *Arch Surg* 1991; 126:997–1001.
13. Taylor E, Feinstein R, Soper N, White PF. Effect of nitrous oxide on surgical conditions during laparoscopic cholecystectomy. *Anesthesiology* 1991;75:541–543.
14. Lonie DS, Harper NJN. Nitrous oxide anaesthesia and vomiting: the effect of nitrous oxide anaesthesia on the incidence of vomiting following gynaecological laparoscopy. *Anesthesia* 1986;41: 703–707.
15. Bailie R, Craig G, Restall J. Total intravenous anaesthesia for laparoscopy. *Anaesthesia* 1989;44: 60–63.
16. Pandit SK, Kothary SP, Pandit UA, Mathai MK. Comparison of fentanyl and butorphanol for outpatient anaesthesia. *Can J Anaesth* 1987;34:130–134.
17. Fragen RJ, Shanks CA. Neuromuscular recovery after laparoscopy. *Anesth Analg* 1984;63:51–54.
18. Kong KL, Cooper. Recovery of neuromuscular function and postoperative morbidity following blockade by atracurium, alcuronium, and vecuronium. *Anaesthesia* 1988;43:450–453.
19. Engbaek J, Ording H, Ostergaard D, Viby-Mogensen J. Edrophonium and neostigmine for reversal of the neuromuscular blocking effect of vercuronium. *Acta Anaesthesiol Scand* 1985;29:544–546.
20. Phillips RS, Goldberg RI, Watson PW, Marshall JR, Barkin JS. Mechanism of improved patient tolerance to nitrous oxide in diagnostic laparoscopy. *Am J Gastroenterol* 1987;82:143–144.
21. Lehtinen AM, Laatikainen T, Koskimies AI, Hovorka J. Modifying effects of epidural analgesia or general anesthesia on the stress hormone response to laparoscopy for in vitro fertilization. *J In Vitro Fertil Embryo Transplant* 1987;4:23–29.
22. Jones MJ, Mitchell RW, Hindocha N. Effect of increased intra-abdominal pressure during laparoscopy on the lower esophageal sphincter. *Anesth Analg* 1989;68:63–65.
23. Peterson HB, Hulka JF, Speilman FJ, Lee S, Marchbanks PA. Local versus general anesthesia for laparoscopic sterilization: a randomized study. *Obstet Gynecol* 1987;70:903–908.
24. Skacel M, Sengupta P. Morbidity after day case laparoscopy: a comparison of two techniques of tracheal anaesthesia. *Anaesthesia* 1986;41:537–541.
25. Smith BE, Suchak M, Siggins D, Challands J. Rectus sheath block for diagnostic laparoscopy. *Anaesthesia* 1988;43:947–948.
26. Edwards ND, Barclay K, Catling SJ, Martin DG, Morgan RH. Day case laparoscopy: a survey of postoperative pain. *Anaesthesia* 1991;46:1077–1080.
27. Vegfors M, Cederholm I, Lennmarken C, Lofstrom JB. Should oxygen be administered after laparoscopy in healthy patients? *Acta Anaesthesiol Scand* 1988;32:350–352.
28. Pandit SK, Kothary SP, Pandit UA, Randel G, Levy L. Dose-response study of droperidol and metoclopramide as antiemetics for outpatient anesthesia. *Anesth Analg* 1989;68:798–802.
29. Kaplan MB, Rogers R. Laparoscopic surgery: a view from the head of the table. *Semin Laparosc Surg* 1994;1:207–210.
30. Ishizaki Y, Bandai Y, Shimomura K, Abe H, Ohtomo Y, Idezuki Y. Changes in splanchnic blood flow and cardiovascular effects following peritoneal insufflation of carbon dioxide. *Surg Endosc* 1993;7:420–423.
31. Ishizaki Y, Bandai Y, Shimomura K, Abe H, Ohtomo Y, Idezuki Y. Safe intraabdominal pressure of carbon dioxide pneumoperitoneum during laparoscopic surgery. *Surgery* 1993;114:549–554.
32. McKenzie R, Wadhwa RK, Bedger RC. Noninvasive measurements of cardiac output during laparoscopy. *J Reprod Med* 1980;24:247–250.
33. Smith I, Benzie RJ, Gordon NLM, Kelman GR, Swapp GH. Cardiovascular effects of peritoneal insufflation of carbon dioxide for laparoscopy. *Br Med J* 1971;14:410–411.
34. Fitzgerald SD, Andrus CH, Baudendistel LJ, Dahms TE, Kaminski DL. Hypercarbia during carbon dioxide pneumoperitoneum. *Am J Surg* 1992;163:186–190.
35. Bongard FS, Pianim NA, Leighton TA, et al. Helium insufflation for laparoscopy operation. *Surg Gynecol Obstet* 1993;177:140–146.
36. van de Bos GC, Drake AJ, Noble MI. The effect of carbon dioxide upon myocardial contractile performance, blood flow and oxygen consumption. *J Physiol* 1979;287:149–161.
37. Williams MC, Murr PC. Laparoscopic insufflation of the abdomen depresses cardiopulmonary function. *Surg Endosc* 1993;7:12–16.
38. El-Minawi MF, Wahbi O, El-Bagouri IS, Sharawi M, El-Mallah SY. Physiologic changes during CO_2 and N_2O pneumoperitoneum in diagnostic laparoscopy: a comparative study. *J Reprod Med* 1981;26:338–346.
39. Leighton T, Pianim N, Liu SY, Kono M, Klein S, Bongard F. Effectors of hypercarbia during experimental pneumoperitoneum. *Am Surg* 1992;52:717–721.
40. Wittgen CM, Naunheim KS, Andrus CH, Kaminski DL. Preoperative pulmonary function evaluation for laparoscopic cholecystectomy. *Arch Surg* 1993;128:880–886.
41. Brampton WJ, Watson RJ. Arterial to end-tidal carbon dioxide tension differences during laparoscopy: magnitude and effect of anaesthetic technique. *Anaesthesia* 1990;45:210–214.
42. Safran D, Sgambati S, Orlando R. Laparoscopy in high-risk cardiac patients. *Surg Gynecol Obstet* 1993;176:548–554.
43. Wittgen CM, Andrus JP, Andrus CH, Kaminski DL. Cholecystectomy: which procedure is best for the high-risk patient? *Surg Endosc* 1993;7:395–399.

44. Johnson D, Lit D, Osachoff J, et al. Postoperative respiratory function after laparoscopic cholecystectomy. *Surg Laparosc Endosc* 1992;2:221–226.
45. Melville RJ, Frizis HI, Forsling ML, LeQuesne LP. The stimulus for vasopressin release during laparoscopy. *Surg Gynecol Obstet* 1985;161:253–256.
46. Solis Herruzo JA, Castellano G, Larrodera L, et al. Plasma arginine vasopressin concentration during laparoscopy. *Hepato-gastroenterol* 1989;36:499–503.
47. Lefebvre G, Thirion AV, Vauthier-Brouzes D, et al. Laparoscopic surgery versus laparotomy: comparative analysis of stress markers. *J Gynecol Obstet Biol Reprod* 1992;21:507–511.
48. Senagore A, Kilbride M, Luchtefeld M, MacKeigan J, Warzynski M, Cortisol and IL-6 response attenuated following laparoscopic colectomy. *Surg Endosc* 1993;7:121(abst).
49. Griffith J, Everitt N, Curley P, McMahon M. Laparoscopic versus ''open'' cholecystectomy: reduced influence upon immune function and the acute phase response. *Surg Endosc* 1993;7:123(abst).
50. Dubelman A. Complications of laparoscopic surgery: surgical and anesthetic considerations. *Semin Laparosc Surg* 1994;4:219–222.
51. Kent RB. Subcutaneous emphysema and hypercarbia following laparoscopic cholecystectomy. *Arch Surg* 1991;126:1154–1156.
52. Doctor NH, Hussain Z. Bilateral pneumothorax associated with laparoscopy: a case report of a rare hazard and review of literature. *Anaesthesia* 1973;28:75–81.
53. Murray DP, Rankin RA, Lackey C. Bilateral pneumothoraces complicating peritoneoscopy. *Gastrointest Endosc* 1984;45–46.
54. Wadhwa RK, McKenzie R, Wadhwa SR, Katz DL, Byers JF. Gas embolism during laparoscopy. *Anesthesiology* 1978;48:74–76.
55. Yacoub OF, Cardona I, Coveler LA, Dodson MG. Carbon dioxide embolism during laparoscopy. *Anesthesiology* 1982;57:533–535.
56. Root B, Levy MN, Pollack S, Lubert M, Pathak K. Gas embolism death after laparoscopy delayed by ''trapping'' in portal circulation. *Anesth Analg* 1978;57:232–237.
57. DePlater RMH, Jones ISC. Non-fatal carbon dioxide embolism during laparoscopy. *Anaesth Intens Care* 1989;17:359–361.
58. Beebe DS, McNevin MP, Crain JM, et al. Evidence of venous stasis after abdominal insufflation for laparoscopic cholecystectomy. *Anesthesiology* 1992;77:A147.
59. Ott DE. Correction of laparoscopic insufflation hypothermia. *J Laparoendosc Surg* 1991;1:183–186.
60. Scott DB, Julian DG. Observations on cardiac arrhythmias during laparoscopy. *Br Med J* 1972;1:411–413.
61. Brantley JC, Riley PM. Cardiovascular collapse during laparoscopy: a report of two cases. *Am J Obstet Gynecol* 1988;159:735–737.
62. Shifren JL, Adlestein L, Finkler NJ. Asystolic cardiac arrest: a rare complication of laparoscopy. *Obstet Gynecol* 1992;79:840–841.
63. Chen S. Anesthesia and thoracoscopic surgery. *Semin Laparosc Surg* 1994;1:211–214.
64. Boutin C, Viallat JR, Cargnino P, Farisse. Thoracoscopy in malignant pleural effusions. *Am Rev Respir Dis* 1981;124:588–592.
65. Millar FA, Hutchison GL, Wood RAB. Anaesthesia for thoracoscopic pleurectomy and ligation of bullae. *Anaesthesia* 1992;47:1060–1062.
66. Miller DL, Allen MS, Trastek VF, Deschamps C, Pairolero PC. Videothoracoscopic wedge excision of the lung. *Ann Thorac Surg* 1992;54:410–414.
67. Page RD, Jeffrey RR, Donnelly RJ. Thoracoscopy: a review of 121 consecutive surgical procedures. *Ann Thorac Surg* 1989;48:66–68.
68. Wakabayashi A. Expanded applications of diagnostic and therapeutic thoracoscopy. *J Thorac Cardiovasc Surg* 1991;102:721–723.
69. Rogers DA, Philippe PG, Lobe TE, et al. Thoracoscopy in children: an initial experience with an evolving technique. *J Laparoendosc Surg* 1992;2:7–14.
70. Menzies R, Charbonneau M. Thoracoscopy for the diagnosis of pleural disease. *Ann Intern Med* 1991;114:271–276.
71. Rodgers BM, Moazam F, Talbert JL. Thoracoscopy in children. *Ann Surg* 1979;189:176–180.
72. Oldenburg FA, Newhouse MT. Thoracoscopy: a safe, accurate diagnostic procedure using the rigid thoracoscope and local anesthesia. *Chest* 1979;75:45–50.
73. Rusch VW, Mountain C. Thoracoscopy under regional anesthesia for the diagnosis and management of pleural disease. *Am J Surg* 1987;154:274–278.
74. Rodgers BM, Ryckman FC, Moazam F, Talbert JL. Thoracoscopy for intrathoracic tumors. *Ann Thorac Surg* 1981;31:414–420.
75. Bagnato VJ. Surgical thoracoscopy: a preliminary report. *J Laparoendosc Surg* 1992;2:131–136.
76. Hazelrigg SR, Landreneau RM, Mack M, et al. Thoracoscopic stapled resection for spontaneous pneumothorax. *J Thorac Cardiovasc Surg* 1993;105:389–393.
77. Faurschou P, Madsen F, Viskum K. Thoracoscopy: influence of the procedure on some respiratory and cardiac values. *Thorax* 1983;38:341–343.
78. Barker SJ, Clarke C, Trivedi N, Hyatt J, Fynes M, Roessler P. Anesthesia for thoracoscopic laser ablation of bullous emphysema. *Anesthesiology* 1993;78:44–50.
79. Schwartz AJ, Hensley FA. Case 6-5—1992: anesthetic considerations for thoracoscopic procedures. *J Cardiothoracic Vasc Anesth* 1992;6:624–627.
80. Wolfer RS, Krasna MJ, Hasnain JU, McLaughlin JS. Hemodynamic effects of CO_2 insufflation during thoracoscopy. *Ann Thorac Surg* 1994;58:404–408.
81. Keller R. Thoracoscopic pleurodesis in persistent and recurrent pneumothorax. *Zentralbl Chir* 1992;117:267–269.

82. Wakabayashi A, Brenner M, Kayaleh RA, et al. Thoracoscopic carbon dioxide laser treatment of bullous emphysema. *Lancet* 1991;337:881–883.

83. Jones DR, Graeber GM, Tanguilig GG, Hobbs G, Murray GF. Effects of insufflation on hemodynamics during thoracoscopy. *Ann Thorac Surg* 1993;55:1379–1382.

84. Drott C, Gothberg G, Claes G. Endoscopic procedures of the upper-thoracic sympathetic chain: a review. *Arch Surg* 1993;128:237–241.

85. Daniel TM, Kern JA, Tribble CG, Kron IL, Spotnitz WB, Rodgers BM. Thoracoscopic surgery for diseases of the lung and pleura. *Ann Surg* 1993;217:566–575.

86. Kaiser LR. Diagnostic and therapeutic uses of pleuroscopy (thoracoscopy) in lung cancer. *Surg Clin North Am* 1987;67:1081–1086.

87. Thermann M, Lodderkemper R, Schroder D. Thoracoscopy: a forgotten endoscopic procedure? *Endoscopy* 1985;17:203–204.

Training and Credentialing

Thomas L. Dent
Department of Surgery
Abington Memorial Hospital
Abington, Pennsylvania 19001

Operative Laparoscopy and Thoracoscopy, edited by
B. V. MacFadyen, Jr. and
J. L. Ponsky. Lippincott-Raven
Publishers, Philadelphia © 1996.

Clinical general surgical privileges are functions and procedures that an institution, usually a hospital, permits a surgeon to perform in the course of caring for patients in that institution. Not too long ago, the clinical privileging process was relatively simple: the general surgeon was assumed to have acquired the knowledge and operative skills within the speciality of general surgery during a period of residency training. Few truly new procedures that required skills different from those acquired during residency training were developed during the postresidency practice of a general surgeon. All abdominal procedures, for example, were performed through an abdominal incision. The same instruments (scalpels, hemostats, scissors, ligatures, sutures, etc.) were used to remove or reconstruct organs or tissue within the abdominal cavity. Most "new" procedures were either new applications of standard general surgical techniques (e.g., highly selective vagotomy rather than truncal vagotomy) or modest technical variations (e.g., stapled rather than sutured intestinal anastomoses, electrocautery rather than ligature for hemostasis) that could be adopted easily once academic centers, either by research or fiat, had deemed them acceptable for general use. Debate over the appropriateness or even the safety of a "new" procedure was limited to the medical and surgical professions, and patients usually were not given any choice as to which procedure variation they would undergo.

The unprecedented publicity generated by the rapid adoption of laparoscopic cholecystectomy by surgeons and patients, and the resultant discussion of the "learning curve" of new procedures (1) have led to a greater scrutiny of the entire surgical training and privileging process by regulatory agencies, the news media, patients, legislators, attorneys, courts, and hospitals.

THE PRIVILEGING PROCESS

The privileging process is intended to ensure that patients receive skillful care by competent practitioners. Although there has been some discussion about "portable privileges" granted by some national surgical organizations (such as the American College of Surgeons) in response to new managed care initiatives (2), the responsibility for the granting of clinical privileges currently belongs to each hospital's governing board (3). The hospital is supposed to develop its own mechanism for the granting of all clinical privileges; frequently, "national" criteria published by speciality boards or specialty societies are adopted. A credentials committee or the chief of a clinical service evaluates each request for clinical privileges by reviewing the requesting physician's credentials (board certification; general and specific training and experience in the privileges requested; and certification of competence by the residency program director, instructors, and/or peers). Competence (i.e., a safe and acceptable level of skill) can refer either to a physician's general ability within a speciality to provide patient care, or to the ability to perform a specific technical procedure or operation. Based on this evaluation by the credentials committee or clinical service chief, each physician's clinical privileges are recommended to and granted by the hospital governing board. Some hospitals initially grant privileges provisionally and/or require that physicians be proctored for a period of time before full privileges are granted, while others do not. Individual hospitals and department chairmen are charged by the Joint Commission on Accreditation of Healthcare Organizations (JCAHO) with assuring the continuing competence of each member of the medical staff. Credentials must be reevaluated and clinical privileges regranted at least every 2 years (3).

In my experience (4,5) the best approach to the initial granting of operative privileges is by organ categories within a specialty, rather than by specific procedures. So, for example, the granting of privileges in "gastric operations" is more logical than separate privileges for "hemigastrectomy," "gastrostomy," "gastrotomy," and "gastric fundoplication." This categorical approach simplifies the privileging process by eliminating the need for an exhaustive list of thousands of procedures and their variations (many procedure codes are changed, deleted, and added to by the Current Procedural Terminology [CPT] Committee of the American Medical Association each year). This categorical approach also recognizes the similarity of the skills necessary to perform the various procedures involving each organ category. The surgeon's competence to perform each category of operations *at the time of application for clinical privileges* is certified by either the director of the surgical residency program and/or the individual's prior chief of surgery, based upon their personal observation and judgment of the skills of the surgeon-applicant.

Residency education in the United States is the most rigorous in the world and is regulated by the Accreditation Council for Graduate Medical Education (ACGME) through Residency Review Committees (RRC) for each recognized medical and surgical specialty and subspecialty. Each RRC has specific requirements as to the amount and content of educational exposure to the specialty and the type of operative procedures that must be performed before a resident is eligible to sit for a board examination in that specialty. Therefore, when a physician becomes certified by his or her respective board, there is reasonable assurance that the physician is competent to perform the procedures included in that specialty's organ-specific procedure list *at the time of board certification.*

NEW PRIVILEGES FOR ESTABLISHED PROCEDURES

Board certification, however, does not certify competence in operative procedures that were either not included in the residency experience or did not exist at the time residency training was completed. If a surgeon applies for clinical privileges to perform a procedure that is already standard or established (i.e., one in which other practitioners already have privileges), but not previously included in his or her residency training, hospitals need only establish that the procedure is appropriate to the clinical knowledge base and practice pattern of the applicant-surgeon and require documentation of additional training, experience, competence, and, possibly, proctoring in the additional procedure during a provisional period, before privileges are granted. The granting of privileges in colonoscopy for a general surgeon whose residency training did not include this procedure is a good example of an established procedure that requires new privileges.

Even for standard or established procedures, however, it can be difficult for a surgeon already in practice to obtain adequate hands-on training. There currently are no nationally or regionally organized postresidency laboratories or training programs where general surgeons can go to master technical skills. Laboratories or preceptorships developed by specialty societies, universities, individual surgeons, and even instrument manufacturers have responded partially to surgeons' educational needs, but these experiences are variable, and their quality is not subjected to the same scrutiny as residency training programs (6).

Despite these shortcomings, once surgeons have obtained appropriate (as defined in hospital criteria) postresidency training in already established procedures, the hospital can determine if the surgeon has fulfilled the previously defined criteria and, if so, grant these additional privileges.

NEW PRIVILEGES FOR NEW PROCEDURES

The privileging process becomes more difficult for a hospital if a procedure is truly new and has never been performed at that hospital. First, the hospital should determine if the proposed new procedure is "sufficiently different" from other similar procedures, because additional privileging for a minor variation of an already established procedure is probably not necessary. A "litmus test" is to decide whether the "new" procedure requires any additional formal training in an animal laboratory. If so, then it is probably a truly new procedure requiring separate privileges.

Before establishing criteria for the granting of new privileges, the hospital also must decide if the new procedure is safe and effective, that is, not experimental or investigational. If the new procedure has not yet been so demonstrated, privileges should not be granted unless the procedure is part of an experimental trial under the supervision of the hospital's institutional review committee or board. This judgment as to the safety and effectiveness of a procedure is a difficult one for hospitals today, because objective data are rarely available before patients and surgeons hear about early promising results of a procedure. Regardless, the hospital, by relying on necessarily imperfect information, must make this judgment. Separate privileging categories should also be considered for certain procedures that are controversial, risky, or of high visibility, and for those procedures that are performed by more than one clinical specialty (4,5).

If the procedure is determined to be new and judged by the hospital to be reasonably safe and effective, the hospital should formulate criteria for obtaining clinical privileges in the new procedure (4,5). The criteria must specify the type of training and credentials required, the necessary didactic and laboratory experience, the method of documenting competence in the procedure, and whether or not proctoring is required prior to the granting of full privileges. Lists of criteria and guidelines for the granting of clinical privileges in new procedures often are available from national specialty organizations, but these criteria and guidelines must be reviewed carefully by the hospital for bias and protectionism, especially if the procedure is performed by more than one specialty group (7).

Privileging lists should be updated periodically. Once a new procedure has become widely accepted, has its safety and effectiveness confirmed by studies, and has been incorporated into all residency training programs, the procedure can then be moved into an organ-specific privileging category, and separate privileging is no longer necessary.

LAPAROSCOPIC SURGERY

Most general surgical procedures performed through laparoscopes are not "new" in the strictest sense, but an extrapolation of established laparoscopic techniques to the treatment of other abdominal organs. Diagnostic and therapeutic laparoscopy of the abdominal cavity have been performed by gynecologists for years; general surgeons are certainly experienced in the performance of abdominal operations. However, the use of small laparoscopic access trocars to remove or alter abdominal organs by manipulating instruments seen on a television monitor are skills that were not learned by most general surgeons during their residency training and are sufficiently different from other operations that additional formal training is necessary (6). In addition, laparoscopic surgery is radically changing general surgical practice with unprecedented rapidity without, as yet, well-defined morbidity, mortality, and outcome data, and thus qualifies as being both controversial and high visibility (1,8). Therefore, until these new procedures are better defined, taught in adequate numbers in all surgical residency programs, and incorporated into the appropriate organ privilege categories, separate privileges are appropriate.

Rather than developing privileging guidelines for every possible laparoscopic procedure, it seems more logical to separate laparoscopy into two categories: basic and advanced. Basic laparoscopic procedures are those that require simple dissection or excisional techniques that can be accomplished with the use of scissors, clips, electrocautery, and staplers, while advanced laparoscopic procedures usually involve more complex surgical maneuvers and require a mastery of laparoscopic suturing and knot-tying.

BASIC LAPAROSCOPIC SURGERY

Basic laparoscopic general surgical procedures include diagnostic laparoscopy, lysis of adhesions, cholecystectomy, and appendectomy. Our hospital modified the Society of American Gastrointestinal Endoscopic Surgeons' (SAGES) guidelines (9) to develop criteria for granting of privileges in basic laparoscopic surgery (4,5). In keeping with the principles published by the American College of Surgeons (ACS), only those surgeons privileged to perform open abdominal surgical procedures were permitted to apply for privileges in laparoscopic general surgery (10, 11). A training course or preceptorship in basic laparoscopic surgery, including both didactic instruction by an experienced faculty and hands-on experience in basic laparoscopic techniques in live animals, is important for surgeons whose residency training did not include laparoscopic experience (6,12). Some (1) have concluded that "weekend courses" alone are not sufficient to train surgeons in a new technique, but, if well designed, they provide an adequate initial training experience that should be supplemented by assisting in operations on humans. SAGES has developed a method of approval of training courses (6) that helps to ensure the quality of the educational experience, and has also published a list of available preceptorships. Laparoscopic surgery is now being incorporated into most general surgery residency curricula, and residents are being trained as in other surgical procedures: by assisting an experienced surgeon and then performing the procedure under gradually decreasing supervision (4,12–16). Residency training in surgical laparoscopy also fulfills one of the criteria of some hospitals.

Once training has been acquired, some hospitals require experience in assisting in human laparoscopic operations to qualify for provisional privileges in basic laparoscopy. Finally, a minimum of five proctored laparoscopic operations must be performed (17). Once the applicant's competence in basic laparoscopic surgery has been certified in writing by the proctor, full privileges can be granted.

ADVANCED LAPAROSCOPIC PROCEDURES

Advanced laparoscopy obviously includes all laparoscopic procedures not included in the basic laparoscopy category. Currently, laparoscopic common bile duct exploration, vagotomy, inguinal herniorrhaphy, bowel resection, gastric fundoplication, and splenectomy are the most common advanced procedures being performed.

Privileging criteria for advanced laparoscopic procedures first must include current competence and privileges in basic laparoscopic techniques. Prior privileges and experience in comparable open procedures are also prerequisites (11). Additional didactic and hands-on training in advanced laparoscopic techniques (by training courses, preceptorships, or in residency programs), participation in advanced cases as an assistant, and written certification of competence by a proctor are necessary before advanced laparoscopic privileges are granted.

NEW LAPAROSCOPIC PROCEDURES

New surgical variations and procedures using laparoscopes are in constant development. Additional training for surgeons to perform these procedures once they are already trained in basic and advanced laparoscopic surgery will probably consist of learning by lecture, videotape, and/or "scrubbing in" with a colleague. Learning by using a laparoscopic "simulator," similar to pilots learning to fly, is an exciting possibility for the future. However, as with other clinical privileges, and in keeping with traditional medical ethics, the surgeon, monitored by the clinical service chief and/or the credentials committee and assisted by responsible national specialty organizations, such as the ACS and SAGES, should recognize when and how much additional training in each new variation is necessary, and when the "variation" is actually a new procedure that requires additional formal training and additional privileges.

ESTABLISHED, LOGICAL, AND INVESTIGATIONAL LAPAROSCOPIC PROCEDURES

Some would like to see all laparoscopic surgery restricted to academic centers that "participate in current or planned prospective studies designed to optimize the technique and carefully refine its indications" (18). As imperfect as our system is, progress would be severely impeded if every logical surgical innovation, such as laparoscopic cholecystectomy, had to undergo extensive prospective randomized trials prior to clinical use. There are many examples of logical procedures that were so obviously superior to prior treatments that they were never scientifically validated by randomized trials before being accepted and performed. Examples include aortic aneurysmectomy and even open cholecystectomy.

Many laparoscopic procedures are almost identical to their "open" counterparts, with the only variation being the method of access to the abdominal cavity. For example, the gallbladder is removed laparoscopically in approximately the same way as during traditional open cholecystectomy, except that different instruments are used. If laparoscopic removal can be shown to be as safe or safer than open, the long-term outcome logically can be assumed to be identical (19–24). However, even for laparoscopic cholecystectomy, some (8,18,25,26) are not yet willing to agree to its unrestricted acceptance, citing more liberal indications for cholecystectomy leading to a higher expenditure of health-care money, increased operating room costs, and a higher incidence of common bile duct injury. The procedure has been shown to be acceptably safe once the learning curve has been passed, and costs are not a privileging issue (4,23,27). As long as the complications and outcomes of laparoscopic cholecystectomy are continually monitored by the hospital, it is appropriate to grant privileges for this "logical" laparoscopic procedure.

Other laparoscopic procedures are also a logical combination of open and laparoscopic techniques. For example, laparoscopic appendectomy, pelvic lymphadenopathy, common bile duct exploration, splenectomy, gastric fundoplication, and highly selective vagotomy (as opposed to posterior truncal and anterior seromyotomy, the open counterpart of which is not accepted worldwide) are virtually identical to open procedures and these techniques can be learned with minimal additional training once basic and advanced laparoscopic surgical techniques are mastered. Therefore, they would not require additional privileges for general surgeons already privileged in advanced laparoscopic surgery. However, *since these procedures have not yet been shown to have any advantages over their open counterparts and their comparative safety is still unknown,* surgeons should choose to use them cautiously, if at all, until more outcome information is available (28–31). This is a very difficult "gray" area for hospitals and credentials committees, and requires cooperation among surgeons, the chief of surgery, and the hospital in deciding when and if a new procedure should replace an established one. Issues of safety, cost effectiveness, experience, volume, and skill must all be considered.

Laparoscopic surgery also is being used to perform some truly new procedures that bear little resemblance to their "open" counterparts. There is an important difference between an individual surgeon performing a procedure that is a logical amalgamation of proven surgical techniques with known outcomes to performing one that is completely new and unproved—the latter amounting to uncontrolled human experimentation. Despite initial enthusiastic reports of "successful" laparoscopic inguinal hernia repair (32,33) and intestinal resection (34,35), these procedures differ significantly from open techniques and warrant more scientific study and standardization before their widespread clinical use is appropriate (36–38). Privileges to perform these procedures should be withheld by hospitals (unless their surgeons are participating in an experimental study or a clinical trial) until more outcome information is available. For example, our hospital's institutional review committee requires that each patient undergoing a laparoscopic herniorrhaphy sign a consent form that explains the experimental nature of the procedure and the lack of scientific data regarding its safety, efficacy, and outcome.

There is no substitute for careful controlled studies of these truly new procedures before they are performed on patients. At all costs, we must renounce the attitude as stated by a vice president of a major instrument company at a recent national meeting of endoscopic surgeons: "Peer review is a nice idea, as long as it doesn't slow up the approval process"!

MONITORING OF QUALITY

The quality of a surgeon's performance in laparoscopic surgery (4,5), as in all other surgical procedures, should be monitored by the Department of Surgery and the hospital's quality improvement programs. Proctoring, additional training, or even restriction of privileges may be necessary if individual poor outcomes or high complication rates are identified. Continuing education in laparoscopic surgery also is important because new variations in technique and equipment are inevitable in this rapidly evolving field.

CONCLUSION

Hospitals in the United States are charged by the Joint Commission on Accreditation of Healthcare Organizations (JCAHO) to evaluate the credentials of and to grant specific clinical privileges to their staff physicians as well as to ensure the quality of care. Each hospital must determine:

1. Whether a new procedure is safe and effective
2. Whether the procedure is sufficiently different from other procedures as to require additional privileges
3. What the privileging criteria should be
4. How the quality of the performance of these procedures should be monitored and assured

Unless general surgeons were taught laparoscopic surgical techniques during their residency training, additional formal training in this new field is necessary before they should be granted privileges to perform these procedures. Criteria for granting hospital privileges for basic and advanced surgical laparoscopy, including didactic and technical education, technical experience, and proctoring, are described.

Some laparoscopic procedures are, except for the laparoscopic approach, identical to their open counterparts and, once deemed safe and effective, similar outcomes can be logically assumed. Other procedures, especially laparoscopic inguinal herniorrhaphy, are markedly different from traditional "open" operations and should be performed only as part of an experimental study until better outcome data are available.

REFERENCES

1. Altman LK. Surgical injuries lead to new rule. *The New York Times* 1992;June 14:1(col 1), 47(col 1).
2. Ebert PA. As I see it. *Bull Am Coll Surg* 1993;78:2–3.
3. Joint Commission on Accreditation of Healthcare Organizations. *The 1994 Joint Commission Accreditation Manual for Hospitals*. Oakbrook Terrace, IL: Joint Commission on Accreditation of Healthcare Organizations, 1993.
4. Dent TL. Training, credentialing, and granting of clinical privileges for laparoscopic cholecystectomy. *Am J Surg* 1991;161:399–403.
5. Dent TL. Training, credentialing, and evaluation in laparoscopic surgery. *Surg Clin N Am* 1992; 72:1003–1011.
6. Greene FL. Training, credentialing, and privileging for minimally invasive surgery. *Prob Gen Surg* 1991;8:502–506.
7. Diethrich EB. The credentialing conundrum. *Endovasc Surg* 1993;1:1–3.
8. Braasch JW. Laparoscopic cholecystectomy and other procedures. *Arch Surg* 1992;127:887.
9. Society of American Gastrointestinal Endoscopic Surgeons. *Granting of Privileges for Laparoscopic (Peritoneoscopic) General Surgery*. Los Angeles, Society of American Gastrointestinal Endoscopic Surgeons, 1992.
10. American College of Surgeons. Statement on laparoscopic cholecystectomy. *Bull Am Coll Surg* 1990;75:22.
11. American College of Surgeons. Statement on laparoscopic and thoracoscopic procedures. *Bull Am Coll Surg* 1991;78:48.
12. Zucker KA, Bailey RW, Graham SM, Scovill W, Imbembo AL. Training for laparoscopic surgery. *World J Surg* 1993;17:3–7.
13. Bailey RW, Imbembo AL, Zucker KA. Establishment of a laparoscopic cholecystectomy training program. *Am Surg* 1991;57:231–236.
14. Sigman HH, Fried GM, Hinchey EJ, et al. Role of the teaching hospital in the development of a laparoscopic cholecystectomy program. *Can J Surg* 1992;35:49–54.
15. Cohen MM. Initial experience with laparoscopic cholecystectomy in a teaching hospital. *Can J Surg* 1992;35:59–63.
16. Schirmer BD, Edge SB, Dix J, Miller AD. Incorporation of laparoscopy into a surgical endoscopy training program. *Am J Surg* 1992;163:46–52.
17. Satava RM. Proctors, preceptors, and laparoscopic surgery: the role of "proctor" in the surgical credentialing process. *Surg Endosc* 1993;7:283–284.

18. Cuschieri A, Berci G, McSherry CK. Laparoscopic cholecystectomy. *Am J Surg* 1990;159:273.
19. Graves HA Jr, Ballinger JF, Anderson WJ. Appraisal of laparoscopic cholecystectomy. *Ann Surg* 1991;213:655–664.
20. Neugebauer E, Troidl H, Spangenberger W, Dietrich A, Lefering R. Conventional versus laparoscopic cholecystectomy and the randomized controlled trial. *Br J Surg* 1991;78:150–154.
21. Airan M, Appel M, Berci G, et al. Retrospective and prospective multi-institutional laparoscopic cholecystectomy study organized by the Society of American Gastrointestinal Endoscopic Surgeons. *Surg Endosc* 1992;6:169–176.
22. Bailey RW, Zucker KA, Flowers JL, Scovill WA, Imbembo AL. Laparoscopic cholecystectomy: experience with 375 consecutive patients. *Ann Surg* 1991;214:531–541.
23. Larson GM, Vitale GC, Casey J, et al. Multipractice analysis of laparoscopic cholecystectomy in 1,983 patients. *Am J Surg* 1992;163:221–226.
24. Soper NJ, Dunnegan DL. Laparoscopic cholecystectomy: experience of a single surgeon. *World J Surg* 1993;17:16–20.
25. Legorreta AP, Silber JH, Costantino GN, Kobylinski RW, Katz SL. Increased cholecystectomy rate after the introduction of laparoscopic cholecystectomy. *JAMA* 1993;270:1429–1432.
26. Diehl AK. Laparoscopic cholecystectomy: too much of a good thing? *JAMA* 1993;270:1469–1470.
27. Ebert PA. As I see it. *Bull Am Coll Surg* 1990;77:2–3.
28. Warshaw AL. Reflections on laparoscopic surgery. *Surgery* 1993;114:629–630.
29. Richards W, Watson D, Lynch G, et al. A review of the results of laparoscopic versus open appendectomy. *Surg Gynecol Obstet* 1993;177:473–480.
30. Schirmer BD, Schmieg RE, Dix J, Edge SB, Hanks JB. Laparoscopic versus traditional appendectomy for suspected appendicitis. *Am J Surg* 1993;165:670–675.
31. Cuschieri AE, Hunter J, Wolfe B, Swanstrom LL, Hutson W. Multicenter prospective evaluation of laparoscopic antireflux surgery: preliminary report. *Surg Endosc* 1993;7:505–510.
32. Dion YM, Morin J. Laparoscopic inguinal herniorrhaphy. *Can J Surg* 1992;35:209–212.
33. Ger R, Mishrick A, Hurwitz J, Romero C, Oddsen R. Management of groin hernias by laparoscopy. *World J Surg* 1993;17:46–50.
34. Schlinkert RT. Laparoscopic-assisted right hemicolectomy. *Dis Colon Rectum* 1991;34:1030–1031.
35. Franklin ME Jr, Ramos R, Rosenthal D, Schuessler W. Laparoscopic colon procedures. *World J Surg* 1993;17:51–56.
36. American Society of Colon and Rectal Surgeons. Colon and rectal surgeons adopt position on laparoscopic cholecystectomy. *Dis Colon Rectum* 1991;34:8A.
37. Nyhus LM. Laparoscopic hernia repair. *Arch Surg* 1992;127:137.
38. Lichtenstein IL, Shulman AG, Amid PK. Laparoscopic hernioplasty. *Arch Surg* 1991;126:1449.

4

Economic and Environmental Considerations

Bruce D. Schirmer
Department of Surgery
University of Virginia Health Sciences Center
Charlottesville, Virginia 22908

Operative Laparoscopy and Thoracoscopy, edited by
B. V. MacFadyen, Jr. and
J. L. Ponsky. Lippincott-Raven
Publishers, Philadelphia © 1996.

During its short existence as a major part of general surgical practice, laparoscopic surgery has probably been more influenced by both economic and environmental factors than has any other technique or procedure performed by surgeons today. Similarly, the rapid adoption of this new technology, particularly in laparoscopic cholecystectomy, is unparalleled in surgical history.

To a great extent, videolaparoscopy has been pushed by industry, patient demands, and the media and has had an impact on the fields of thoracic surgery, urology, and gynecology. This chapter discusses the significant economic and environmental considerations in both the adoption and evolution of laparoscopic procedures since 1989, and their influence on the current and future performance of laparoscopic procedures.

ECONOMIC ASPECTS OF THE EXPLOSION OF LAPAROSCOPIC SURGERY

Beginning in late 1989, there was a rapid proliferation of laparoscopic cholecystectomy among general surgeons in this country. By December 1989, fewer than 100 surgeons had successfully performed laparoscopic cholecystectomies with a total experience below 1,000 cases. In 1992, it was estimated that at least 50% of the annual volume of 750,000 cholecystectomies were performed laparoscopically, and this increased to 85% by 1993.

The Media and Public Opinion

Mass media fueled the emergence of this new technology. Early publicity frequently emphasized laser technology with laparoscopic cholecystectomy, and this procedure was funded by economically interested parties. Public perceptions were very important in advancing the acceptance of laparoscopic cholecystectomy, especially that it is minimally invasive, requires short hospitalization, permits early return to work, and reduces postoperative pain. These perceptions have been corroborated by large clinical studies showing a low morbidity and mortality equivalent to the open operation.

The Surgeon in Private Practice

General surgeons in private practice felt tremendous economic pressure to learn the technology of laparoscopic cholecystectomy, since biliary surgery accounted for 25% of their practice. During 1990, institutions offering training courses in laparoscopic cholecystectomy were often overwhelmed with requests by surgeons to learn the technology. Safer guidelines on training, privileging, and credentialing were issued in 1990, and guided the institutions to develop strong teaching courses and proper control of the clinical application of this technology.

The Academic Surgeon

In general, academic surgeons were slower to adopt the technology. Initially, chairmen of academic surgical departments were skeptical of the procedure. However, as with private practitioners, academic surgeons soon appreciated the value and benefits of laparoscopic cholecystectomy to their patients and joined the ranks of surgeons now using the technology.

The Role of Industry

The role of industry has been prominent in fueling the fire of change toward laparoscopic surgery. Since 1989, when only one major exhibit on laparoscopic cholestectomy was seen at the American College of Surgeons Meeting, the great preponderance of industrial exhibits at that annual meeting now display various aspects of laparoscopic surgery. Development of laparoscopic equipment has occurred nearly as rapidly as the adoption of the technique for a variety of other general surgical procedures as well as gynecologic, urologic, and thoracic surgery.

In 1990, one of the major problems for general surgeons to successfully perform laparoscopic cholecystectomy was the lack of appropriate laparoscopic instruments. At that time, the majority of reusable laparoscopic instruments were manufactured by hand in Germany and large-volume production was difficult. It was not uncommon for general surgeons to wait 6 to 8 months for delivery of a set of reusable laparoscopic instruments. This stimulated the manufacturing of disposable instruments and one medical instrument company reported sales growths of 100% during the years 1990–1992. Since that time, many newly formed instrument companies have started the production and further development of all types of laparoscopic instruments. It is difficult to estimate the economic impact of laparoscopic surgery on the economy in general, but it has been responsible for the creation of a significant number of jobs.

The major medical instrument companies, most notably United States Surgical Corporation and Ethicon Corporation, have assumed a significant role in training general surgeons to perform laparoscopic procedures in this country. Training centers have been developed for surgeons, and their educational role should not be underestimated. It is of some concern that the current environment of cost containment may significantly decrease the ability of industry to support such teaching efforts. Therefore, the individual surgeon or the individual medical center will have to assume the costs of such further training, and the availability of these training opportunities will most likely significantly decrease.

Hospital Administration Aspects

Hospital administrators quickly realized the importance of performing laparoscopic cholecystectomy. It decreased hospitalization days, and it was an attractive advertisement for the hospital to demonstrate its involvement in the latest surgical techniques. Some hospitals were willing to reimburse the expenses for training surgeons in order to obtain qualified staff. Hospital budgets were adjusted so that laparoscopic instruments and videotelescopic equipment could be purchased, and these charges were most frequently recouped by increasing patient charges for laparoscopic cholecystectomy as compared to open cholecystectomy.

Another major concern for the hospital administration and clinical staff was that of credentialing for laparoscopic surgery. In academic medical centers, credentialing has been accomplished through the recommendation of the chairman of a given department, and it was usually based on the documentation and/or demonstration of adequate training. However, in private hospitals, economic motives among surgical groups created problems, and credentialing often became a turf battle. This type of economically driven credentialing has resulted in close scrutiny of operative results by surgeons as they were initiating their experience in laparoscopic surgery.

Bile Duct Injuries

During 1991 and 1992, reports began appearing in the lay press and the surgical literature of an increased incidence of bile duct injuries wherein inexperienced surgeons performing laparoscopic cholecystectomy were much more likely to injure the common bile duct. Other complications of laparoscopic surgery were also reported, including major vascular injuries and unrecognized bowel injuries. However, the increased incidence of bile duct injuries (greater than 1% in a few series), compared to the open operation rate of 0.1% to 0.5%, created excessive media reaction and public alarm. The New York State Health Authority went so far as to suspend the privileges of any surgeon in that state incurring such a complication. A requirement was established of either probation with monitoring or the need for further training before full reprivileging could be reinstituted. Bile duct injuries had an obvious economic and societal impact, particularly in the area of malpractice.

CURRENT PRACTICES IN LAPAROSCOPIC SURGERY

Other Laparoscopic Procedures

General surgeons now perform a variety of laparoscopic procedures besides cholecystectomy. The adoption of these other procedures has been less rapid than for cholecystectomy for reasons that include a decreased public and professional demand to perform these procedures laparoscopically, lack of instrument development, and insufficient data substantiating the benefits. Although the data for laparoscopic inguinal herniorrhaphy demonstrate recurrence rates less than 1%, the follow-up has been short and the morbidity and mortality rates are similar to the open operation. While it seems probable that parameters such as patient discomfort, postoperative pain, and return to normal activity may prove to be favorable for laparoscopic herniorrhaphy when compared to the open technique, it is used for only 15% of all herniorrhaphies performed. Another example of a procedure that did not initially produce better results by the laparoscopic performance is appendectomy. Our initial experience with laparoscopic appendectomy showed it was as good as open appendectomy, with some advantages. A recently completed multicenter trial has shown decreased wound infection rate and lessened time to return to normal activity for laparoscopic appendectomy versus open appendectomy. Another advantage of laparoscopic appendectomy includes the improved ability to make a diagnosis when acute appendicitis is not present. The emergent nature of appendicitis, however, tends to decrease a patient's ability to seek out a surgeon who performs a laparoscopic appendectomy. Consequently, there is much less economic pressure on a practicing surgeon to incorporate this procedure into his or her practice.

Laparoscopic Nissen fundoplication and laparoscopic colon resection are more advanced laparoscopic procedures that have achieved less rapid proliferation among general surgeons. Currently, data are lacking comparing the potential benefits of performing these procedures laparoscopically to the open approach. However, initial series suggest a potential for benefits similar to those seen with laparoscopic cholecystectomy. Since fundoplication and colon resection are performed significantly less frequently than appendectomy, herniorrhaphy, or cholecystectomy, there is a decreased economic incentive to perform them laparoscopically. In addition, these procedures involve markedly increased technical skills when compared to cholecystectomy and thus require additional training and commitment on the part of the surgeon to obtaining the skills necessary to safely perform them. Unless the procedures are performed frequently, the economic rewards for such time and training efforts are few, particularly if laparoscopy requires increased operative time. Despite lessened economic incentive, most general surgeons are obtaining advanced laparoscopic training so as to perform more advanced laparoscopic procedures.

Cost Effectiveness of Individual Laparoscopic Procedures

As each new laparoscopic procedure has been successfully performed, there has usually been some comparison cost analysis between the open and laparoscopic technique. In most cases, the available data have focused on hospital charges and not the true cost, and surgeons' fees have been excluded in these analyses. A cost factor that is poorly quantitated to date is the recuperative time needed before return to work. This may be influenced by a variety of factors such as patient expectation and corporation requirements; corporations should set standards of expected return to work, which should be similar to patterns seen in the self-employed population.

Several studies clearly confirm the cost effectiveness of laparoscopic cholecystectomy compared to open cholecystectomy. Hospital charges are uniformly lower, since length of stay is decreased, whereas operating room charges are higher, but not enough to offset the savings in length of stay. Differences in charges of approximately $600 to $800 per patient can be realized through the use of laparoscopic cholecystectomy (Table 1). In a study of total charges to patients covered by Blue Cross/Blue Shield of Virginia in 1991 and 1992, total charges for patients undergoing open cholecystectomy were significantly higher than those for patients undergoing laparoscopic cholecystectomy (Fig. 1). Bailey's series of patients treated with laparoscopic cholecystectomies returned to work an average of 21 days sooner than patients with open cholecystectomy. In their study, Deloitte and Touche found a potential total cost savings of over $2,000 per patient when the laparoscopic technique was used. Return to work is faster, but studies comparing

Table 1. *Charges for laparoscopic versus open cholecystectomy*

Charges	Laparoscopic	Open	p
Total hospital	$4831 ± 142	$5056 ± 505	.13
Operating room	$2684 ± 142	$2197 ± 115	.07
Operating room as a percentage of total hospital	56.3 ± 1.9%	41.2 ± 1.5%	<.05

From Schirmer and Dix, ref. 2, with permission.

populations in the United States and France have shown that the length of allowed worker sick leave is probably the single largest determinant as to when people actually return to the job.

Laparoscopic appendectomy can be cost effective compared to open appendectomy, but studies addressing this question have been mixed in terms of results, and no clear pattern has emerged. Other procedures performed by the general surgeon that are not yet confirmed as being cost effective, but hold significant promise for achieving such status, include laparoscopic Nissen fundoplication and perhaps laparoscopic colectomy. The latter currently takes 25% to 30% longer time to perform than open colectomy according to some reports, thus minimizing the cost savings. However, with increasing skill and speed of the surgeons, operative time should decrease.

It appears unlikely that laparoscopic inguinal herniorrhaphy will be a cost-effective procedure, since most open herniorrhaphies are performed on an outpatient basis. The increased cost of the equipment to perform the procedure make it less likely to be cost effective unless significant and quantifiable monetary savings in terms of return to work and activity can be demonstrated.

Deloitte and Touche recently published a study comparing the hospital cost (not charges) of four procedures using the laparoscopic and open approaches. Findings revealed that laparoscopic cholecystectomy and thoracoscopic lung biopsy or wedge resection were cost-effective procedures, while laparoscopic-assisted hysterectomy was slightly costlier but potentially comparable to open ab-

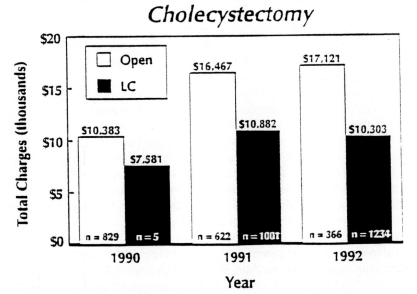

Figure 1. Total charges for patients covered by Blue Cross/Blue Shield of Virginia undergoing open cholecystectomy were significantly greater than those for patients undergoing laparoscopic cholecystectomy. (From Eggleston JM, London SD, Glasheen WP, et al. A retrospective analysis of 6,387 cholecystectomies. Medical Progress Through Technology, in press.)

Table 2. *Hospital cost savings of laparoscopic versus open surgery*

Procedure	Cost savings	
	Average	"BestPractices"
Cholecystectomy	+$1545	+$1957
Hysterectomy	−$936	+$352
Herniorrhaphy	−$1518	−$1311
Pulmonary wedge resection or biopsy	+$2809	+$4114

dominal hysterectomy. On the other hand, laparoscopic inguinal herniorrhaphy was more costly (Table 2).

Other than laparoscopic lung resection and hysterectomy, few laparoscopic procedures performed by surgical subspecialists have been analyzed for their cost effectiveness. However, it is likely that laparoscopic pelvic lymph node dissection for staging prostate cancer may prove to be cost effective as well.

There are a number of factors that contribute to the costs of laparoscopic procedures, which include operator skill, operative setting, such as in a teaching or nonteaching environment, and the continuity of the surgical team, including the skills of the assisting personnel. Finally, more controllable cost aspects of the procedure include instrument choice (reusable versus disposable) and selection and standardization of technology.

Disposable Instruments

The conversion of surgeons to laparoscopic techniques occurred rapidly along with a large demand for instruments, which was initially met by manufacturers of disposable instruments. Today, the use of disposable instruments is widespread among most surgeons, and the majority of laparoscopic cholecystectomies involve the use of at least some disposable instrumentation, including trocars, Veress needles, and scissors. The advantages of sharp cutting edges and consistent sterilization make the disposable instruments desirable. On the other hand, reusable instruments are initially more expensive and there is a reprocessing cost for cleaning and resterilizing the instruments after each procedure.

There is ongoing debate about the relative additional cost of disposable instrumentation for laparoscopic procedures. In addition, disposable instruments more easily accommodate a surgical schedule where more than one laparoscopic procedure is performed sequentially, thus avoiding the potential delays from waiting for instruments to be processed and resterilized.

Resterilization of the video equipment used in laparoscopic surgery is also a major concern regarding effectiveness and lost operating time. Disposable camera covers are now in widespread use to prevent the necessity for resterilizing the camera after each use. At our institution, we found resterilization led to a high incidence of damage to the camera, requiring frequent costly repairs. Since using disposable camera covers, few cameras have required repair and the cost savings in repair bills appears to clearly justify the cost of the covers themselves.

Technology has been developed to resterilize the videotelescopic equipment safely within 30 minutes between cases using peracetic acid sterilizing instead of steam autoclaving. Such technology has also been important to preserving the life of videotelescopic equipment and yet allowing its frequent use for multiple procedures throughout any one day. We currently use such a system to resterilize the telescope, light cord, and cautery cord attachments of our laparoscopy instruments.

Opponents of disposable instrumentation have cited the prohibitive costs for the use of disposable instruments for each case. It has been estimated that disposable instruments for a typical laparoscopic cholecystectomy may cost $300 to

$500, and in laparoscopic herniorrhaphy, estimates have reached $565 to $700 per case. In the era of managed care, reimbursement will more than likely be based on a global fee for each procedure, and the need to minimize the expense for instrumentation becomes apparent. Therefore, the economics of the times will likely dictate that fewer disposable instruments be used or that semidisposable instruments be developed in order to decrease instrument costs.

Laser Technology

Early reports of laparoscopic cholecystectomy involved using the laser to perform parts of the operation. However, surgeons who did not have lasers available or found them unaffordable proceeded to use monopolar or, at times, bipolar cautery. It has been estimated that the lasers used in these procedures can cost $500 to $600. By the end of 1990, those surgeons with extensive laparoscopic experience reported no significant differences in results, operating time, or complication rates when either laser or cautery was used.

Reimbursement

The issue of reimbursement for laparoscopic procedures has been variable. During 1989 and 1990, most general surgeons were required to increase their training and skill in this new technique, and therefore they felt that reimbursement at a level higher than traditional cholecystectomy was indicated. In general, most private insurance companies began reimbursing surgeons' fees by the late 1990s.

In 1991, the American Medical Association (AMA) created the first Current Procedural Terminology (CPT) codes for laparoscopic cholecystectomy and cholangiography, and only recently have more CPT codes become available for other commonly performed laparoscopic procedures. On the other hand, Nissen fundoplication and colon resection have not yet been assigned such codes. With the adoption of the RBRVS reimbursement scale by Medicare in 1993, the surgeon's payment in Virginia in 1993 has decreased from $2,000 to $2,200 for private insurers to $550 under the RBRVS Medicare system. In addition, under the RBRVS system of reimbursement, open cholecystectomy is currently reimbursed at a higher rate than laparoscopic cholecystectomy. Therefore in 1993, there was no economic incentive for a general surgeon to perform a laparoscopic cholecystectomy on a patient over age 65. Nevertheless, general surgeons perform most of their cholecystectomies laparoscopically because of the clear benefits to their patients.

Surgical Subspecialties

Thoracic surgeons have also adopted laparoscopic technology for the performance of certain noncardiac procedures such as pulmonary wedge resection, pleurodesis, and pulmonary biopsy. In general, the number of these cases relative to the number of vascular and cardiac cases in the average thoracic surgeon's practice make the economic incentive for performing thoracoscopy somewhat limited. Nevertheless, the obvious patient benefits of avoiding an open thoracotomy have encouraged many thoracic surgeons to adopt these techniques.

Gynecologists were performing laparoscopic surgery in significant numbers long before most general surgeons considered using the procedure. Infertility surgery, treatment of ectopic pregnancy, assessment and treatment of pelvic pain and endometriosis, and, more recently, hysterectomy are all procedures that can be performed laparoscopically. Most gynecologists have incorporated videolaparoscopy into their practice and have been stimulated by general surgeons to adopt laparoscopic-assisted hysterectomy.

Urologists have also adopted laparoscopic techniques for lymph node dissection in the treatment and staging of prostate cancer and for laparoscopic nephrectomy. The economic aspects of these procedures have been less dramatic than with general surgery, but decreased patient morbidity and mortality have been observed.

ECONOMIC CONSIDERATIONS AND THE FUTURE OF LAPAROSCOPY

Surgeons face a variety of factors that will influence their decision to expand the use of videolaparoscopy. Patient outcome and performance factors as well as economic and environmental considerations are extremely important. The spread of laparoscopy to nations outside the United States and Europe has been somewhat slower owing to regional medical practices, cultural differences, and economic factors. In Japan, there has been a conservative approach to new technology, while in Latin America, the cost of technology has been a major deterrent. In addition, availability of equipment, personnel, and adequate training have also limited the adoption of these techniques.

A recent report recorded data gathered from a Pennsylvania HMO U.S. Health Care. They found that the incidence of cholecystectomy had increased from 1.35 to 2.15 per 1,000 population from the years 1988 to 1992 for the patients covered under their plan. Therefore, in spite of cost savings of 25% for laparoscopic versus open cholecystectomy, the HMO found their total expenditures for gallbladder disease rose 11.4% during these four years. Other surveys have also confirmed that the number of cholecystectomies increased in 1992. Although it was felt this could be attributed to a backlog of symptomatic but untreated patients, it now appears this pattern may be continuing. Potential reasons for this pattern may include a decreased reluctance of patients to seek appropriate surgical treatment for symptomatic gallstones or a tendency of surgeons to liberalize the criteria for surgical candidates. It is hoped that future data will clarify this issue.

The Future

As health care changes in the United States, cost savings and efficiency by the surgeon, hospitals, and employees will be further refined. The cost/benefit analysis of videolaparoscopy will be continually evaluated. Industrial competition will allow the cost of instrumentation and technology to decrease, and as surgeons develop better techniques, hospitalization, morbidity, and mortality rates will decrease. However, the paramount goal is improved patient care and safety, and the challenge for the future will be to strive for this goal cost effectively.

RECOMMENDED READING

1. Meyers WC, Branum GD, Farouk M, et al. A prospective analysis of 1518 laparoscopic cholecystectomies. *N Engl J Med* 1991;324:1073–1078.
2. Schirmer BD, Dix J. Cost-effectiveness of laparoscopic cholecystectomy. *J Lapaoendosc Surg* 1992;2:145–150.
3. Bass EB, Pitt HA, Lillemoe KD. Cost-effectiveness of laparoscopic cholecystectomy. *Am J Surg* 1993;165:466–471.
4. Deloitte & Touche. *Economic impact of laparoscopic surgery.* 1993.
5. Voyles CR, Petro AB, Meena AL, et al. A practical approach to laparoscopic cholecystectomy. *Am J Surg* 1991;161:365–370.
7. Diehl AK. Laparoscopic cholecystectomy: too much of a good thing? *JAMA* 1993;270:1469–1470.
8. State of New York Department of Health. Memorandum. New York: Department of Health, 1992.
9. Apelgren KN, Blank ML, Slomski CA, et al. Reusable instruments are more cost-effective than disposable instruments for laparoscopic cholecystectomy. *Surg Endosc* 1994;8:32–34.
10. Petere JH, Ellison EC, Innes JT, et al. Safety and efficacy of laparoscopic cholecystectomy: a prospective analysis of 100 initial patients. *Ann Surg* 1991;213:3–12.

11. Kavic MS. Laparoscopic hernia repair. *Surg Endosc* 1993;7:163–167.
12. Mowschenson PM. Improving the cost-effectiveness of laparoscopic cholecystectomy. *J Laparo-endosc Surg* 1993;3:113–119.
13. Voyles CR. The laparoscopic buck stops here! *Am J Surg* 1993;165:472–473.
14. MacFadyen BV, Arregui MD, Corbitt JD, et al. Complications of laparoscopic herniorrhaphy. *Surg Endosc* 1993;7:155–158.
15. Bernarde HR, Hartman TW. Complications after laparoscopic cholecystectomy. *Am J Surg* 1993; 165:533–535.
16. Bailey RW, et al. Laparoscopic cholecystectomy: experience with 375 consecutive patients. *Ann Surg* 1991.
17. Vitale G, Collet D, Larson GM, et al. Interruption of professional and home activities after laparoscopic cholecystectomy among French and American patients. *Am J Surg* 1991;161:396–398.
18. Hunter J, Ortega A, Peters J, et al. A prospective, randomized comparison of laparoscopic appendectomy with open appendectomy. *Am J Surg* 1995;169:208–213.
19. Phillips EH, Franklin M, Carroll BJ, et al. Laparoscopic colectomy. *Ann Surg* 1992;216:703–707.
20. Weerts JM, Dallemagne B, Hamoir E, et al. Laparoscopic Nissen fundoplication: detailed analysis of 132 patients. *Surg Laparosc Endosc* 1993;3:359–364.

Equipment Disinfection and Sterilization*

David W. Duppler
Department of Surgery
Appleton Medical Center
Appleton, Wisconsin 54911

Operative Laparoscopy and Thoracoscopy, edited by
B. V. MacFadyen, Jr. and
J. L. Ponsky. Lippincott-Raven
Publishers, Philadelphia © 1996.

LAPAROSCOPIC EQUIPMENT

At the core of any set of laparoscopic instruments is the video imaging equipment. The laparoscopic revolution would not have been possible without the development of the high-resolution videolaparoscopic camera. This allows all members of the surgical team to view the operative field simultaneously. The original cameras were single-chip cameras. The "chip" is a *charged coupled device* (CCD), which simply refers to the element that receives the light and converts it into a video signal. These cameras would commonly provide resolution in the range of 300 lines. Newer cameras, using either larger single chips or multiple chips, have improved resolution to 600 lines and beyond. In general, the multiple-chip cameras provide not only greater resolution, but improved color and light sensitivity. They are also more expensive.

Exciting new developments in the field of video imaging include the three-dimensional laparoscopic video system and high-definition television. Three-dimensional video imaging systems are just now becoming available in the marketplace and may help improve the efficiency of surgeons performing complicated movements and manipulations, such as laparoscopic suturing and knot-tying.

---

* Excerpts from this chapter can be found in *Surgical Clinics of North America*, Vol. 72, No. 5, October 1992, pp. 1021–1032.

These systems are significantly more expensive than basic video imaging systems. The use of high-definition television in laparoscopic surgery is still in its infancy. The camera is large and quite unwieldy for use during laparoscopic procedures and is also prohibitively expensive. Surgeons who have used this technology, however, have reported the video images are clearly superior to anything they have used previously. Both three-dimensional and high-definition television technology are expected to continue to evolve, with the hope they may become more affordable in the future.

Laparoscopes come in various sizes, ranging from 2 to 10 mm in diameter. In addition, various angled scopes are available from 0- to 90-degree orientation. Angled scopes, although somewhat more difficult to learn to use, generally provide the surgeon with more flexibility in viewing internal structures. Angled scopes

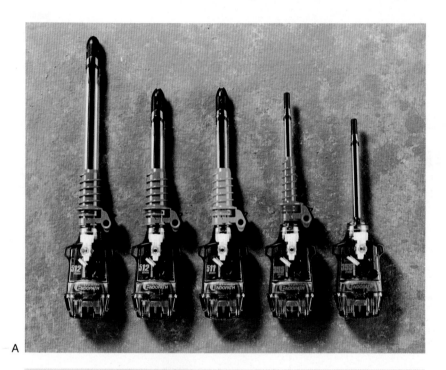

A

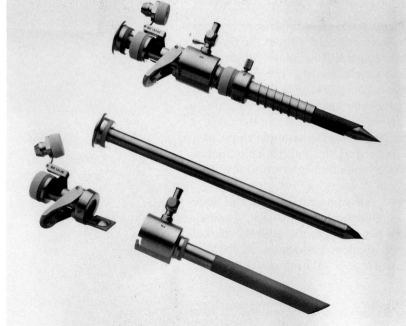

B

Figure 1. Various types and sizes of disposable laparoscopic trocars **(A)** and reusable trocars **(B).** (Courtesy of Ethicon Eudo-Surgery, Inc., New Brunswick, N.J. and Karl Storz Endoscopy/America Inc., Culver City, C.A.)

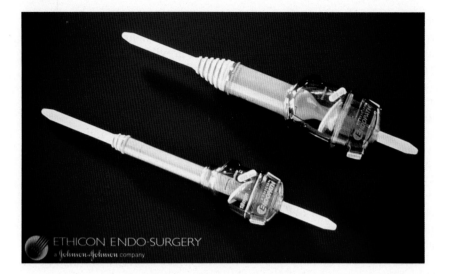

Figure 2. Access and conversion trocars for enlarging laparoscopic incisions. (Courtesy of Ethicon Endo-Surgery, Inc., New Brunswick, N.J.)

often provide access to areas that would be "blind" to 0-degree scopes. The flexible laparoscope is based on the same principle, to allow the surgeon more variability and access to areas not accessible with more traditional laparoscopes. Operative laparoscopes that have an operating channel are occasionally helpful in therapeutic laparoscopic procedures. Newer laparoscopes can withstand heat sterilization, making them more readily available in a sterilized form.

Many different types of laparoscopic trocars are available, all designed to provide various means of accessing the peritoneum or thorax (Fig. 1). Many disposable trocars are equipped with so-called "safety shields" designed to decrease the risk of internal injury. None of these instruments has been proved to be safer than nonshielded trocars. The safety of trocars is determined primarily by the way they are used and not by the way they are manufactured. In addition, there are various access trocars, which can be used to convert standard trocars into larger openings, either for inserting larger instruments or extracting tissue (Fig. 2).

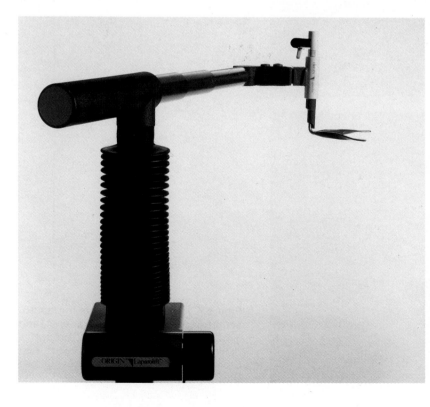

Figure 3. The Laparolift system for gasless laparoscopy. (Courtesy of Origin Medsystems, Inc., Menlo Park, C.A.)

Laparoscopic insufflators and light sources have become reasonably standard, with improvements over earlier equipment. Laparoscopic light sources now routinely contain xenon instead of halogen, which was previously used. Xenon provides a brighter light for improved visualization and resolution. The most important aspect of insufflators is their ability to provide high flow, ≥6 l per minute, so that an adequate pneumoperitoneum can be maintained during complex procedures involving the exchange of multiple instruments.

Several Japanese surgeons have pioneered the use of an abdominal wall suspension system, which obviates the need for a laparoscopic insufflator. An abdominal wall suspension system that is somewhat more sophisticated than the original devices is commercially available (Fig. 3). This system allows for a closer regulation of the abdominal wall tension and can be provided through a single abdominal wall puncture. Any method of abdominal wall suspension allows the surgeon to use standard surgical instruments as opposed to laparoscopic instruments, since concern about maintenance of a pneumoperitoneum does not exist.

Many different types of laparoscopic graspers, tissue dissectors, and scissors are available, both in reusable and disposable forms. There are also some curved

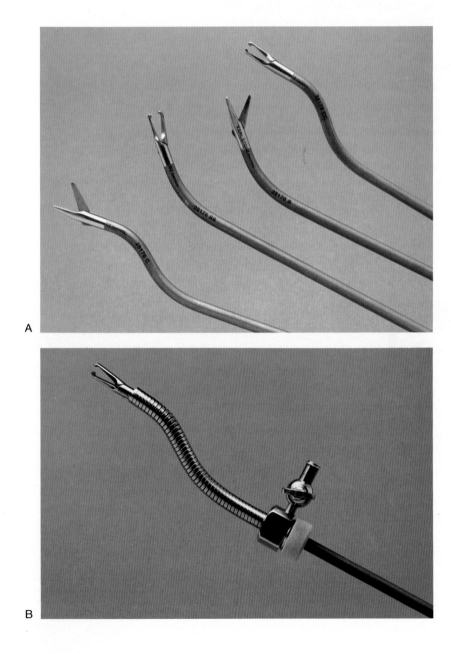

A

B

Figure 4. Curved instruments for laparoscopic and thoracoscopic surgery **(A)** and a curved instrument placed through a malleable trocar **(B).** (Courtesy of Karl Storz Endoscopy-America, Inc., Culver City, C.A.)

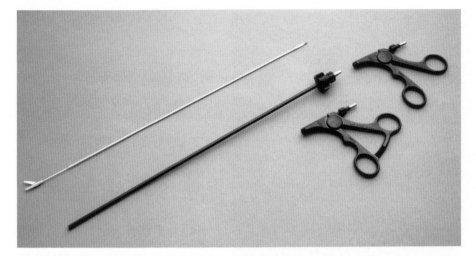

Figure 5. The disassembled components of a reusable laparoscopic scissors. (Courtesy of Karl Storz Endoscopy-America, Inc., Culver City, C.A.)

instruments that have been developed, which give the surgeon more versatility of movement within the peritoneal or pleural cavities. These are generally inserted through pliable trocars (Fig. 4). Reusable instruments now come in easily assembled and disassembled components, and some parts may even be discarded after each procedure. This facilitates cleaning and handling of the instruments (Fig. 5). Laparoscopic suturing has led to the manufacture of various forms of needle holders (Fig. 6), also available in disposable forms (Fig. 7), suturing devices for assisting in closure of the fascial trocar incision (Fig. 8), tissue retractors (Fig. 9), clip appliers, specimen retrieval bags, suction/irrigation devices, and tissue morcellators in various forms. Innovative stapling devices are available for hemostasis and to facilitate gastrointestinal anastomoses and resections (Fig. 10).

There are also various forms of laparoscopic ultrasonic probes that can be used for staging of malignancies, detecting choledocholithiasis, and assisting in

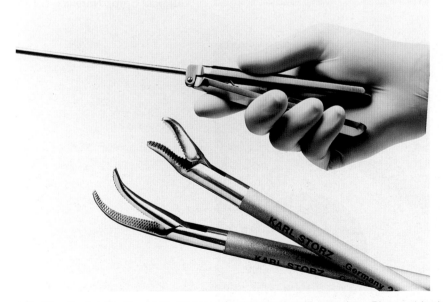

Figure 6. The Szabo-Berci needle holders for laparoscopic suturing. Pictured is the handle *(above),* the parrot beak needle holder *(middle),* and the flamingo tipped tissue grasper *(bottom).* (Courtesy of Karl Storz Endoscopy-America, Inc., Culver City, C.A.)

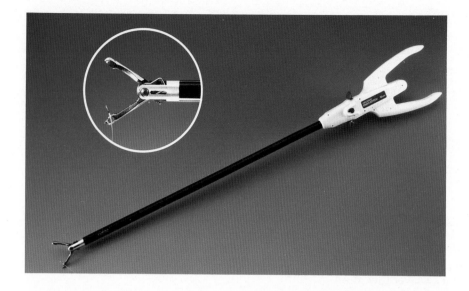

Figure 7. The Endo Stitch instrument, a disposable laparoscopic suturing system. (Courtesy of U.S. Surgical Corp., Norwalk, C.T.)

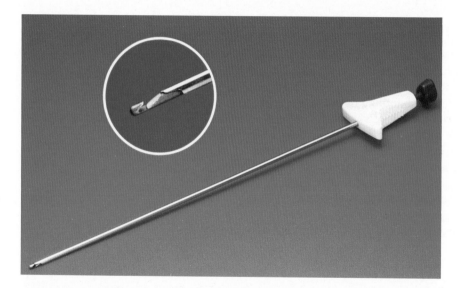

Figure 8. The Endo Close instrument for fascial suturing. (Courtesy of U.S. Surgical Corp., Norwalk, C.T.)

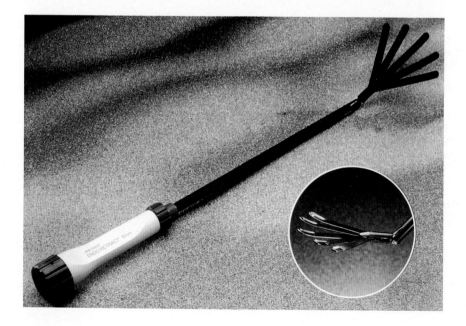

Figure 9. One of the types of tissue retractors available. (Courtesy of U.S. Surgical Corp., Norwalk, C.T.)

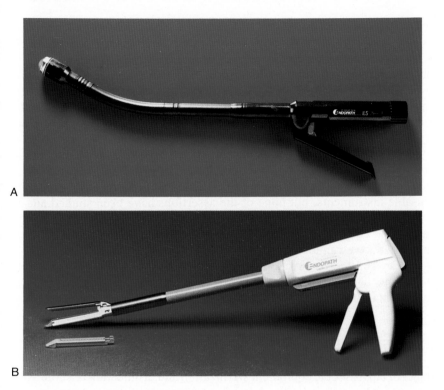

A

B

Figure 10. Stapling devices designed for laparoscopic use: an intraluminal stapler **(A),** and a linear stapler **(B).** (Courtesy of Ethicon Endo-Surgery, New Brunswick, N.J.)

the identification of vascular structures during dissection. The role of these devices has not yet been clearly defined.

Various means of achieving hemostasis are available. This is commonly achieved with some type of thermal cautery or application of clips, ligatures, sutures, or topical agents. Many types of laparoscopic instruments have been designed for monopolar cautery, which is still the most commonly used form of thermal cautery (Fig. 11). When used laparoscopically, monopolar cautery has all the dangers associated with its use during open surgery or intraluminal procedures, such as collateral injury from disseminated energy as well as spark-gap injury. Bipolar cautery instruments have been devised to avoid some of these dangers, but their use is still somewhat limited. There are also various types of lasers that

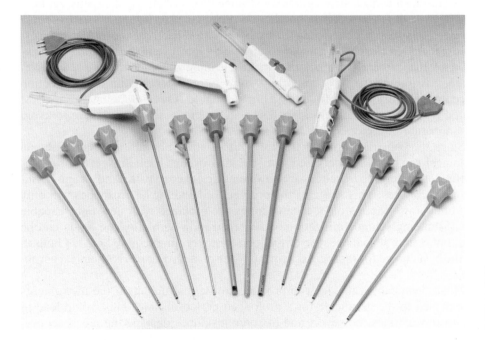

Figure 11. Various tips and attachments for use with monopolar cautery. (Courtesy of Ethicon Endo-Surgery, New Brunswick, N.J.)

can be used in operative laparoscopy. In general, lasers have superior cutting capabilities when compared to monopolar electrocautery but inferior coagulation. These characteristics may vary between types of lasers and laser fibers.

The debate regarding reusable versus disposable laparoscopic instruments is unlikely to be settled at any time soon. At the core of the debate is the question as to which type of instrument is more cost effective. It is important to remember that there are hidden costs involved with the of both disposable and reusable instruments, and these hidden costs will vary among institutions (1). Therefore, it is important for each institution to determine which type of instruments may be most cost efficient in its situation. Manufacturers of disposable instruments contend their instruments are more likely to be sterile and function appropriately than the reusable instruments, but none of the assertions have been studied adequately to confirm or refute these contentions.

As laparoscopic equipment continues to evolve we will undoubtedly be exposed to instruments we cannot even dream of today. Just as it would have been impossible for Dr. Halsted to envision laparoscopic cholecystectomy, so it may be difficult for many of us to comprehend robotics and telepresence surgery, which is clearly on the horizon (2).

EQUIPMENT DISINFECTION AND STERILIZATION

The subject of laparoscopic equipment sterilization and disinfection is a confusing and controversial one. It is best to begin by defining the differences between sterilization and disinfection.

Sterilization is the complete elimination or destruction of all forms of microbial life. Sterilization is achieved by steam, gas, or liquid chemical sterilants. *Disinfection* is a relative term and is divided into three levels, depending on the amount of microorganisms eliminated: *high, intermediate,* and *low level.* High-level disinfection refers to the elimination of all microbial organisms, with the exception of bacterial spores. Intermediate- and low-level disinfection destroys fewer organisms. When it comes to surgical instruments, only high-level disinfection is applied. This is usually achieved by using a chemical sterilant but exposing the surgical instruments for less time than needed for sterilization (3,4).

Most laparoscopic equipment, such as graspers, scissors, and trocars, are safely sterilized using a steam autoclave. Since this is relatively inexpensive, fast, and effective, it is the preferred method for achieving sterilization. Laparoscopic cameras, however, will be damaged by heat. The repeated exposure of laparoscopic cameras to chemical germicides can cause damage, and the irregular configuration of the camera's surface can make cleaning difficult and unpredictable. Cleaning is one of the most important steps in any sterilization or disinfection procedure, and also very difficult and unpredictable. Therefore, cameras are best treated with the use of a barrier, such as a sterile enclosed plastic sleeve to avoid contamination of the operative field.

Since the camera should be treated with a barrier and all other laparoscopic equipment can be steam-sterilized, only the laparoscope itself presents a problem. Fortunately, many laparoscopes are now being designed to withstand steam-sterilization procedures. This suggests the problem of handling laparoscopes will only be a temporary one, as older laparoscopes are replaced with new ones capable of withstanding steam sterilization. Gas sterilization with ethylene oxide can be used, but is impractical because of the long turnover time required (12–24 hours). So, the best choice for reprocessing these types of laparoscopes is chemical germicides.

Most chemical germicides can produce sterile instruments if the instruments are exposed to the germicide for a prolonged period of time. This would lead to long turnover times, however, and in some instances damage the laparoscopes.

Since this is impractical, most hospitals that use liquid germicides for processing the laparoscopes use shorter exposure times, with the aim of achieving high-level disinfection. The germicides that can be used for sterilization or high-level disinfection include 2% glutaraldehyde-based formulations, peracetic acid, demand-released chloride dioxide, and various forms of hydrogen peroxide (4). Chloride dioxide has not been commonly used in this country. A new sterilization process using hydrogen peroxide was recently developed, but there is little clinical information regarding its use. Therefore, 2% glutaraldehyde and peracetic acid are the only two choices left for processing lensed instruments such as laparoscopes.

Glutaraldehyde formulations are the most popular chemical sterilant used for disinfection of medical equipment in the United States (5,6). They are popular because of the advantages of excellent biocidal activity in the presence of organic contamination, noncorrosive action on endoscopes or equipment, and noncoagulation of proteinaceous material (4). High-level disinfection can be accomplished only with solutions having no less than 1% concentration of glutaraldehyde. More dilute formulations are ineffective. Most manufacturers of glutaraldehyde currently recommend a minimum of 20 minutes of exposure to provide high-level disinfection. Although the use life of 2% glutaraldehyde solution is generally accepted as 28–30 days, this can be decreased with heavy use or inadvertent dilution or contamination. The potency and use life of a chemical sterilant are determined by the use pattern, not by time. Test kits are available to determine if the solution is still sufficiently potent for high-level disinfection. These chemical concentration monitors should be used routinely to determine the appropriate intervals for germicide replacement and replenishment. When all the above factors are controlled and the instrument is adequately cleaned, such that bacterial spores are not present, the end result could, in theory, be a sterile instrument. Each of the above factors adds a variable to the disinfection process that may be difficult to control and the absence of bacterial spores cannot always be assured.

A new sterilization process marketed under the brand name Steris has become available over the past several years. It has the advantage of being a closed system that controls a number of the factors mentioned above that can limit the efficacy of a germicide (7). The active ingredient of the system, peracetic acid, is a strong germicide that reportedly has little harmful effect on optical equipment. The manufacturer claims that the Steris system provides sterile instruments, a claim supported by the laboratory testing data provided by the manufacturer (8). This would appear to be a promising option for the reprocessing of laparoscopic equipment but independently conducted and published studies confirming the manufacturer's claim are lacking at this time.

It is important to remember that the efficacy of whatever chemical germicide is being used is influenced by several factors, including the organic load on the instrument (i.e., the efficacy of cleaning), the type and level of microbial contamination, the concentration of and time of exposure to the germicide, the physical configuration of the instrument (e.g., hinges, lumens), and the temperature and pH of the disinfection process (4).

There are no data to suggest that high-level disinfection, when properly performed, increases the risk of infection during laparoscopy. There continues to be concern, however, about the use of instruments treated with high-level disinfection rather than sterilization. Unfortunately, there are not many scientific data to definitively answer the question regarding the safety of disinfection versus sterilization.

There have been only two studies that have attempted to look at this problem in a prospective fashion. A study by Huezo and coworkers (9) analyzed 3,903 women undergoing laparoscopic tubal sterilization; 58% of the procedures were performed with equipment sterilized with ethylene oxide, and 42% of the procedures were performed with equipment disinfected with 2% glutaraldehyde. When 2% glutaraldehyde was used, all of the surgical instruments, not just the laparoscope, were treated in this fashion by soaking the instruments in glutaraldehyde for 10 to 15 minutes. No difference in wound infection rates could be seen between the two groups of patients.

In the other prospective study, 100 consecutive patients undergoing laparoscopy, conducted in 1979 by Corson and colleagues (10), the laparoscope was soaked for 15 minutes in 2% glutaraldehyde before the procedure. After a standard skin preparation with povidone iodine, cultures were obtained from the umbilical skin, the pelvic peritoneum, and the laparoscope: 61% of the umbilical and 29% of the peritoneal cultures were positive. The organisms cultured from the skin and peritoneum were similar. Of the laparoscope cultures, 22% were also positive for organisms, but these organisms were different from those cultured from the umbilicus and peritoneum. This suggested that the peritoneum was being contaminated by skin flora and not by the laparoscope. No cross-contamination was noted between patients, and there were no clinical infections in any of the patients.

Other retrospective reviews also support the safety of high-level disinfection. Loffer (11) conducted a retrospective review of 3,258 patients undergoing laparoscopy. All laparoscopes underwent high-level disinfection with 2% glutaraldehyde prior to use, and only three wound infections were encountered, all minor and treated with local care. None of the infections could be traced to contaminated equipment.

The 1975 membership survey of the American Association of Gynecologic Laparoscopists included 117,705 patients who underwent diagnostic laparoscopy or laparoscopic tubal sterilization (5). The majority of surgeons used high-level disinfection for their equipment. The incidence of infectious complications was 0.3%, with seven cases supposedly traced to contaminated instruments. None of these cases could be documented on follow-up, however. The authors concluded that high-level disinfection with 2% glutaraldehyde between patients was adequate.

The Ad Hoc Committee on Infection Control in the Handling of Endoscopic Equipment of the Association for Practitioners in Infection Control has proposed the following guidelines for the preparation of laparoscopic instrumentation (12):

1. Meticulous care should be taken in mechanically cleaning all of the parts of the laparoscopic instrument. This is the most important step in the reprocessing of laparoscopic equipment, no matter what type of disinfection or sterilization is being used.
2. High-level disinfection or sterilization are acceptable methods of preparing instruments for use. All metal instruments or parts that can undergo sterilization using a steam autoclave should be handled in this manner. When ethylene oxide is used for sterilization, the recommendation of the manufacturer should be followed for both sterilization and aeration.
3. High-level disinfection, when chosen, should be performed with a chemical germicide capable of killing all microorganisms (gram-positive and gram-negative bacteria, fungi, mycobacteria, lipophilic and hydrophilic viruses) except bacterial spores and should be used in accordance with the disinfectant manufacturer's instructions.
4. Aseptic technique should be used in transferring the disinfected or sterilized endoscope and other instruments to the sterile surgical field.
5. When procedures are to be performed on patients who are at increased risk of infection because of a compromised immune system, particular attention must be paid to all aspects of infection control. Under these circumstances, sterilization of the instruments is recommended.

It is also important to note additions to the prescribed protocol are not necessary to deal with HIV or hepatitis B-contaminated equipment. Since laparoscopic equipment is used on patients with both recognized and unrecognized infections, it should be reprocessed in the same manner after each patient use. Both hepatitis B and HIV are inactivated by high-level disinfection.

As mentioned previously, the current concern regarding sterilization versus high-level disinfection really applies to laparoscopes only, as other instruments can be processed differently. High-level disinfection is effective on laparoscopes because of the smooth surfaces and configuration of the instrument. This makes thorough cleaning and thorough exposure to liquid chemical germicides much simpler and more reliable. As more complicated laparoscopic instruments are developed, their disinfection and sterilization may become more complicated. Such instruments include laparoscopes with irrigating channels, the semiflexible laparoscope, flexible small-caliber choledochoscopes, and any instrument with multiple pieces or channels that would make cleaning difficult. Careful attention to cleaning and disinfection or sterilization of these instruments is imperative in order to lessen the risk of postlaparoscopic infections. Even traditional sterilization methods may prove ineffective or too toxic for these more complex laparoscopic instruments. Gas sterilization with ethylene oxide, for example, has been shown to be effective in sterilizing simple instruments such as a rigid laparoscope, but failures have been seen when used on more complex instruments such as flexible endoscopes (13).

Historically, laparoscopic procedures have had low infection rates, partly because most of the laparoscopies have been diagnostic—short procedures that create little devitalized tissue. As laparoscopic surgery continues to evolve into more complex and time-consuming procedures, greater contamination of laparoscopic equipment may occur than we have seen in the past. Whether the use of instruments that have undergone disinfection rather than sterilization will lead to an increase in infectious complications remains to be seen.

> **SURGICAL PEARLS**
> Most laparoscopic equipment is easily and safely sterilized using a steam autoclave. Delicate instruments, such as the laparoscope, pose unique disinfection and sterilization problems. All equipment should be sterilized. However, when sterilization is not feasible, high-level disinfection is adequate.

REFERENCES

1. Reichert M. Laparoscopic instruments: patient care and cost issues. *AORN J* 1993;57:637–655.
2. Satava RM. High tech surgery: speculation on future directions. In: Hunter JG, Sackier JM, eds. *Minimally invasive surgery.* New York: McGraw-Hill; 1993:339–347.
3. Favero MS, Bond WW. Chemical disinfection of medical and surgical materials. In: Block Social Services, ed. *Disinfection, sterilization, and preservation,* 4th ed. Philadelphia: Lea & Febiger; 1991:617.
4. Rutala W. APIC guideline for selection and use of disinfectants. *Am J Infect Control* 1990;18: 99–117.
5. Phillips J, Hulka B, Hulka J, et al. Laparoscopic procedures: the American Association of Gynecologic Laparoscopists' membership survey for 1975. *J Reprod Med* 1977;18:277–232.
6. Rutala WA, Clontz EP, Weber DJ, et al. Disinfection practices for endoscopes and other semicritical items. *Infect Control Hosp Epidemiol* 1991;12:282–288.
7. Crow S. Peracetic acid sterilization: a timely development for a busy healthcare industry. *Infect Control Hosp Epidemiol* 1992;12:2.
8. STERIS System 1. *Technical data monograph.* Cleveland, OH: STERIS Corp., 1988.
9. Huezo CM, et al. Risk of wound and pelvic infection after laparoscopic tubal sterilization: Instrument disinfection versus sterilization. *Obstet Gynecol* 1983;61:598–602.
10. Corson SL, Block S, Mintz C, et al. Sterilization of laparoscopes: is soaking sufficient? *J Reprod Med* 1979;23:49–56.
11. Loffer FD. Disinfection vs. sterilization of gynecologic laparoscopy equipment: the experience of the Phoenix SurgiCenter. *J Reprod Med* 1980;25:263–266.
12. Ad Hoc Committee on Infection Control in the Handling of Endoscopic Equipment (Association for Practitioners in Infection Control). Guidelines for preparation of laparoscopic instrumentation. *AORJ J* 1980;32:65–76.
13. Vesley D, et al. Significant factors in the disinfection and sterilization of flexible endoscopes. *AJIC* 1992;20:291–300.

6

Video Imaging

George Berci
Departments of Surgical Endoscopy and Surgery
USC School of Medicine
Los Angeles, California 90024; and
EndoCare Center
Midway Hospital
Los Angeles, California 90036

Margaret Paz-Partlow
EndoCare Center
Midway Hospital
Los Angeles, California 90036

Operative Laparoscopy and Thoracoscopy, edited by B. V. MacFadyen, Jr. and J. L. Ponsky. Lippincott-Raven Publishers, Philadelphia © 1996.

Television is possibly the most dramatic and influential single facet of the new minimally invasive surgery (MIS), opening what was previously the surgeon's exclusive realm to the entire operating team. Video imaging can be viewed as a blessing or a curse, given one's experiences and reservations about the medium. Most hospitals now have at least a basic setup for laparoscopic surgery, including the ubiquitous video cart. That equipment may still be functional, but due to the dizzying proliferation of imaging breakthroughs, it is probably already obsolete. In the current climate of fiscal constraints, we must choose acquisitions carefully. A better understanding of these emerging technologies can help us delve through a morass of offerings, and thus assemble a compendium of equipment that will work for us.

HISTORY

Research leading to modern video dates back to the 1880s. Among the many who expended their efforts, Zworykin, who evolved the principles of the iconoscope in 1923 and Farnsworth, who developed the electronic scanning system in 1930 initiated television as we know it today. For any operator who has complained about the excruciating weight of a 4-oz camera inhibiting his mobility, we bring to mind the first closed-circuit videobronchoscopy, performed in 1957 by Soulas in France (Fig. 1). The camera, a studio model, weighed a modest 180 lb. By 1962, the senior author (G.B.) developed and clinically tested a miniaturized black and white model weighing only 12 oz (Fig. 2). The 1970s spawned color cameras with vidicon tubes to replace the passé orthicons. As image quality and light sensitivity improved exponentially, adapting television to endoscopic uses became more feasible. Still, when videoarthroscopy was introduced at our institution in 1980, the complex arrangement of cantilevered arm, articulated beamsplitter, and hulking 2-lb camera, its position and performance constantly fine-tuned by a special techni-

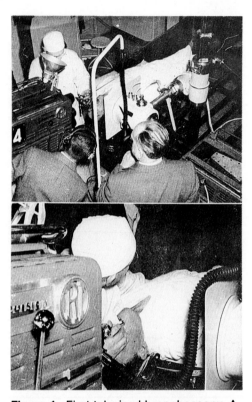

Figure 1. First televised bronchoscopy, A. Soulas, M.D., 1956. (From De Montreynaud JMD. *Traité Practique de Photographie et de Cinématographie Medicales.* Paris: Publications Photo-Cinéma/Paul Montel, 1960.)

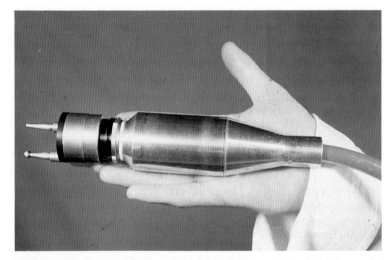

Figure 2. Miniature black and white television camera. 1.8 in. × 4.8 in.; wt. 12 oz. (Developed by G. Berci and Davids, 1962.)

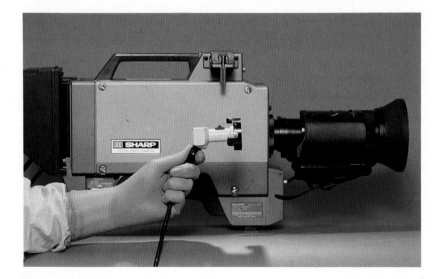

Figure 3. Size comparison by Circon MOS chip camera and Sharp studio camera, 1984.

cian, orthopaedic surgeons rained maledictions as often as compliments upon our heads (Fig. 3).

VISUAL PERCEPTION

The subjectivity of human vision is influenced partly by cognitive responses and partly by the eye's construction. As a sensory perception, vision feeds environmental images into our brains, which are stored as memories. We use these imprints to rationalize our world and to interpret new perceptions. A videocamera has neither the ability to imprint nor to rationalize. Our vision is binocular and imprints perspective and depth clues to help us walk, drive, and reach for objects. Up to now, cameras were seldom binocular, rather single ocular in design. When observing a monitor image, one must rely on these imprinted clues as guides to depth perception. The eye's sensitivity varies in its consistency across the retina, but a charge couple device (CCD) is constant across its pickup surface. This is a dominant factor as to why CCDs have greater sensitivity to light than tubes and produce better transmissions under low light situations.

The eye's lens, which is clear and is shaped and oriented something like a camera, collects light reflected from the object when the surgeon looks at an organ, after it passes through the cornea and aqueous humor, on through the pupil of the iris and into the lens. Light rays must bend so that they converge at the retina's center, the fovea, in order to focus the image (Fig. 4). Visual sensation results

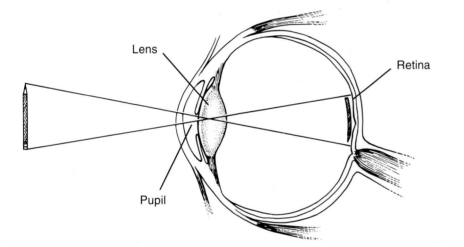

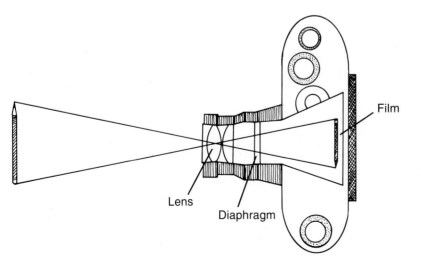

Figure 4. Camera/eye analogy: the diaphragm of a camera and the iris of the eye adjust the amount of light traveling to the interior. In both, the lens causes the image to appear inverted on the light-sensitive surface. In the eye the image is righted in the process of interpretation by the brain.

when the retina is stimulated by light. The human eye's retina can detect electromagnetic radiation limited to wavelengths between 400 and 700 nm (visible spectrum). The optic nerve acts as a pathway from the eyes to the brain. The primary sensory neurons are the rods and cones located in the retina. Rods and cones are sensitive to light stimuli. They relay impulses to a second neuron in the retina, which in turn transmits the impulse to a second neuron in the retina, which in turn transmits the impulse to a third neuron, the fibers of which make up the optic nerve. After the optic nerves leave the two orbital cavities, they fuse at the optic chiasma, then separate at the optic tracts, which encircle the midbrain and pass to the lateral geniculate bodies. The optic nerve is actually a tract of the brain rather than a peripheral nerve. Where the optic nerve attaches to the eyeball, the dura mater fuses to the sclera (Fig. 5).

Cones are sensitive to color, but rods control dark adaptation. Night vision is achromatic (black/white) vision. Similarly, a typical half-inch camera will lose color as light is diminished. Visual perception may hinge on the concurrent processing of multiplexed temporal messages from all visual areas. We enhance the endoscope's monocular view and add acuity to the viewer's visual adaptation and perception by supplying a binocular picture at an optimal viewing distance from a suitably bright video screen. Thus, surgeons are better able to execute intricate techniques from this well-illuminated, binocular, albeit two-dimensional, video image.

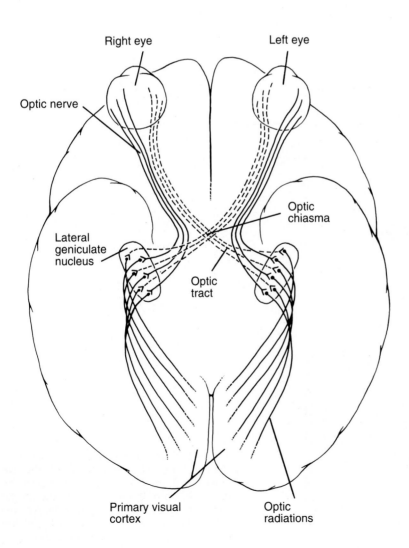

Figure 5. Schematic of the optical pathways.

OPTICS

Telescopes have not changed significantly since Hopkins introduced his revolutionary rod-lens design in the mid-1950s. Given the particular specialty, variable sizes are needed for optimal vision. In an effort to bring more light into the upper abdomen, laparoscopes with bigger rod lenses have been introduced. Additional brightness is a trade-off for depth of field and visual acuity. Light conducting fiber attributes have been upgraded, leading to improved light transmission.

LIGHT SOURCE

The culmination of multiple generations of halogen filament lamps, various flash globes, and sundry assorted lamps, an automatic xenon high-intensity light source introduced during the mid-1980s is still our standard workhorse. This light unit, with its 300-W lamp is the brightest, most dependable unit available for use with rigid endoscopes (Fig. 6). Xenon short-arc technology linked with special ceramic-to-metal sealing techniques comprise the lamp's core. Its prealigned internal reflector effects a large collection angle around the arc, maximizing output efficiency. Moreover, it has excellent transmission from the ultraviolet to the infrared. This unit dispenses automatic light control for video while also functioning as a flash generator adequate for still photography (35mm slides).

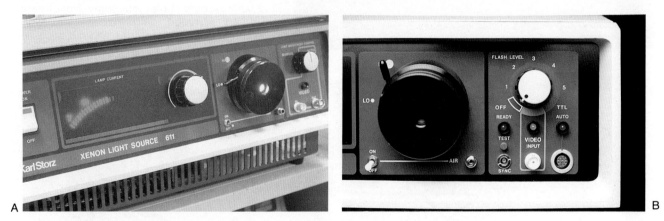

Figure 6. A: Xenon automatic light source. **B:** Close-up of flash settings and video connection. (Karl Storz Endoscopy.)

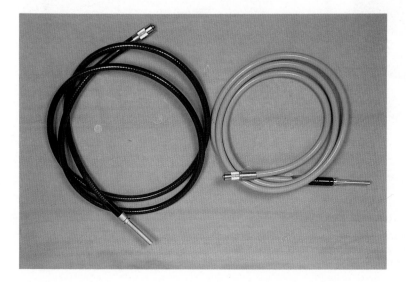

Figure 7. Light cables, fluid on the left, fiberoptic to the right.

Smaller, less expensive sources based on 170-W xenon lamps have been developed for those applications that require less light. Recently, extremely inexpensive units with highly efficient metal halide globes and ingenious electronics have become available for use in tandem with the more light-sensitive CCD technology.

Light is transmitted from the light source to the telescope through light cables, either fiberoptic or fluid-based. Fiberoptic cables are more flexible, but compress the spectrum, suppressing the blue end, and their illumination has a yellow tinge. Fluid cables transmit the full spectrum and about 30% more light, but are more inconvenient to use due to their rigidity. Also, they turn yellow if gassed, so they

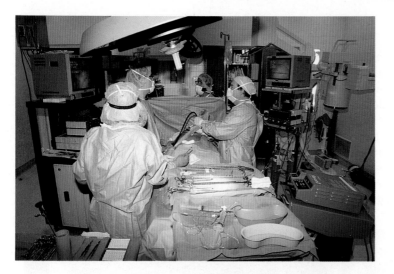

Figure 8. View of the operating room during a laparoscopic cholecystectomy. Note that the primary surgeon performs ambidextrously, wielding both the telescope and left accessory grasper.

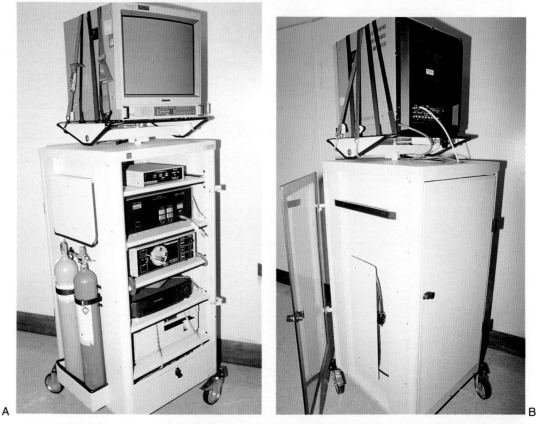

A   B

Figure 9. Video cart. **A:** Front view shows enough shelf space to house control unit, insufflator, light, video recorder, and hardcopy printer. **B:** Back view shows full access to coaxial connections and convenient side AC cable storage (Seitz Corp.).

can only be sterilized through soaking. A cable must be carefully inspected before a procedure to determine its condition. A fiberoptic cable with more than 15% broken fibers is not adequate for video. A fluid cable that is yellowed or has a cracked quartz end must also be replaced (Fig. 7). After such herculean labors, surgeons expect not only to see well, but to obtain permanent endoscopic records both superior in quality and fairly uncomplicated to procure.

OPERATING SUITES

Operating rooms come in varying dimensions. Their physical layout must be carefully studied and apparatus arrayed in a manner that is acceptable to the operating team, yet does not compromise the aseptic field. One must keep in mind the logistical requirements of an adequate traffic flow pattern while integrating other ancillary equipment (i.e., xenon light, insufflator, irrigation pump) into the available floor space (Fig. 8). Video carts designed specially for the operating room environment are available from many manufacturers at varying prices. Easy access to coaxial cable connections in the back, compact profile, and generous wheels are desirable features (Fig. 9).

Up to now, most minimally invasive surgery suites have been furnished with such carts for flexibility of usage. The time has come to consider dedicated rooms

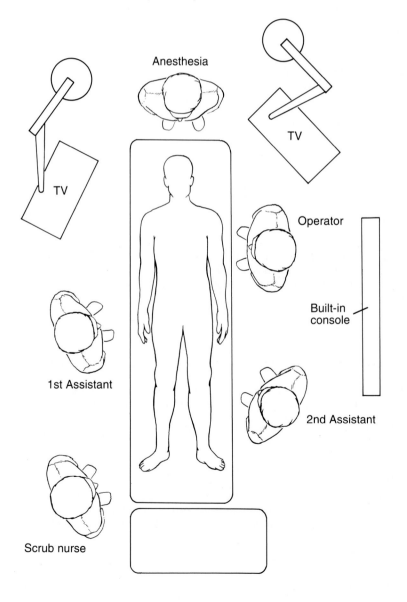

Figure 10. Ceiling suspended fixtures holding video monitors and cameras could be adjusted to any position necessary. Built-in wall consoles would hold the remaining ancillary equipment, freeing floor space to the circulating nurse.

Table 1. *Laparoscopic instrumentation and technology: planning and intervention*

I. Preoperative preparation
   A. Check procedure/surgeon reference card
   B. Assemble all necessary instrumentation
   C. Critical pieces, spares in the room
II. Room layout
   A. Determine TV carts' placement according to surgeon's preference
   B. Arrange all equipment around operating table before patient is brought into the room
III. Insufflation
   A. *Scrub*: Check Veress needle's patency
   B. *Circulator*: Set up insufflator
      1. Tank full? (spare 2nd tank)
      2. Tank on? (wrench)
      3. Insufflator on?
      4. Set pressure, flow rate, zero volume
      5. Tubing kinked?
      6. Luer locks blocked?
      7. Trocar inflow closed? in line obstructed?
IV. Irrigation/suction
   A. Peristaltic pumps
   B. Endoflow
   C. Suction
V. Optics/light
   A. *Scrub*: Visually inspect telescope
      1. Foggy?
      2. Scratched?
      3. Bent?
      4. Broken light bundles? (>25% replace)
   B. *Scrub*: Check light cable
      1. Fluid
         a. Bent?
         b. Quartz ends cracked?
         c. Fluid yellowed?
         d. Casing cracked?
      2. Fiber
         a. Torn cover?
         b. Broken fibers? (>25% replace)
         c. Yellowed?
VI. Video endoscopy/documentation
   A. Cart setup
      1. Label all coaxial cables
      2. Paste connections diagram on cart door
      3. Keep spare cables for quick replacement
      4. Consolidate AC cords with UL multioutlet strip/isolation transformer
   B. Basic setup
      1. Plug in main power cord
      2. Turn on
         a. Monitor
         b. VCR
            (1) If cart contains ¾-in. VCR, red RECORD button must be pressed to display TV image
            (2) Check that ¾-in. tape cassette has red disk inserted in back
            (3) ½-in. cassettes should have unbroken tab to record; if broken, cover with scotch tape
            (4) Review previously recorded tapes to ensure against involuntary erasure
               (a) Use visual search
               (b) Search by logged numbers/times
            (5) Keep spare cassettes on hand
            (6) Press "Record" and "Play" simultaneously
            (7) Press "Pause"; use foot pedal to record intermittently
            (8) Determine who is responsible for recording: circulator or surgeon
         c. Character generator
         d. Still video printer
      3. Connect camera control unit to cart via coaxial cable labeled "Camera"

Table 1. *Continued*

    4. Connect automatic xenon light source to cart using coaxial cable labeled "Light"
    5. If camera sensor is unsterile, plug into camera control unit
       a. Do not bend prongs, match dot/dot
       b. Grasp at connector, not cable
    6. Turn on power to camera control unit
 C. Monitor
    1. "Live" camera image should be visible when "Line A" is selected
    2. Mavigraph will be fed into "Line B, RGB, or CMPTR"
 D. Camera
    1. *Circulator*: Confirm camera connected to cart, power on, camera sensor connected (unsterile)
    2. *Scrub*: If sensor is sterile, check for fog behind cover plate, hand connecting end to circulator
    3. *Scrub*: Sensor unsterile, have circulator feed camera sensor into sterile plastic bag
    4. *Scrub*: Attach cable to endoscope, hand distal end of sterile field to couple with xenon
    5. *Circulator*: Ensure that cable is firmly coupled
    6. *Scrub*: Attach camera sensor to laparoscope with light source on
    7. Aim scope at 4 × 4 gauze and reduce light (source/back of scope) to control highlights
    8. *Circulator*: White balance camera, press button/toggle
    9. Adjust camera zoom and focus for optical image
 E. Still video printer
    1. *Circulator*: Confirm unit on, right line selected
    2. Press "Remaining ribbon," number extant prints appear on screen
    3. Keep spare ribbon/paper packet on hand
    4. Press "Full/Split," page breakup
    5. Press "Input/Memory," camera image appears
       a. "No Input" message, unit not getting video signal
       b. Check connections
       c. Press "Input Select" until "Video" appears
    6. Record-press "Memory"; toggle back to live with "Input/Memory"
    7. Print
       a. More than one print-use "+/−"; number will display on screen (Q1)
       b. Press green "Print" button, 60-sec dev.
       c. Do not try to remove print, it will eject

with fixed video installations that would maximize space and efficiency. At a recent national conference, examples of custom built suites were on show, featuring monitors and cameras on ceiling-suspended arms that could be moved to diverse locations around the operating room table according to surgeon preference. Ancillary equipment resided in built-in niches away from the table, all coaxial and electrical cables fed through the ceiling (Fig. 10). Imagine traversing an operating room without having to dodge carts and trip over cables. Any surgeon who has been plagued by a stiff neck after assisting at a laparoscopic procedure may appreciate the potential for physical comfort and increased efficiency this idea extends (Table 1).

MONITORS

The operative team is reliant on the video image throughout all phases of the procedure. It is agreed a priori that the monitor on which the laparoscopic image is viewed should be of the highest quality. The picture should be flicker-free, with enhanced black performance for better contrast, and efficient white balance circuitry that can deliver more stable color and high resolution. Most commonly, a 19-in. high-resolution color video monitor is placed opposite the primary surgeon, and a second monitor before the assistant. Both monitors should supply

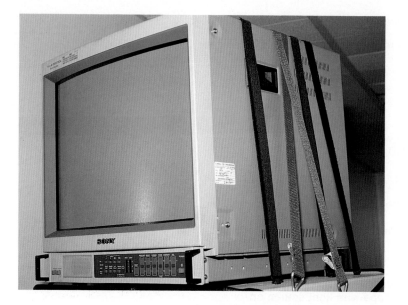

Figure 11. A 19-in. high-resolution monitor; horizontal resolution, 700 lines. (Sony Corp.)

approximately 700 lines of horizontal resolution, almost twice the 350 lines on a standard consumer monitor (Fig. 11).

CAMERA SYSTEMS

All aspects of laparoscopic surgery, from operator performance and comfort, and team participation, to data storage, are facilitated joining a solid-state camera to an endoscope. In more complicated procedures, such as laparoscopic colon resection or splenectomy, it is mandatory that the assistant operate from the same

Table 2. *TV Monitors*

Poor termination can be responsible for many "gremlins" on your TV monitor, among them:
- *Poor color*
- *Highlight detail lost* in a phosphorescent "bloom"
- *Visual "noise"*—electrical interference from other equipment, especially ESUs.

The video image originates at a source, usually a camera control unit. The electronic signal is *looped* through a series of additional devices—character generator, VCR, perhaps a mavigraph, and video monitor(s). The *looping circuits* on these devices have both video IN and OUT connectors.

To prevent the above symptoms from appearing, the *final* video output must be TERMI- NATED. A 75-ohm resistor is put on the last VIDEO OUT to prevent the output connector (and any cable attached to it) from acting like an antenna, pulling extraneous electri- cal interference back into the circuit.

Most of our older monitors (Sony 1900, 1910, and 2030) have termination *switches*, which should be in the ON or 75Ω position on the last monitor (or input) in the circuit.

The new Sony 1943 and 1343 MD monitors in use in lap choles and other areas *do not have these switches*. Instead, the monitor is *automatically* terminated *when nothing is connected to the video out jack*. With these monitors, the following rules need to be followed:
1. Be sure input coaxial cable is connected to VIDEO IN.
2. Make certain there is *nothing* connected to VIDEO OUT on the *last monitor in the series*.

Confirm that all video equipment connections are firm and, with BNC-type (bayonet) connecters, turned clockwise to lock.

monitor image as the primary surgeon, thus assuring precision of execution and an expeditious procedure.

Developed by engineers at Bell Laboratories in 1970, the silicon CCD was originally intended for military, aerospace, and machine vision applications. Its impact on endoscopic video was momentous. If video usage was to become the standard rather than the exception, then small, rugged, sterilizable cameras were vital to any endoscopic suite. The light sensitivity of silicon is responsible for the unique attributes of the integrated image sensor. Electrical resistance abates as light strikes the surface of a silicon device, propagating current carriers. Packets of amplifiable electrical charges store and transfer information on the photosensitive silicon elements. The chip's surface is covered with a compact grid of photocell receptors, each of which creates a pixel (smallest unit of picture elements of an image). The number of pixels on a chip's surface determines its resolution. Typical ⅔-in. and/or ½-in. chips used in solid-state cameras today contain 250,000 to 380,000 pixels.

One of the most recent modifications is a hole accumulator diode (HAD) sensor that is capable of broader dynamic range and lower dark current, combined with a new electronic shutter that executes charge separation within each individual pixel. Light levels up to 600% of normal exposure can be controlled by an HAD sensor. By using this sensor in an endoscopic camera, for example, one amply illuminated views of pericolic gutters while the camera simultaneously controls excessive highlights from the falciform ligament or stomach. In a newer version, known as the HyperHAD, almost 100% of the light reaches the sensor's imaging area. Capping each pixel with its own convex lens augments sensitivity one full f-stop. Vertical smear is eradicated due to the reduction of stray light reflection from insensitive imager elements because OCL focuses almost all incident light. Pixel size decreased so that the ½-in. HyperHAD chip bears an identical number to their prior ⅔-in. chip (768 × 493 pixels = 378,624).

Until recently, the camera we constantly employed with satisfactory results was built on a ⅔-in. CCD chip. This has been superseded by a HyperHAD-based model, for it blends outstanding color rendition with superb light sensitivity. The sensor is a 6.4 × 4.8 mm interline transfer CCD chip. Horizontal resolution is listed as greater than 450 lines with a signal-to-noise ratio of 52 dB. It maintains accurate dimensional detail and gives edge detection precision. It is offered as a detachable camera with a built-in zoom lens that ranges from 25 to 38 mm. The camera head weighs 4 oz, its dimensions 1.1 in. in diameter by 2.7 in. in length. The present automatic shutter is more accurate than previous models, preventing blooming or streaking under extreme lighting conditions. The camera head and connecting cable may be cold-soaked or gas-sterilized (Fig. 12).

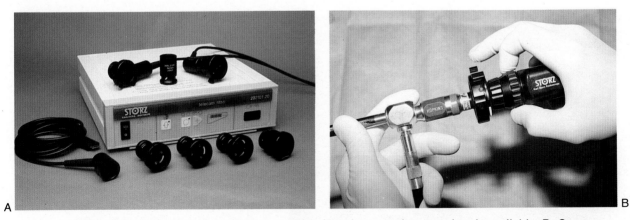

A   B

Figure 12. A: Endoscopic camera control unit and assorted camera heads available. **B:** Camera coupled to endoscope. (Karl Storz Endoscopy.)

The HyperHAD has also been incorporated into three-chip camera designs. Basically, they consist of three interline transfer CCDs and an F5.6 ultraminiature, primary color (RGB) separation system. Variable focal length lenses are not available for these cameras. Endoscopic lenses in fixed focal lengths ranging from 22 mm to 40 mm can be obtained. The sensing area is equivalent to the ½-in. optical format. Each color channel has 768 (H) × 493 (V) picture elements for a total of 1,135,782 pixels in the American NTSC format and 1,369,998 pixels in the PAL European format. Horizontal resolution (luminance) can vary >600 to >800 lines (Fig. 13). In those we have observed, automatic gain control is fast and precise. Clean, bright, sharp camera images are the norm when viewed on an RGB monitor.

There are drawbacks to 3-CCD technology. They cost nearly twice as much as most one-chip cameras, placing them beyond the reach of current capital equipment funds of most hospitals. Camera heads weigh noticeably more than those of single chips and can lead to fatigue for the camera operator. There are a variety of supporting arms that can be used to hold cameras, ranging from mechanical to fully computerized, but this means additional expense. Fiscally and physically a single-chip camera that could deliver an image comparable with that of three-chip cameras would resolve these issues.

Contrast enhancement, which to the observer dramatically sharpens the image by straightening the edges on picture elements, is an adjunct being offered by several manufacturers. Through two-dimensional filtering, pixel by pixel, a digitally processed image can have corrected edges and enhanced highlight details; it can help visual recognition of patterns in images to reveal subtle and obscured details. A one-HyperHAD chip camera boosted with edge enhancement compares favorably visually with a three-chip (also HyperHAD) model.

By coupling the sensor to the ocular "glass to glass," eliminating a space where condensation and subsequent fogging might transpire, several manufacturers have submitted cameras that do away with the conventional eyepiece. They can also tender a sharper, more radiant image.

Flexible electronic endoscopes with a CCD imaging chip at the distal end were introduced in gastroenterology about ten years ago. After multitudinous revisions, electronic endoscopes with their superior images and light transmission, dominate gastrointestinal flexible endoscopy. Along the same lines, several companies have presented an electronic laparoscope, advertising truer color and less distortion than traditional rigid telescope/camera systems. Because their only optical components are the distal lenses, they purport to be less damage-prone (Fig. 14). As they incorporate more features such as VCR remote control on an ergonomic handle, longer light cables, and smaller light sources, they become more attractive to surgeons and nurses looking for a simpler approach.

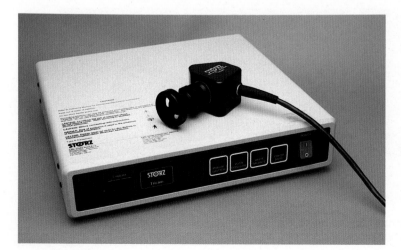

Figure 13. A 3-chip camera and control unit. (Karl Storz Endoscopy.)

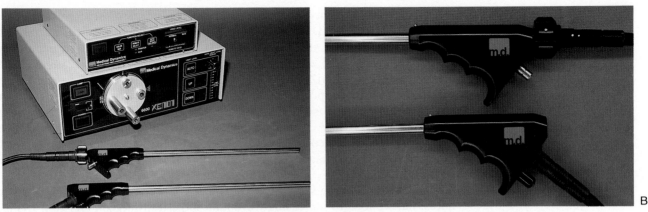

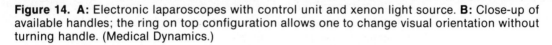

Figure 14. A: Electronic laparoscopes with control unit and xenon light source. **B:** Close-up of available handles; the ring on top configuration allows one to change visual orientation without turning handle. (Medical Dynamics.)

Some major companies are observing their competitors' initial results in this area while continuing research before their own versions are proffered to the marketplace. In this way they can profit from the collected experience. For example, one major manufacturer has introduced a flexible laparoscope aimed primarily at thoracoscopy as they progress developing a videoscope. The scope tip can be flexed over 100 degrees, a propitious feature in the thoracic cavity's circumscribed space. Coupled with a ½-in. chip camera for added light sensitivity, it gives an adequate picture but cannot equal the visual acuity of a rigid telescope.

At times, during more advanced procedures, such as laparoscopic common-duct exploration, one wishes to utilize a second camera on the flexible choledocho-scope, while preserving the abdominal image through the laparoscope for dilatation of the cystic duct and scope introduction and orientation. One option is to use a digital mixer, which can split the screen and bring in the two video images side by side rather than bring yet one more cart into an already crowded operating room. The mixer's joystick allows the surgeon to see both images or only one, as needed, once the unit has been programmed with one's choice. Although the surgeon can only view one camera image at a time, there are also some camera control units that power two camera heads simultaneously. Best of all, the newest option is a processor that accommodates two heads and provides the picture-in-picture feature (Fig. 15).

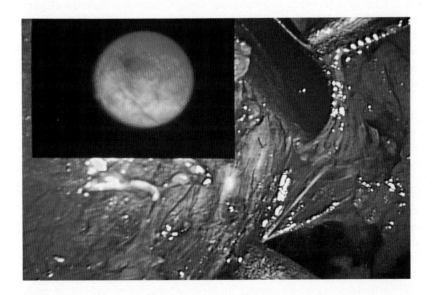

Figure 15. Example of picture-in-picture feature during CBD exploration.

In Japan, experiments have been conducted in ear microsurgery using a high-definition television (HDTV) system that is computer-enhanced for documentation. At the prototype stage is a new HD camera system with an endoscopic adaptor, which may be coupled to standard endoscopes. The 1,125-line HDTV display can provide horizontal resolution about five times that of standard video output. Some limited, promising clinical trials have been performed. Given the strides in research, a closed circuit environment, such as an operating room might shortly be using HDTV. Already available for computerized design applications are workstations that incorporate HDTV display with almost 2 million pixels worth of information, more than six times the relative size of standard NTSC television or VGA graphics.

Our current imaging systems are adequate for the more basic surgical procedures, but we foresee increasingly arduous surgeries. Surgeon and staff training must turn unremittingly intensive to foster these endeavors. To prevent us from inflicting unwitting injuries, it is just as crucial that the caliber of our instrumentation improve. Tools with which we will labor more dependably in a remote fashion than we do in open surgery today are being developed internationally. Stereoscopy research indicates that there are remote control tasks that are very difficult, prone to error, and time-consuming using a two-dimensional display, but are relatively easy using a three-dimensional display.

Our visual comprehension of the world is established on two-dimensional images; flat patterns of varying light intensity and color falling on a single plane of cells in the retina. Yet we come to perceive solidity and depth. We can do this because a number of cues about depth are available in the retinal image: shading, perspective, occlusion of one object by another, and stereoscopic disparity.

One can display stereoscopic images with a standard interlaced television system using alternate fields for the left and right eye image. The correct image is conducted to the correct eye through a selection device. Commonly used selection devices include shutter glasses and switchable polarizing screens. This method is referred to as field-sequential display. To reinforce monocular depth cues, binocular disparity is employed on field-sequential stereoscopic displays. Because of the influence of accommodation and convergence, although predicted apparent depth may be estimated using geometric equations, the actual apparent depth may not follow predictions. Viewing distance vitally sways subject depth ratings. Given this effect of viewing distance on apparent depth, distance must be specified for a given application to ensure veridical depth perception by the viewer.

New PC boards, appropriate software, and two cameras make stereoscopic video procurable right now. As a training tool, endoscope images are easily grasped when articulated in three dimensional stereo. Benefits include clearer visualization and better understanding of data, and easier recognition of form and pattern. One can achieve three to six times greater accuracy for rudimentary psychophysical measures like stereoacuity and depth scaling, and 20% to 75% savings in time to completion of manipulator tasks. Stereoscopic video can facilitate remote manipulation tasks that incorporate unfamiliar objects and lack monocular cues.

Diverse investigators have reported on the bearing of stereopsis on enhanced viewer performance. In field-sequential stereoscopy the display presents left and right perspectives, alternating rapidly (60 times per second per eye) so that each eye sees only its own viewpoint. The viewer must wear special glasses with high-performance liquid crystal glasses synchronized to the video field rate. An infrared emitter in the monitor broadcasts the synchronization data picked up by the battery-powered glasses. Because it operates at twice the rate of traditional video arrays (30 frames per second), one perceives a flicker-free stereoscopic image if each eye can behold 60 fields per second of its primary viewpoint.

As a telescope is rotated along its longitudinal axis in the abdomen, one needs to maintain image orientation, another impediment in calibrating stereoscopy to endoscopy. Nevertheless, systems aimed at laparoscopic surgery are already being marketed. One design produces three-dimensional images in real time through alternating frame technology. A single camera is affixed to a telescope in which images from two separate viewpoints are combined through folded optics and transmitted along a single light path. The projected three-dimensional picture is autostereoscopic, for both eyes view the same screen on a standard monitor. A surgeon experiences momentary disorientation if given a two-dimensional image on which he or she must perform three-dimensional tasks. A true stereoscopic display would alleviate the problem. How does one document a three-dimensional image? One may acquire any of an assortment of moderately economical devices for capturing, editing and displaying field-sequential 60-cycle stereoscopic video. Multiplexers that change the output of any two genlockable (synchronized signals) cameras into field-sequential video can used. Standard recorders and customary techniques can be implemented when editing the videotapes.

Stereoscopic video systems are at an experimental stage. More clinical experience is required in evaluating their merits. Do they significantly augment efficacy in a surgeon's performance of laparoscopic surgery? Are they cost efficient? These and other questions are yet to be answered.

RECORDING MEDIA

One's budget and intent in documenting a procedure will dictate what type of media will be suitable. Today's state-of-the-art method would be to digitize images

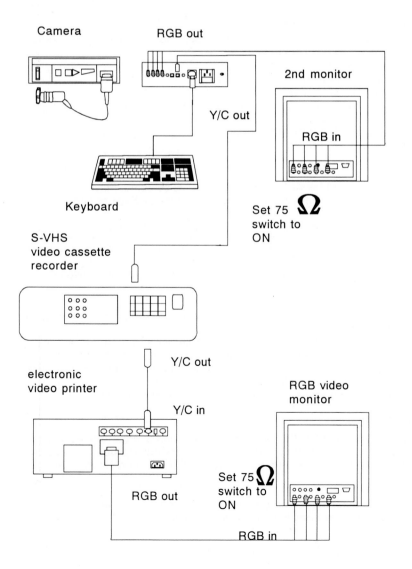

Figure 16. Diagram showing one way to connect several documentation sources and multiple monitors.

for storage on magnetic or optical disc media. But one can also preserve images on videotape, on still video disks, or on film in an analog form. Digitized pictures will make it possible to integrate specimen or operating room photographs with computed tomography (CT) scans, radiographs, and other test results into patients' written records on photographic compact disks (photo CDs), forming the core of a database that could be accessible to researcher and clinician alike. Hard copies can be made using electronic or digital printers of visual data stored on CD or transmitted over phone lines via modem, then displayed on computer or video screens in conferences for consultation and education. Often, one will both moving media and hardcopy documentation. Multiple units and monitors can be interconnected on the video carts for this purpose (Fig. 16).

There are multitudinous technological alternatives to paper processing including microforms and data processing. Electronic document management links all options in a resourceful solution to patient data storage. Data can be merged, its original format or origination device notwithstanding, through graphical interfaces and interapplication data sharing and communication tools. Under these conditions, images are a data type and integrated as a natural extension of desktop

Table 3. *Video endoscopy procedure*

Basic Setup

1. Plug in main power cord.
2. Turn on POWER to
   (a) Monitor.
   (b) Video Cassette Recorder (VCR).
       [Note: If stack contains a ¾-in. Sony VCR (5600 or 5800), the red RECORD button must be pressed to display image.]
   (c) Character Generator.
   (d) Still Video Printer (Mavigraph), if present.
3. Connect Camera Control Unit to stack via coax cable labled CAMERA.
4. Connect 610 automatic xenon light source (if applicable) to video stack using coax cable labeled LIGHT SOURCE.
5. If camera is unsterile, plug into camera control unit.
6. Turn on power to camera control unit.

Monitor

"Live" camera image should be visible when "Line A" is selected. Mavigraph will be fed into one of the following, depending on monitor: "Line B, RGB or CMPTR."

Sony Monitor	Live	Mavigraph	Comment
2030	Line A	Line B, CMPTR	Press CONTROL to access line selections.
1910	Line A	Line B, RGB	
1943MD	Line A	Line B, RGB	Press ANALOG (EXT) for RGB display.

Camera

1. Confirm that camera is connected to stack, power is on, and camera connected.
2. Attach camera to endoscope with light source on.
3. Aim endoscope at 4 × 4 gauze and reduce light (either at source or by backing off endoscope) to eliminate any "bloom" or glare wiping out highlight details.
4. White balance camera. On some camera control units this is a separate button. On others, press the power toggle switch *past* the ON position to W/B.
5. Adjust camera zoom and focus to optimum image size and sharpness.

Video Cassette Recorder

All video stacks are provided with ½-in. VHS VCRs. Some units are additionally equipped with ¾-in. machines used primarily when higher quality tapes are required for editing of teaching tapes. The ½-in. machines are the standard for most applications.

The two primary ½-in. machines are the Sharp XA 100 or 300 and the Panasonic AG 6300MD. The ¾-in. VCRs are Sony 5800 or 5600 machines.

VCR Type/Model	Record Function	Foot Pedal?
½-in. panasonic AG 6300MD	Press and *hold* RECORD Press PLAY	Yes
½-in. Sharp XA 100 or XA 300	One touch record Press RECORD only	No
¾-in. Sony 5600 & 5800	Press and *hold* RECORD. Press PLAY	Yes

To stop recording, press PAUSE or STOP.

[*Note:* After several minutes, most VCRs will leave the PAUSE mode to prevent damage to the tape and/or recording heads. For long periods, where no recording will be desired, it is best to use the STOP function.]

A *visual search* may be conducted on any VCR using the following controls:

VCR Type/Model	Visual Search Control Functions
½-in. Sharp XA 100 & 300	Press PLAY and use FF (Fast Forward) and REV (Reverse) to search.
¾-in. Sony 5800 ½-in. panasonic AG 6300MD	Press SEARCH and rotate *knob* (lower right) to search.
¾-in. Sony 5600	Press FWD (Search Forward) and REV (Reverse) *buttons*.

Still Video Printer (MAVIGRAPH):
Confirm that Mavigraph Power is on, and appropriate monitor line has been selected (see *Monitor* section in this table.)

Initial monitor image will be white screen with Mavigraph information printed along bottom:

Q 1 1A1B 2A2B M

The M indicates ''Memory.'' The printer defaults to page one (1A1B is highlighted in red on screen).
1. Press the FULL/SPLIT key once to select four images, twice to select nine, thrice to return to full screen. Four or nine asterisks (*) indicate number of screen divisions; *red* asterisk indicates next still picture recording position. It may be moved using *arrow* keys.
2. Press the INPUT/MEMORY button. Camera image should appear, and M on bottom right is replaced with I (Input).
3. If a NO INPUT message appears on screen, the mavigraph is not getting or does not recognize a video input:
   (a) Confirm that camera control unit power is on and unit is connected to stack via CAMERA coaxial cable. If a ¾-in. VCR is on cart, check that red RECORD button is on.
   (b) Press the mavigraph INPUT SELECT button until the word VIDEO appears on screen. Live image should appear.
4. To *record* a still image, press the red MEMORY button. Image will record and display on the MEMORY screen. Press IMPUT/MEMORY to return to live image.
5. When all still positions have been filled, recording may be continued by going to the *second* page of memory:
   (a) Press MEMORY PAGE button; red high light moves from 1A1B to 2A2B.
   (b) Check MEMORY screen by pressing INPUT/MEMORY; screen should be blank.
6. Printing ribbon and paper supply may be checked by pressing REMAINING RIBBON button; number of remaining prints will be displayed on screen.
7. To print:
   (a) If more than one print is desired, use '' + −'' under print quantity; number of prints will display following the Q at lower left of screen.
   (b) Press green PRINT button. Green ''printing'' light will flash on front of mavigraph. Q number will flash and change color on screen.
8. Finished print will emerge in approximately 1 minute.

[*Note:* Print will pass through compartment during printing cycle. Do not attempt to remove until it is ejected cleanly.]

applications. One electronic "folder" could hold a patient's complete medical history including his progress notes, pathology reports, and endoscopic pictures.

SCANNERS

Scanners play a part in this process by allowing us to translate printed material to an electronic signal computers can store in relational databases. One needs a scanner, processing software and a compatible computer in which to store images. A scanner contains a light source that transmits and reflects a narrow strip of the page being scanned by the scan head (optical sensor). Intercepting light as it passes over the item, the head then relays to the unit's CCDs. Each CCDs electrical charge is then converted from analog to digital for processing and storage.

On the market now, one rapid film scanner can digitize and display representative color images in 18 seconds from any 35mm film source, color negative, color transparency, or black and white negative. Image compression technology can achieve ratios up to 24:1 so that up to 300 images can be stored on an 80-megabyte hard drive.

To augment the resolution and color depth of electronic images, flatbed scanners use new microlenses with better linear arrays. Varying sizes of both reflective and transmitive copy may be scanned with a flatbed. An inexpensive overhead video unit has a 300,000-pixel, ½-in. CCD sensor head positioned over the baseboard by a single column.

SLIDES

The best quality endoscopic 35mm slides for lecturing and publication are obtained through a 35mm single-reflex camera with an endoscopic zoom lens attached directly to a telescope eyepiece. While the surgeon wrestles with the camera's bulk as he or she photographs the scene, the rest of the team cannot follow the progress visually, making it difficult to follow requests for assistance. Often, the surgeon will wish to procure progressive views of the procedure. During this logistical challenge the team strives, not always successfully, to maintain the sterility of the surgical field. Three telescopes are employed: the surgeon attaches one scope to the 35mm camera and shoots; the scrub has a second sterile scope ready to exchange as soon as the surgeon is through shooting; a third scope lies soaking in Cidex to minimize delays. The camera can be bagged, but the controls are hard to handle by a gloved operator. The sync cord that connects the flash unit to the camera is short, another offense against sterility. The surgeon must "double-glove" incessantly. This is not the easiest documentation method. There are light sources that combine continuous illumination with automatic flash. The flash can be discharged in either manual or automatic mode when the surgeon presses the release button. One should make all setting adjustments (shutter speed, film ASA, flash mode) when testing the system prior to the procedure. Film processing will normally take 24 hours, depending on what laboratory facilities are accessible to the institution.

While no one would dispute the superior caliber of 35mm film documentation over that of video, the difficulties inherent in the former make us look to more convenient methods. Electronic photography is an alternative. Slides may be made from the video signal using a still video recorder with a 35mm back. A built-in digital memory captures a field of a moving video image, then photographs it on a small CRT tube. A more complex version digitizes the video image and stores it on a magnetic-optical disk. The end user sends the disk to a central laboratory that generates 35mm slides or prints from the digital data. This system provides excellent slides but is considerably more expensive than more basic units. Digital

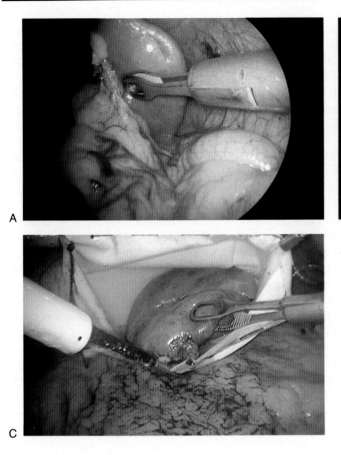

A

B

C

Figure 17. Laparoscopic splenectomy. **A:** 35mm film slide obtained by coupling a 35mm camera directly to the laparoscope (note resolution). **B:** Freeze frame from analog video signal, recorded on 35mm Ektachrome (shot with Polaroid Freezeframe Video Image Recorder). **C:** Freeze frame from RGB video signal stored on Bernoulli disk, transferred to 35mm negative film, printed as 35mm slide. (Courtesy of Dr. B. Carroll and Dr. E. Phillips.)

imaging makes it conceivable to manipulate, transmit, and extract information in new, more productive, ways (Fig. 17).

VIDEOTAPE RECORDERS

Given the escalating resolution of endoscopic cameras, Super VHS (S-VHS) has supplanted ¾-in. U-matic videotape format in our routinely recorded procedures for consultation, lectures, and teaching. S-VHS has a resolution of over 400 horizontal lines with an improved signal to noise ratio. By separating luminance *(Y)* and chrominance *(C)*, S-VHS abolishes signal interference and enhances picture quality. One major advantage of S-VHS recorders is that either S-VHS or conventional VHS tapes may be recorded and/or played back on the same unit. Since either entire procedures or selected highlights can be documented fairly inexpensively, videotaping is popular. The videotape record may be analyzed at length and may be edited for lectures and presentations. Most surgeons maintain VHS recorders in their offices and for routine applications employ ordinary VHS cassettes. They preserve these tapes for consultation and patient education. Real-time counters and variable visual search are professional features found on many units. A momentary contact foot switch has been attached to the recorders so that the surgeon or circulator can activate the pause/record function during a case. Some cameras have this feature incorporated in the housing via a button. Anyone wishing to begin a video library has to consider the necessary space in which to store it and the expense of a librarian to properly maintain its contents.

A digital tape system was first introduced in 1986. It was primarily designed to capture computer graphics for use in video without the signal degradation of analog tape. With analog recording, each duplication generation adds about 15% noise to the observed image. Analog video is a continuous electronic signal that oscillates with the brightness (luminance) and color (chrominance) of the video signal. In contrast, digital recording converts the analog signal to a bitstream of 1's and 0's, (binary code) then processes this stream into a low-bandwidth signal for recording. The digital video recorder (DVR) virtually eliminates dropouts (errors) because its method of error correction is superior to that used for analog video. The performance levels of a digital system are much more constant, which surmounts most of the performance drawbacks that have always plagued magnetic and optical recording. Given the many advantages of a digital system, the decision to use it instead of an analog system would seem self-evident. The expense of digital equipment is a definite factor influencing one's choices; operating it and even building a facility within a medical center to accommodate it would entail a much larger fiscal commitment than analog suites, and thus it is beyond the reach of most hospitals today.

The quality of digital replicas is not lessened through copying or duplicating as is the case with analog video recordings. Therefore, digital image copies will be as good in resolution as the original exposure. Prompt conversion of electronic information to digital signals means less opportunity for other parts of the electronic image environment to interject image-degrading signals. Perhaps the most pronounced significance of digital imaging is that image data can be sharpened, cleaned up, expanded, processed, manipulated, and enhanced through methods that are unthinkable with analog images.

Digital audiotape (DAT) offers single-cassette capacity, data-transfer speeds, quick file recovery, and cost effectiveness. A 400-megabyte (per side) optical disk costs more than $200.00 each, compared to only $30.00 for a 1.2-gigabyte DAT cassette.

DISK RECORDERS

Another practical option for storing endoscopic images is a disk recorder that utilizes either floppy or optical disks as its recording medium. Optical-memory disk recorders that record still pictures or full-motion video onto a laser disk with a resolution of approximately 580 horizontal lines are the highest quality recording media obtainable. More economic units are offered in the guise of floppy disk recorders, which allow one to record up to 25 video frames or 50 fields (2 field = 1 frame) on a two-sided 2-in. floppy disk, but with reduced resolution of 380 lines. Retrieving stored data from earlier examinations is a rapid, uncomplicated process, and disks take up far less storage room. Images stored on disk can be previewed after a procedure, and specific frames can be selected and printed using a still video printer. Prints have become prevalent in patient education, since physicians will frequently show these prints to patients and relatives directly after an examination to illustrate findings prior to adding them to the patient's chart.

But the 2-in. floppy disk may not be able to squeeze all the electronic information essential for more complex disk images into a required disk sector, as camera sensors gradually approach 35mm film quality. It may be conceivable to decrease the number of exposures on one disk and join several disk sectors into one image, or crowd more information into less space by manipulating electronic data compression techniques. On a more expensive level, a system which permits the recording of 14,000 high-resolution still images on a single 2-hour S-VHS tape has also been designed. New photo-CD technology is just being introduced. A CD could contain 100 images from varying sources and could be played internationally across all broadcast standards (NTSC, PAL, SECAM), thus offering portability as well as outstanding photographic-based images.

STILL VIDEO PRINTERS

As with other capital outlays, budget is a factor in making a choice. Exceptional high-resolution hardcopy devices are costly, prices commencing at $20,000. There are more frugal, lower resolution color hardcopy printers, differing in technique and price, from ink jets and thermal dye transfer to dry electrostatic-charge printers. As with chip technology, printers have proceeded through myriad inceptions, each fine-tuning and refining the printing process.

Graphic digital information sources can be linked to a new digital continuous tone printer that produces photograph-quality full color or black and white prints. It transfers cyan, yellow, and magenta from its ribbon to the thermal medium. Individual heating elements control each pixel's dye density by modulating electrical impulses. A true continuous tone print is the result.

FUTURE

You cannot fight against the future. Time is on our side.
——Gladstone, 1866

We now travel from the realm of what is to that of what will be, inspiring age-old debates between pragmatists and visionaries. Given the amazing changes surgery has seen in the past decade, arguing against change would seem inane; one question might be: change at what price? As we examine the many demands on our dwindling resources, where are the latter best spent? There must always be experimental research forging ahead of everyday applications or there will be no progress.

As the surgical community ponders how best to conduct continuing training, other disciplines grapple with this issue as well. Gastroenterologists have been designing computer simulation training modules for several years, although no one model has been universally adopted. How do we simulate bleeding, respiration, or other physiologic parameters? Equivalency is also a concern. How does an interactive computer module equate with traditional hands-on instruction? Orthopaedic surgeons are viewing and manipulating a model of the human leg within a virtual environment scheme. The value of a head-coupled stereo display and direct three-dimensional manipulation for a surgical simulation application are being assessed. Forays into computer simulator programs especially adapted for laparoscopic surgery have already been published.

VIRTUAL REALITY

Rather than revise assorted aspects of laparoscopic surgery separately, some propose a consummately novel environment in which surgeons may operate autonomously with new-found visual acuity and dexterity. Artificial realities allow users to interact with computers in an intuitive and direct format and to increase the number of interactions per unit of time. The ultimate objective is to devise a simulated reality that not only seems as real as the reality it depicts, but allows us to go beyond reality to overcome problems that presently defeat us. As researchers conceptualize advanced surgical applications, radiologists already employ magnetic resonance imaging and computed tomography three-dimensional digital scanning to outline treatment before administering to patients. The same gloves that our children don to battle the intergalactic hordes can be worn by surgeons to translate hand and finger movements into electrical signals that will guide remotely placed instruments. Microrobots will execute delicate surgery within the body cavities directed by operators sitting at remote workstations, possibly on the other side of the world. This is the unstoppable future.

For the present, new imaging technology has transformed general surgery forever. Operative techniques and instrumentation fluctuate wildly as surgeons strive to find conclusive answers to the technical and ethical dilemmas confronting them. It is incumbent upon the surgical community to evaluate meticulously before decreeing which technology will be retained as true innovations and which will be discarded as fads.

SURGICAL PEARLS

Catalog all media with date, procedure, patient hospital number, surgeon name, length (if a videotape).

Keep extra coaxial cable on hand in video carts to allow quick replacement during a case, if necessary.

Prepare a clear, concise troubleshooting guide for all video components and hang it on the video carts.

Do not place videocamera heads or telescopes in an ultrasonic cleaner.

Before a procedure, visually inspect camera lenses and telescopes for chips, scratches, and other damage.

RECOMMENDED READING

1. Berci G. Television and endoscopy. In: Berci G, ed. *Endoscopy*. E. Norwalk, CT: Appleton & Lange; 1976:271–279.
2. Paz Partlow M. Video imaging and photo documentation. In: Cuschieri A, Buess G, Perissat J, eds. *Operative manual of endoscopic surgery*. Berlin: Springer-Verlag; 1992:34–37.
3. Satava MR. Hi tech surgery: speculation on future directions. In: Hunter J, Sackier J, eds. *Minimally invasive surgery*. New York: McGraw-Hill; 1993:339–347.
4. Robinson R. *The video primer*. New York: Perigee Books–Putnam, 1983.

Electrosurgery and Laser Application

William S. Laycock
Department of Surgery
Dartmouth–Hitchcock Medical Center
Lebanon, New Hampshire 03756

John G. Hunter
Department of Surgery
Emory University School of Medicine
Atlanta, Georgia 30322

Operative Laparoscopy and Thoracoscopy, edited by B. V. MacFadyen, Jr. and J. L. Ponsky. Lippincott-Raven Publishers, Philadelphia © 1996.

The growth of laparoscopic surgery as a therapeutic tool has inevitably led to the development and adaptation of energy sources for use in the laparoscopic environment. A theme common to energy sources is the conversion of energy, usually electrical, to heat at the tissue level. The various ways in which the heat is delivered to tissue are what allows the surgeon to perform dissection, cutting, or coagulation in a controlled and predictable fashion. The two main energy sources currently used in laparoscopic surgery are electrosurgery and laser.

Although a degree in biomechanical physics is not prerequisite for using these devices, a basic understanding of laser and electrosurgical principles is needed for the safe and effective performance of therapeutic laparoscopic surgery. The objectives of this chapter are to explain the biophysical properties behind electrosurgical and laser energy, discuss the methods of energy delivery, and emphasize techniques to minimize complications from their use in laparoscopic surgery.

ELECTROSURGERY

Pioneered by the work of William Bovie and Harvey Cushing, the use of electrosurgical generators for cutting and desiccating tissue has origins in the 1920s. Today electrosurgical units are ubiquitous in the operating room. Although the "Bovie" is used at some point in most open abdominal procedures, it is safe to say that many surgeons do not have a clear understanding of the physics responsible for the tissue effects produced by various electrosurgical settings. Although it may be possible for these surgeons to safely use electrocautery in the open abdomen, the laparoscopic environment is less tolerant of errors. In addition, there are a number of potential perils with electrosurgery that are unique to the laparoscopic domain. More than ever, a conscientious surgeon needs a background in the biophysical principles and inherent dangers of electrosurgery.

Electrosurgical Current

A surgeon has two main choices by which to deliver electrosurgical current to tissue: monopolar or bipolar. With monopolar units, a circuit consists of an active electrode (laparoscopic hook, blade, spatula, etc.) delivering the current that passes through tissues and returns to the generator through the indifferent electrode (grounding pad). With bipolar electrosurgery, tissue to be treated is placed directly between two electrodes so that current flows only through tissue contiguous with both electrodes, eliminating the need for a grounding pad and, in general, decreasing the hazards of stray current.

For monopolar electrosurgery the eˊectrosurgical generator has two modes of operation: cutting or coagulation. It is often assumed that the name of the waveform will determine the clinical effects produced. In reality, other factors related to how the electrode is used will influence the actual tissue effect and misconceptions can lead to serious errors in electrosurgical technique. Cutting, a vaporization mode, is characterized by a high-current, low-voltage, continuous sine waveform without intervening pauses (see Fig. 1A). The goal is to heat the tissue quickly, such that cell water is converted to steam, causing the cell to explode. Heat is dissipated in the steam with minimal lateral thermal tissue damage but poor thermocoagulation. If the electrode is allowed to remain stationary, pressing into tissue, the tissue temperature rises and the width of thermal damage increases. This tissue effect is called desiccation (see below). During normal operation, a series of electrical sparks between active electrode and tissue create a steam bubble producing the sensation of floating through the tissue with little resistance. The electrode should not be allowed to contact tissue directly.

Coagulation, the fulguration mode, utilizes a high-voltage, low-current, interrupted waveform (see Fig. 1B). Coagulation occurs by spraying high-current density bursts, like lightning bolts, to tissue, with intervening pauses that will drive electrons across a high-resistance, nonionized air gap between tissue and the electrode. This results in rapid surface heating with a superficial eschar and shallow depth of necrosis. Significant cutting does not occur because the heat is more widely dispersed by the long sparks and interrupted waveform. Coagulation mode is often helpful on a diffusely oozing surface, such as the gallbladder bed, without

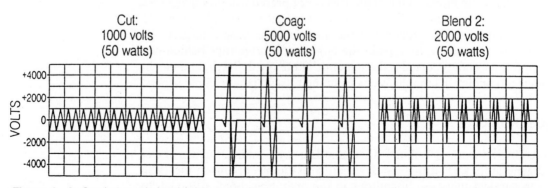

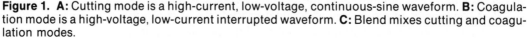

Figure 1. A: Cutting mode is a high-current, low-voltage, continuous-sine waveform. **B:** Coagulation mode is a high-voltage, low-current interrupted waveform. **C:** Blend mixes cutting and coagulation modes.

a discrete bleeding vessel. This is also a noncontact mode and relies on sparking between electrode and tissue.

The blend option mixes cutting and coagulation waveforms by interrupting the sine wave current and increasing the voltage, affecting advantages of both waveforms (see Fig. 1C). Interruption of current will manifest as a slower rate of cutting and additional lateral tissue heating, resulting in better hemostasis and a greater width of tissue necrosis. Blend 1 produces the least amount of hemostasis, blend 3 a greater amount. Blend, like cut and coagulation, is a noncontact mode, so the electrode should be activated prior to tissue contact.

Desiccation is the only true contact electrosurgery. This results in nearly complete transfer of energy to tissue with the greatest degree of temperature elevation and necrosis. The direct contact makes the particular waveform less critical, but in general the cut waveform is optimal to avoid sparking through the coagulated tissue (1). As tissue temperature rises, water is evaporated producing "desiccation." As desiccation increases, tissue resistance increases until with complete desiccation current stops flowing due to very high resistance. Clinically one observes the tissue turn brown then bubble and steam. Hemostasis is achieved as a result of fibrous binding between dehydrated, denatured cells of vessel endothelium (1). Because there is a significantly deeper zone of necrosis with desiccation, one should be careful to avoid electrode contact with tissue and its use unintentionally, as it has been shown to be associated with a greater degree of inflammation and interference with wound healing (2).

Tissue Effects

A property of the electrolyte composition of cells is that tissues can function as electrical conductors. Direct current (DC) applied to tissue results in depolarization of cell membranes. If depolarization occurs in neuromuscular tissue the result is neural impulse conduction and vigorous tetanic muscular contraction, commonly known as "shock." With alternating current (AC) the effect can vary depending on the frequency of current. Frequencies below 100,000 cps will produce depolarization of tissue that is rapidly counteracted due to reversal of the current. The subject will experience fasciculations in neuromuscular tissue. With very high-frequency current (>100,000 cps) ions within cells will be pulled back and forth with such speed that depolarization does not occur, but rather kinetic energy results in heat that raises the temperature of the cell, causing not an electrical effect (a "shock") but a thermal one (a burn). Frequencies in the range between 100,000 and 4,000,000 cps will produce electrosurgical effects. Most generators produce current in the 500,000–750,000 cps range. These frequencies are characteristic of radiowaves. Therefore, electrosurgical energy is known as radiofrequency (RF) electricity. As the electrical current produces heat, the tissue temperature rises. At 44°C, tissue necrosis begins. Between 60 and 100°C coagulation is seen with collagen converted into glucose. Above 100°C tissue water is vaporized and above 200°C carbonization occurs resulting in black eschar formation (1).

Tissue heating is dependent upon the square of the current density

$$T = \left(\frac{A}{cm^2}\right)^2$$

with current density defined as the amount of current flowing through a cross-sectional area of tissue. Current density

$$I = \frac{V}{R}$$

is directly proportional to applied power (voltage), and inversely proportional to tissue resistance (impedance). In general, at a fixed-energy setting the size of the active electrode in contact with the tissue will determine the rate of heating. The smaller the contact area, the faster the heating. The large size of the grounding pad makes for a low-current density and minimal heating. The grounding pad should not be bent, or placed on hairy skin, bony prominence, or scars, all of which can cause a decrease in the contact surface area and increase the risk of a burn to the patient.

Hazards of Electrosurgery

Because of an unacceptable incidence of intestinal perforation with monopolar electrosurgery during tubal ligation, gynecologists abandoned it, favoring bipolar or mechanical methods for tubal sterilization (3). Despite histologic evidence that some of these complications were a result of mechanical rather than electrosurgical trauma, aversion to monopolar electrosurgery continued (4). In contrast to open surgery, where the electrode and the abdominal viscera are all within the surgeon's view, the use of electrosurgery in the laparoscopic environment has several distinctive potential hazards. The central theme is current division; when current, following the path of least resistance, passes through unintentional pathways.

The first hazard is insulation failure. An electrode passed through a trocar into the peritoneal cavity is insulated along its entire length, save the distal tip. Unfortunately, the laparoscopic video image does not view most of the electrode, and insulation failure, with subsequent division of current to adjacent tissue, can occur outside the surgeon's field and without his or her knowledge (see Fig. 2). Such an injury may be totally unseen or manifested only by tissue blanching. This may result in full-thickness bowel wall coagulation with subsequent necrosis and

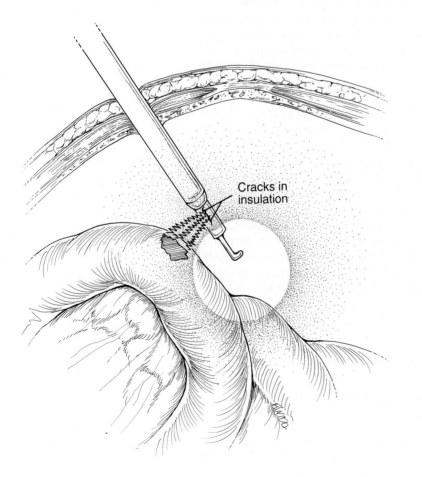

Cracks in insulation

Figure 2. Insulation failure could result in tissue injury outside the surgeon's field of view.

perforation. All electrodes must be carefully inspected at the start of each case, particularly the portion that contacts the flapper valve of the trocar, as this is usually the first point of failure due to repeated mechanical trauma. Experimentally, it has been shown that defects of insulation not visible can deliver nearly 100% of available electrical energy to sites outside the laparoscopic field of view (5).

The second potential problem is capacitive coupling between active monopolar electrodes and trocars. A capacitor is defined as two conductors separated by an insulator. This involves transfer of current from the laparoscopic instrument through its insulation to a metal guide, a telescope or the trocar, and can be greater than 40% of the available power. If the trocar is all metal, this energy will return to the ground plate through the abdominal wall without consequence because of the very large contact surface between trocar and body wall allowing low-current density at all points. A dangerous situation can arise if a metal trocar is used with a plastic screw anchor at the skin level. This will electrically isolate the trocar from draining its capacitively coupled charge (electrons) into the abdominal wall, and if bowel is contacted a thermal injury could result (see Fig. 3). In a dog model, as little as 21 W of capacitive-coupled power applied to bowel for 5 seconds can cause full-thickness burns (5). The capacitive charge is greatest with a long length of cylinder and when trocar and electrode are of similar diameter (1). When operative laparoscopes were used in gynecologic procedures with needle-tip electrodes in the operating channel, up to 80% of available power could be transferred to the laparoscope when the electrode was activated but was not in contact with conductive tissue. With a metal trocar this current is drained into the abdominal wall, but with plastic or fiberglass trocars the laparoscope became a "highly charged weapon." For safety reasons it is best to use either all metal or all plastic trocars to reduce the capacitive effect. Capacitive coupling can also occur when crossing the active electrode with another laparoscopic instrument. The energy

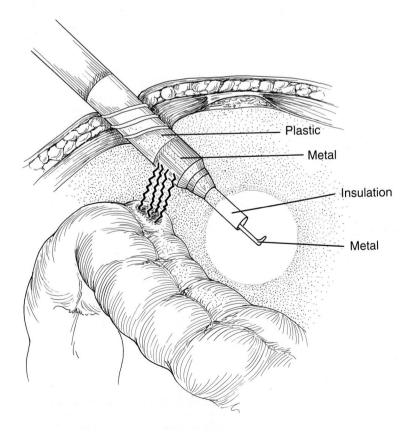

Plastic

Metal

Insulation

Metal

Figure 3. Capacitive coupling injury can occur when a plastic screw anchor is used to hold a metal trocar.

transfer in this setting can be as high as 10% of the power set on the electrosurgical generator (1).

A third hazard is unintended direct coupling. This can occur when the active electrode comes into contact with other metal instruments, cannulas, or the laparoscope. If a grasper holding bowel is contacted by the active electrode, a thermal injury is likely. A metal trocar that comes into contact with the electrode is not a dangerous situation, provided a plastic screw anchor is not used, as electrons will pass harmlessly into the abdominal wall and return to the grounding pad. Contact with the metal laparoscope can be a perilous condition. If an all metal trocar is used the current should pass safely into the abdominal wall. Use of a plastic trocar to pass the laparoscope could allow current to transfer to bowel or other viscera out of the laparoscopic field of view (see Fig. 4). Experimentally, arcing from a laparoscope in contact with an active electrode was observed at 20 W when plastic screw anchors were used at the cannula-abdominal interface (5). The use of an all-metal trocar without a plastic screw anchor to pass the laparoscope is the optimal situation from a safety standpoint.

A final dangerous condition can occur when current is allowed to pass through an unintentionally narrowed return circuit. This will increase the local current density and therefore tissue heating and thermal burn can result. Tissue temperature elevation as high as 82°C has been documented several centimeters from the point of electrode contact (6). An example of this is heating the end of the appendiceal stump that has been ligated with a ligature. The laws of physics dictate that if the ligature narrows appendiceal diameter by 50% and an electrode is applied to the cut end of the appendix, the temperature at the ligature will be 16 times greater than at the point of contact (see Fig. 5) (7). This could result in postoperative sloughing of the appendiceal stalk with fecal fistula development.

One advantage that the laparoscopic approach has over the use of open electrosurgery is a decreased risk of secondary sparking. When the relative humidity is increased from 0% to 100%, the voltage required to push a spark across a gap is increased by 3.5%. Despite the use of dry CO_2, the pneumoperitoneum has a

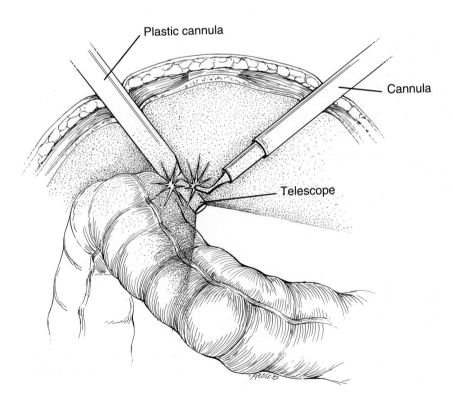

Figure 4. Direct coupling between the electrode and laparoscope can cause unrecognized tissue injury.

relative humidity of nearly 100%, as the use of carbon dioxide further impedes sparking (6). This should dispel the misconception that uncontrolled sparking makes monopolar electrosurgery unsafe in laparoscopic surgery.

As alluded to earlier, the advantage of bipolar electrosurgery is that many of these current division problems are avoided. An additional concept to remember is that the output of the electrosurgical generator must be decreased in bipolar mode. Current flow will be through a much smaller volume of tissue, unlike the high-resistance circuit present in monopolar surgery. This lower energy requirement has been shown to produce less lateral tissue damage and necrosis when compared to monopolar electrosurgery (8). Use of bipolar electrosurgery in laparoscopy has been essentially limited to coagulating forceps. Recent advances in bipolar technology have led to the development of bipolar scissors and other dissection devices. Production of bipolar devices may give the laparoscopic surgeon many options for tissue manipulation with a greater level of safety than currently available, but it is unlikely that monopolar electrosurgery will be totally replaced.

Electrosurgery has been used successfully for over 60 years. Laparoscopic application of this modality can be performed safely and with great therapeutic benefit. Knowledge of basic biophysical properties and awareness of potential hazards in electrosurgery empowers the surgeon with an extremely versatile and useful tool with which to perform a wide range of minimally invasive procedures.

LASERS

The current enthusiasm for laparoscopic surgery by general surgeons was initiated by reports of laser laparoscopic cholecystectomy. Initial enthusiasm for the

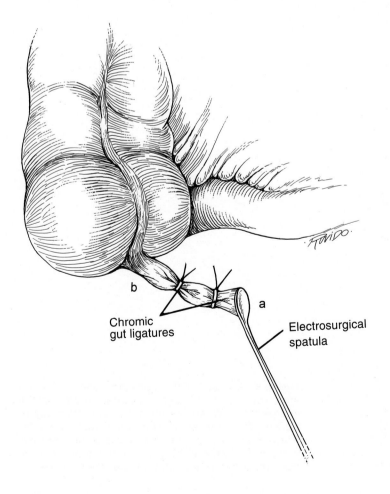

b
Chromic
gut ligatures

a
Electrosurgical
spatula

Figure 5. The temperature at point *b* will be 16 times the temperature at point *a* if the diameter at point *b* is one-half the diameter at point *a*.

laser has diminished following reports concerning the lack of advantages in laser use and its potential dangers in the hands of novice laparoscopic surgeons (13). Nevertheless, lasers are still useful for endoscopic surgery. With a foundation in the physical and biophysical properties of lasers, the surgeon is better equipped to make sound judgments regarding their utility and not be intimidated by this beneficial energy source.

Laser Physics

The term laser is an acronym for *l*ight *a*mplification by *s*timulated *e*mission of *r*adiation. The first successful application of lasers occurred in the early 1960s. Since that time much research and effort have gone into further development of

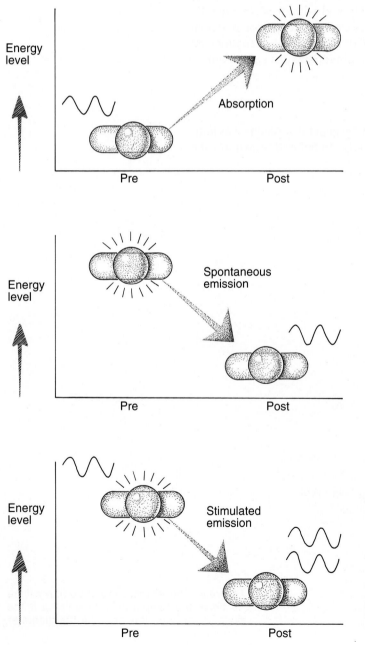

Figure 6. An electron in its ground state receives energy from the pump and is elevated to an unstable energy state. When the electron spontaneously returns to its ground state, a photon of light, characteristic of that atom, is emitted. When this photon strikes a second excited electron, a stimulated decay occurs, resulting in two photons that are in phase.

this technology. An understanding of laser physics is based on the idea that light acts both as a particle and a wave. The light particle (photon) is responsible for initiating and amplifying a beam of light in which all light waves are synchronized in time and space—the laser beam.

Many different types of materials are used as the active medium in lasers: liquid, gas, and solids. The name of a given laser is derived from the active medium: CO_2, Nd:YAG, argon (see the next section). A power source, or pump, stimulates the laser medium with either electric, thermal, or optical energy. Once this energy contacts the laser medium, electrons are "pumped" to higher energy (valence) levels. Following excitation, an electron will spontaneously return to its ground state releasing the absorbed energy as a photon of light that has a specific wavelength unique to the material of the laser medium. This process is called spontaneous emission. If a greater amount of energy is applied to the laser medium a larger number of electrons will be in the unstable excited state at any one time. When a photon collides with an excited electron a "stimulated" event occurs, releasing a second photon of identical wave and particle characteristics to the first photon (see Fig. 6). When more electrons in the medium are in an excited rather than ground state a population inversion has occurred, and this is necessary for the lasing action to take place. The photon/electron collision cascade produces light in which all photons are of the same wavelength and all wavefronts are in phase with each other across time and space. This is called coherent light and is the feature uniting all types of lasers (see Fig. 7) (9). The reason a laser beam has a greater ability to heat tissue than an equivalent amount of noncoherent light is that the crests of all the light waves traveling together create a wave amplitude that is the sum of the individual wave energies.

The power of the laser beam is determined by the number of waves that are marching in rank. This number is determined by the number of unstable electrons available for stimulated emission. The number of unstable electrons is determined by the chemical and physical properties of the laser medium and the amount of energy applied to the electrical power source.

The laser medium is contained within an optical cavity with parallel mirrors at either end. One mirror is modified to allow a small fraction of the light energy out, but most of the energy is reflected back into the medium for further stimulation and hence amplification of the process (see Fig. 8). Photons emitted in directions away from the laser cavity are not amplified and are dissipated as heat. In some laser systems, more than 99% of energy input is dissipated as heat. Because of such inefficiency, most lasers require complex power sources and cooling systems.

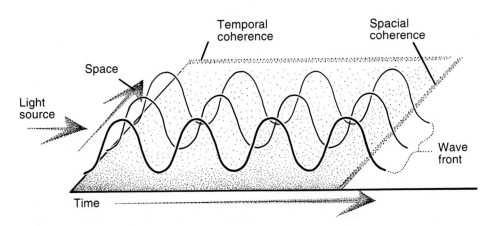
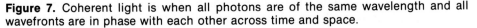

Figure 7. Coherent light is when all photons are of the same wavelength and all wavefronts are in phase with each other across time and space.

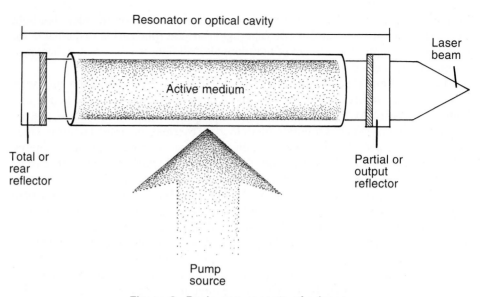

Figure 8. Basic components of a laser.

Tissue Interaction

Lasers can interact with tissue to cause biologic, photochemical, photomechanical, or thermal reactions. Most medical lasers affect tissue by heating it. The amount of heat generated is determined by power density of the laser beam (how many photons per square centimeter), concentration of chromophores (melanin, water, hemoglobin) within the tissue, and the wavelength of the laser. A chromophore is a cellular component capable of absorbing a specific wavelength of light. For example, water highly absorbs light in the ultraviolet and infrared portions of the spectrum. Therefore, lasers designed to vaporize tissue with a high water content would best utilize a wavelength in the ultraviolet or infrared portion of the spectrum. This is selective absorption. In the visible spectrum, light is absorbed by tissue chromophores complementary to the beam of light. Thus a red lesion is well treated with a green laser such as the KTP.

A laser should be chosen that will be most absorbed by the target tissue and least absorbed by the background tissue. With dark-colored target tissue, where almost any laser will be absorbed, the main choice of laser should be determined by the background tissue to spare it of injury.

Current laser wavelengths cover the entire visible light spectrum as well as portions of the ultraviolet and infrared spectrum (10). At the present time there are four main types of lasers used for medical purposes. The CO_2 laser ($\lambda = 10..6$ μm) produces light in the far-infrared portion of the electromagnetic spectrum and is highly absorbed by water. Because tissue is 70% to 90% water, 98% of CO_2 energy is absorbed at a tissue depth of roughly 0.17 mm (11). The CO_2 laser's major advantage is the ability to vaporize a very thin surface of tissue. The argon laser ($\lambda = 488,514$ nm) emits a blue-green light in the visible spectrum. It is primarily absorbed by melanin and hemoglobin and can be used selectively to photocoagulate a hemangioma of the skin or ablate an endometrial deposit in the pelvis. The neodymium-doped yttrium aluminum garnet laser (Nd:YAG) ($\lambda = 1,064$ nm) is in the near-infrared spectrum. It is poorly absorbed by water and hemoglobin and therefore penetrates deeply into tissues. It has been used successfully to control gastrointestinal bleeding and in thermal ablation of bulky tumors (11). The potassium-titanyl-phosphate laser (KTP) ($\lambda = 532$ nm) is a wavelength-halved Nd:YAG laser with a green light in the visible spectrum. It has an absorption spectrum similar to the argon laser. Applications that take advantage of selective absorption to improve clinical outcome are the key to laser use (7). When the laser is used as a generic heater of tissue without making use of selective absorption it is not clear there are benefits over less expensive technology capable of heat generation (7).

Laser Delivery

Once a laser light has been produced, it must be delivered to the tissue in some manageable fashion. For laparoscopic surgery, fiberoptic delivery through quartz glass fibers with high internal reflectance is the most practical method. Wavelengths shorter than 250 nm and longer than 2,500 nm will not be transmitted through quartz fibers. For long- and short-wavelength lasers, such as the CO_2 laser, rigid articulated arms with lenses and mirrors are used. The only advantage of this system is the ability to focus the laser beam to a small spot. This system is used by many gynecologists for vaporization of endometriosis.

As light emerges from the tip of a quartz fiber it will diverge. Divergence is a measure of how much the beam will increase in diameter over distance from the fiber tip. Therefore, the power density (in watts per square centimeter) will depend on how far the fiber tip is from the tissue and falls off exponentially with increasing distance. Several contact tips have been developed that may be placed at the end of the quartz fiber. The simplest contact tip is the cleaved quartz fiber that is placed in contact with the tissue until a layer of carbon builds up on the tip. The laser light energy is converted to heat by absorption at the tip and allows the fiber to function in contact with tissue much like an electrosurgical electrode in the desiccation mode. The disadvantage of contact glass tips is that they remain hot for 5 to 10 seconds after removal from tissue that could result in inadvertent injury to surrounding tissue (12).

Hazards of Lasers

Because lasers do not rely on the completion of an electrical circuit to function, the dangers of current division are eliminated. The main danger associated with using lasers laparoscopically is when the laser is operated in a noncontact mode. If the laser is turned on and careful attention not given to the orientation of the quartz fiber, a thermal injury can result to a nearby structure or one outside the laparoscopic field of view but in the path of the laser. As mentioned previously, a danger exists with glass contact tips because they can remain hot for several seconds after use, and, if placed in contact with abdominal viscera, a thermal injury could result. A common precaution with lasers in the open environment is the use of protective eye wear. For laparoscopic applications, protective goggles are not necessary because the laser should not be activated unless the fiber is inside the abdominal cavity. At most, a filter may be needed between the laparoscope and the camera to protect the CCD ''chip'' from the intense monochromatic laser light.

LASER OR ELECTROCAUTERY?

There is a divergence of opinion regarding the superiority of laser or electrosurgery energy for laparoscopic surgical procedures. The first reports of laparoscopic cholecystectomy in the United States were on those performed using laser energy. Subsequent to this, many institutions made significant capital investments in laser technology that, combined with the efforts of marketing managers, resulted in a media blitz touting the benefits of laser surgery. In the mind of the public, laparoscopic surgery became equated with ''laser surgery.''

In an attempt to answer some of the questions concerning the safety and efficacy of lasers and electrosurgery for laparoscopic cholecystectomy, Hunter and colleagues (13) performed a prospective randomized trial comparing these modalities. A total of 103 patients were randomized: 52 to monopolar electrosurgery and 51 to Nd:YAG laser dissection. Dissection time was significantly longer in the group undergoing laser resection: 23.56 minutes vs 19.24 minutes ($p < .02$). The estimated blood loss was also significantly greater in the laser group. The incidence of gallbladder perforations, liver injuries, and postoperative liver function tests failed to reach a significant difference. In one retrospective analysis of 50 cholecystectomies comparing KTP laser with electrosurgery, the KTP laser was 20 minutes slower and $500 more expensive (14).

Many different laparoscopic procedures have been performed using laser technology. The principle of selective absorption, choosing a laser with tissue absorption and effects specific for the target tissue, is the essential factor to bear in mind when trying to decide whether laser technology is appropriate for a given application. This is a feature unique to light energy and is the basis for the versatility of lasers. Electrosurgery is sensitive only to water content and cannot discriminate by color. Because lasers are expensive to build, maintain, and operate, it would seem prudent to limit their use to applications in which their particular features improve clinical outcome. If selective tissue absorption is not critical, and there is no evidence for a statistically significant difference in safety or efficacy, it is difficult to justify the additional expense of laser over alternative technology.

SUMMARY

In just a short period of time, laparoscopic surgery has gone from being an orphan of general surgery to the most exciting and rapidly expanding area of new development. In order to stay current in this field, a laparoscopic surgeon must be able to understand new technologies and place them in the proper context with regard to his or her clinical practice for optimal patient care and safety.

To fully comprehend an energy source it is helpful to break it down into four parts:

1. How is the energy created (light, electricity, shockwaves)?
2. How is the energy transported from the generator to the tissue (electrode, fiberoptics, mirrors, fluid)?
3. How does the energy interact with tissue (thermal, mechanical, photochemical)?
4. How does the energy source interact with the environment in which it is used (division of current, lateral thermal diffusion injury potential, anesthetic complications)?

When these questions can be answered completely, then the surgeon can use an energy source to its full capacity and with maximal safety to the patient.

REFERENCES

1. Odell RC. Laparoscopic electrosurgery. In: Hunter JG, Sackier JM, eds. *Minimally invasive surgery.* New York: McGraw-Hill; 1993:33–41.
2. Rappaport WD, Hunter GC, Allen R, Lick S, Halldorsson A, Chvapil T, et al. Effect of electrocautery on wound healing in midline laparotomy incisions. *Am J Surg* 1990;160:618–620.
3. Deaths following female sterilization with unipolar electrocoagulating devices. *MMWR* 1981;30: 149.
4. Soderstrom RM, Levy BS. Bowel injuries during laparoscopy: causes and medicolegal questions. *Cont Obstet Gynecol* 1986;41–45.
5. Voyles CR, Tucker RD. Education and engineering solutions for potential problems with laparoscopic monopolar electrosurgery. *Am J Surg* 1992;164:57–62.

6. Saye WB, Miller W, Hertzman P. Electrosurgery thermal injury. *Surg Laparosc Endosc* 1991;1: 223–228.
7. Hunter JG. Laser use in laparoscopic surgery. *Surg Clin North Am* 1992;72:655–664.
8. Tucker RD, Platz CE, Sievert CE, Vennes JA, Silvis SE. In vivo evaluation of monopolar versus bipolar electrosurgical polypectomy snares. *Am J Gastroenterol* 1990;10:1386–1390.
9. Hunter JG. Laser physics and tissue interaction. In: *Minimally invasive surgery*. New York: McGraw Hill; 1993:23–31.
10. Fuller TA. Fundamentals of laser surgery. In: *Surgical lasers*. New York: Macmillan.
11. Fuller TA. Fundamentals of lasers in surgery and medicine. In: Diton GA, ed. *Surgical application of lasers*. Chicago: Year Book Medical Publishers; 1987:16–33.
12. Hunter JG. Laser or electrocautery for laparoscopy? *Am J Surg* 1991;161:345–349.
13. Bordelon BM, Hobday KA, Hunter JG. Laser versus electrosurgery in laparoscopic cholecystectomy. *Arch Surg* 1993;128:233–236.
14. Voyles CR, Petro AB, Meena AL, et al. A practical approach to laparoscopic cholecystectomy. *Am J Surg* 1991;161:365–370.

8

Basic Techniques

Mohan C. Airan
Department of Surgery
Chicago Medical School
Finch University
Lombard, Illinois, 60148–5396

Operative Laparoscopy and Thoracoscopy, edited by B. V. MacFadyen, Jr. and J. L. Ponsky. Lippincott-Raven Publishers, Philadelphia © 1996.

KEY WORDS

Insufflation   Trocar-cannula

Pneumoperitoneum   Veress needle

⊙ ANATOMY

Umbilicus

The thinnest portion of the abdominal wall is the central scar in the pit of the umbilicus (Fig. 1). The peritoneum is always attached to the central scar due to the resolution of the umbilical cord following birth.

Gynecologists have traditionally selected an infraumbilical approach to enter the abdomen. This sometimes causes the Veress needle to strip the peritoneum during insertion because the needle is pointed toward the pelvis, which necessitates using a longer Veress needle or a deeper insertion. However, if the central scar of the umbilicus is used to enter the abdomen the length required never exceeds 1½ to 2 in., which rarely will injure underlying structures.

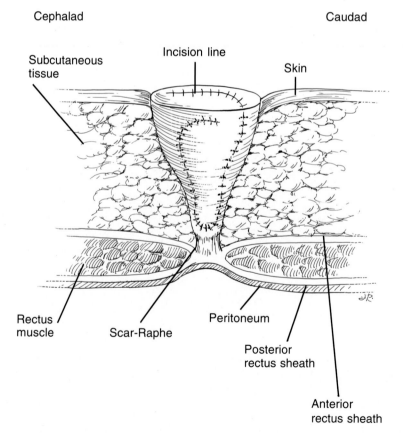

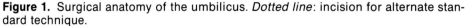

Figure 1. Surgical anatomy of the umbilicus. *Dotted line*: incision for alternate standard technique.

The conical funnel of the umbilicus can vary from being almost flat to 6–7 in. in depth. However, even in the deepest funnel the central scar area is always 1½ to 2 in. in depth. This surgical anatomic quirk has allowed me to successfully perform Veress needle insertions without a single mishap in over 2,000 consecutive insertions.

Pneumoperitoneum

Pneumoperitoneum is designed to prevent injury to underlying viscera and vascular structures. The commonest injury sites are located immediately below the umbilicus and happen during the initial puncture with the Veress needle and during the initial insertion of the trocar-cannula. Blind insertion of trocar-cannulas without attention to the monitors may cause injuries. The sites of injury are depicted in Fig. 2. Pneumoperitoneum provides a large pocket of CO_2 in the greater peritoneal sac into which sharp surgical instruments can be advanced with care without damaging underlying viscera.

Epigastric Arteries

Figure 3 depicts the approximate course of the epigastric arteries. These arteries are in the rectus sheath embedded in the posterior aspect of the rectus muscle inferiorly and almost in the middle of the rectus muscle superiorly.

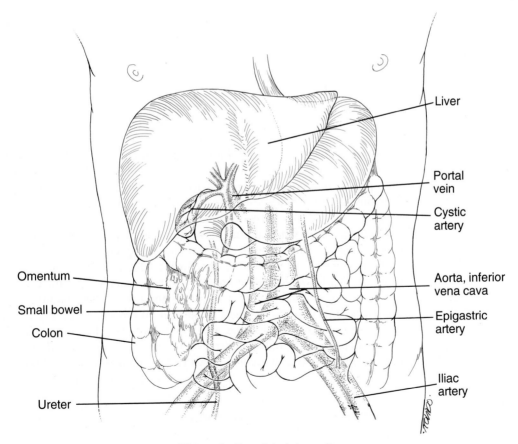

Figure 2. Possible injury sites.

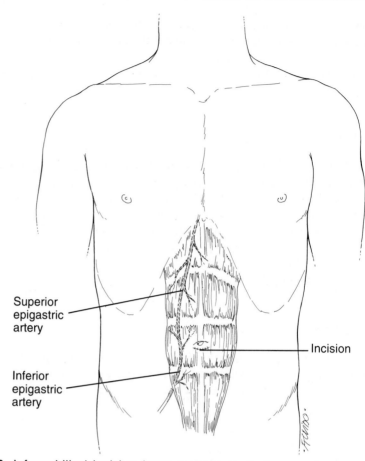

Figure 3. Infraumbilical incision (open technique). Surface anatomy: approximate course of inferior and superior epigastric arteries.

▶ **PREOPERATIVE PLANNING**

A detailed history of previous intraabdominal operations should be obtained. Previous abdominal surgery is not necessarily a contraindication for classical insertion of the Veress needle into the abdominal cavity. Surgeons who are not comfortable with the classical technique of Veress needle insertion should perform the open technique to gain access to the peritoneal cavity. When patients have previous abdominal incisions, alternate site entry using the standard Veress needle may be attempted by surgeons who are familiar with Veress needle technique.

Older patients who take many medications have problems in evacuating the colon. These patients may benefit from a colon preparation. Patients should have an enema before they come to the hospital for a laparoscopic procedure, and, rarely, a full bowel preparation may be necessary to ensure a collapsed small and large bowel. The patient should fast the night before admission. To prevent accidental injury to the stomach or bladder and to minimize the risk of aspiration pneumonia, a nasogastric tube and Foley catheter should be placed before the Veress needle is inserted. If alternate site entry is contemplated, mechanical colon preparation should be mandatory. A Fleet's enema and/or a Dulcolax suppository should be given 2–3 hours before surgery to ensure an empty colon.

Open Technique Versus Closed Technique

The decision to use open or closed technique depends on the experience of the operator. Open technique is the safest for surgeons who do not perform closed

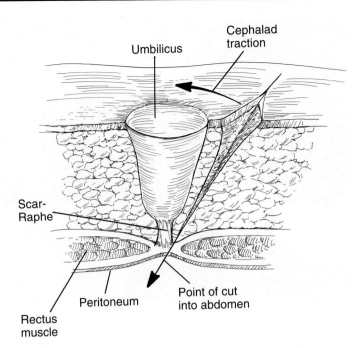
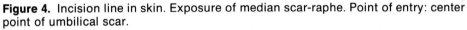

Figure 4. Incision line in skin. Exposure of median scar-raphe. Point of entry: center point of umbilical scar.

technique routinely (Fig. 4). However, even the highly experienced practitioners of the closed technique may have to use the open technique in the following instances:

1. History of multiple intraabdominal operations in the past
2. History of peritonitis in the past
3. Large incarcerated umbilical hernia
4. Distended abdomen, ileus, and possible small bowel obstruction where lysis of adhesions is anticipated
5. History of extensive endometriosis
6. Trauma laparoscopy
7. History of multiple intraabdominal adhesions
8. Pregnancy

An ultrasound slide test to determine underlying adhesions has been described in the literature, but I have no experience with this test.

▼ INTRAOPERATIVE MANAGEMENT/SURGICAL TECHNIQUE

Position of Patient

A supine or Trendelenburg position is used to create the pneumoperitoneum. When a satisfactory pneumoperitoneum has been created, the operating table may be tilted to a head-up or head-down (Trendelenburg) position or may be tilted to the right or left to visualize structures on the opposite side of the tilt. Care must be taken to position the arms properly to prevent ulnar nerve and brachial plexus injuries. There should be a footboard to prevent the patient from slipping downward toward the foot (Fig. 5). A safety belt should be placed on the torso to prevent the patient from sliding sideward. If extreme Trendelenburg position is anticipated, as in pelviscopy or colon surgery, sufficiently padded shoulder restraints should be available to prevent the patient from slipping cranially.

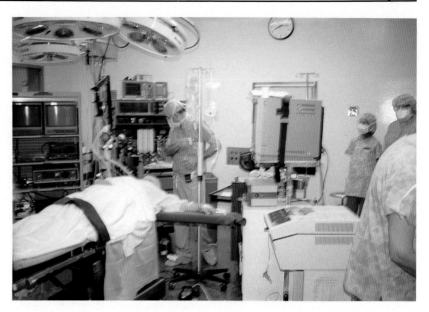

Figure 5. Positioning of patient in the operating room.

Monitor Placement

Generally, the monitor should be located opposite the operator with the camera pointed toward the monitor. However, a large monitor may be placed in a middle position either at the head or foot end of the table. Experienced laparoscopic surgeons usually can manage to correct for the manipulative aberrations caused by working against the camera.

Return Electrode Placement

Care must be exercised in placing the return electrode. If the patient has a hairy body, the site selected for placement should be shaved. The return electrode should never be placed on a limb that has a metal prosthesis in it, as this may cause prosthetic failure and burn injuries. Return electrode monitoring systems should be used on all patients undergoing laparoscopic monopolar electrosurgery to ensure that alternate-site burn injuries do not occur.

Electrosurgical Unit

The audible tone generator on the electrosurgical unit should *never* be turned off. This audible tone is specifically designed to alert operating room personnel to a failure in the return electrode monitoring system and also if the unit is accidentally switched on, thereby possibly avoiding an injury.

The setting of the electrosurgical unit should rarely exceed 30 W in the coagulation mode. Occasionally, a fulguration mode may be necessary to coagulate a vein in the gallbladder bed. In this mode, the tip of the active electrode should not touch the tissues. Most of the laparoscopic cholecystectomies can be adequately performed using 25 W of power in the coagulation mode.

Insufflators

Insufflators should have a capacity of at least 10 L/min, and they should have a sensitive pressure monitoring system that is easy to read, preferably a digital readout. The audible alarm on the insufflators should never be turned off.

Insufflation of the Peritoneal Cavity

Carbon dioxide is the gas of choice for most operative laparoscopy; it does not support combustion and is readily expelled following absorption from the peritoneal cavity or if accidentally injected into a blood vessel. All patients should have expired gas CO_2 monitors during anesthesia to detect accidental CO_2 air embolism. Automatic CO_2 insufflators are available and should be used instead of the old-fashioned manual insufflators. The modern automatic insufflator can handle a flow of 10 L/min. The rate of flow is usually limited by the resistance in the port through which it flows. A Y connector with double hookups to ports would enable a larger volume to be insufflated to compensate for CO_2 loss during suction and irrigation. Smoke evacuation systems may be cost effective.

Placement of Veress Needle

The commonest method of induction of pneumoperitoneum is by means of the Veress needle.

In the standard technique, preferred by most gynecologists, the Veress needle is most often inserted at the subumbilical site with the abdominal skin held taut with a towel clip or the hand of the operator. A No. 11 blade is used to make a small incision at the infraumbilical point of insertion (Fig. 6). The needle should

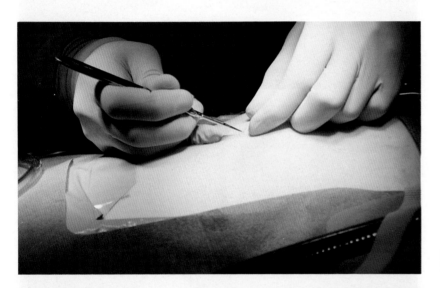

Figure 6. Infraumbilical insertion point incision.

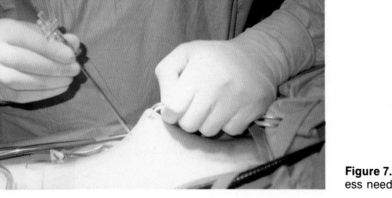

Figure 7. Correct method of holding Veress needle.

be held like a pen between the thumb and index finger and supported by the middle finger (Fig. 7). The needle is inserted into the peritoneal cavity carefully (Figs. 8 and 9). A definite click is felt when the needle penetrates the midline fascia. The passage of the needle into the peritoneum can be difficult to assess as the peritoneum tends to tent and the "feel" is less distinct. This "feel" is least distinct with the disposable Veress needles because they are very sharp. The reusable Veress needle gives a better "feel." Once the Veress needle is placed in the peritoneal cavity, standard tests for placement are performed before starting the insufflation.

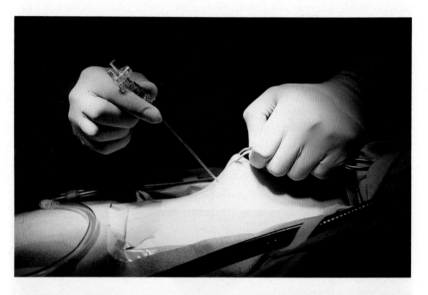

Figure 8. Gentle advancement of Veress needle into fascia.

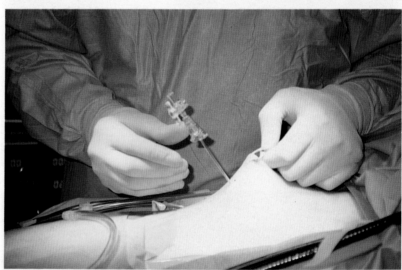

Figure 9. Gentle advancement into peritoneal cavity.

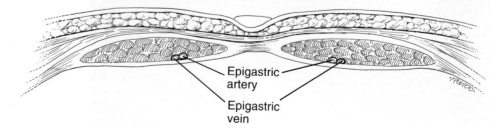

Epigastric artery

Epigastric vein

Figure 10. Umbilical scar, thinnest part of anterior abdominal wall.

In the *alternate standard technique* the Veress needle is introduced into the thinnest portion of the anterior abdominal wall, which is the scar in the pit of the umbilicus (Figs. 1, 10, and 11) (1). The side of the funnel of the umbilicus is grasped by two sharp towel clips (Fig. 12). A No. 11 blade is used to make an incision in the pit of the umbilicus (Figs. 1 and 13). A reusable Veress needle is placed into the abdomen (Fig. 14). The needle should never advance more than 1 to 1½ in. into the abdominal cavity. Insufflation is begun after the standard tests for proper placement are performed.

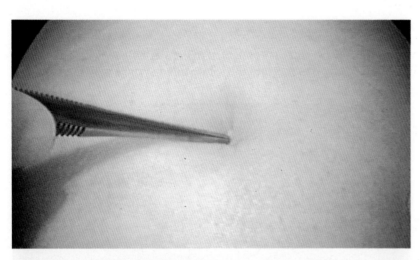

Figure 11. Umbilical scar, thinnest part of anterior abdominal wall.

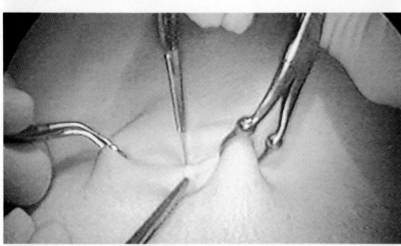

Figure 12. No. 11 blade incision into midpoint umbilical scar.

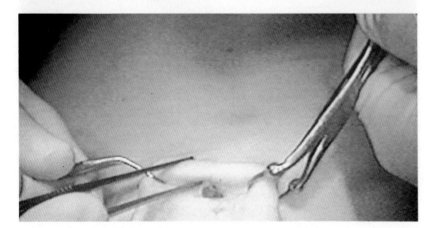

Figure 13. S-shaped extension into cone of umbilicus.

At the end of insufflation, the incision is extended inferiorly and horizontally toward the upper portion of the skin of the umbilicus (Fig. 1). The trocar-cannula can then be inserted directly through this thin portion of the abdomen with the least force into the abdomen.

Tests For Checking Proper Veress Needle Placement

The following tests should be performed to check the correct placement of the Veress needle:

Aspiration Test

A saline- or water-filled syringe is connected to the Veress needle and aspirated (Fig. 15). Aspiration of blood or gas into the saline-filled syringe may indicate that

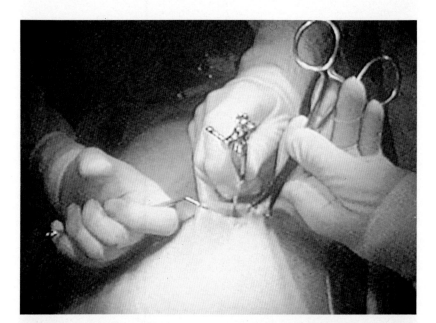

Figure 14. Penholder grip—Veress needle—introduction into peritoneal cavity.

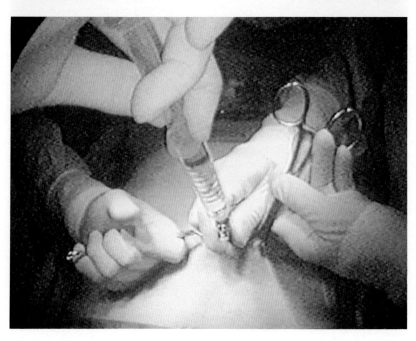

Figure 15. Placement tests, aspiration, injection.

the needle may have been placed into a blood vessel or a hollow viscus accidentally. This is considered a positive test. If this test is negative, then fluid is gently injected into the Veress needle. Negative pressure in the syringe should not aspirate the injected fluid back into the syringe. Return of injected fluid into the syringe may indicate a preperitoneal placement of the Veress needle.

Drop Test

A drop of saline is placed on the top of the opening into the Veress needle and the shut-off valve is opened (Fig. 16). The drop should readily disappear into the peritoneal cavity if the needle tip is lying free in the peritoneal cavity due to the negative pressure in the abdomen. Elevation of the towel clips sometimes facilitates this disappearance of the drop by dislodging the tip from underlying structures and creating a negative pressure in the abdomen.

Immediate Insufflation Pressure Test

When the aspiration and drop tests are performed, the insufflation tube is connected to the Veress needle (Fig. 17). The insufflation pressure should not

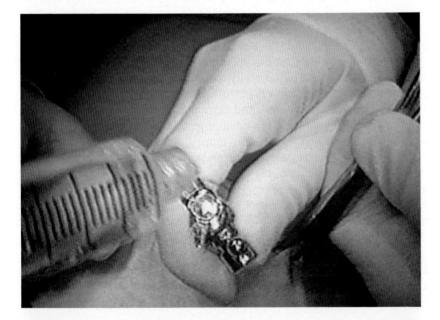

Figure 16. Hanging drop placement test.

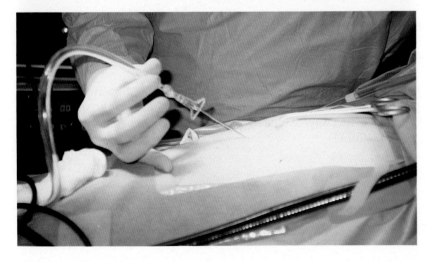

Figure 17. Starting insufflation following placement tests.

exceed 5 to 6 mmHg at 1.0 L/min flow of CO_2. If in doubt, static pressure can be obtained. This should not exceed 3 to 5 mmHg if CO_2 has already been insufflated, otherwise it should be "0" mmHg or negative when the towel clips attached to the abdominal wall are elevated. Pressure exceeding this indicates a preperitoneal placement of the needle tip in a virgin abdomen. In an abdomen that has been operated on previously, it may also indicate placement into an underlying structure (i.e., adhesions or bowel).

The initial insufflation should always be carried out slowly: 1.0 L/min. Once the placement is ensured, then the rate can be advanced to 6–10 L/min. The pressure in the peritoneal cavity is usually set between 10 and 15 mmHg. The abdomen should be percussed to confirm uniform distribution of the gas in the peritoneal cavity. Lopsided distribution of gas should make one suspect preperitoneal placement. This lopsided distribution can occur in an abdomen that has been previously operated on and should not cause concern.

Problems During Insufflation

If, during induction of pneumoperitoneum, the previous tests suggest incorrect placement, the Veress needle is simply withdrawn, reinserted, and retested.

If blood is withdrawn on aspiration test and fountains back into the Veress needle when the syringe is disconnected, major vessel injury is likely and an immediate laparotomy should be performed to ascertain the source of the bleeding.

If bowel contents are aspirated, the needle should be withdrawn and the open technique performed. Upon successful pneumoperitoneum, the site underlying previous insertion effort should be carefully visualized to ascertain the injury to the bowel. Simple, single, small bowel perforations without persistent leak can be observed with irrigation, antibiotics, and close postoperative follow-up. Colon injuries should be repaired immediately and appropriately. More extensive or tangential bowel injuries should be repaired by immediate laparotomy.

If large preperitoneal space is created by preperitoneal insufflation, the open technique should be used to gain access to the abdominal cavity after total decompression of the preperitoneal space, using the same Veress needle.

Sometimes during the course of a procedure the insufflator indicator shows a pressure higher than the set limit. The most common cause for this is an occlusion of the insufflation line. If the line is completely open, then the cause is usually a patient who is too lightly anesthetized and is about to wake up. Proper adjustment of the anesthetic agent corrects the problem. All sharp instruments should be withdrawn from the abdomen immediately when the preset pressure alarm sounds to prevent injury to intraabdominal structures.

PNEUMOPERITONEUM IN A PREVIOUSLY OPERATED-ON ABDOMEN

Alternate Site Entry

I have been successful with the alternate site technique; however, the safest approach may be the open cutdown technique. A point close to the rib margin in the left midclavicular line approximately at the lateral edge of the rectus muscle is chosen (Figs. 18–20) (1).

Position of Patient

Reverse Trendelenburg position is advocated to drop the colon down. A nasogastric tube is placed in the stomach for decompression. It is assumed that the patient's colon has been mechanically prepared.

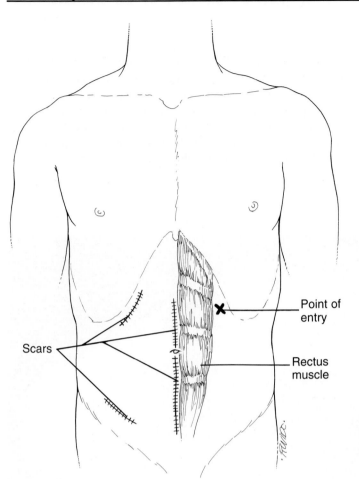

Figure 18. Patient is in the Trendelenburg position. The preferred point of alternate site entry is close to the costal margin on either side and away from previous incisions.

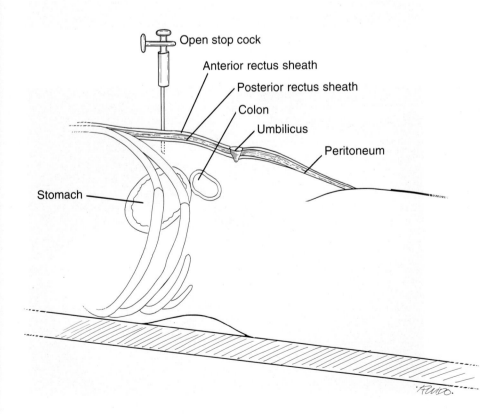

Figure 19. Lateral view: reverse Trendelenburg position. The rib margin holds the abdominal wall up anteriorly. Veress needle with open stop cock allows air to rush into potential negative pressure in abdomen allowing underlying structures to fall away due to gravity.

Insertion of Veress Needle

An incision is made with a No. 11 blade into the recommended site (Fig. 21). A reusable Veress needle is passed into the abdomen gently with an open stopcock. Anterior rectus sheath, posterior rectus sheath, and peritoneum are usually felt as the Veress needle enters the peritoneum. A hiss of air going into the peritoneum can be heard upon entry into the abdomen if the operating room is quiet (Fig. 22). Following this, the standard tests for placement of the Veress needle can be carried out (Figs. 15 and 16) and insufflation is begun if the placement is deemed proper (Fig. 23).

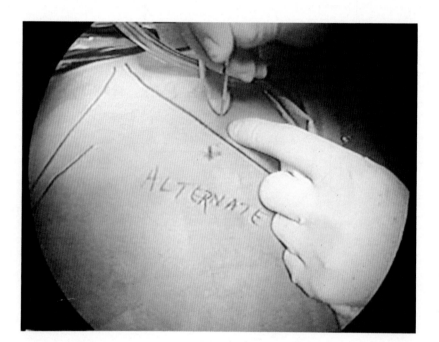

Figure 20. Preferred alternate entry site: left subcostal margin.

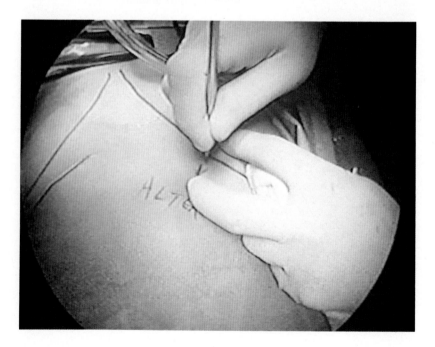

Figure 21. No. 7 blade incision of skin.

Insertion of Primary "Look in 5-mm Telescope" Following Alternate Site Entry: Intraperitoneal Sounding Test

Following pneumoperitoneum, a sounding test for adhesions should be carried out at the selected point of insertion of the 5-mm inspection telescope (Figs. 24–26). A No. 22-gauge spinal needle attached to a 5-ml syringe half-filled with saline is inserted vertically into the abdominal cavity at the preselected site. Slight negative pressure is applied to the syringe. The point of aspiration of gas into the syringe is marked with a hemostat on the needle. This gives the distance to the peritoneum from the skin surface. The needle is then withdrawn and reinserted several times at 45-degree angles in a 360-degree arc. If the bubbling of air is not observed, or is sporadic at a certain point in the arc, it denotes the presence of omental adhesions and/or bowel at the point of interruption of air bubbling.

Several such insertions will help determine the area of air pocket into which a 5-mm trocar-cannula can be inserted safely. A skin incision wider than the trocar-cannula is made at this point, and the trocar-cannula is inserted carefully to the

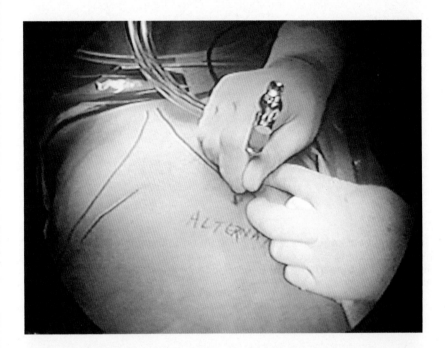

Figure 22. Penholder grip, Veress needle insertion into abdominal cavity.

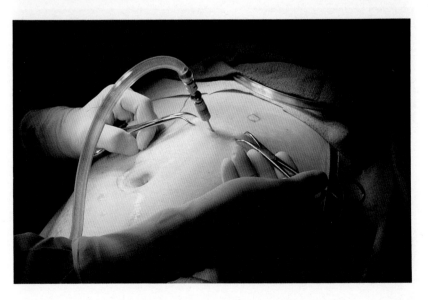

Figure 23. Insufflation following placement tests.

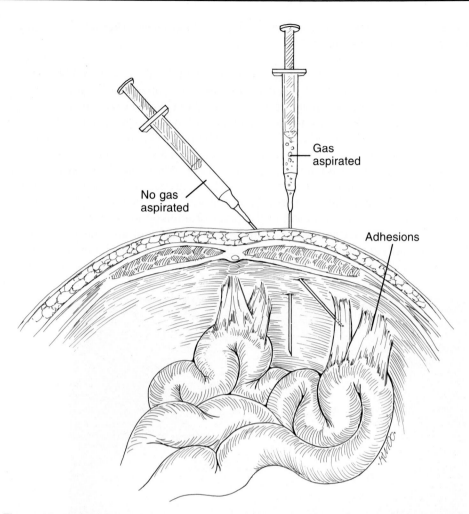

Figure 24. Intraperitoneal sounding test. *1*, Constant bubbling in areas that are clear of adhesions. *2*, No bubbling or sporadic bubbling in areas of bowel or omental adhesions. *3*, Safe area (pneumoperitoneum) to introduce 5-mm telescope through the 5-mm trocar-cannula.

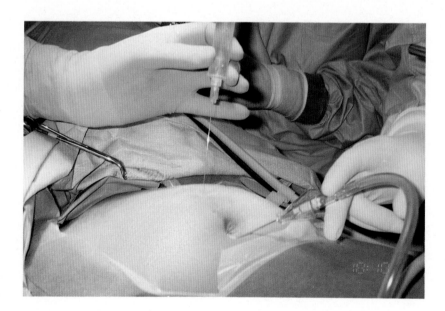

Figure 25. Intraperitoneal sounding test.

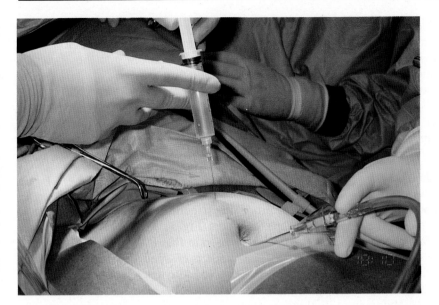

Figure 26. Intraperitoneal sounding test: change of direction.

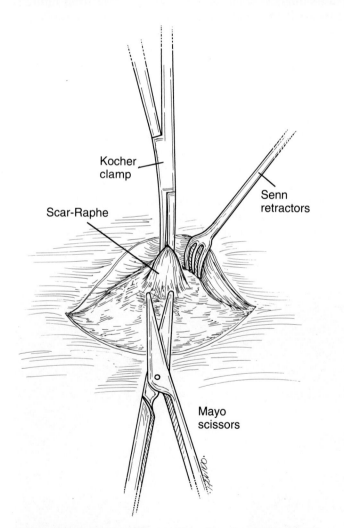

Figure 27. Open technique. Skin is retracted upward. Kocher clamp is placed on the anterior portion of the median scar. Clamp is elevated anterosuperiorly to put raphe on tension. Mayo scissors cut into abdomen through raphe (without spreading), incising attached peritoneum.

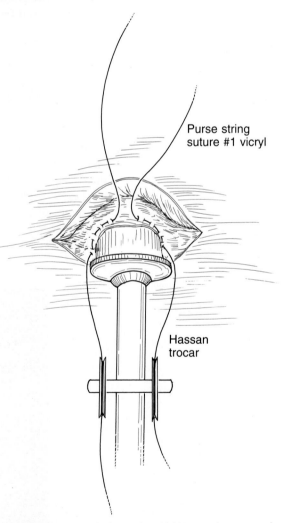

Figure 28. Open technique. Insert Hasson trocar and secure in place with pursestring suture.

measured length. The trocar is withdrawn and the stopcock on the cannula opened. A hiss of air denotes insertion into the air pocket in the abdominal cavity.

A previously "whited out" 5-mm telescope is introduced into the abdomen and complete exploration of the abdominal contents is carried out. The site of Veress needle insertion and the space directly underneath it are carefully examined. The size, nature, and location of adhesions are determined prior to insertion of a larger trocar-cannula to perform necessary adhesiolysis and permit the main planned operation.

Open Technique

The open technique is safest for producing pneumoperitoneum. A horizontal incision is placed 0.5 cm inferior to the umbilicus (Fig. 3). The incision is deepened until the fascia is reached (Fig. 4). The upper skin flap is stretched cranially to locate the scar of the umbilicus. This scar-raphe is grasped with a Kocher clamp and retracted cephalad to stretch the scar. Curved Mayo scissors are used to cut directly posterior into the abdomen (Fig. 27). *Do not spread the scar.* The cut will enter the abdomen at its thinnest point. A No. 1 Vicryl pursestring suture is then placed to retain and secure the blunt Hasson trocar-cannula into the abdomen (Fig. 28) (2).

TROCAR-CANNULA INSERTION

Position of Patient

The patient should be placed in the Trendelenburg position if standard insertion technique is used. The trocar-cannula should be aimed toward the pelvis. The index finger should be extended parallel to the shaft of the trocar and pointed in the direction of insertion to stop the penetration of the trocar-cannula beyond 2 in. (Fig. 29). The assistant should further support the trocar-cannula shaft to limit the depth of penetration of the trocar-cannula (Fig. 30) and prevent accidental deep insertion, which may produce serious injuries. The abdomen should be fixed at the insertion level with two towel clips on either side of the insertion site to

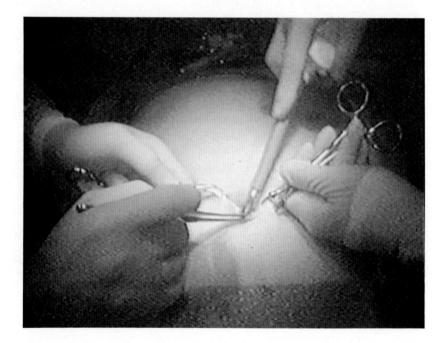

Figure 29. Extended index finger to limit penetration of the trocar-cannula.

stabilize it. The opening in the skin *must be slightly larger than the actual outer diameter of the trocar-cannula.* This is best achieved by dilating the skin opening with a hemostat. The force used to enter the abdomen should never deform the abdominal wall so much that it reduces the effectiveness of the pneumoperitoneum. Check the trocar setting if excessive force is necessary to penetrate the abdominal wall with a disposable trocar-cannula. Most commonly the trocar is not *armed* properly. If the trocar is *armed properly* then the reason for excessive force is usually due to a small skin opening. Widening the skin opening will facilitate the insertion of the trocar-cannula without excessive force. Always check disposable trocar-cannulas if excessive force is necessary. The trocar arming mechanism has been known to fail.

The safety shields of most disposable trocar-cannulas cannot be relied upon to prevent organ injury. Disposable trocars should always be inserted with straight perpendicular force into the abdominal wall, using the previously mentioned precautions.

Nondisposable trocar-cannulas should be inserted with a twisting, rotating motion. The least traumatic trocars have a conical tip without cutting edges. Most disposable and nondisposable trocars have a cutting edge and therefore should not be placed in the path of superior or inferior epigastric arteries.

Z Technique for Insertion of Conical Diagnostic Trocar-Cannula (Semm)

For diagnostic laparoscopy the Z technique is particularly useful. It provides a secure gastight insertion point, and the fascia need not be repaired to prevent trocar-site hernias. A *conical reusable trocar-cannula* is placed through a small infraumbilical incision (Figs. 31 and 32), with the trocar pointing toward the pubis. The trocar travels the length of the conical tip in the subcutaneous tissues. A 90-degree change in the direction of travel is undertaken (Fig. 33). The trocar is rotated 90 degrees for perpendicular insertion into the rectus sheath and muscle (Fig. 33), aimed posteriorly. The trocar-cannula is then advanced into the rectus muscle.

A second 90-degree rotation toward the central point of pelvis is now accomplished. The trocar penetrates the posterior rectus sheath and is pointed into the

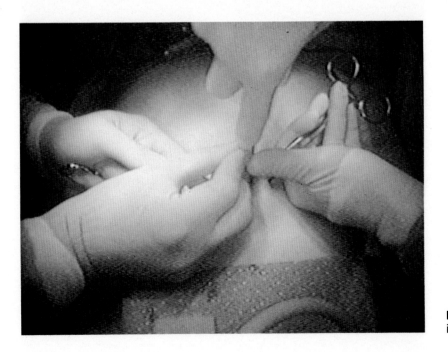

Figure 30. Assistant's finger further limits penetration of the trocar-cannula.

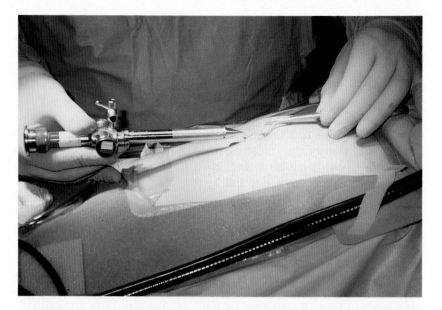

Figure 31. Conical reusable trocar-cannula in Semm's Z technique.

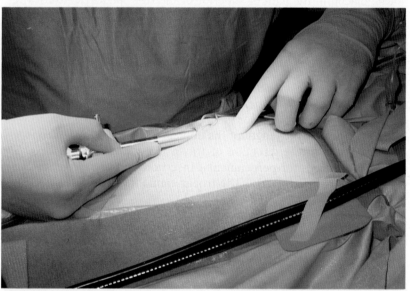

Figure 32. Subumbilical incision, subcutaneous insertion.

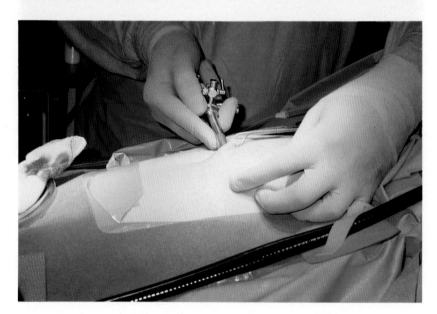

Figure 33. A 90-degree change in direction with penetration rectus sheath.

pelvis caudad (Figs. 34 and 35) and inserted smoothly into the abdomen. The depth of penetration is always limited to the tip of the extended index finger (Fig. 35). Insufflation (Fig. 36) is started after standard tests for placement are performed.

Figure 37 shows the atraumatic entrance of the conical tip trocar cannula through the rectus muscle. These wounds do not need to be repaired to prevent trocar-site hernias. The rectus muscle gives a very snug fit so that gas leak is minimized. The rectus muscle closes promptly upon withdrawal of the trocar. This technique is only useful in diagnostic situations and the port cannot be used to extract gallbladder and appendixes due to invasion of the potential rectus sheath space. There are commercially available disposable, conical, dilatable trocar-cannulas in different sizes that duplicate the performance of reusable conical trocar-cannulas. These are nontraumatic and do not cut muscle or fascia and therefore cause less pain. These rarely require repair of underlying fascia.

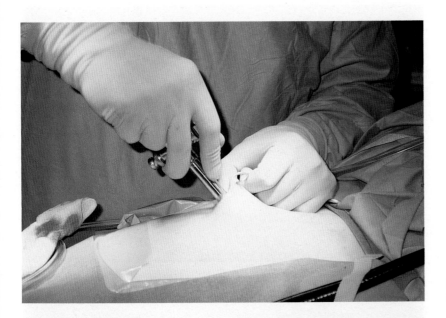

Figure 34. Second 90-degree change in direction, penetrating rectus muscle.

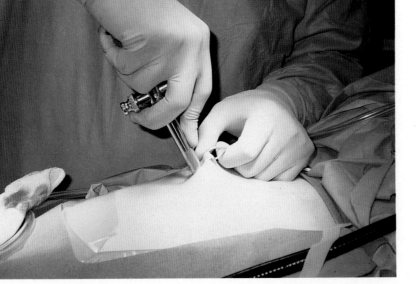

Figure 35. Caudad change angle of insertion to penetrate into abdominal cavity.

Secondary Trocars-Cannulas

Secondary trocar-cannulas should be placed under direct vision following transillumination of the abdominal wall to check for epigastric arteries. Transillumination is successful only in thin abdominal wall configurations. Direct visualization of the inferior epigastric artery prior to insertion prevents injuries (Figs. 38 and 39).

Inspection of Abdominal Contents

Immediate inspection of the possible areas of injuries should be undertaken with a 0-degree telescope. Structures underlying the Veress needle insertion site should be checked.

Following this initial "quick check," a thorough anterior abdominal inspection should be carried out with a 30-degree telescope. To visualize pelvic structures

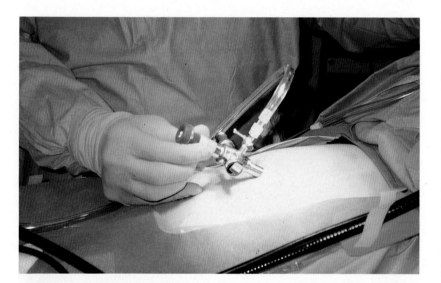

Figure 36. Start of insufflation.

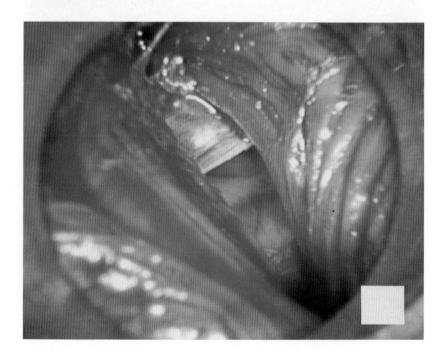

Figure 37. Atraumatic insertion site of conical tip trocar-cannula laparoscopic view.

properly, a uterine manipulator, such as a Hulka catheter, may be necessary. If a uterine manipulator is not used a 5-mm assist trocar-cannula should be placed in the lower midline, avoiding the bladder, to elevate the uterus and examine the ovaries. Patient positioning by operating table rotation can assist in visualizing most of the anterior abdominal contents. Angled telescopes and flexible telescopes provide better visualization of the liver and spleen.

Additional Ports

Additional assist ports should be created as needed (Figs. 40 and 41). Figure 42 shows a configuration for laparoscopic cholecystectomy; however, the ports can be adjusted to the procedure planned. The principle should be to avoid epigastric arteries and the hernial orifices in the lower abdomen. For two-handed tech-

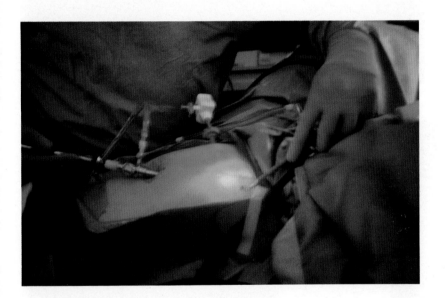

Figure 38. Transillumination of abdominal wall to locate vessels.

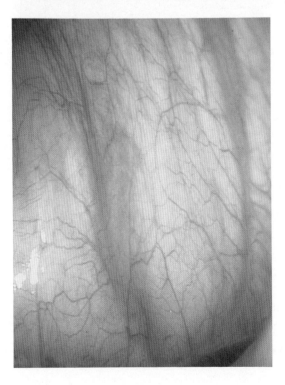

Figure 39. Direct visualization of inferior epigastric artery.

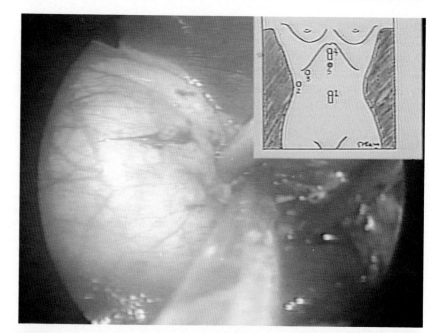

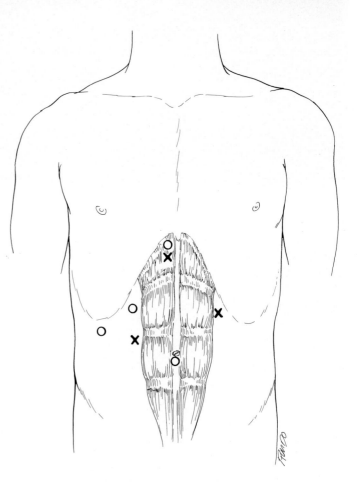

Figure 40. Secondary, additional, parallel epigastric port.

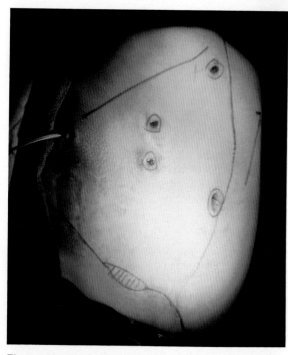

Figure 41. Secondary, additional, right midclavicular parallel port.

O Primary sites
X Secondary sites

Figure 42. Sites of ports in laparoscopic cholecystectomy: primary and secondary.

niques, the parallel assist ports should be at least 2½ in. apart to facilitate ease of dissection.

Sudden massive bleeding can occur in Calot's triangle. To control this bleeding laparoscopically an additional parallel port can be inserted 2½ in. inferior to the operating epigastric or the right midclavicular port. Two-handed dissection with precise ligation of a bleeding cystic artery can be achieved safely without opening the abdomen (6).

CAMERAS

Most laparoscopic cholecystectomies can be performed with a single-chip camera. However, advanced procedures such as fundoplications, colon resections, and esophageal resections may require a three-chip camera to obtain better resolutions of the picture. Large 19- to 21-in. monitors specifically designed to be integrated with these cameras provide a superior picture and reduce eyestrain. Superior cameras have longer depth of field and require fewer adjustments of focus. Cameras can only adjust the position of viewing but not the angle of viewing.

LIGHT CORDS

Light transmission from the light source to the laparoscope can be severely restricted by damaged fibreoptic bundles or, in the case of liquid cables, damaged glass optical ends. These ends are damaged frequently by careless handling at the close of procedures, and these ends should be checked before plugging them into the light source at the beginning of procedures.

TELESCOPES

Although 0-degree telescopes (Figs. 43 and 44) are satisfactory, 25- to 30-degree telescopes (Fig. 45) are recommended because they can peer around structures and are very valuable in the precise dissection of Callot's triangle window. Also, 45-degree telescopes are valuable in laparoscopic hernia repairs. The problem with the angled telescope is that it requires a trained camera-holder who is part of a team to precisely aim the camera. The field of view changes *opposite* to the position of the light cord, that is, when the light cord attachment to the laparoscope is tilted to the right, the field of view is tilted to the left. The angled laparoscopic telescope has the ability to look up or down and, depending on the position of the lens, the ability to peer into corners is enhanced. The 0-degree telescopes cannot perform these maneuvers.

COMPLICATIONS RELATED TO LAPAROSCOPIC EQUIPMENT

Electrical Burns

Undetected catastrophic intraabdominal burns can occur due to insulation failure of active instruments in monopolar surgery. Wire electrodes and insulated reusable scissors, graspers, and dissectors should be checked for cracked insulation before each use.

The second cause of accidental burn is failure to visualize the active tip of the instrument at *all times* in the monitor. During complicated procedures, the long uninsulated scissors tip or grasper tip may not be visualized during activation of the current, leading to accidental burn of the adjacent small bowel or colon. Setting electrosurgical unit output at high settings, and activating the current for long periods of time, may cause electrical burn, which is not seen at the time of surgery. Laparoscopic procedures can be successfully performed using 25W–30W of coagulation setting.

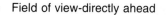

Field of view-directly ahead

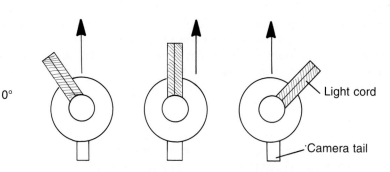

Light cord

Camera tail

0°-no change in view-rotation of light cord

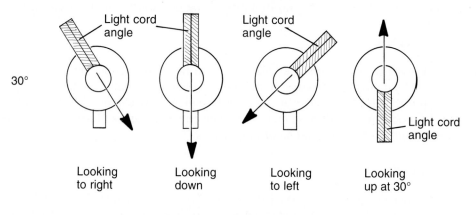

Field of view-tilted opposite light cord

Light cord angle

Light cord angle

Light cord angle

30°

Looking to right

Looking down

Looking to left

Looking up at 30°

Arrows represent field of view

Figure 43. Telescopes: 0°–30°. Line of sight is opposite the light cord insertion into laparoscope.

Division of Current–Alternate Site Burns

In all monopolar surgery the patient is placed in the path of the electrons, that is, the patient is a conductor of electricity; therefore, if another conductor of electricity touches the patient, the current flow could be divided and, depending on the resistance at the point of contact, he or she may sustain a burn. To prevent alternate site injuries *only* electrostatic units with *isolated surgical outputs* should be used. Return electrode pads should be monitored for their effectiveness and *this feature should be part of the electrosurgical unit*. If the return electrode malfunctions during the course of the operation, the circuit inside the electrosurgical unit will sound an alarm and shut it off to protect the patient. It is recommended that all laparoscopic surgeries should be performed with newer, modern electrosurgical units incorporating the above features.

Hot Light Cords

Light cords get hot when in use, therefore they should not be unplugged after use and left to hang loose. There have been operating room fires with severe burns to the patient when, at the end of the procedures, light cords were unplugged and left dangling close to draperies. When starting a procedure the light cord should

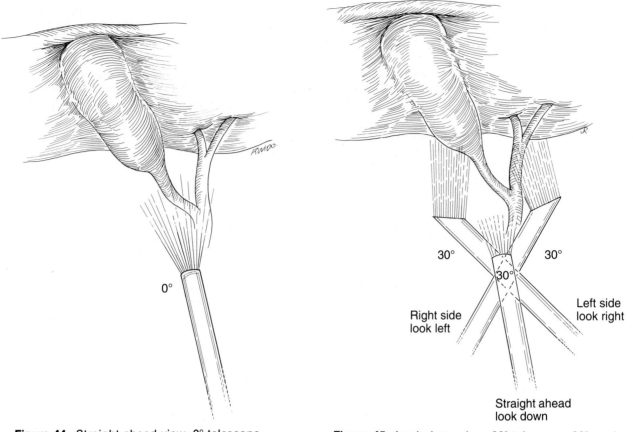

Figure 44. Straight-ahead view, 0° telescope.

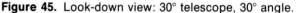

Figure 45. Look-down view: 30° telescope, 30° angle.

always be plugged into the laparoscope before turning on the light. The end of the laparoscope should not touch the draperies. The practice of turning on the light with the light cords attached lying on the draperies should be abandoned.

BASIC THORACOSCOPY

In 1922 Jacobaeus (5) reported on the importance of thoracoscopy in surgery of the chest. He mainly used it for the treatment of pulmonary tuberculosis and, eventually, the thoracoscope was retired for use only as a diagnostic tool due to the advent of modern antimicrobial treatment of tuberculosis. The development of minimally invasive surgery and improvement in the video endoscopic equipment renewed interest in thoracoscopic procedures.

Equipment

The endoscopic equipment developed for laparoscopic procedures can be used successfully for thoracoscopic procedures. Dual video monitors are positioned on both sides of the operating table. For most procedures, a 0-degree 10-mm rigid telescope is used. Angled 30- or 45-degree telescopes are useful in the various recesses of the thoracic cavity.

The unique anatomy of the thoracic cage may preclude the use of pneumothorax to provide compression of the lungs. Adequate collapse of the lung can be provided by selective bronchial entubation with double-lumen endotrachael tubes. These tubes can be properly placed with the help of flexible bronchoscopes by anesthesiologists.

When the use of double-lumen endotrachael tubes is impossible or unsuccessful, then selective entubation of the bronchus with insufflation of the desired thoracic cavity and Fogarty balloon occlusion of the opposite bronchus can be performed (Fig. 46). If pneumothorax is selected to compress the lung, the pressure should not exceed 10 mmHg to avoid the cardiovascular consequences of diminished venous return and compression of the heart, due to a tension pneumothorax. Continuous blood pressure monitoring through a radial artery catheter is mandatory in cases where lung collapse has to be achieved by pneumothorax. Pneumothorax may be indicated in pediatric cases or patients requiring lung biopsies who are already on mechanical ventilation.

Patient Position

The patient is usually positioned in a full lateral decubitus position (Figs. 47 and 48). The position can be modified to treat a specific pathology. The upper arm and forearm are suspended properly to access the axilla. The table is broken to enhance the opening of the ribs. A roll is placed under the opposite axilla to avoid brachial plexus compression. The patient may be placed on a beanbag to help rotate the patient to a desirable position.

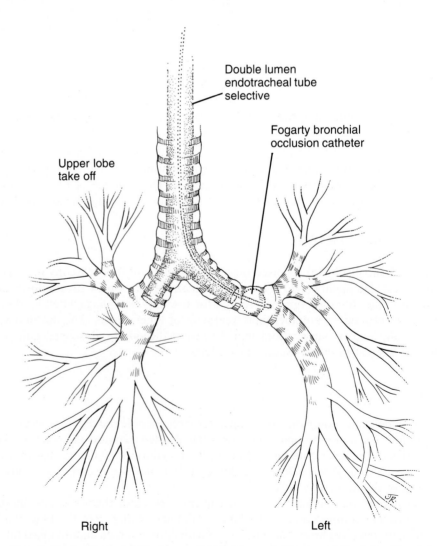

Figure 46. Anatomy of trachea and bronchus: right upper lobe takeoff point.

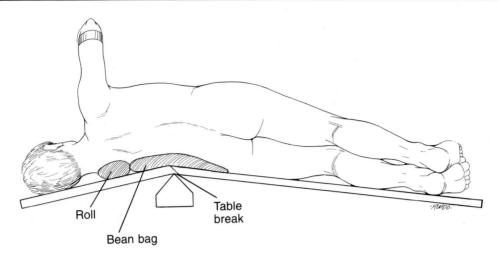

Roll

Bean bag

Table
break

Figure 47. Left lateral decubitus view. Patient's arm suspended at table break.

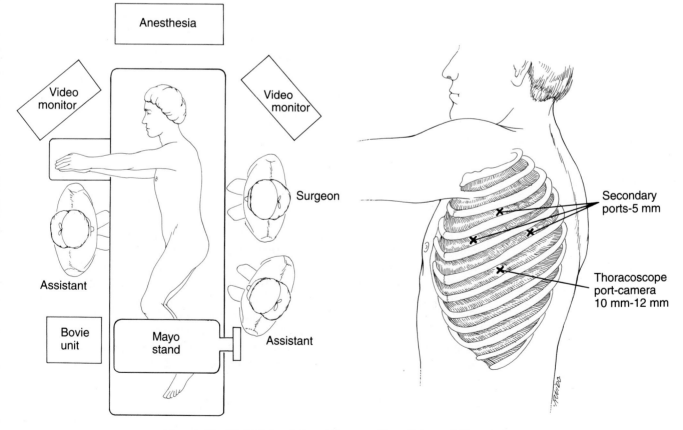

Anesthesia

Video
monitor

Video
monitor

Surgeon

Assistant

Bovie
unit

Mayo
stand

Assistant

Secondary
ports-5 mm

Thoracoscope
port-camera
10 mm-12 mm

Figure 48. Right lateral decubitus position. Triangulating ports.

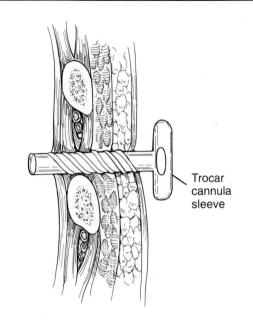

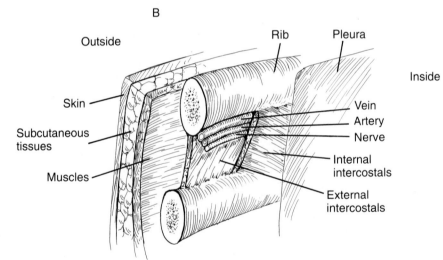

Figure 49. A,B: Placement of port, superior to the rib.

Ports

The ports are always placed above the rib margin to prevent injury to the intercostal artery, vein, and nerve that travel in a groove below the rib between internal and external intercostal muscles (Fig. 49). Disposable ports are available commercially and can be tailored to the thickness of the chest wall. These have either screw-in threads or suture points to maintain position in the chest wall. They also have one-way flap valves in case pneumoperitoneum is used.

The visualizing port should always be in the middle of the triangulated operating ports for the best view of the operative site (Fig. 48). The operating ports may be 5 or 10 mm, depending on the contemplated procedure.

▲ COMPLICATIONS

We conducted a national survey of 4,292 hospitals performing laparoscopic cholecystectomies in 1990. There was a 40.8% response rate (3).

Bowel injury rate of 0.14% included punctures from Veress needle, trocar insertions, and thermal burns.

Vascular injury rates were reported to be 0.25%. Aortic, venacaval injuries were reported during insertion of trocar-cannulas. Injury to the inferior epigastric vessels can be significantly decreased if the trocar is inserted in the midline or lateral to the rectus muscle. However, these injuries occurred during the initial rush of surgeons unfamiliar with laparoscopic techniques.

Strict credentialing guidelines almost eliminated these injuries (4). The most frequent complications now seen are due to trocar-cannulas causing trocar site bleeding. The majority of small bowel transmural injuries can be safely managed conservatively if the site of puncture is identified during immediate exploration following insertion. However, injuries unrecognized at the time of insertion usually are diagnosed when the patient presents with sepsis, peritonitis, and/or intra-abdominal abscess.

Monopolar electrical injuries are usually not recognized until the third or fourth postoperative day and present with signs of peritonitis.

Bleeding from thoracoscopic trocar insertion sites can be profuse if an intercostal artery is injured.

☑ CONCLUSIONS

Insertion of the initial trocar-cannula is the single most risky maneuver during laparoscopy. This is significantly reduced if the open technique or the standard alternative technique is used. Minimal force should be used to place the trocars. Conical trocar-cannulas are the most atraumatic and should be used if possible. Initial thoracoscopic ports should be placed high up in the fifth or sixth intercostal spaces to avoid injury to liver, diaphragm, and spleen.

Strict credentialing guidelines and concurrent monitoring of all laparoscopic procedures should reduce injury rates and make laparoscopy safer (6). I believe that laparoscopic operating teams reduce operating time and complications (7).

ACKNOWLEDGMENTS

I thank Vipal Arora, M.D., Gynecologist, Good Samaritan Hospital for Semm's Z technique slides.

RECOMMENDED READING

1. American College of Surgeons Scientific Exhibit. *Specific techniques in laparoscopic general surgery,* October 20–25, 1991.
2. Hasson HM. Modified instrument and method for laparoscopy. *Am J Obstet Gynecol* 1971;110: 886–887.
3. Deziel DJ, Millikan KW, Economou SG, Doolas A, Ko ST, Airan MC. Complications of laparoscopic cholecystectomy: a national survey of 4,292 hospitals and an analysis of 77,604 cases. *Am J Surg* 1993;65:9–14.
4. Airan MC, Ko ST. Effectiveness of strict credentialing and proctoring guidelines on outcomes of laparoscopic cholecystectomy in a community hospital. *Surg Endosc* 1994;8:396–399.
5. Jacobaeus HC. The practical importance of thoracoscopy in surgery of the chest. *Surg Gynecol Obstet* 1922;34:289–296.
6. Ko ST, Airan MC. Review of 300 consecutive laparoscopic cholecystectomies: development, evolution, and results. *Surg Endosc* 1991;5:103–108.
7. Airan MC, Ko ST. Assessment of quality of care in laparoscopic cholecystectomy. *J Am Coll Med Qual* 7:85–87.

SURGICAL PEARLS

The single most effective way to prevent trocar-cannula insertion injuries is to extend the right index finger to limit the penetration depth and also to have the assistant further limit the insertion depth with fingers around the shaft of the cannula.

Visualization of the inferior epigastric artery with a 30-degree telescope prior to insertion of lateral lower abdominal ports will prevent injury to this artery.

Precise dissection of the junction of cystic duct with Hartmann's pouch of the gallbladder is facilitated by using a 25- to 30-degree telescope.

9

Suturing and Knot-Tying Techniques

Daniel B. Jones and Nathaniel J. Soper
Department of Surgery
Washington University
Barnes Hospital
St. Louis, Missouri 63110

Operative Laparoscopy and Thoracoscopy, edited by
B. V. MacFadyen, Jr. and
J. L. Ponsky. Lippincott-Raven
Publishers, Philadelphia © 1996.

Suturing and knot-tying are essential surgical skills requiring practice to master. Developing these basic skills is not less important for the laparoscopic surgeon simply because stapling devices and clip appliers are available in the operating room. Occasionally, the surgeon may want to tie an extracorporeal knot and advance the knot within the abdominal cavity. After suturing on delicate tissue, most surgeons prefer to instrument-tie intracorporeally. No one technique is applicable in all situations, and a surgeon performing advanced laparoscopic operations should know several methods to ligate vessels, reapproximate tissue surfaces, and reconstruct organs.

Experienced surgeons who throw a square knot with ease after an open incision find that laparoscopic suturing and knot-typing rely on a different set of skills. Difficulty with knot-tying during laparoscopic surgery results mainly from operating with only a two-dimensional video-projected image. The screen lacks depth perception. Furthermore, long laparoscopic instruments with restricted movements allow little tactile feel of the suture. Moreover, the 15-fold magnification requires a corresponding 15-fold reduction in speed and enhanced efficiency in movement for completion of tasks in a reasonable period of time. The surgeon may understand how to instrument-tie, but only a serious dedication to practice will develop one's laparoscopic dexterity.

SUTURING

Port Placement

Careful planning and proper trocar placement simplifies laparoscopic suturing. Ideally, the shaft of the needle holder should be placed parallel to the line of incision being reapproximated. The tip of the needle driver should easily reach the working area with only half (approximately 15 cm) of the instrument's length within the abdominal cavity. The assisting grasping forceps should also comfortably reach the line of incision from the opposite side, and together the two instruments should form a 60- to 90-degree angle from the axis of the laparoscope (Fig. 1). At a minimum, three port sites are necessary. The most "natural" video projection occurs with the camera positioned between and behind the grasper and needle driver (Fig. 2). This ideal positioning is sometimes impractical, and an acceptable alternative position is for the laparoscope to approach the operative field from one side of the two working instruments. The camera should never approach the operative field opposite to the vector of the working instruments, as the video image will be reversed (mirror image), and it becomes virtually impossible to precisely manipulate the instruments. Also, ports inserted too closely together (< 7 cm) will result in a scissoring ("sword-fighting") of instruments and obscured camera visualization.

Because suturing requires both hands, a free hand is not available to stabilize the working port. The port must be secured to prevent dislodgment either by screw threads on the shaft or by suturing the trocar to the skin. After the trocars have been placed, the assistant can simplify laparoscopic suturing by presenting tissue to the tip of the needle at right angles whenever possible. Atraumatic instruments should be used to prevent inadvertent tissue injury. If the surgeon is struggling with a particular angle, an additional port may be inserted. Being mindful of trocar placement at the beginning of the operation is especially important when a considerable amount of suturing is anticipated during a case.

Suture Materials

Selection of suture materials (catgut, silk or synthetics, monofilament or braided, permanent or absorbable) is not different from open surgery. A disadvantage of catgut is that the suture may catch and get caught up in the port as the surgeon advances a throw. This problem is usually avoided with synthetic sutures (2-0 or 3-0 polydiaxanone), which slide easily during knot advancement. Although newer synthetic fibers have greater tensile strength and memory, monofilament strands such as polypropylene also are more likely to loosen. Consequently, synthetics require more throws to prevent an individual knot from unraveling. For intracorporeal knotting, only 8–15 cm of suture is used to ease suturing by minimizing the amount of suture dragged through tissues. During extracorporeal knotting, longer suture lengths (60–90 cm) are required to reach the operative field and return out the same port.

Needle

A variety of needle curvatures are available from which the surgeon may choose: for example, straight, ski tip, or curved (Fig. 3). Straight needles are easiest to position and hold within the jaws of the needle driver but are difficult to drive through tissue in an arc. When using a straight needle the assisting grasper must position adjacent tissue to include an appropriate purchase by the needle (Fig. 4). Ski needles (straight in the shaft, curved near the tip) load like straight needles but with the added advantage of the curve near the tip, allowing it to arc

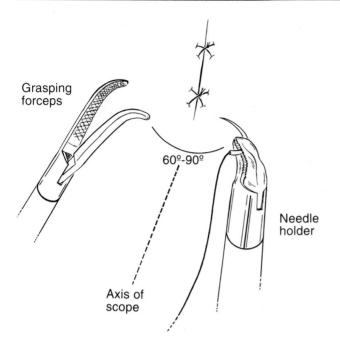

Figure 1. Relationship of the needle driver and assisting grasper to the suture line forms a 60° to 90° angle.

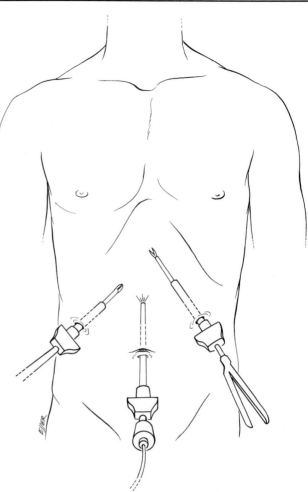

Figure 2. Ideal position of working ports and scope. The laparoscope is centered behind suturing instruments.

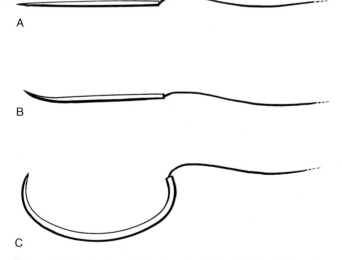

Figure 3. Basic needle types. **A:** straight, **B:** ski tip; **C:** curved.

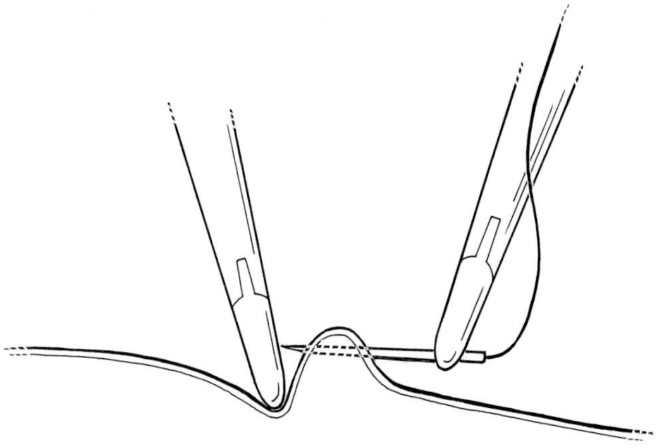

Figure 4. Suturing with straight needle.

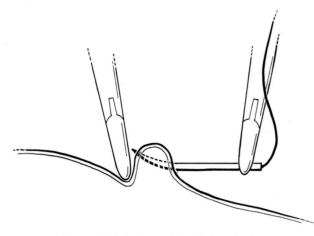

Figure 5. Suturing with ski tip needle.

Figure 6. Suturing with curved needle.

through tissues with minimal damage (Fig. 5). The curved needle is the most difficult to position properly within the jaws of the needle driver. The benefit of the curved needle is that the bite of tissue is the same as the surgeon is accustomed to during open surgery (Fig. 6). By supinating the wrist, the needle cleanly passes through tissues without tearing. Some needles are blackened to limit reflective glare during laparoscopy.

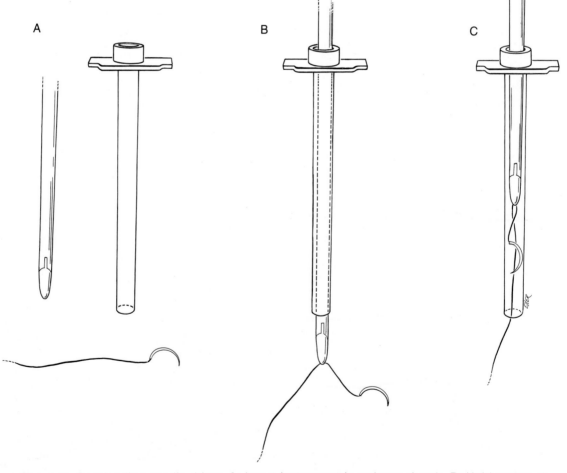

Figure 7. Backloading needle driver. **A:** Insert instrument in reducer sheath. **B:** Hold suture at least 5 mm behind needle base. **C:** Withdraw instrument and needle into sheath.

The suture may be backloaded into a reducing sheath prior to being introduced into the abdominal cavity (Fig. 7). Using a reducer facilitates passage of the needle through the trocar and protects the port's valve from ripping. When passing suture through the port, the suture should be grasped at least 5 mm behind the needle and swage point. Obviously, pop-off needles are avoided in laparoscopic procedures as they may detach prematurely. Large curved needles may not fit through a 10-mm port. If a large needle is necessary, either the port size can be enlarged, or the port temporarily removed and the needle introduced directly through the skin incision. The surgeon should be familiar with the advantages and disadvantages of all three types of needles.

Needle Holder

Needle holders should be capable of grasping the needle firmly, positioning the needle at a 90-degree angle, releasing the needle smoothly, and grasping suture without destroying the braid. Most current needle-holder designs are suboptimal in one or more of these properties. The handles of most needle holders are awkward to manipulate, being oriented at 90 degrees to the shaft. The pistol grip restricts movement and may cause digital cutaneous nerve injury. The ideal needle-driver handles are in-line with the shaft (coaxial) and rotate easily (Fig. 8). The in-line position allows the surgeon to perform precise surgical maneuvers and operate unencumbered. Many surgeons prefer needle holders with two moveable, serrated, diamond-shaped jaws that provide more grasping strength. Spring-oper-

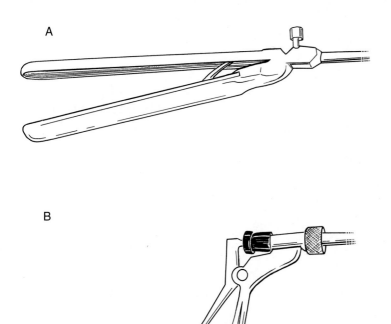

Figure 8. Needle holders with inline shaft **(A)** and pistol grip **(B)**.

ated needle holders are available at predetermined angles (45 degrees right, 45 degrees left, or 90 degrees), but fixed angles limit suturing flexibility and are not suited for intracorporeal knot-tying. Newer prototypes magnetically set the needle within the jaws of the needle driver.

A well-designed complementary assisting forceps facilitates intracorporeal suturing and knot-tying. Assisting instruments with curved tips simplify looping the suture during intracorporeal knot-tying. The smooth tapered end of the forceps prevents the loop from catching on the instrument's shaft. A pointed tip warrants caution, though, as it may puncture the liver or spleen, and sharp jaws may fray suture. Control of the instrument tips under constant camera visualization prevents iatrogenic injury. One popular assisting instrument, the Szabo-Berci ''flamingo'' (Karl Storz, Culver City, CA), is useful.

The surgeon should be relaxed while operating. During laparoscopic suturing the arms will quickly tire if the elbows or shoulders are abducted and neck muscles tensed. Most surgeons will palm their instruments at waist level. For more delicate suturing control, the instruments may be held at shoulder level and manipulated with the fingertips. Operating table height and position is adjusted to keep the surgeon as comfortable as possible. For example, during procedures involving upper abdominal organs it is often convenient for the surgeon to stand or sit between the abducted legs of a patient in the lithotomy position.

Needle Loading

Correct positioning of the needle in the jaws of the needle holder is one of the most difficult actions to perform with monocular vision. When properly per-

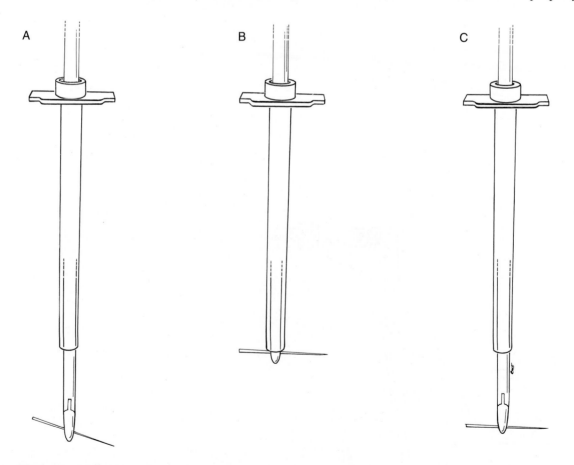

A   B   C

Figure 9. Straight needle is aligned perpendicular to needle driver using reducer sheath. **A:** Oblique needle angle. **B:** Abut sheath. **C:** Reintroduce needle at 90-degree angle.

formed, the surgeon's assisting grasper quickly introduces the needle and hands it off at a perfect 90-degree angle. More often though, the surgeon should be prepared to adjust the angle after grasping it initially. If care and time are not taken to position the needle properly, the needle may slip in the jaws or tear tissue.

Several different methods work well for adjusting the needle within the needle holder's jaws. A straight needle that is held loosely at an oblique angle is easily positioned at 90 degrees by slowly withdrawing the needle driver until the needle abuts the edges of the reducer sheath (Fig. 9). A curved needle's direction may be changed by gently tugging on the suture tail while the needle driver holds the needle loosely and allows it to swivel (Fig. 10). Grasping the suture too firmly

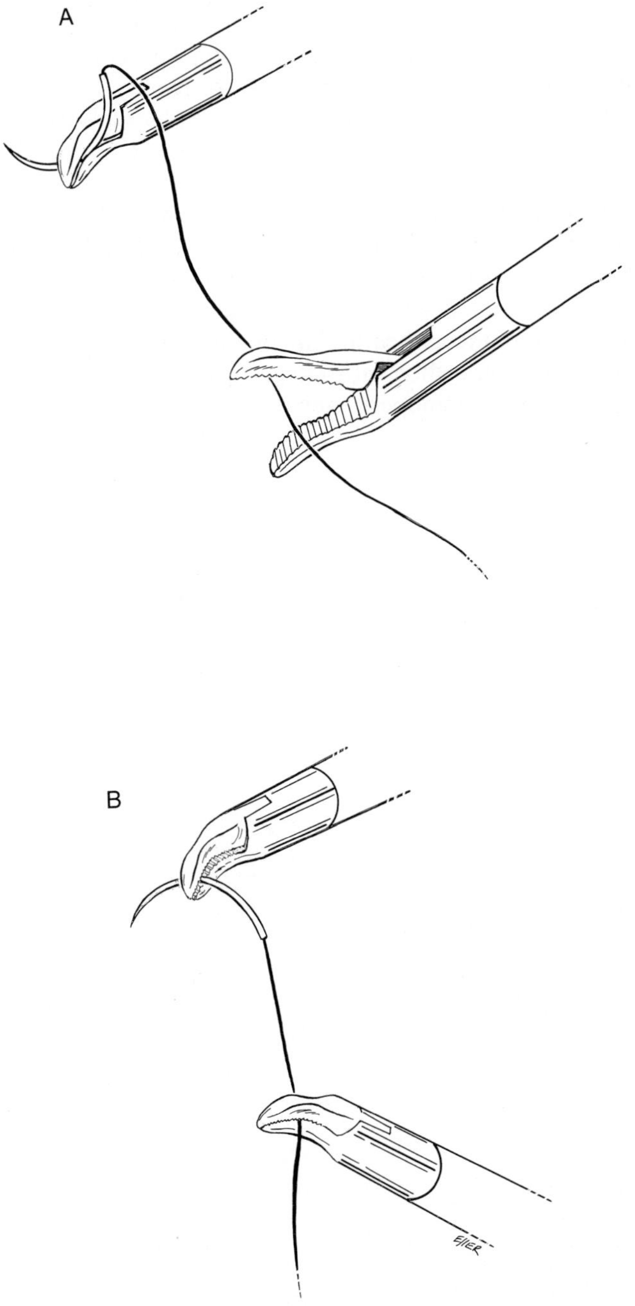

Figure 10. Reversing needle direction. **A:** Assisting grasper pulls suture while needle pivots within needle holder's jaws. **B:** Needle loaded in opposite direction.

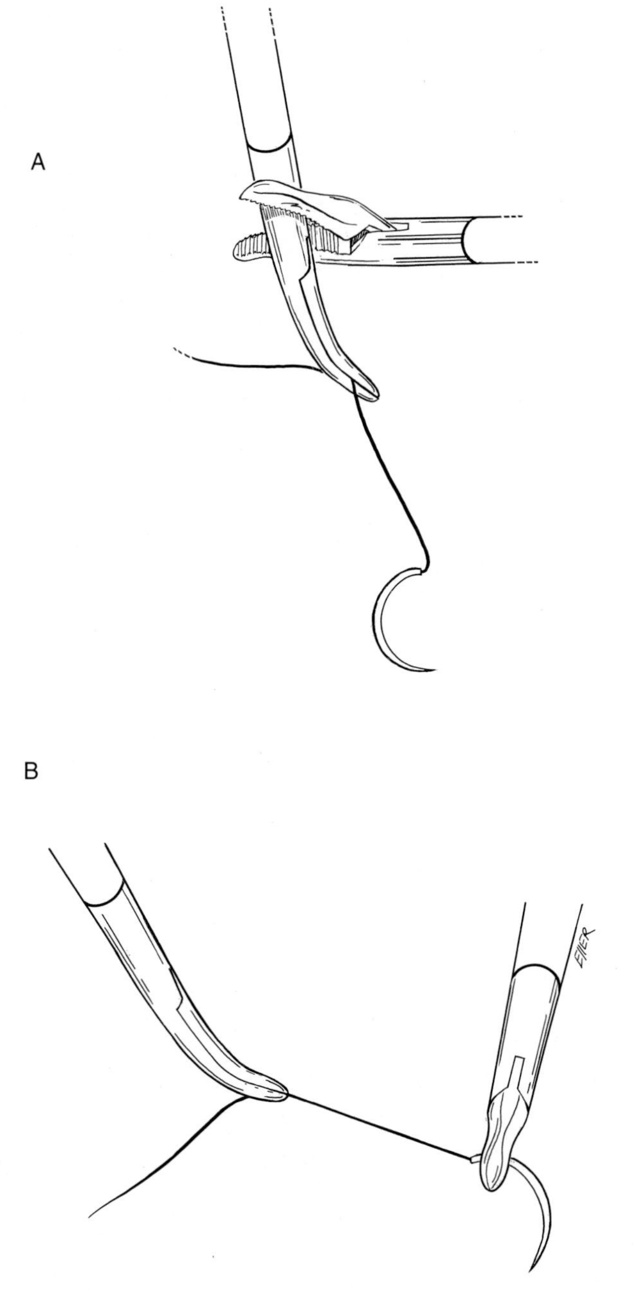

Figure 11. Locating suture in two dimensions. **A:** Grasp assisting instrument. **B:** Slide down shaft with jaws opened to locate the needle.

may fray and weaken it. Rather than passing the needle to the needle holder, many surgeons rest the needle on the surface of the liver or stomach, and pick up the needle at the intended angle without the need to coordinate the movements of both the needle holder and assisting grasper. One way to quickly locate the needle in space is by opening the needle driver jaws around the shaft of the·assisting instrument which holds the suture. The jaws then slide down the shaft and suture to load the needle (Fig. 11). The assisting grasper lightly taps the needle into final position.

EXTRACORPOREAL KNOTTING

Extracorporeal techniques can be used to ligate vessels, approximate tissue, reconstruct organs, and suture anastomoses. Extracorporeal knot-tying refers to knots that are tied outside the abdominal cavity and then advanced into the operative field with a knot-pusher instrument. Preformed knots are readily available today, but with practice an extracorporeal knot can be completed by the surgeon in a timely manner. A square knot or sliding loop knot is the most frequently thrown extracorporeal knot.

Several disadvantages of extracorporeal knot-tying limit its application. For one, a significant amount of suture is drawn through tissue before being brought back out the port for knot-tying. Lengthy suture may saw through tissue as the knot is formed and cinched. Second, an air leak occurs whenever introducing or withdrawing the suture through the reducer sheath. Any ongoing air leak is minimized by an assistant sealing the reducer orifice with a fingertip during extracorporeal knot-tying. The sudden loss of pneumoperitoneum is offset somewhat by

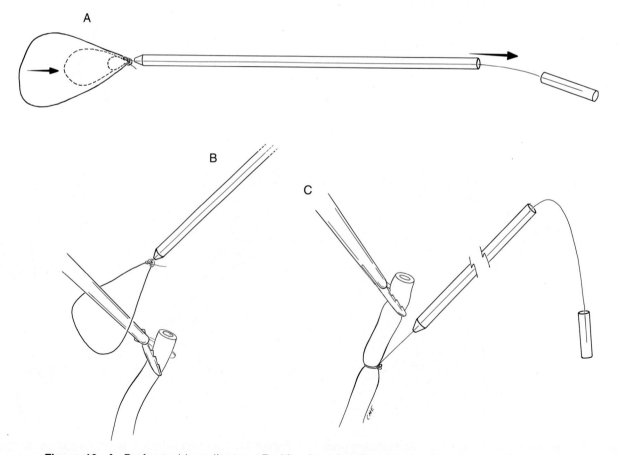

Figure 12. A: Preformed loop ligature. **B:** After lassoing the grasping instruments, the pedicle is isolated. **C:** The loop is slid to proper position and tightened.

the use of newer high-flow insufflators that rapidly replace escaping gas. A third common problem is tearing tissues during advancement of the extracorporeal knot with the knot pusher. To avoid disruption, the knot pusher should be envisioned as an extension of the surgeon's finger. Like standard knot-tying, the knot is pushed down to the tissue without pulling up on the suture. It may be helpful for the assistant to hold the suture with a forceps near the tissue during knot advancement and in this manner dampen suture tension.

Preformed Knots

The Endoloop (Ethicon, Inc., New Brunswich, NJ) and Surgite (U.S. Surgical, Inc., Norwalk, CT) are preformed sliding knots used to tie off a pedicle such as a blood vessel, cystic duct, or appendiceal base. Loop ligatures also close openings in cystic structures and prevent spillage (e.g., from a ruptured gallbladder). The preformed loop is introduced after backloading into a 3-mm reducer sleeve. A grasping forceps is passed through the loop and stabilizes the pedicle of tissue (Fig. 12). The loop is slid off the grasping instrument and encircles the pedicle.

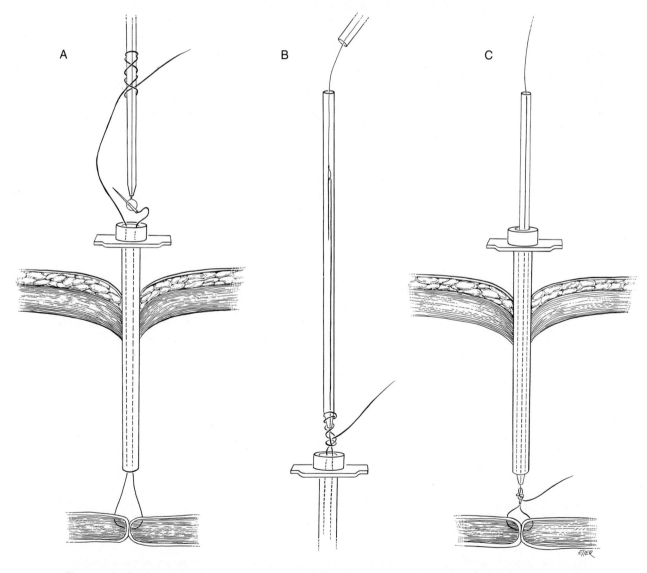

Figure 13. Preformed knot. **A:** After suturing, the needle and suture are withdrawn through the port. The needle is passed through a wire ring at the tip of the push-bar. **B:** The knot is slid off the plastic pusher apparatus. **C:** The knot is advanced through the reducer sheath.

The proximal plastic end of the push-bar apparatus is snapped, the suture pulled, and the loop is closed snugly around the pedicle. Finally, the suture is cut with a hook scissors leaving a ¼-in. tail. The key to proper loop ligature placement is to place the tip of the knot pusher exactly where the knot should finally rest.

The Pre-Tied Endoknot (Ethicon, Inc.) and Suture Applier (Laparomed Corp., Irvine, CA) are preformed knots with an attached needle. After passing the suture through tissue, the needle and suture are withdrawn from the abdominal cavity out of the same port. A pretied knot is slipped off a disposable knot pusher and advanced intracorporeally with the knot-pusher instrument (Fig. 13). The pre-formed knot is a modified Roeder-type knot, which is secure and reliable, particularly when using chromic catgut, which swells after hydration. Other devices, such as the Suture Applier, carry the needle through two preformed loops attached to the tip of the apparatus. The handle is pulled to fasten the knot before the apparatus is withdrawn.

The Roeder Knot

With practice a Roeder knot can be thrown quickly and more economically than commercially packaged pretied knots. The Roeder knot was originally used for tonsillectomies in children, and now has been adapted for application in laparoscopic surgery. A needle that is attached to a long suture (60–90 cm) is used. After suturing the tissue, the two ends of the suture material are withdrawn from the abdomen through the same port. An assistant places a finger over the reducer to minimize air leak and to separate the suture ends. A half-hitch is thrown and the knot may be held in place with the surgeon's thumb and third finger (Fig. 14A). The free end is wrapped three times around both suture strands (Fig. 14B). The tail of the suture then is passed through the last loop (Fig. 14C). A variation of this knot next passes the tail through the loop formed by the initial half-hitch (Fig. 14D). This step is probably advantageous with newer synthetic suture materials, which have a tendency to loosen. Catgut and silk suture swell with hydration

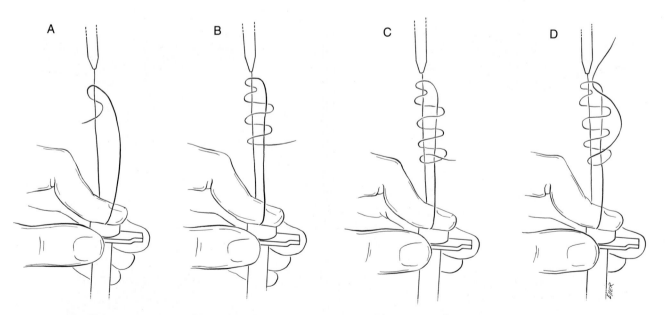

Figure 14. Roeder knot. **A:** After suturing, both ends of suture are withdrawn and separated by an assistant's finger. **B:** A half-hitch is formed. **C:** Three wraps around both suture ends are made before inserting the long end through the last loop. **D:** The long end may also be inserted through the initial loops.

and form a strong knot without adding the extra step. Pulling gently on the tail will complete the knot. A 5-mm tail is cut and the knot is advanced with a knot pusher. Most surgeons find the Roeder knot trustworthy.

Square Knot

An extracorporeal square knot is the most simple yet secure knot to tie through a laparoscope. After suturing the tissue, both ends of suture material are exteriorized through the same port. The square knot is created by separately advancing two half-hitches with a knot pusher (Fig. 15). Care is taken to throw the second half-hitch in the opposite direction to the first half-hitch in order to create a square knot. If both half-hitches are thrown in the same direction, a slip knot is formed rather than a square knot. To advance the square knot, both half-hitches can be converted first into a sliding slip knot configuration by lightly pulling above and below the knot on the same side (right or left side) (Fig. 16). With the slip knot, the throws are easily advanced with the knot pusher to the desired tension. The locking square-knot configuration is again formed by pulling the two limbs of suture in opposite directions. The surgeon can reconvert a square knot to a slip knot and back again intracorporeally until the knot is cinched down. As with open

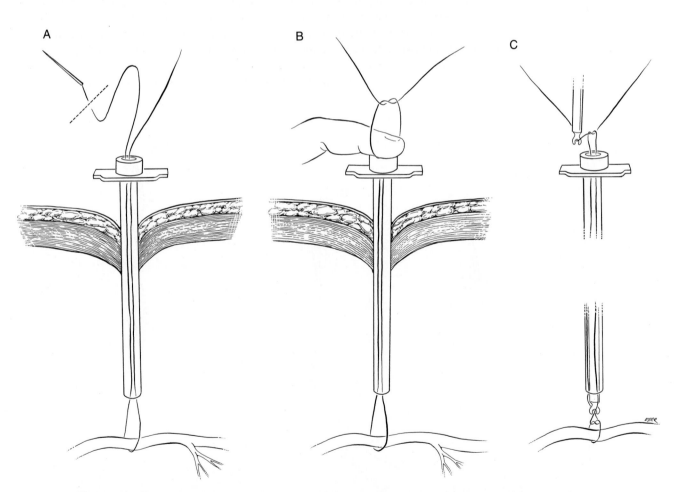

Figure 15. Extracorporeal square knot. **A:** The needle end of the suture is withdrawn through the suture introducer. **B:** An assistant's finger separates suture ends while the surgeon forms a half-hitch. **C:** The first throw is advanced with a knot pusher. A second half-hitch in the same fashion forms a slip knot, while a second half-hitch thrown in the opposite direction creates a square knot.

surgery, additional half-hitches are formed and advanced to complete the knot. Rapid loss of pneumoperitoneum is frequently a problem during the period of extracorporeal knot tying. Methods to simplify and speed knot tying will help reduce air leak. For this reason, some surgeons space all individual half-hitches 1 cm apart sequentially before pushing each down with a knot pusher.

The most significant drawback of extracorporeal square knotting is that a long length of suture must be dragged through tissue, and some tension on the tissue is inevitable; thus, this technique should be used with simple sutures placed in resilient tissue such as the stomach during fundoplication. Many surgeons have found that improper suture selection will hinder knot-tying as well. As previously mentioned, synthetics are particularly well suited for extracorporeal suturing, since the knots will slide down easily and cause minimal tissue tearing.

INTRACORPOREAL KNOTTING

Intracorporeal suturing is favored for delicate structures or after completing a running suture line. There are many instances in which intracorporeal suturing is needed, for example, choledochotomy, reinforcement of stapled bowel anastomoses, and closure of gastric seromyotomies. Working within the abdomen avoids the seesaw effect and tugging on tissues that occurs during extracorporeal knot-tying while carrying long segments of suture material through tissue and out the same port. The major disadvantage to intracorporeal suturing is its degree of difficulty, especially in tight spaces. Under greater than 15-fold magnification, all movements are exaggerated and require the surgeon to be intentional and precise; otherwise, considerable operative time is lost. Intracorporeal knot-tying, while difficult to master, is an important skill in the laparoscopic surgeon's armamentarium.

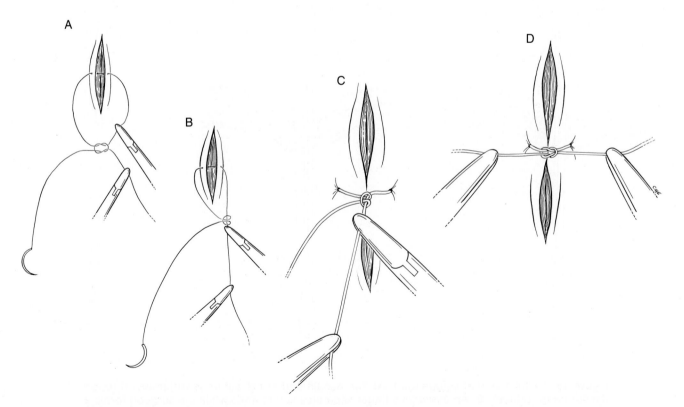

Figure 16. Converting a square knot to a slip knot intracorporeally after introducing an extracorporeally formed knot. **A:** Square knot. **B:** Slip knot. **C:** Advancement of slip knot. **D:** Reconverting to a square knot.

Square Knot

The square knot is achieved in a similar fashion to the "instrument tie" performed during open surgery (Fig. 17). The suture length should be between 8 and 15 cm. Shorter and longer suture will complicate looping suture around the instruments. Needle and sutures are backloaded through a reducer. After incorporating a bite of tissue, the suture tail is best kept short and strategically placed next to the knot where it can be readily grasped.

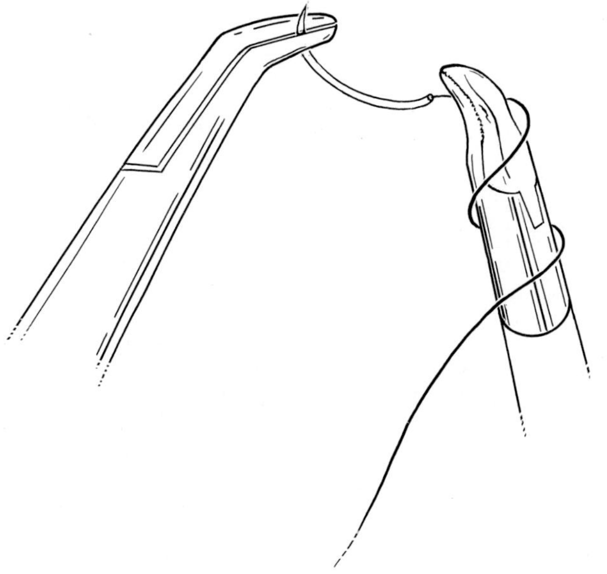

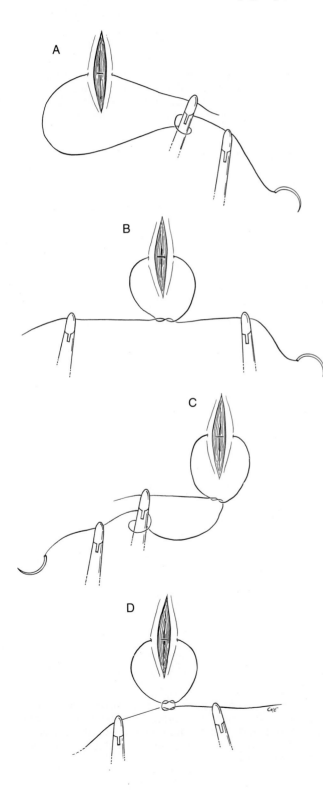

Figure 18. Holding needle at tip simplifies looping suture during intracorporeal suturing by improving the angles between needle driver and assisting grasper.

Figure 17. Intracorporeal instrument tie. **A:** Initial loop. **B:** First half-hitch. **C:** Second loop with loop in opposite direction. **D:** Square knot.

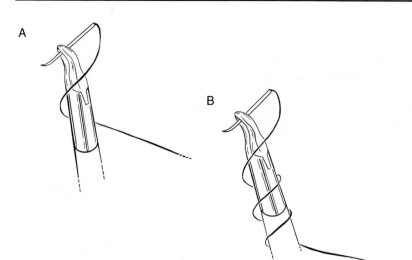

Figure 19. Triple-twist knot. Formed by holding needle within the needle driver jaws and rotating the needle driver 360° four times to create three loops on its shaft.

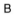

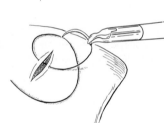

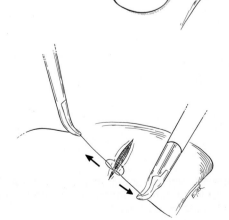

Figure 20. Insert knot. **A:** Suture on tissue surface. **B:** Suture crossed. **C:** An instrument is inserted through the loop and grasps the suture tail. **D:** The first half-hitch is tightened. Subsequent half-hitches are formed in a similar fashion alternating direction of crisscrossing suture.

There are several ways to loop a suture around an instrument. To begin, two loops are fashioned around one instrument similar to a traditional twice-thrown surgeon's knot. Double winding for the first half-knot enables a certain amount of locking. Whether the suture is looped once or twice, the wrapped instrument holds the short end of the suture and carries it through the loop. Grasping the tail as near to the tip as possible will facilitate passing the suture through the loop. The second half-hitch is begun by looping the long end about the instrument, but in this instance the wrap is in the opposite direction to square the knot. As before, the instrument wrapped with suture grasps the short end of the suture and pulls it through the loop. Alternating the direction of further loops ensures that the knots will be squared.

When attempted laparoscopically, the loops are frequently difficult to throw because of the angle that the instruments enter the abdomen. Holding the tip of the curved needle perpendicular to the needle driver's shaft will improve the angle and facilitate loop placements (Fig. 18). Inserting additional trocars or placing the camera in a different port should also be tried. Angled scopes and three-dimensional technology may improve visualization and orientation. It should be remembered that altering the suture length, using curved assisting-grasper instruments, and effectively planning trocar placement is sometimes all that is necessary to make intracorporeal instrument tying manageable.

An alternative method to forming loops is the triple-twist knot. With the needle held at its tip, the needle holder is rotated 360 degrees four times as the suture wraps around the instrument's shaft (Fig. 19). The needle is then dropped. Next, the needle holder grasps the tail of the suture and passes it through the loops. The throw is completed in the usual fashion by pulling the ends of the suture apart to form a surgeon's knot. Additional ties are thrown for greater knot security.

Sometimes it is difficult to maneuver instruments within a given port angle. In this situation, the suture may be positioned to form a loop upon itself while lying on adjacent tissue (Fig. 20). A grasping instrument then picks up the suture

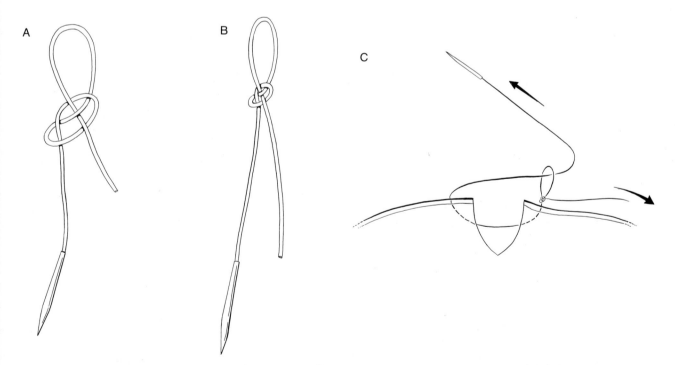

Figure 21. The "Dundee" knot may be used to start a running suture line. **A:** External component of knot. **B:** Adjusting loop size by pulling on tail. **C:** Needle is passed through loop. (From Cuschieri A. Tissue approximation. *Probl Gen Surg (Laparoscopic Surgery)* 1991;8:366–377, with permission.)

where it crosses itself or the loop may remain lying on the tissue surface. A second instrument is inserted through the loop and grasps the short tail of the suture to complete the throw. The second half-hitch is similarly formed but in the opposite direction. This technique is particularly easy with the depth perception gained from three-dimensional laparoscopes.

Dundee Knot

An externally formed slip knot at the end of a suture can be used to initiate a running suture line without an intracorporeal knot. By crossing over and then under itself, a double loop is formed resembling a figure-of-eight (Fig. 21). The

A
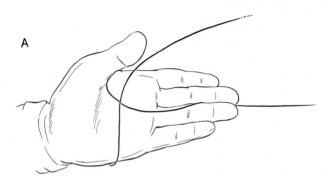

B
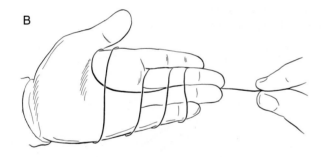

C
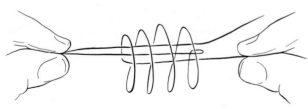

D
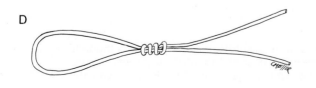

Figure 22. Quick slip knot. Suture is wrapped around the hand four times and slipped over a loop of suture to form a slip knot.

suture is passed in and out through both loops. Leaving a 1.5-cm tail, the knot is introduced through a reducer to the operative field. After running the first stitch, the needle and suture are passed through the loop of the slip knot. The suture is pulled into the loop and impinges on the tissue. The Dundee knot is tightened by pulling the tail in the opposite direction to the suture, thereby jamming the knot. The suture line can then be completed in the standard fashion.

Quick-Slip Knot

Rather than a Dundee slip knot, a slip knot may be formed quickly about the surgeon's hand. With the short end of the suture held between the middle and ring finger, the suture is wrapped once around the palm and three times around the fingers (Fig. 22). The short end is then stabilized by the other hand, and the middle and ring finger carry the long end of the suture as a loop through the wraps. The wraps are tightened around the loop to finish the knot. The loop slides easily to the desired size.

There are several advantages to using a Dundee or Quick-Slip knot. For a running suture, the first knot is completed by simply inserting the needle through the noose. For interrupted suturing, a second tie is made to the short end of the suture. A preformed knot at the tail of the suture is unlikely to slip inadvertently through the tissue during suture manipulation. Often considerable operative time is saved with continuous sutures and the needle-through-the-noose technique.

Aberdeen Knot

The Aberdeen knot may be used to complete a running suture line (Fig. 23). An initial loop is brought beneath the previous throw. A second loop is passed through the initial loop and tightened. The tail of the suture is inserted through the second loop to clinch the knot. The assistant should keep tension on the suture and prevent gaps in the suture line. This may require rubber-shod atraumatic instruments to avoid damage to the suture.

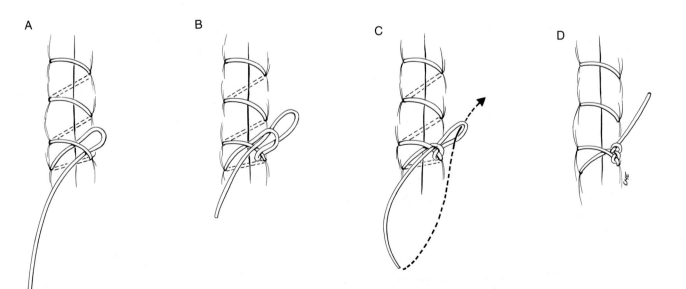

Figure 23. The Aberdeen knot is used to finish a running suture line. **A:** Initial loop. **B:** Second loop. **C:** Tightened loop. **D:** Completed knot.

ALTERNATIVES TO SUTURING

Other manufactured devices are available for the surgeon to ligate vessels and approximate tissue. Some techniques have wide applications, while others are still investigational. Linear staplers divide bowel and can almost instantaneously perform an anastomosis. Vascular staplers divide vessels, and articulating fascial staplers may secure mesh to the abdominal wall during hernia repairs.

Clip appliers ligate small blood vessels and ductal structures and are especially popular when dividing the cystic artery and cystic duct during cholecystecomy. Various clip sizes accommodate pedicle width. Absorbable clips are available for small vessels. Titanium clips are used for medium-size vessels. Fastening the clip at a 90-degree angle helps prevent slippage and delayed bleeding. Structures such as arteries are commonly doubly clipped for added insurance. Catheters within ducts may likewise be secured with temporary clips. While individual clips can be positioned manually, preloaded clip appliers are less likely to shear tissue. The disadvantages of metal clips and staples are their high cost and thermal damage conducted to adjacent tissue during the use of monopolar electrocautery. Clip appliers and stapling instruments are, moreover, relatively inflexible and may not articulate to the necessary angle for application.

The Lapra-Ty (Ethicon Inc., NJ) is a system of synthetic clips that are affixed to suture and form a temporary "knot" to resist slippage through tissue (Fig. 24). They are analogous to lead sinkers on a fishing line. These work well for temporary knots (absorbed after 10 days) or for finishing an intracorporeal square knot when the suture length is inadequate for traditional knots. In addition, a loose throw may be salvaged and tightened by placing a Lapra-Ty around both suture strands beneath the knot.

Well-established principles of surgical technique do not change with the advent of new technology. A properly formed knot should approximate equal depths of tissue edges without undue tension. A suture line that is too tight causes necrosis, while incorporating different amounts of tissue causes overlap of the two sides. Wound healing goals may be more easily achieved in the future with further technological advances. For example, anastomotic welding with laser, bipolar cautery technology, ultrasonic coagulation and fibrin glue sealants may become common practice in laparoscopy. In the meantime, surgeons must develop their skills at suturing and knot-tying in order to successfully perform complex and varied laparoscopic operations. *Practice makes perfect.*

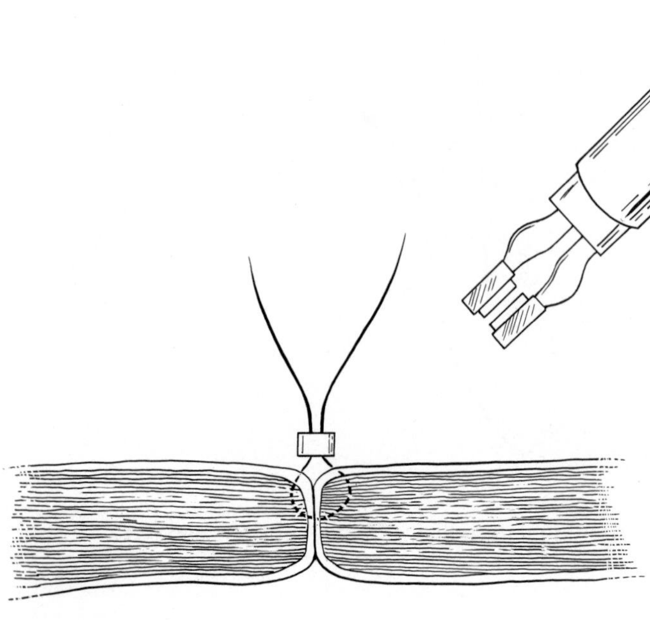

Figure 24. Lapra-Ty clipped to suture.

ACKNOWLEDGMENTS

We thank The Washington University Institute for Minimally Invasive Surgery and Ethicon Endosurgery for their support, and Ms. Judy A. Schmidt for secretarial assistance.

EXERCISES

Suturing and knot-tying is demanding for even the most experienced laparoscopic surgeon and requires extensive training. In order to avoid the humiliation of video ineptitude while trying to grasp the needle, suture, and tie a knot as the operating room nurse shudders, the clock ticks, and the patient suffers, we strongly advise practicing suturing techniques outside the operating room. The following suggested exercises are listed in order from simplest to most difficult. Progressing in an orderly fashion will help alleviate some of the frustration associated with learning a large number of new laparoscopic skills at one sitting. Preferably a simulation device should be used with a video camera and monitor to recreate actual working conditions. In the near future, computerized "virtual reality" simulators may allow the performance of complete operations in an inanimate setting. With practice the surgeon will become facile and confident in his or her ability. Similar drills may be used by program directors to assess resident performance, and by hospital credentialing committees to determine a surgeon's proficiency with advanced laparoscopic techniques.

PRACTICE EXERCISES

1. Clip applier
2. Loop ligature
3. Simple suture (straight, ski tip, curved needles)
4. Pretied knot
5. Extracorporeal Roeder knot
6. Intracorporeal square knot (instrument tie, triple-twist knot)
7. Dundee jamming knot
8. Aberdeen knot
9. End-to-side and side-to-side anastomoses (using foam organs or tissue specimens)

RECOMMENDED READING

1. Meilahn JE. The need for improving laparoscopic suturing and knot-tying. *J Laparoendosc Surg* 1992;2:267.
2. Kennedy JS. A technique for extracorporeal suturing. *J Laparoendosc Surg* 1992;2:269–272.
3. Pietrafitta JJ. A technique of laparoscopic knot tying. *J Laparoendosc Surg* 1992;2:273–275.
4. Soper NJ, Hunter JG. Suturing and knot tying in laparoscopy. *Surg Clin North Am* 1992;72: 1139–1152.
5. McDougall EM, Soper NJ. Laparoscopic suturing and knot tying. In: Soper NJ, Odem RR, Clayman RV, McDougall EM, eds. *Essentials of laparoscopy.* St. Louis: Quality Medical Publishing; 1994: 148–183.
6. Ko S, Airan MC. Therapeutic laparoscopic suturing techniques. *Surg Endosc* 1992;6:41.
7. Laws HL. Credentialling residents for laparoscopic surgery: a matter of opinion. *Curr Surg* 1991; 48:684–686.
8. Hasson HM. Suture loop techniques to facilitate microsurgical and laparoscopic procedures. *J Reprod Med* 1987;32:765–767.

SECTION II

EXPLORATORY LAPAROSCOPY

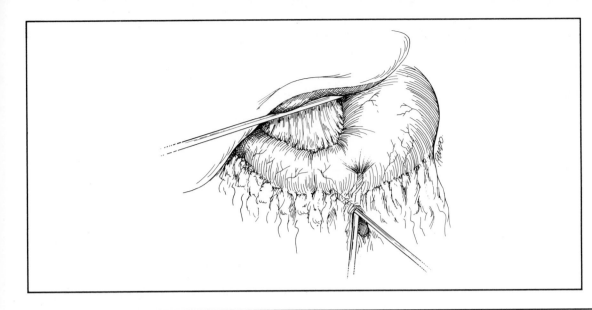

10

Diagnostic Exploratory Laparoscopy

Frederick L. Greene and E. Dwayne Lett
Department of Surgery
University of South Carolina
School of Medicine
Columbia, South Carolina 29203

Operative Laparoscopy and Thoracoscopy, edited by
B. V. MacFadyen, Jr. and
J. L. Ponsky. Lippincott-Raven
Publishers, Philadelphia © 1996.

KEY WORDS

Abdominal lymphoma   Electrocautery

Biopsy   Pneumoperitoneum

Celiotomy

Diagnostic laparoscopy has proved to be an excellent tool for the diagnosis, staging, and therapeutic management of certain disease processes. When used in conjunction with more conventional diagnostic studies such as ultrasound, computed tomography, and magnetic resonance imaging, information obtained can be quite specific and helpful. Preoperative planning as well as selection of either curative or palliative procedures is facilitated through a laparoscopic evaluation. Probably the primary importance for abdominal laparoscopy is to help the surgeon decide whether an open operation is appropriate for the patient.

● ANATOMY

The laparoscopic approach to the patient requires the same basic knowledge of anatomy as possessed by the surgeon who performs open celiotomy. The major difference, of course, is that laparoscopic retraction of certain areas of the abdominal cavity is much more difficult than the "hands-on" approach used in open exploration.

The main anatomic areas in the *greater omental bursa* include the colonic gutters and the region of the diaphragm on both the right and left upper quadrants. Anatomically, the spleen may be difficult to evaluate but can be mobilized more effectively using the right-side-down lateral position on the operating table as well as placing the patient in reverse Trendelenburg position. Since the small bowel is tethered to the retroperitoneum at the base of the mesentery, gravity is important in mobilizing these areas for better exploration of the pelvis as well as the left and right paracolonic gutters. Anatomically, the area of the portal hepatis and the gastrohepatic omentum are easy to approach if 30- or 45-degree laparoscopes are used. When the 0-degree laparoscope is used, the liver must be retracted effectively in order to view the subhepatic space more readily.

The most difficult area to gain anatomic perspective during laparoscopy is the retroperitoneum. Knowledge of the *lesser omental bursa,* which extends from the porta hepatis to the tail of the pancreas, will ensure a complete investigation once the gastrohepatic omentum or gastrocolic omentum is entered. As in open exploration, the greater omentum may be teased off the transverse colon with the knowledge that the blood supply of the greater omentum comes from the gastroepiploic vasculature. Any laparoscopic exploration is more difficult in the obese patient, since the fat will obscure the vessels at the base of the mesentery. Ideally, the constant location of the inferior mesenteric vein will achieve a more definitive and easier dissection of the paraaortic area, especially when lymph node biopsy is performed. Routine identification of the pelvic anatomy in the female may be difficult because of adhesions to the fallopian tubes or ovaries. The most important anatomic relationships of the pelvis include identification of the ureter, as both the right and left ureters cross their respectively common iliac arteries at the bifurcations. Full identification of the ureters is important before any definitive pelvic node dissection or colonic resection.

▶ PREOPERATIVE PLANNING

Preoperative preparation is important and must include laboratory evaluation with special attention to coagulation factors. In addition, radiographic examination of the chest and electrocardiography, if indicated, are necessary. As with any open procedure, all material risks and potential benefits must be explained to the patient. Also, the patient must be informed of the possibility that laparoscopy may be terminated and the procedure converted to an open celiotomy. Having preoperative informed consent is most important if the procedure is planned under general anesthesia.

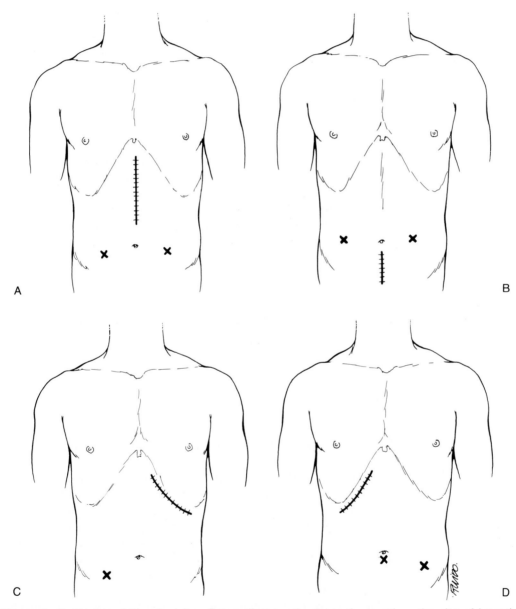

Figure 1. A: Upper midline incision. Depending on the type of operation, the site of insertion can be in either the left of the right lower quadrant (umbilicus-iliac crest line, lateral third). **B:** Left subcostal incision. The approach of choice is in the right lower quadrant (umbilicus-iliac crest line, lateral third). **C:** Lower midline incision. Depending on the nature of the previous operation, a left or right approach at the level of the umbilicus along the linea semilunaris (the lateral edge of the rectus muscle) is used. **D:** Right subcostal incision. The site of insertion is either in the midline below the umbilicus or in the left lower quadrant (umbilicus-iliac crest line, lateral third).

A thorough history must be obtained preoperatively. The surgeon must elicit information regarding a patient's cardiopulmonary status. Dysrhythmias may be initiated or exacerbated with the production of pneumoperitoneum. Patients with borderline pulmonary function are at increased risk, as carbon dioxide pneumoperitoneum tends to increase pulmonary dead space. It is recommended that the patient undergo cardiac monitoring throughout the entire procedure. Patients who are not candidates for open procedures are generally considered poor risk for closed procedures as well. Of particular importance is the history of prior operations. The surgeon should be aware of the extent of all previous intraabdominal procedures so that he or she may avoid or manage associated adhesions during trocar placement (Fig. 1). A history of chronic liver disease or coagulopathy must be obtained.

The physical examination should be thorough. Cardiopulmonary evaluation must be performed to evaluate any abnormalities. The abdomen must be inspected for the presence of previous surgical scars. Prelaparoscopic ultrasound may be used to map the intraabdominal adhesions in order to facilitate introduction of pneumoperitoneum and subsequent trocar placement. The surgeon should inspect the abdomen for evidence of portal hypertension, including a *caput medusa* and should palpate the abdomen for any evidence of organomegaly. If either hepatic or splenic enlargement is identified, the extent of the intraabdominal viscera should be marked on the anterior abdominal wall to prevent injury at trocar placement. Finally, a history of hiatal hernia should be obtained, as the patient with a large hiatal hernia sac that distends with the introduction of pneumoperitoneum is at greater risk for cardiorespiratory embarrassment.

Most of the contraindications to laparoscopy are relative, but there are at least two absolutes. The first is the patient with an obvious acute surgical abdomen with indications for open celiotomy. The second is the patient with abdominal wall sepsis who is at great risk for contamination of the peritoneal cavity with laparoscopy. Generalized illnesses that preclude an operative procedure or general anesthesia may be absolute or relative contraindications. Additional relative contraindications include obstruction or ileus with significant bowel distention. Obesity can be an eliminating factor due to inadequate instrument length. The full effects of pneumoperitoneum on the pregnant patient and her fetus have yet to be delineated. Finally, patients with penetrating abdominal injury and possible diaphragmatic injury are at risk for intraoperative tension pneumothorax. Tube thoracostomy before abdominal insufflation may be indicated to prevent this complication.

▼ INTRAOPERATIVE MANAGEMENT/SURGICAL TECHNIQUE

The patient is prepared for laparoscopy in a fashion similar to that for traditional celiotomy. Sedation and amnestics are given intravenously. If the procedure is to be performed under a general anesthetic, a muscle relaxant must be given as well. Although some have advocated local or regional anesthetic techniques for diagnostic laparoscopy, we prefer general anesthesia, which allows for better patient compliance and an opportunity for a more complete endoscopic examination. Preoperative antibiotics are usually indicated, and we prefer a second-generation cephalosporin.

The minimum instrumentation for diagnostic laparoscopy includes a 10-mm diameter 0- or 30-degree telescope, one or two 5-mm diameter grasping devices, a coagulation device, and a suction irrigating device. Other useful instruments include the 5-mm 30-degree laparoscope and core needle biopsy device. The patient should have the stomach and bladder evacuated with a nasogastric tube and Foley catheter. The abdomen and lower chest should be prepped and draped as for an open celiotomy. Trocar placement depends on the patient's body habitus, surgeon preference, or preoperative diagnostic imaging studies. The surgeon is usually standing at the patient's left and the first assistant on the patient's right. The patient's initial position is supine with variations depending on intraoperative needs.

The greatest number of patients undergoing diagnostic laparoscopy are those with known or suspected malignancy. Laparoscopy can provide information about disease stage, metastases, and resectability. Laparoscopy can provide information that relates to a variety of other benign disease processes as well. Although it is possible to perform laparoscopy in the emergency room, outpatient clinic, or some other location rather than the operating room, we prefer laparoscopic evaluation in the controlled environment of the operating suite. If diagnostic laparoscopy is performed using local anesthesia, one should maintain the pneumoperitoneum in the range of 7 to 10 mmHg pressure, have a variety of scopes available, and perform most of the examination with the patient in the supine position. Conversion to general anesthesia and change of venue to the operating room may be indicated if laparoscopic findings and patient compliance dictate. As indicated, we perform diagnostic laparoscopy in the operating suite under general anesthesia using carbon dioxide pressures in the 12- to 14-mmHg range. A muscle relaxant may be given and the patient's position may be varied.

Before placing trocars, a general rule for intraabdominal visualization is to plan triangulation of ports with at least three trocars placed into the peritoneal cavity (Fig. 2). We routinely place our initial trocar for the laparoscopic camera in the infraumbilical position with secondary and tertiary trocar placement based

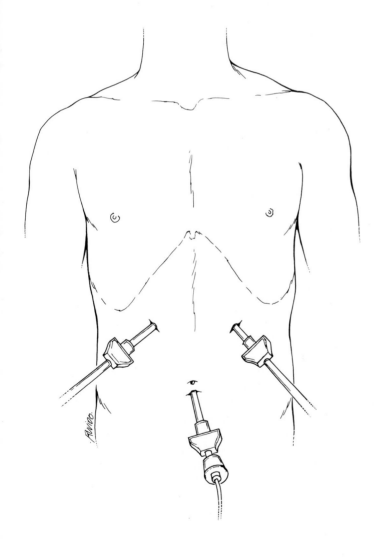

Figure 2. Sites of insertion of the main and accessory trocars for infragastric examination of the pancreas. The main trocar is introduced through a sub-umbilical stab incision, the first accessory trocar along the left linea semilunaris above the umbilicus and the second accessory trocar through the equivalent site on the right side.

on preoperative studies as well as initial abdominal inspection. The midline infra-umbilical position is the usual position for our primary trocar placement. A 10-mm port is usually placed in this position after establishment of an adequate pneumoperitoneum. Although we prefer an open technique, using a Hasson cannula, one may insufflate the abdomen using the Veress needle technique. If this technique is to be used, the skin of the abdomen on either side of the midline is grasped and lifted upward, the skin incision is made, and the Veress needle is advanced until the fascia and the parietal peritoneum have been pierced. Peritoneal entrance should be ensured by injecting saline. Low-flow CO_2 insufflation is begun to ensure proper intraperitoneal gas introduction. The abdomen is palpated to ensure that proper pneumoperitoneum is being obtained prior to the introduction of a 10-mm trocar after removal of the Veress needle. When using the open method to establish pneumoperitoneum, the Hasson cannula is placed through the linea alba in the infraumbilical position. Either a vertical or a transverse incision is made just inferior to the umbilicus and dissected to the level of the fascia. The fascia is then incised and a suture is placed on either side of the fascia to help with traction and to secure the Hasson cannula if desired. The parietal peritoneum is incised and digital exploration through the incision is performed. The Hasson cannula is placed in the incision and secured into position. Carbon dioxide is then insufflated with a low flow rate initially and then increased as pneumoperitoneum is affirmed. The telescope is then introduced through the Hasson cannula. If the patient has evidence of hepatobiliary disease and portal hypertension with abdominal wall venous distention, the Veress needle can be placed in the left upper quadrant, lateral to the rectus muscle, using the previously described techniques of insufflation of the abdominal cavity. The alternatively placed open technique may also be advisable in certain situations. If the patient has ascites, the laparoscopic camera may be placed through the infraumbilical port. Aspiration of the ascites is not performed until placement of the second trocar. Pneumoperitoneum is initiated prior to aspiration, but instillation of gas must be achieved above the area of abdominal fluid to avoid the nuisance of intraabdominal bubbling.

For the patient with presumed hepatobiliary disease, the 10-mm diameter 0-degree laparoscope is placed through the umbilical port. A 5-mm diameter port is placed in the left upper quadrant in the midclavicular line for grasping and lifting. Other accessory trocars may be placed in the subxiphoid and right upper quadrant positions. The laparoscope is used to evaluate the appearance of the liver and to identify the presence and character of any ascites that may be present. If any liver mass is noted to be present, its size, location, and fixation to surrounding structures can be assessed. Arteriovenous malformations must be correctly interpreted prior to a decision to biopsy any hepatic mass. If ascites is present, aspiration of fluid through accessory trocar sites should be performed to facilitate proper culture and cytologic investigation. If an exudate, the ascitic fluid may indicate tuberculosis or brucellosis. A transudate may indicate either nephrotic syndrome, congestive heart failure, or even Meigs syndrome. Chylous ascites has a characteristic milky appearance and may be confirmed by lymphocyte count or triglyceride levels. The ascites associated with peritoneal mesothelioma has a characteristic thickness similar to white syrup.

Hepatic metastases may be palpated using a 5-mm diameter grasping forceps to determine whether these lesions are solid or cystic. The liver may be lifted to view the undersurface. This is especially important in assessing the left lateral lobe. The gastrohepatic and gastrocolic ligaments may be divided to further visualize the underside of the liver or the lesser curvature node-bearing regions of the stomach, esophagus, and pancreas. Unusual anatomic variance may be noted as well. Finally, biopsies of solid lesions may be obtained with laparoscopic assistance. A core biopsy needle may be placed through a separate stab wound in the anterior abdominal wall, allowing the needle to be directed into the mass to facilitate a biopsy (Fig. 3). Hemostasis must be confirmed using electrocautery devices to control bleeding from the biopsy site. To better evaluate the dome of the liver and the subdiaphragmatic space on the right, the patient is placed in steep reverse Trendelenburg position, and a 30-degree laparoscope may be placed. The patient may also be turned to the right lateral position to view the left subdiaphragmatic space, the spleen, and the greater curvature of the stomach.

Retroperitoneal masses may be evaluated by division of the gastrohepatic (Fig. 4) and gastrocolic attachments (Fig. 5). This will facilitate the approach to the periaortic nodal area if biopsy of this region is indicated. To achieve complete inspection of the pelvis, the laparoscope should be introduced at the umbilical position, and the patient should be placed in steep Trendelenburg position to allow the bowel to fall from the pelvis (Fig. 6). A 5-mm suprapubic trocar should be placed. The bladder should be at minimal risk, since it was decompressed preoperatively by Foley catheter placement. Depending on suspected pathology, tertiary trocars may be placed in the right or left iliac fossae lateral to the rectus muscle. From this position, iliac node biopsies can be performed. This approach is appropriate for the evaluation of patients with chronic pain. In patients with a history of pelvic inflammatory disease, this position allows excellent visualization of the pelvic structures and facilitates evaluation of adhesions secondary to inflammation or endometriosis. If there is evidence of an infectious process, lavage to obtain cultures may be performed. The liver may be evaluated for evidence of Fitz-Hugh and Curtis syndrome in this same patient with a history of previous right upper quadrant pain. In the patient with a history of previous abdominal operations,

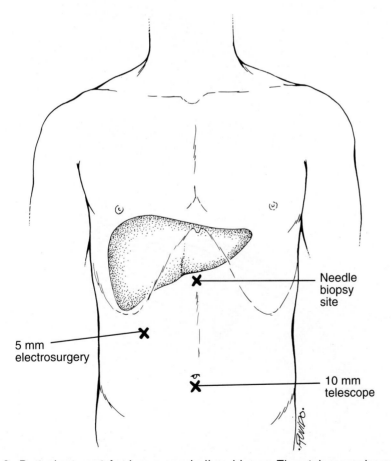

Needle biopsy site

5 mm electrosurgery

10 mm telescope

Figure 3. Port placement for laparoscopic liver biopsy. The stab wound necessary for the core biopsy may be made anywhere beneath the costal margin that allows the best access to the liver lesion requiring biopsy. In a diffusely cirrhotic liver, biopsy of the lateral segment of the left lobe can be made through a stab wound, high in the midline.

adhesions may be a cause of chronic pain. Preoperative ultrasound may identify these adhesions to make entry into the abdominal cavity less risky.

Once the laparoscope and accessory trocars are in position, adhesions may be divided using sharp dissection or cautery. The patient with chronic abdominal pain must be evaluated for identification of occult Crohn's disease or Meckel's diverticulum. This will involve mobilization of small bowel using nontraumatic grasping forceps to allow for complete intestinal inspection. To assess more acute pain syndromes, potentially secondary to appendicitis or pelvic inflammatory disease, the laparoscopic camera is placed in the infraumbilical position. A secondary trocar is again placed in the suprapubic position and a 10- to 12-mm port is placed

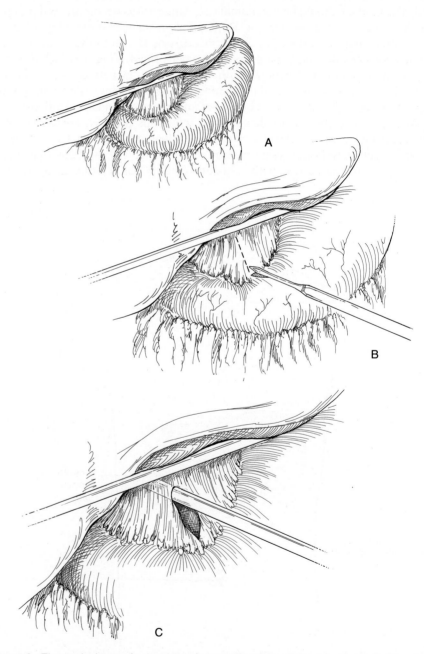

Figure 4. The technique of supragastric examination of the pancreas. **A:** The liver is elevated by the first palpating probe to expose the lesser omentum and lesser curvature of the stomach. **B:** Through a second accessory cannula the laparoscopic scissors are used to a hole in an avascular area of the omentum. **C:** The hole is enlarged by the second palpating probe and the telescope is then inserted into the lesser sac.

in the left lower quadrant. An additional 5-mm trocar may be placed in the right pararectus position as needed. Similar trocar placement is performed if a right colonic lesion is suspected. Trocars are placed in a mirror-image fashion if a left lower quadrant or left colonic lesions is suspected. If the surgeon is entertaining a suspicion of ischemic bowel in a patient with severe atherosclerotic cardiovascular disease, the laparoscope may be used in conjunction with colonoscopy to assist in the diagnosis. Intraoperative Doppler may be used to assess blood flow to the bowel, and techniques using intraoperative fluorescein have been recommended. For patients who will not tolerate unnecessary celiotomy, diagnostic laparoscopy may be the procedure of choice to evaluate an acute abdominal process. Laparoscopy can be useful for the identification of acute acalculous cholecystitis in the intensive care unit patient with respiratory failure or sepsis of unknown etiology. In addition, patients undergoing bone marrow transplantation will many times present with acute abdominal findings due to immunosuppressive conditions that cause unusual gastrointestinal manifestations. These patients will need to be treated medically and will not benefit by open celiotomy.

In the patient with blunt abdominal trauma, laparoscopy may give more direct information than diagnostic peritoneal lavage. Computed tomography provides better evaluation of the retroperitoneum than laparoscopy, but may be deficient in localizing the source of abdominal blood. Laparoscopy should be used as an adjunct along with imaging studies to decrease the number of negative celiotomies. We, again, advocate that this laparoscopic evaluation be performed in the operating room under controlled conditions of patient monitoring and airway control.

For trauma evaluations, a 10-mm diameter camera is placed in the infraumbilical position. Accessory trocars are placed in the right and left lower quadrant areas. The small bowel is completely inspected and evaluated for hematoma or perforation. The abdominal cavity is evaluated for enteric fluid, evidence of hemorrhage, and retroperitoneal hematoma. The liver and spleen are examined thoroughly, and the diaphragm is thoroughly inspected. The 30-degree laparoscope may be used to better evaluate the posterior portion of the diaphragm. Gastric or small bowel injuries may be repaired using the laparoscope if the surgeon is familiar

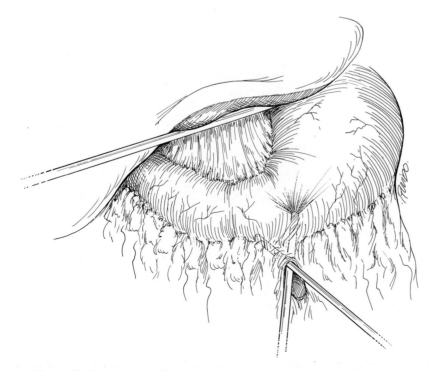

Figure 5. Technique of infragastric approach to retroperitoneum.

with suturing techniques. If formal celiotomy is indicated, since the patient is already under general anesthesia, conversion to an open abdominal procedure is easily accomplished.

Penetrating trauma, especially stab wounds, can be evaluated with the laparoscope. The camera is introduced through the umbilical site and the abdomen evaluated for peritoneal breech. Small wounds may be repaired laparoscopically or the patient may be formally explored as indicated. If the surgeon finds no evidence of intraabdominal injury, the patient should be observed for 12 to 24 hours to assess for missed injury. Patients with blunt abdominal trauma are at risk for occult injury of the diaphragm and may develop tension pneumothorax when pneumoperitoneum is introduced. The chest, therefore, should be prepped and the surgeon must be prepared to perform rapid thoracostomy tube placement as indicated. Patients with penetrating injury are at risk for gas embolization in the face of major venous or hepatic injury. The surgeons must keep this in mind if there

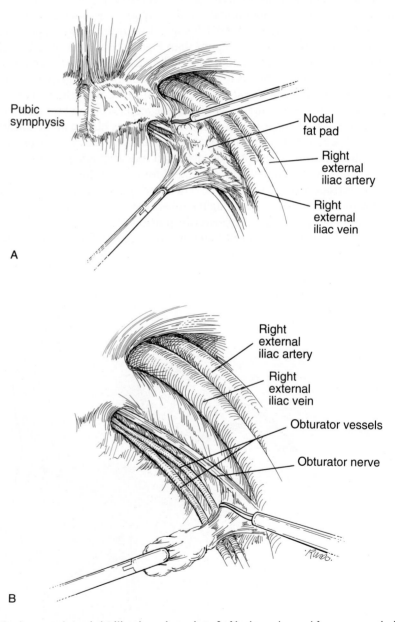

Figure 6. Approach to right iliac lymph nodes. **A:** Nodes released from around obturator vein and nerve. **B:** Node packet divided at apex.

is evidence of cardiac decompensation or sudden fall in end-tidal CO_2 early in the procedure.

Other potential uses of diagnostic laparoscopy for abdominal disease include "second-look" evaluation in patients with previously treated intraabdominal malignancy. Those patients with a history of colonic cancer and rising levels of carcinoembryonic antigen or patients with known ovarian cancer undergoing adjuvant therapy may be good candidates for "second-look" laparoscopic evaluation.

Laparoscopy has been especially helpful in the evaluation and staging of patients with Hodgkin's lymphoma. Preoperative and intraoperative monitoring are similar, as described in other scenarios. We generally employ a three- to four-trocar technique using the infraumbilical approach for placement of a 10-mm diameter 0-degree laparoscopic camera. Right and left upper quadrant 5-mm trocars are utilized for routine evaluation of liver, spleen, and retrogastric nodal areas. While we do not recommend or perform splenic biopsy or splenectomy in the evaluation of patients with Hodgkin's disease, the spleen is fully inspected by turning the operating table into a right-side-down position and employing steep reverse Trendelenburg. Small areas of metastases on the splenic capsule may be identified and hilar adenopathy may be assessed using this technique. Liver biopsy is performed using a core biopsy technique through a separate stab wound incision as well as wedge biopsy along the right or left lobar edge. If specific lesions are noted, biopsies are taken from these areas. The challenge for diagnostic exploration and staging of abdominal lymphoma is to fully evaluate the retroperitoneum. The most fruitful area for biopsy is in the lower aortic and parailiac arterial regions. To facilitate this, intraabdominal fan retractors are passed through a 10-mm port placed in the right lower quadrant. The patient may be turned, using the table position, into a right-side- or left-side-down position, depending on the iliac region to be assessed. The retroperitoneum is opened, using electrocautery techniques, and isolated nodes are identified. It is important to be aggressive in clipping efferent and afferent lymphatics when dissecting the retroperitoneal space to obtain nodes for staging. Failure to secure the lymphatics in these areas will lead to chylous ascites, which may be managed with difficulty and is a truly unwanted complication in the laparoscopic assessment in the retroperitoneal area. As in the biopsy of any tissue in the abdominal cavity, it is especially important not to produce crush artifacts, which will render the tissue unacceptable for pathologic interpretation. While best results are obtained by removing entire lymph nodes, partial biopsy of node-bearing areas is acceptable as long as the tissue is handled gently and significant cautery artifact is avoided. It is also extremely important to send this tissue in a fresh state directly to the pathologist for appropriate pathologic testing and immunochemical assessment as indicated.

Full diagnostic exploration in the assessment of abdominal lymphoma, when done properly, will prepare the surgeon-laparoscopist for the assessment of any intraabdominal process. Using appropriate techniques of trocar placement, establishment of pneumoperitoneum, hepatic and nodal biopsy, and full assessment of retroperitoneum, the surgeon will play a major role, not only in the management of patients with lymphoma, but in providing full information to allow the application of appropriate local or systemic treatment.

▲ COMPLICATIONS

Complications of diagnostic exploratory laparoscopy include both physiologic problems related to cardiopulmonary manifestations of general anesthesia and the resultant effects of creating a pneumoperitoneum. Studies have clearly demonstrated that cardiac output and venous return are affected adversely as intraabdominal pressure is increased above the level of 15-mmHg pressure. In addition, the unfavorable cardiopulmonary consequences are enhanced when patients are

SURGICAL PEARLS
Irrigation through the laparoscope should be performed with warm Ringer lactate solution, since saline may increase adhesion formation.

In the presence of ascites, a Veress needle should be placed with the patient in the *reverse* Trendelenburg position to allow the intestine to float out of the pelvis.

Significant gas embolization during establishment of pneumoperitoneum is associated with a *fall* in end-tidal CO_2 levels because of associated pulmonary outflow obstruction.

Inspection of the small bowel should begin at the ileocecal valve and progress to the ligament of Treitz.

Tension pneumothorax may be rapidly produced in performing diagnostic laparoscopy for blunt trauma in the presence of associated diaphragmatic injury.

placed in reverse Trendelenburg position. For these reasons, careful monitoring using pulse oximetry and end-tidal monitoring of carbon dioxide are mandatory during the diagnostic study. The mechanical effects of diagnostic laparoscopy may lead to bleeding from the abdominal wall due to trocar puncture, intraabdominal bleeding secondary to trocar penetration, barotrauma secondary to dissection of air into the subcutaneous space, and perforation of the gastrointestinal tract or other hollow viscus during trocar insertion or biopsy. For these reasons, the careful placement of the initial trocar into the abdomen is mandatory and may be facilitated by the open or Hasson technique.

As in any operative procedure, positioning of the patient is important to avoid pressure effects or neurologic injury due to inappropriate positioning. Placement of a footboard is important, especially if the patient will be placed in steep reversed Trendelenburg position. It is to be remembered that the feet must be at a right angle and flush against the footboard in order to avoid an inversion or eversion injury during the procedure. This may, in fact, create a footdrop, which will be incapacitating for the patient.

In addition to the previously mentioned physiologic or mechanical complications, infection may always be a consequence of abdominal exploration, whether performed laparoscopically or in an open manner. The use of prophylactic antibiotics is appropriate when nodal dissection is performed in a patient who is already immunocompromised by cancer or other disease. Careful attention to soft tissue techniques when closing trocar sites will also lessen the degree of infectious problems in the abdominal wall and reduce the possibility of hernia through the trocar site.

☑ CONCLUSION

It is a truism that postoperative complications begin preoperatively. Careful consideration of all facets of the patient's metabolic and physiologic needs will reduce the consequences of adverse outcome in patients undergoing diagnostic exploratory laparoscopy.

RECOMMENDED READING

1. Greene FL. Laparoscopic surgery in cancer treatment. In: DeVita VT, Hellman S, Rosenberg SA, eds. *Important advances in oncology—1993*. Philadelphia: JB Lippincott; 1993:157–166.
2. Clayman RV, McDougall EM, Kavoussi LR. Laparoscopic pelvic lymphadenectomy. In: Hunter JG, Sackier JM, eds. *Minimally invasive surgery*. New York: McGraw-Hill; 1993:279–289.
3. Spinelli P, DiFelice G. Laparoscopy in abdominal malignancies. *Prob Gen Surg* 1991;8:329–347.
4. Gill B, Traverso LW. The acute abdomen and laparoscopy. *Gastrointest Clin North Am* 1993;3: 271–281.
5. Klaiber C, Metzger A, Petelin JB. Laparoscopic adhesiolysis. In: *Manual of laparoscopic surgery*. Seattle, WA: Hogrefe and Huber, 1993.

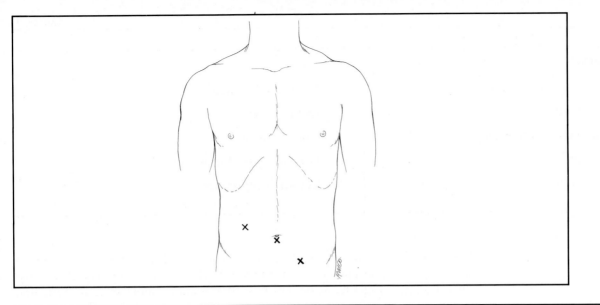

11

Management of the Acute Abdomen

Mark W. Roberts and Bruce M. Wolfe
Department of Surgery
University of California
Davis Medical Center
Sacramento, California 95817

Richard Graves
Department of Obstetrics and Gynecology
Division of Gynecology
University of California at Davis School of Medicine
Sacramento, California 95818

Operative Laparoscopy and Thoracoscopy, edited by
B. V. MacFadyen, Jr. and
J. L. Ponsky. Lippincott-Raven
Publishers, Philadelphia © 1996.

KEY WORDS

Laparoscopic appendectomy

Acute cholecystitis

Laparoscopic cholecystectomy

Acute abdomen

Perforated duodenal ulcer

Perforated gastric ulcer

Laparoscopy

Diverticulitis

Ovarian cyst, torsion of

Ectopic pregnancy

The presentation of patients with acute abdominal pain continues to be a common occurrence in clinical practice. The differential diagnosis is extensive. A tentative clinical diagnosis can be made, but this often requires surgery for confirmation. Initially, it must be determined whether an operation is required. Then, the surgeon must decide where the incision will be made. Until recently, the role of laparoscopy was limited to diagnosis. The laparoscope was introduced to determine whether laparotomy would be required. With the development of new techniques, it has become possible to perform definitive therapeutic procedures under videoendoscopic control in the setting of the acute abdomen. Because of these advances it is usually appropriate to proceed with the laparoscopic approach except in cases of trauma or unstable vital signs and shock.

Advantages of using a laparoscopic or minimally invasive approach to the acute abdomen include the ability to examine the entire peritoneal cavity and perform a definitive procedure. Two to four incisions will accommodate 5- to 12-mm trocars, thereby reducing postoperative pain and disability, hospitalization, and disfigurement by scar formation. Potential disadvantages include the possibility of incorrect assessment of the laparoscopic findings, complications specific to the laparoscopic approach, inability to perform the operative procedure as it would be performed with a conventional incision, and increased cost owing to expensive equipment and longer operative time. Carefully controlled studies will ultimately be necessary to determine the overall advantages (or disadvantages) of the laparoscopic approach.

Many of the causes of the acute abdomen can be managed laparoscopically (Table 1). The decision whether to proceed using laparoscopic techniques should be based on the skill and experience of the surgeon. The therapeutic approach in these patients is based on clinical suspicion and on the results of diagnostic laparoscopy. Each procedure is begun by performing diagnostic laparoscopy to determine the specific abnormality present. A pneumoperitoneum is obtained with either the Veress needle technique or by incision and placement of an open trocar. A 10-mm trocar is used and a 30-degree forward oblique telescope is inserted. Complete visualization of the abdominal viscera is then performed. It may be necessary to place additional trocars to aid in dissection of adhesions and organ

Table 1. *Laparoscopy for the acute abdomen*

Condition	Accurate diagnosis	Definitive procedure
Appendicitis	+	+
Acute cholecystitis	+	+
Perforated duodenal ulcer	+	+
Perforated gastric ulcer	+	+/−
Pelvic disease	+	+
Diverticulitis	+/−	+/−
Pancreatitis	+/−	+/−
Ischemic intestine	+	+/−

manipulation to accomplish complete visualization. Once the specific abnormality is identified, additional trocars are placed as appropriate for completion of the definitive procedure.

APPENDICITIS

◉ ANATOMY

The appendix is found in the right lower quadrant of the abdominal cavity. It is positioned on the inferior aspect of the cecum. The taeniae of the colon coalesce to form the outer longitudinal muscular coat of the appendix. The inner circular layer is a continuation of the same muscular layer of the cecum. The ileum joins the cecum just medial to the appendix. The base of the appendix is constant in its location, but the tip is variable in its orientation in relation to the cecum. It may be found retrocecal, pelvic, or lying adjacent to the distal ileum. In the adult, the appendix measures 8 to 12 cm in length. Its blood supply is from branches of the appendicular artery, which courses through the mesoappendix. The appendicular artery is a branch of the ileocolic artery.

▶ PREOPERATIVE PLANNING

Appendicitis is a common condition, occurring in 250,000 patients per year in the United States. The appropriate role of laparoscopic appendectomy remains to be defined as a straightforward appendectomy through a muscle-splitting incision produces relatively little morbidity and disability in contrast to an open cholecystectomy. A laparoscopic approach to suspected appendicitis is recommended in cases in which the diagnosis is uncertain, perforation is suspected, or the patient is obese. This procedure accommodates more extensive abdominal and/or pelvic exploration in cases in which the appendix appears to be normal or to have secondary peritoneal inflammation. Excessive retraction or extension of the incision is often necessary to exclude other diagnoses in these cases, whereas adequate exploration from the upper abdomen to the pelvis can be accomplished with a 10-mm port for the laparoscope and one or two trocars for organ manipulation. Appendicitis occurs more commonly in males by a ratio of 1.4:1 but incidental appendectomy occurs more frequently in females by a remarkable ratio of 12.1:1. These data underscore the difficulty of establishing an accurate preoperative diagnosis of appendicitis in reproductive age females, in whom the diagnostic error rate is 35–46%. The accuracy of the clinical diagnosis of appendicitis is lower for the very young and the old. The role of laparoscopy in children is unclear, but laparoscopy can well be applied to the elderly with abdominal pain in whom the indications for abdominal exploration are often not well defined.

Laparoscopic management of perforated appendicitis may prove to be superior to open appendectomy. Dissection of adherent intestine and irrigation of the entire peritoneal cavity can be accomplished without extension of the incision. Drainage can be done, and a lesser exposure of the wound to infected tissue can be obtained as the appendix is removed. An alternative cause of acute abdomen can be identified and operatively managed. Obese patients have an increased wound infection rate and require larger incisions for standard exposure. Further advantages of the laparoscopic approach include decreased exposure of subcutaneous tissue to the infected appendix and therefore a lower wound infection rate.

In the past, the application of laparoscopy in appendicitis was limited to a diagnostic role; however, the description of laparoscopic appendectomy by Semm and subsequent reports of larger series of laparoscopic appendectomies have established appendectomy as a logical extension of diagnostic laparoscopy. Appen-

SURGICAL PEARLS
Indications for laparoscopic appendectomy include patients with an uncertain diagnosis (i.e., reproductive age females and the elderly), obese patients, and those with suspected perforated appendicitis.

We also urge performing appendectomy even if the appendix appears normal.

Many times appendiceal inflammation is not detectable without microscopic evaluation.

dectomy is indicated unless there are other findings that require operative intervention or show that appendectomy is not indicated. Appendectomy is also recommended in cases of clinically suspected appendicitis in which the appendix appears normal, as this procedure will only marginally increase morbidity and postoperative disability, if at all. Many of the conditions that are often confused with appendicitis may recur. In addition, a false-negative interpretation of the findings may mistakenly lead to retention of an inflamed appendix. The primary circumstance in which appendectomy is not indicated occurs when the laparoscopic findings of a condition other than appendicitis mandate operative intervention.

▼ INTRAOPERATIVE MANAGEMENT/SURGICAL TECHNIQUE

The patient is positioned to aid in intestinal retraction: Trendelenburg for removal of small intestine from the pelvis and left lateral decubitus for right lower quadrant exposure. Laparoscopy is then performed through an umbilical trocar, which is versatile for examining the entire peritoneal cavity. It is also helpful to tuck the left arm because that is the side where the surgeon stands. A second 5-mm trocar (or 10-mm trocar, depending on the instruments to be used) is placed in the left lower quadrant well above the bladder (Fig. 1). A third 10-mm trocar is placed to the right of the umbilicus. A 12-mm trocar is needed if an endoscopic stapler is to be used. A fourth trocar is placed if needed to aid retraction or exposure. Preference regarding location of this fourth trocar varies from the right lower quadrant laterally to the left of the midline midway between the umbilicus and the symphysis. Placement of a trocar directly over the appendix is not recom-

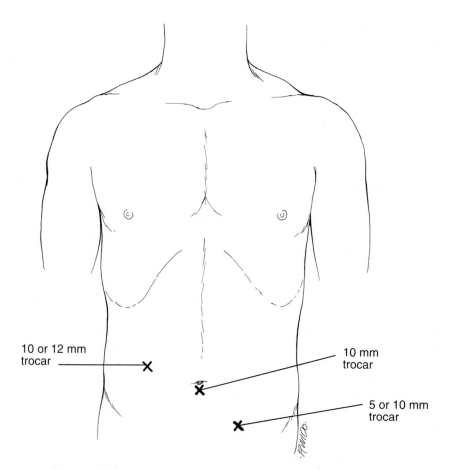

Figure 1. Trocar placement for laparoscopic appendectomy.

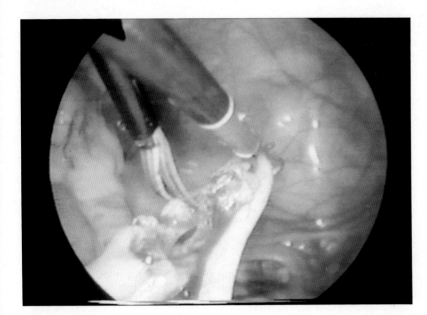

Figure 2. Control of the vessels allows division of the mesoappendix.

mended, as such placement makes videoendoscopic hand-eye coordination more difficult.

Exposure of the appendix is aided by the use of endoscopic intestinal instruments for grasping, manipulating, or retracting intestine. The peritoneal reflection of the lateral aspect of the cecum and ascending colon may require division for cecal mobilization. The mesoappendix is divided with control of the vessels by application of endoscopic clips, ligatures, staples, or coagulation (Fig. 2). Several forms of energy to produce heat for coagulation are satisfactory, including standard electrocautery, argon beam coagulation, and lasers. The base of the appendix may be secured before division with loop ligatures passed over the length of the appendix or around the appendix with subsequent knotting (Fig. 3). An endoscopic linear stapling-cutting device may alternatively be used to secure and divide the base of the appendix (Fig. 4). In cases in which dissection of an adherent or retrocecal appendix is difficult, it may be advantageous to divide the base of the appendix initially and dissect the appendix in a retrograde fashion. Application of monopolar electrocautery to the appendix or appendiceal stump after dissection

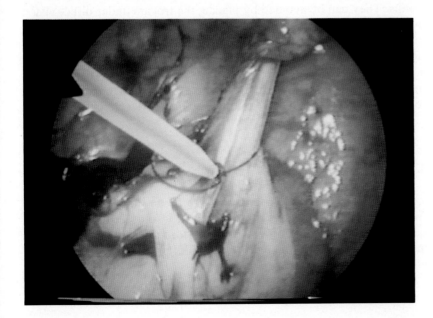

Figure 3. Loop ligatures and subsequent knotting secure the base of the appendix.

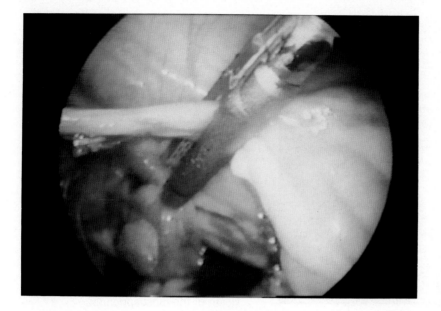

Figure 4. An option for dividing and securing the base of the appendix is with endoscopic linear staple-cutting.

and ligation of the stump should be avoided, as the constricted cross-sectional area of the ligature may produce exaggerated resistance to electron flow and excessive heating at the site, possibly leading to necrosis at the level of the ligature. Inspection for bleeding and whatever irrigation is to be done are accomplished before specimen removal. The specimen is removed by pulling it into the 10-mm trocar if this can be easily accomplished (Fig. 5). Alternatively, the specimen can be placed in a plastic bag and removed. The finger of a glove may also be satisfactory for this purpose.

▲ COMPLICATIONS

Bleeding from trocar sites can be troublesome if the trocar is placed through the rectus muscle and the inferior epigastric vessels are lacerated. This can be avoided by placing the trocars close to the midline or lateral to the rectus muscle. Bowel perforations can be disastrous for the patient if they are not recognized. These perforations commonly occur either with trocar placement or during dissection of adhesions. They can be avoided by placing the trocars under direct vision and with careful dissection while lysing adhesions. Breakdown of the appendiceal stump is a problem in both the open and laparoscopic appendectomy. One way of preventing this is to refrain from cauterizing the appendiceal stump after it has been ligated. In that way the tissue beneath the ligature will have less of a tendency to become necrotic. In the situation where the base of the appendix is necrotic from disease, it is possible to use a laparoscopic stapling device across the cecum (Fig. 6).

✓ CONCLUSIONS

Laparoscopic appendectomy has been shown to be an effective therapeutic modality. There may be advantages to this approach in those patients with an uncertain diagnosis, obese patients, or in cases of perforation with abscess formation. It is important to routinely remove the appendix unless specific operative findings contraindicate its removal.

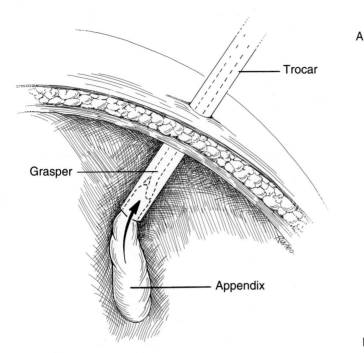

Figure 5. Removing appendix through a trocar.

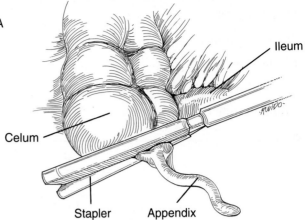

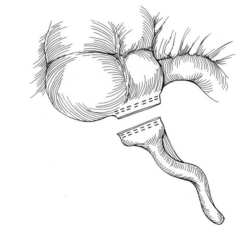

Figure 6. Using the linear-cutting stapler to remove the base of the cecum and a necrotic appendix.

ACUTE CHOLECYSTITIS

● ANATOMY

The gallbladder is found on the dorsal surface of the liver. It is a tubular structure that contains 40 to 50 ml of bile. It has a bulbous fundus that tapers through its body to a narrow neck. The cystic duct continues from the neck of the gallbladder to join with the common hepatic duct. The cystic duct is 3 to 4 cm in length and contains several spiral valves of Heister. The common bile duct is distal to this junction and drains into the second portion of the duodenum at the ampulla of Vater. The common bile duct travels down the hepatoduodenal ligament. The triangle of Calot is bounded by the cystic duct, the common hepatic duct, and the inferior border of the liver. The cystic artery travels through this space to supply the gallbladder. There can be considerable anatomic variability in this region.

▶ PREOPERATIVE PLANNING

The diagnosis of cholelithiasis with acute cholecystitis is generally made preoperatively, but acute cholecystitis may present as an acute abdomen without localized findings, especially if the gallbladder is gangrenous or perforated or the patient has associated cholangitis.

▼ INTRAOPERATIVE MANAGEMENT

General anesthesia is necessary because multiple trocars and operative manipulation may be required for performance of a definitive procedure. The telescope is inserted into the abdominal cavity through an umbilical trocar and complete visualization of the viscera is completed. A 10-mm trocar is placed in the midline below the xiphoid process. Two 5-mm trocars are placed in the right anterior axillary line below the costal margin and at the level of the umbilicus, respectively. These trocars are placed under direct vision to avoid injury to other organs and blood vessels. At this time the fundus of the gallbladder is grasped with an instrument placed through the right-sided inferior trocar (this should be a locking grasper), and the neck of the gallbladder is grasped in a similar fashion through the right-sided superior trocar. Grasping the gallbladder can be difficult when an acute inflammatory state is present. Decompression of the gallbladder can make it possible to grasp a thickened (not necrotic) gallbladder. This is accomplished by percutaneously passing a needle on a syringe (at least 17-gauge) into the fundus of the gallbladder (Fig. 7). When the needle is inserted into the gallbladder an attempt should be made to make a submucosal tunnel to help prevent leakage. Then the contents of the gallbladder can be aspirated with the syringe. The hole that has

SURGICAL PEARLS
Do not hesitate to decompress the gallbladder to improve your ability to grasp an acutely inflamed organ.

Use extra caution in performing ductal dissection beginning at the junction of the neck of the gallbladder and the cystic duct.

Be prepared to convert to open cholecystectomy.

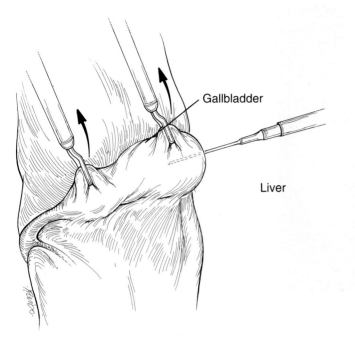

Gallblader

Liver

Figure 7. Decompression of an enlarged gallbladder using a large (at least 17-gauge) needle on a syringe. This can be done percutaneously or the needle can be passed through a trocar. The needles that are used for aspirating ovarian cysts are very useful for gallbladder decompression.

been made can be closed with a suture placed before the needle is inserted, or it can be simply incorporated into the bite of a large-toothed grasper. If the gallbladder is thickened to such an extent that it cannot be grasped, placement of one or two large sutures may be used for grasping. If the gallbladder is necrotic or otherwise cannot be grasped and successfully elevated anteriorly and superiorly, adequate exposure of the triangle of Calot cannot be accomplished, and the procedure should be converted to open cholecystecomy.

The gallbladder should be grasped and retracted in such a way that the triangle of Calot is splayed so that dissection may begin (Fig. 8). This can be accomplished by retracting the neck of the gallbladder in the direction of the patient's right leg and pushing the fundus of the gallbladder over the top of the liver superiorly. Blunt dissection is then begun at the junction of the cystic duct and the gallbladder, with dissecting forceps placed through the subxiphoid trocar. With an inflamed gallbladder, the anatomy in this area may be severely distorted. It is important

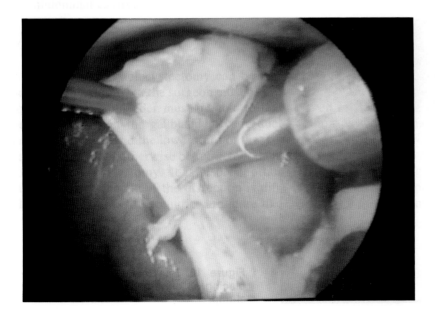

Figure 8. The gallbladder should be grasped and retracted so that the triangle of Calot is splayed out for dissection to begin.

KEY WORDS

Stomach   Perforation

Adhesions   Sutures

Trocars   Omental patch

Insufflation

Perforated Gastric and Duodenal Ulcer

⊡ ANATOMY

The stomach is divided into four areas. The cardia is located at the gastroesophageal junction. The fundus lies cephalad to the gastroesophageal junction. The body or corpus of the stomach is the area that lies between the cardia and fundus proximally, and the antrum distally. The corpus is the largest portion of the stomach. The angularis incisura is found on the lesser curvature of the stomach and marks the beginning of the antrum. The pylorus is the portion of the stomach between the corpus and the duodenum. The corpus produces most of the acidic secretions of the stomach. The pyloric region, containing the antral G cells, produces and secretes gastrin.

The stomach has a rich blood supply. The lesser curvature is supplied by the right and left gastric arteries. The greater curvature is supplied by the right gastroepiploic vessels (a branch of the gastroduodenal artery) and the left gastroepiploic vessels (a branch of the splenic artery). The duodenum is supplied by the gastroduodenal artery (a branch of the celiac plexus), the superior pancreaticoduodenal artery (a branch of the gastroduodenal artery), and the inferior pancreaticoduodenal artery (a branch of the superior mesenteric artery). The venous drainage of the stomach is by way of the coronary, splenic, and gastroepiploic veins before emptying into the portal venous system.

The right (posterior) vagus nerve sends off branches to the celiac region and the posterior stomach after it passes through the esophageal hiatus. The left (anterior) vagus nerve also branches after it passes through the esophageal hiatus. It has hepatic, anterior stomach, and antral branches. The nerves of Latarjet are terminal antral branches of the left vagus nerves. They form the so-called crow's foot distal to the angularis incisura, which innervate the pylorus and are involved with gastric motility.

▶ PREOPERATIVE PLANNING

The preoperative diagnosis is usually fairly well established on the basis of the preoperative evaluation, even though in 30% of the cases there is no evidence of free air on the abdominal films. The indications for operation in all respects are the same as in the conventional operation. The patient will usually have peritoneal irritation, free air in the abdomen, moderate leukocytosis, and significant abdominal pain. The contraindications to the laparoscopic approach are the same as in any laparoscopic procedure. A relative contraindication would be previous gastric surgery, in that the patient may have dense supracolic adhesions. In this instance, it would seem reasonable to begin the operation laparoscopically and convert to laparotomy if the adhesions were too significant to perform the operation safely. If the patient has significant intestinal distention, the umbilical trocar placement and insufflation should be carried out using the open technique.

▼ INTRAOPERATIVE MANAGEMENT

The 30-degree forward oblique telescope is inserted through the umbilical trocar and complete visualization of the abdominal viscera is performed. The three accessory trocars are then placed under direct vision (Fig. 11). A trocar is placed in the right subxiphoid position and a second trocar is placed in the right anterior axillary line at the costal margin. The third trocar is placed on the left side at the junction of the lateral edge of the rectus muscle and the costal margin. The trocars are placed in such a configuration that suturing at the proximal duodenum may be performed. The perforation is then viewed by retracting the liver edge superiorly and applying inferior traction on the pylorus. The perforation is generally on the anterior surface and is easily seen (Fig. 12). If it is not seen, intraoperative gastroduodenoscopy with insufflation of air may aid in locating the defect. Bubbling will be seen at the site of perforation when submerged in fluid. To proceed with the operation, the patient should be placed in the reverse Trendelenburg position. This will improve the exposure by allowing the colon, small bowel, and omentum to fall toward the pelvis.

When exposure is obtained and the perforation is identified, we are ready for repair of the perforation. If the perforation is small (<5.0 mm) and has healthy surrounding tissue, it is possible to perform direct suture closure using 3-0 polyglactin or polydioxanone suture on atraumatic needles (Fig. 13). It is best to close the defect in a transverse direction to prevent narrowing of the lumen. The sutures are to be introduced through a sleeve that fits through a 10-mm trocar. This will prevent the needle from getting snared in the trocar. Usually, two sutures are sufficient to close the defect (Fig. 14). These sutures should be tied as they are placed to prevent tangling of the suture tails. When performing endoscopic sutur-

SURGICAL PEARLS

Suture closure with an omental patch works well, and is our preferred closure.

It is important to copiously irrigate the entire peritoneal cavity.

Vagotomy can be performed at the surgeon's discretion.

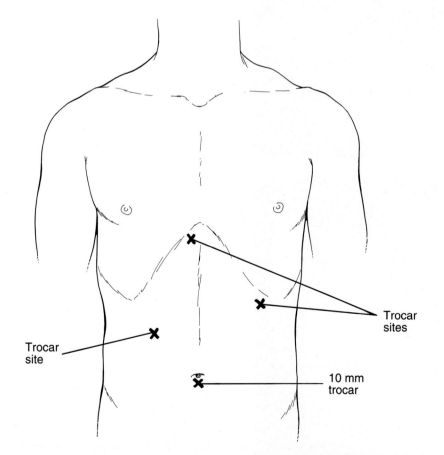

Trocar sites

Trocar site

10 mm trocar

Figure 11. Trocar placement for repair of perforated duodenal ulcer.

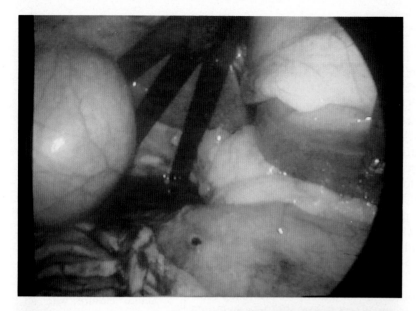

Figure 12. The perforated gastric ulcer is viewed by retracting the liver edge superiorly and applying inferior traction on the pylorus.

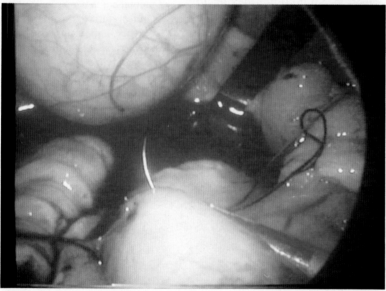

Figure 13. A direct suture closure is used when the perforation is small and there is healthy surrounding tissue.

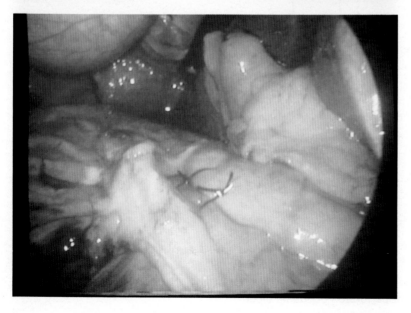

Figure 14. The defect is closed using two sutures.

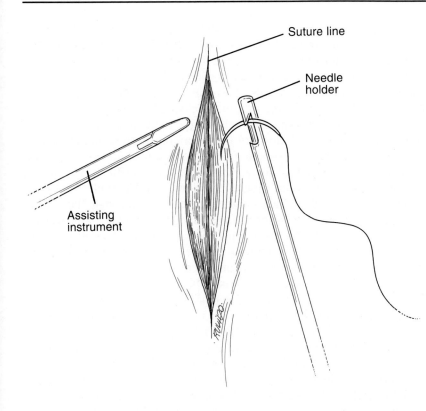

Suture line

Needle
holder

Assisting
instrument

Figure 15. Orientation of the needle driver
to the line of suturing.

ing techniques it is best to have your needle driver in a plane parallel to the suture
line, while your assisting instrument is at a right angle to the suture line (Fig. 15).
This will allow you to place your sutures smoothly because it is in the natural
orientation for rotation of your wrist. Laparoscopic vagotomy may be employed
at this stage of the operation if it is felt to be indicated. The details of this operation
are described in Chapter 32. The risks and benefits of definitive repair must always
be considered in the acute setting.

The surgeon will generally elect to lay an omental flap over the closed perforation to protect the closure. This can be done by dragging a small section of adjacent
omentum over to the defect. It is then secured in place with two or three absorbable
interrupted sutures (Fig. 16).

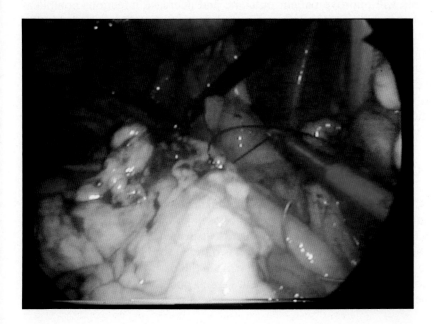

Figure 16. Absorbable interrupted sutures secure the omental flap over the
defect.

Large perforations (>5.0 mm) or those with a large amount of surrounding tissue friability and edema can be closed with an omental plug. An omental flap is fashioned as described above. The apex of the flap is then placed into the defect. The edges of the omentum are then secured to surrounding healthier tissues with several absorbable seromuscular sutures. This will keep the plug in place.

After completion of the repair, the peritoneal cavity must be thoroughly irrigated with warm saline solution. This is usually begun in the right upper quadrant and then the left upper quadrant followed by the pericolic gutters and the pelvis. It is helpful to place the patient in steep Trendelenburg position to irrigate the pelvis. This position is also helpful for aspiration of the irrigant by placing the suction device over the right lateral lobe of the liver. Food particles and other debris must also be removed; if they cannot be removed through the suction device, they must be grasped with forceps and removed through one of the trocars. The suction device will deflate the pneumoperitoneum if it is activated when the tip is not submerged in fluid. The aspiration process can be accomplished more quickly if the pneumoperitoneum is not deflated and the suction device is not set too high, thereby causing fat and other debris to become stuck in it.

Perforated gastric ulcers are approached in much the same manner. Identification of the ulcer may require gastroscopy with insufflation while submerged in fluid. If the ulcer is on the posterior surface of the stomach, the lesser sac is opened using sequential clipping while retracting the stomach superiorly and the transverse colon inferiorly. Definitive repair of perforated gastric ulcers differs from repair of perforated duodenal ulcers in that limited resection to partial gastrectomy is usually preferred in the former. It is up to the judgment of the surgeon whether to convert to open laparotomy to manage this problem.

▲ COMPLICATIONS

Inadequate closure can lead to a leak with subsequent abscess formation. If this occurs, reoperation will be necessary. It is probably best to proceed with conventional laparotomy for drainage and repair. Anastomotic leak can be prevented by careful placement of sutures and placing an omental patch over the closure. A delayed abscess can develop as a result of peritoneal contamination from the initial insult or inadequate peritoneal irrigation. It is vital to get the patient to the operating room as soon as possible once the diagnosis of acute abdomen has been made. Decreasing the amount of time the patient is exposed to the intraluminal contents will improve patient outcome and decrease infectious complications. It is also possible to develop gastric outlet obstruction from closure of the duodenal perforation. Patients often develop edema and local scarring from ulcer disease, which will make them more susceptible to this complication. Gastric outlet obstruction can be minimized by closing the defect in a transverse direction. Kissing ulcers can occur in which there is an anterior perforation and posterior penetration with bleeding. This is managed with an anterior duodenotomy with suture ligation of the bleeding point and closure of the perforation. If there is inadequate visualization, it may be necessary to convert to laparotomy.

☑ CONCLUSIONS

Laparoscopic techniques can successfully manage most of the conditions encountered in patients with an acute abdomen. It is important to position the trocars for suturing the duodenum if perforated ulcer is suspected. Endoscopy with insufflation can be very helpful if the perforation is difficult to find. It is imperative to arrive at the operating room promptly and irrigate the peritoneum well to prevent infectious complications. Tilting the table in various positions helps with irrigating the entire peritoneal surface.

ring
is to
are
red
tim
bow

☑

ultr
out
it is

KEY WORDS

Diverticulitis	Stents
Free perforation	Endoscopic stapler
Obstruction	Mesentery
Trocars	Anastomosis

COLON DISEASE

⦿ ANATOMY

The colon is derived embryologically from the midgut and the hindgut. It extends from the ileocecal valve to the rectum. The cecum, ascending colon, and proximal two-thirds of the transverse colon are derived from the midgut and are supplied by branches of the superior mesenteric artery (the ileocolic, right colic, and middle colic arteries). The distal one-third of the transverse colon, descending colon, sigmoid colon, and proximal rectum are supplied by branches of the inferior mesenteric artery (the left colic, sigmoidal, and superior hemorrhoidal arteries). The ascending colon and descending colon are retroperitoneal structures. The lower rectum is below the peritoneal reflection, and is therefore a retroperitoneal structure.

The colon is made up of an inner mucosa, submucosa (the strongest layer in the bowel wall), muscularis, and serosa. The muscularis has an inner circular layer and an outer longitudinal muscle that completely encircles the colon. In three points around the colon this outer longitudinal muscle is gathered up into bands that are called taeniae. The caliber of the colon is greatest in the cecum and decreases to its smallest diameter in the rectum.

The sympathetic innervation of the right colon is from T10 to T12, and travels in the thoracic splanchnic nerves to the celiac plexus. From the celiac plexus they go to the superior mesenteric plexus, where the postganglionic fibers travel to the colon with the branches of the superior mesenteric artery. The sympathetic innervation of the left colon arises from L1 to L3, where they synapse in the paravertebral ganglia. The efferent fibers from the paravertebral ganglia travel to the colon with branches of the inferior mesenteric artery. The parasympathetic innervation of the right colon is from the right vagus, and travels with the sympathetic fibers. The parasympathetic innervation of the left colon is from S2 to S4 (the nervi erigentes).

▶ PREOPERATIVE PLANNING

When the colon is the source of the acute abdomen it usually is related to diverticulitis, free perforation, or obstruction. The diagnosis of diverticulitis is typically made preoperatively by the patient's history and physical examination in conjunction with pelvic computed tomography (CT) scans and ultrasound. The diagnosis of colon obstruction is similarly made preoperatively, whereas the preoperative diagnosis of patients with free perforation of the colon is often uncertain prior to operation. Free perforations of the colon occur from perforation of a right-sided diverticulum, obstruction due to cancer or diverticulitis, Ogilvie syndrome, trauma, or foreign bodies inserted through the rectum.

Laparoscopy is a valuable tool for diagnosis and definitive therapy in this setting. The indications for operation are the same as in conventional laparotomy.

PELVIC DISEASE

⦿ ANATOMY

The uterus is found in the pelvis. It is connected to the cervix and vagina distally and the fallopian tubes superolaterally. Several ligamentous structures support these pelvic organs. The infundibulopelvic ligament attaches the ovaries and fallopian tubes to the pelvic side wall. It also contains the ovarian vessels. The broad ligaments are lateral attachments of the uterus to the pelvic side wall. The uterine artery passes through the midportion of the broad ligament to supply the uterus, cervix, and fallopian tubes. The fallopian tubes are found in the superior portion of the broad ligament. They receive their blood supply from the uterine artery and the ovarian artery. The ureter is a retroperitoneal structure that passes beneath the infundibulopelvic ligament in the pelvic side wall. The ovaries are suspended between the uterus medially by the ovarian ligament, and the pelvic side wall laterally by the infundibulopelvic ligament. The ovaries receive their blood supply from the ovarian vessels.

▶ PREOPERATIVE PLANNING

Acute abdominal pain from gynecologic sources is a common problem in surgery. The etiology of this pain in reproductive age females is often obscure. The question of appendicitis versus torsion of the ovary or salpingitis is often posed. The answer, on the basis of the patient's history and physical examination, is not always clear. Laparoscopy has been commonly used in the past for chronic pelvic pain. It was not until more recent years that this modality has been used for diagnosis and definitive therapy in patients with acute pelvic pain. Many of the gynecologic sources of acute abdominal pain can be managed laparoscopically.

The clinical findings in acute gynecologic conditions are often very similar to other abdominal conditions. Salpingitis presents with gradual onset lower abdominal pain, fever, leukocytosis, possibly peritoneal signs, severe cervical motion tenderness, and sometimes a vaginal discharge. Patients with a ruptured ovarian cyst typically have sudden onset, sharp, midcycle pain. The pain is usually localized to the right or left, but generalized peritonitis can occur if there is free intraperitoneal hemorrhage. Patients with torsion of an ovary have pain that remains localized to the involved ovary and often a palpable, tender, pelvic mass. Ectopic pregnancy can often be diagnosed preoperatively on the basis of a history of irregular menstrual bleeding, lower abdominal pain, a positive urine β-HCG test, and a confirmatory ultrasound showing an extrauterine gestational sac. The pain experienced in ectopic pregnancy may become generalized with the development of peritoneal signs if there is rupture and free intraperitoneal hemorrhage.

The indications for operation are the same whether it is to be done open or laparoscopically. Laparoscopy is indicated when the diagnosis is uncertain, the patient is obese, and the definitive operative management can be handled with the laparoscopic technique. There are no specific contraindications other than the patient not be in hemorrhagic shock.

▼ INTRAOPERATIVE MANAGEMENT

The pneumoperitoneum is developed using one of the standard techniques. A 0-degree laparoscope is placed through a 10-mm umbilical trocar. Complete visualization of the abdominal viscera is performed as previously described. If salpingitis is found to be the cause of the abdominal pain, no further intervention is required. It is appropriate to take a small piece of involved fimbria for culture purposes. The pelvis can be irrigated and the procedure terminated. Antibiotic therapy is all that is required.

Torsion of the ovary will usually require oophorectomy for definitive management (Fig. 18). At least two accessory trocars will need to be placed. A 12-mm trocar is placed under direct vision approximately four generous fingerbreadths lateral to the umbilicus on the right or the left, on the same side as the torsion (Fig. 19). Care must be taken to avoid damage to the inferior epigastric vessels and the superficial epigastric vessels by transilluminating the abdominal wall, puncturing lateral to the obliterated umbilical artery, and visualizing the abdominal peritoneum, beginning at the round ligament and following the course of the inferior epigastric vessels as they move cranially. The ovarian ligament and fallopian tube are grasped at their junction with the uterus. A linear cutting vascular stapler is then used to ligate and divide these structures proximally. The cautery scissors are used to divide the broad ligament starting on the medial edge and dissecting laterally. The ovary is mobilized in a similar fashion. The infundibulopelvic ligament is then taken down with the cautery scissors. The suspensory ligament of the ovary is then divided using the linear cutting vascular stapler. The specimen is removed through one of the trocar sites.

Salpingostomy is the procedure of choice in the majority of tubal pregnancies because they usually occur in the ampullary portion of the tube (Fig. 20). Trocar placement is the same as described previously. In this procedure the tube is grasped proximally, and a small incision is made over the most distended portion of the tube on the antimesenteric surface. This can be done with cautery, scissors, or laser. The products of conception are then evacuated by gentle traction. Bleeding is controlled with electrocautery. The opening is left to close by secondary intent. Some surgeons close the defect by placing 5-0 to 7-0 Prolene sutures. There is no compelling evidence that this produces improved outcome in terms of later fertility.

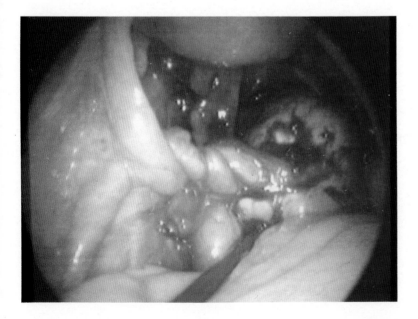

Figure 18. Torsion of the ovary.

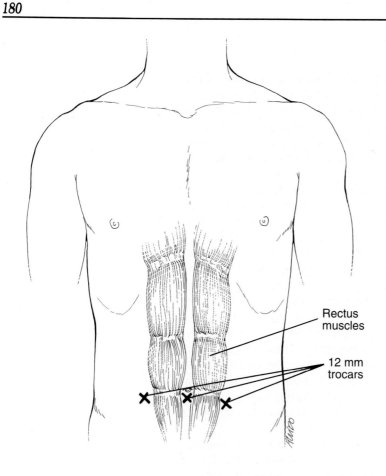

Figure 19. Trocar placement for pelvic operations.

For most isthmic pregnancies segmental excision is preferred because the narrow lumen in this area will tend to occlude even if an operation is used in an attempt to preserve patency. In segmental resection the tube is divided with cautery immediately proximal and distal to the ectopic pregnancy. The cautery scissors are then used to divide the mesosalpinx and remove the involved segment of tube. Cautery may be needed to control bleeding of the mesosalpinx. Primary

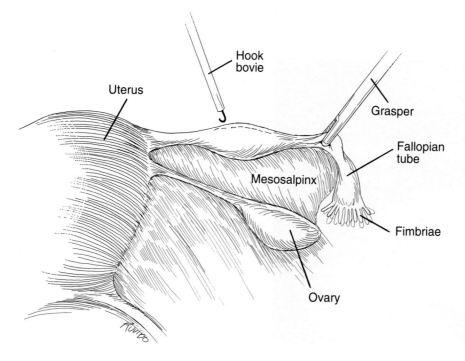

Figure 20. Linear salpingostomy using hook bovie. The incision is made on the antimesenteric border.

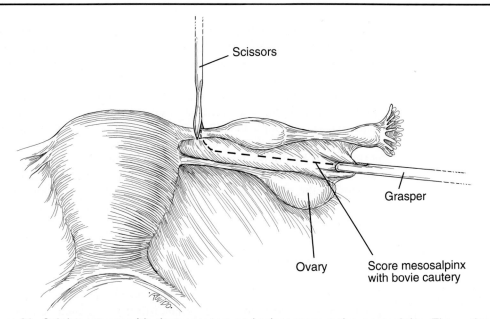

Figure 21. Salpingectomy with electrocautery and scissors score the mesosalpinx. Then scissors are used to divide the fallopian tube and mesosalpinx. The proximal fallopian tube is cauterized prior to its division.

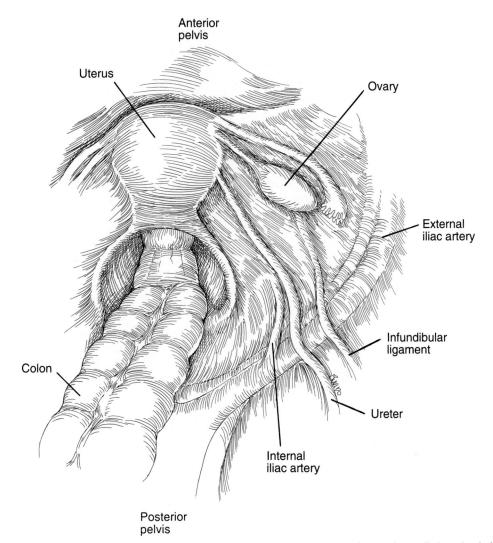

Figure 22. The ureter is a retroperitoneal structure that runs posterior and parallel to the infundibulopelvic ligament at the pelvic rim.

anastomosis is generally not attempted because the tissues are too edematous and friable. Subsequent healing and scarring may also narrow the repair to a significant degree. Patients who are interested in further fertility can have tubal anastomosis at a second procedure.

Salpingectomy should be performed in patients who are not interested in subsequent fertility or have a ruptured ectopic pregnancy with uncontrolled hemorrhage. This is accomplished by grasping the fimbrial end of the tube and cauterizing the mesosalpinx and then dividing it with scissors (Fig. 21). The tube is then ligated at the uterus by doubly ligating the tube with endoloops placed over the fallopian tube. Alternatively, an endoscopic linear-cutting vascular stapler can be used for division of the tube at the uterus. The tube with the ectopic pregnancy is then removed through one of the trocar sites. Salpingectomy can also be performed using the endogastrointestinal vascular stapler.

▲ COMPLICATIONS

SURGICAL PEARLS
To avoid injury to the ureter, it must be identified before ligation of the infundibulopelvic ligament.

Bleeding from trocar sites can be avoided by placing them in the midline or lateral to the rectus muscle.

Bleeding accounts for most of the complications of laparoscopic surgery in the pelvis. Most of these injures are related to trocar placement. Injury to the major vessels in the abdominal wall can be avoided by following the steps as outlined in the discussion on trocar placement (see "Intraoperative Management" section). For bleeding of intrabdominal or retroperitoneal vessels, electrocautery is usually effective. Endoloops can be used satisfactorily for larger vessels. If hemorrhage cannot be controlled, the operation must be converted to laparotomy. Ureteral injury is another potential complication of laparoscopic operations in the pelvis. The course of the ureter runs in close proximity to the ovarian vessels. The ureter must be identified before ligation of the infundibulopelvic ligament during salpingectomy or oophorectomy (Fig. 22).

✓ CONCLUSIONS

Laparoscopy in gynecology is a safe technique when practiced by an experienced surgeon. Bleeding complications in pelvic laparoscopic surgery can be avoided by careful trocar placement and dissection. Trocars should not be placed laterally in the suprapubic region.

KEY WORDS

Diagnostic laparoscopy   Endoscopic intestinal instruments

Appendectomy   Trocars

OTHER CAUSES OF ACUTE ABDOMEN

Pancreatitis can be a cause of acute abdomen that is not identified before operation. The diagnosis is made by opening the lesser sac with sequential clips and scissor dissection. Endoscopic ultrasound will be helpful in localizing areas of inflammation and edema. If areas of necrosis or abscesses are found, the operation should be converted to an open procedure. Preference regarding cholecystecomy, bile duct drainage, or gastrostomy and jejunostomy is left to the surgeon. If the patient does not require debridement of the pancreas, CT scanning with vascular enhancement is useful for following the pancreas for the development of necrosis.

Ischemic bowel can be found at laparoscopy for an acute abdomen. It depends on the judgment of the surgeon to determine if it is a hopeless situation. If the bowel is ischemic and not necrotic, the patient should have emergency mesenteric angiography.

Other causes of acute abdomen include primary peritonitis secondary to bacterial infection with liver disease, tuberculosis, and malignancy involving the peritoneum. Biopsy can be done for other diffuse lesions of the peritoneum. Bowel injuries and hemoperitoneum are common in the trauma patient. The role of laparoscopy in these patients is evolving. Gasless laparoscopy may have an advantage in this setting because of the enhanced ability to use suction to evacuate blood.

RECOMMENDED READING

1. Asbun HJ, Rossi RL, Lowell JA, Munson JL. Bile duct injury during laparoscopic cholecystectomy: mechanism of injury, prevention, and management. *World J Surg* 1993;17:547–552.
2. Hunter JG. Avoidance of bile duct injury during laparoscopic cholecystectomy. *Am J Surg* 1991; 162:71.
3. Hurd WW, Pearl ML, Delancey JO, Quint EH, Garnett B, Bude RO. Laparoscopic injury of abdominal wall blood vessels: a report of three cases. *Obstet Gynecol* 1993;82:673–676.
4. Mouret P, Francois Y, Vignal J, Barth X, Lombard-Platet R. Laparoscopic treatment of perforated peptic ulcer. *Br J Surg* 1990;77:1006.
5. Nathanson LK, Easter DW, Cuschieri A. Laparoscopic repair/peritoneal toilet of perforated ulcer. *Surg Endosc* 1990;4:232–233.
6. Pier A, Gotz F: Laparoscopic appendectomy. *Prob Gen Surg* 1991;8:416–425.
7. Reiertsen O, Rosseland A, Hoivik B, et al. Laparoscopy in patients admitted for acute abdominal pain. *Acta Chir Scand* 1985;151:521.
8. Richards W, Watson D, Lynch G, et al. A review of the results of laparoscopic versus open appendectomy. *Surg Gynecol Obstet* 1993;177:473–480.
9. Thompson JD, Rock JA. *Te Linde's operative gynecology*, 7th ed. Philadelphia: JB Lippincott, 1992; P. 361.
10. Whitworth C, Whitworty P, Sanfillipo J. Value of diagnostic laparoscopy in young women with possible appendicitis. *Surg Gynecol Obstet* 1988;167:187–190.

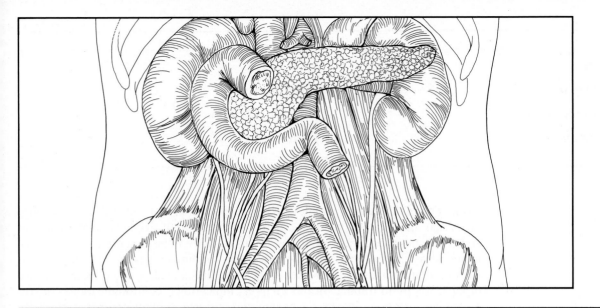

12

Trauma

Nancy L. Furumoto
Department of Surgery
University of Hawaii
Honolulu, Hawaii 96817

Jonathan M. Sackier
Department of Surgery
George Washington University
Washington, DC 20037

Operative Laparoscopy and Thoracoscopy, edited by
B. V. MacFadyen, Jr. and
J. L. Ponsky. Lippincott-Raven
Publishers, Philadelphia © 1996.

KEY WORDS

Ambulatory laparoscopy   Missed injury

Blunt abdominal trauma   Penetrating trauma

Hemoperitoneum   Trauma triage

Evaluation of the trauma patient with laparoscopy was first performed over twenty years ago and has evolved since then to include both diagnosis and treatment (1,2). The more accurate diagnosis obtained allows the potential avoidance of unnecessary laparotomy. Additionally, the "minimally invasive" approach to treating trauma injuries is another advantage that is leading to an increasing use of laparoscopy in trauma. In this chapter, indications, contraindications, instrumentation, location, anesthesia, technique, and use in blunt and penetrating abdominal trauma are considered. The "trauma" that may be caused by laparoscopy itself is also discussed. With knowledge of the uses and possible complications of laparoscopy in trauma patients, the trauma surgeon's skills in diagnosing and treating patients will be enhanced.

With an increasing population has come an increase in trauma victims due to motor vehicle accidents, civilian violence, and industrial accidents. Therefore, a more efficient and accurate method is needed to decide who needs emergent surgical treatment and who can be observed in order to maximize resources. Diagnostic peritoneal lavage, introduced in 1965 by Root and associates (3), is useful in diagnosing intraabdominal bleeding in blunt trauma, but a false-positive rate of 11% to 25% has been reported (4,5) where there was a positive lavage but normal laparotomy findings or bleeding that had ceased.

Computed tomography (CT) scanning has also been a useful diagnostic tool; however, it is not very helpful in borderline cases where there is some free fluid but the source and type of fluid are not known (6). Currently, ultrasound imaging is being evaluated for the same purpose.

Laparoscopy is now added as a diagnostic and, increasingly, a therapeutic tool in the 1990s. One can visualize the peritoneal cavity better and then can act expeditiously if needed (i.e., laparotomy, laparoscopic-guided therapeutic intervention or merely observation) at the time of laparoscopy. To be cost-effective, laparoscopy should result in fewer negative laparotomies, quicker diagnosis and treatment if needed, and, in equivocal cases, more efficient use of hospital resources (i.e., CT scanning, operating room, and intensive care unit). In addition, further studies need to be undertaken in a prospective randomized fashion to compare laparoscopy, computed tomography, and peritoneal lavage in sensitivity and specificity, as well as from the perspective of cost in both penetrating and blunt trauma. Such studies are currently underway by these and other authors. Some investigators are studying the use of laparoscopy as a triage tool performing this endoscopic test first and then proceeding to laparotomy.

◙ ANATOMY

Laparoscopic evaluation of the abdominal cavity in trauma patients requires a thorough knowledge of the anatomy and how to gain adequate exposure of the intraabdominal organs. Sites of bleeding are most often related to the liver and spleen (Fig. 1) and secondarily to the intestinal mesentery and the retroperitoneum (Fig. 2). The retroperitoneum is difficult to evaluate, and occasionally it may be necessary to mobilize the right or left colon to assess ureteral or vascular injury.

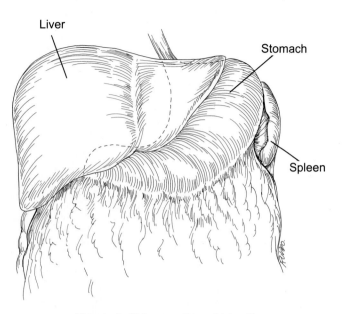

Figure 1. Primary sites of bleeding.

The entire small and large intestines must be observed from the esophageal hiatus to the rectum as it penetrates the pelvic floor. The posterior aspects of these organs may be hard to visualize, but careful observation is mandatory. The use of a 30- and 45-degree laparoscope will help in this assessment as well as the evaluation of the liver and the spleen. The ligament of Treitz can be found at the base of the transverse colon mesentery (Fig. 3). This landmark is important, since mesenteric bleeding may indicate plenic, intestinal, or pancreatic injury. Finally, the head, body, and tail of the pancreas can be observed by entering through the gastrocolic ligament (Fig. 4).

The use of laparoscopy for trauma is limited to the hemodynamically stable patient. Therefore, if one sees an expanding abdomen or a penetrating wound with clear evidence of evisceration, laparoscopy has no role, and the patient should be transferred directly to the operating room.

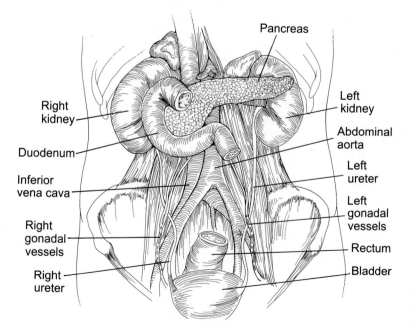

Figure 2. To gain adequate exposure, knowledge of the intestinal mesentery and retroperitoneum is important.

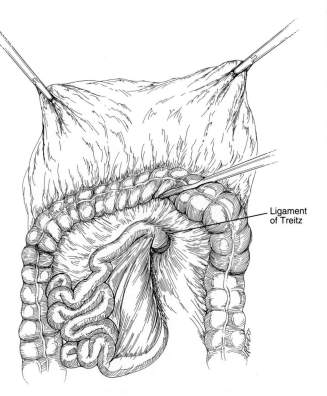

Figure 3. The ligament of Treitz, which is a band of smooth muscle extending from the junction of the duodenum and jejunum to the crus of the diaphragm. Bleeding along this landmark may indicate splenic, intestinal, or pancreatic trauma.

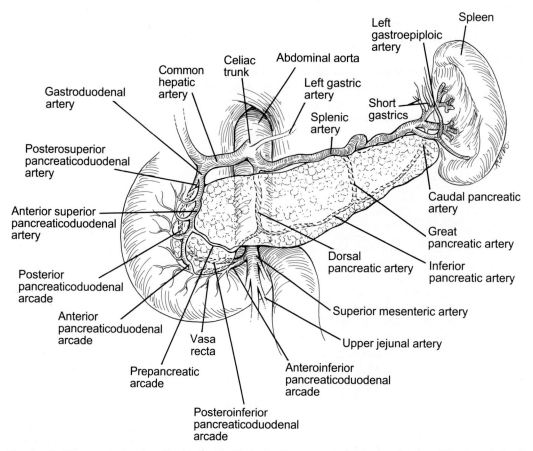

Figure 4. The pancreas is attached anteriorly to the curve of the duodenum. The head, body, and tail can be observed by entering through the gastrocolic ligament.

The choice of whether to insufflate with a Veress needle or Hasson cannula is a personal one, but if there is an umbilical hernia, then the open technique is preferred. In the presence of prior surgical incisions, other sites may be elected for Veress needle insertion (Fig. 5).

The patient should be placed in Trendelenburg position to allow the pelvis to empty and thereby limit the chance of iatrogenic injury.

Additional cannulas should always be inserted under vision and with careful control because trauma can result even when a safety shielded device is used (Fig. 6). The positioning of such cannulas is to accommodate blunt probes to lift organs (Fig. 7) or to irrigate and suction fluid. Ideally, all instruments should be inserted at right angles to the line of sight (Fig. 8).

Obviously, if therapeutic procedures are to be performed (such as suturing) other cannulas may be required. Access to an area by tilting the patient allows

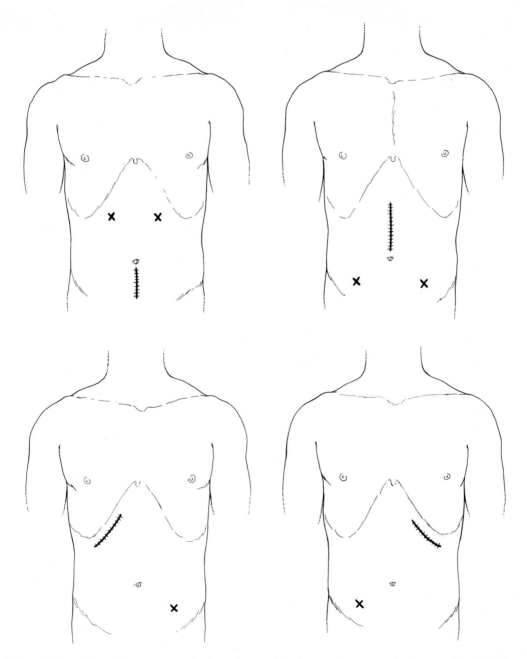

Figure 5. Location of Veress needle insertion points in the presence of prior surgical incisions.

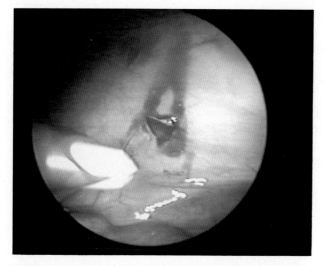

Figure 6. A safety-shielded trocar has been inserted too forcefully, and before the shield could deploy, the device has injured the ''other side'' of the abdominal wall.

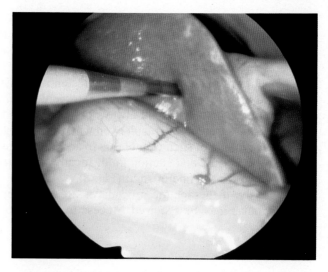

Figure 7. A blunt probe is used to raise the liver.

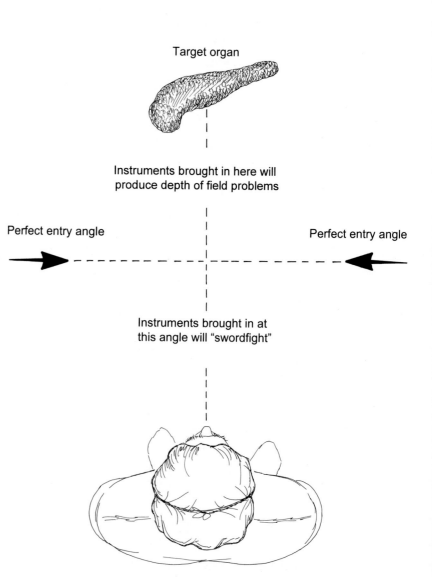

Target organ

Instruments brought in here will produce depth of field problems

Perfect entry angle

Perfect entry angle

Instruments brought in at this angle will "swordfight"

Figure 8. All accessory instruments should be inserted at right angles. If the angle is too acute, one will ''swordfight;'' if too obtuse, depth of field is lost.

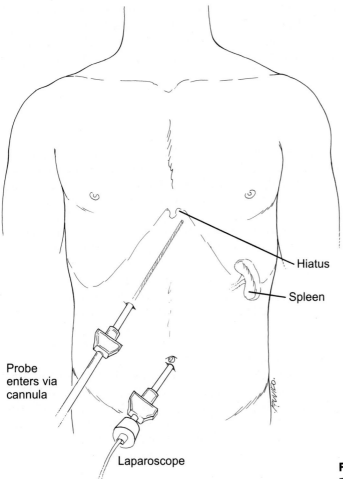

Hiatus

Spleen

Probe
enters via
cannula

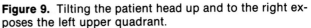

Laparoscope

Figure 9. Tilting the patient head up and to the right exposes the left upper quadrant.

one to see most of the abdomen. For instance, placing the patient head-down will allow the pelvis to be examined, and tilting the patient head-up will expose the upper abdominal organs. By tilting the patient to the left, the right side of the abdomen can be viewed, and, conversely, tilting the patient to the right exposes the left side of the abdomen (Fig. 9). Flexible laparoscopes were used earlier and are now enjoying a renaissance.

▶ PREOPERATIVE PLANNING

The indications for a trauma-induced laparoscopy are the same for a peritoneal lavage. The patient may present with an obscure clinical picture demonstrating questionable physical signs, such as an impaired level of consciousness (head injury, alcoholism, or drug ingestion), evidence of a blunt or penetrating abdominal trauma, unexplained hypotension, or the conscious patient may display equivocal signs during an abdominal examination.

Contraindications

Contraindications depend on the surgeon's experience and judgment but are generally the following: pregnancy, ileus, general peritonitis, morbid obesity, advanced cirrhosis with ascites, and portal hypertension. Obviously unstable patients or those with clear abdominal catastrophe merit immediate laparotomy. It is important for the surgeon to ascertain the goal of the laparoscopy and not waste time if other injuries or medical problems merit immediate attention. Indeed, the surgeon should consider performing the laparoscopy at the time of other interventions, for instance, urgent thoracotomy for bleeding or penetrating wound of the heart.

Instrumentation

Due to the emergent nature of trauma, the required instruments and equipment should be ready at all times and easily accessible, including an endoscopy cart and an instrument tray that is ready at the bedside and is portable so the procedure can be done in the emergency room, intensive care unit, or operating room (7,8).

The centerpiece of the equipment is a mobile cart on which is placed a color video monitor securely bolted in place. Below this is the insufflator with manometer, to which is attached a carbon dioxide cylinder on the back of the cart. A spare cylinder is also on the cart, along with gaskets and a wrench. A xenon light source (150–300 W) is placed on the next shelf along with a half-inch video recorder and, if available, a hard-copy photographic printer for documentation purposes. An irrigation source may also be needed and should be available on the cart. A coagulation device, most commonly monopolar electrosurgery, should also be on the cart or available separately. Finally, spare bulbs, fuses, videotapes, and instrument trays can be kept in the drawer of the cart.

The instrument tray consists of a Veress needle, one 11 and several 5-mm trocars and a 10- and 4-mm laparoscope (preferably a 30-degree forward oblique viewing laparoscope to inspect around corners and up, over, and behind structures). Additionally, a light cable, insufflator, tubing, video camera, coagulation/suction/irrigator probe with required cables and tubing, blunt probe, coagulating forceps, bowel grasping forceps, needle holders, spare suction devices, and sutures for closure.

Location of the Procedure

The procedure can be performed in the emergency room, intensive care unit, or operating room. However, careful patient selection is needed if the operative location is in the emergency room or intensive care unit, as the procedure is more likely to be performed under local anesthesia, and a cooperative patient and knowledgeable staff are required.

Laparoscopy can be performed under local or general anesthesia depending on the patient, the disease process, and location of procedure (9). If local anesthesia is administered, sedation is required, along with a lower pressure pneumoperitoneum (<12 mmHg) and less manipulation of the peritoneal structures to reduce visceral pain stimulation. Frequent monitoring of the patient's blood pressure, pulse, respiration, oxygen saturation, and electrocardiogram (ECG) is mandatory. Generous infiltration of the trocar insertion sites, including the skin, subcutaneous tissue, and peritoneum, with xylocaine or a xylocaine/marcaine mix is done before insertion.

Local anesthesia should not be used in the very young, very old, overly anxious, or uncooperative patient. In these patients, general anesthesia is used, which will secure the airway, thereby allowing for reliable ventilation and end tidal carbon dioxide monitoring. In patients with a history of marginal cardiac or pulmonary function, a pulmonary artery catheter and arterial catheter should be inserted so that the effects of pneumoperitoneum (i.e., decreased cardiac output and increased carbon dioxide) can be monitored.

▼ INTRAOPERATIVE MANAGEMENT/SURGICAL TECHNIQUE

Initial decompression of the stomach with a nasogastric tube and bladder with a Foley catheter is, we feel, mandatory. If the patient is being prepared in the operating room, then sequential compression stockings should also be placed. Antibiotics should be used in conjunction with the normal presentation of the patient.

Generally, in a patient with no previous abdominal surgery, a Veress needle is inserted at the lower border of the umbilicus after a small skin incision is made. The needle is inserted until the top is seen to rise and fall and a click is seen, felt, and heard. The needle position is first checked by aspirating with a syringe to ensure there is no return, injecting saline, which should go in freely with none aspirated back, indicating correct placement within the free peritoneal cavity.

If 10 mm of frank blood or intestinal contents are obtained, the patient should go directly to laparotomy, as in the indications for peritoneal lavage. Insufflation with carbon dioxide is then initiated to a pressure of 10 to 12 mmHg at a flow rate not exceeding 1.51 per minute, the needle is withdrawn, the incision enlarged, and either a 5- or 11-mm trocar is inserted. The latter accommodates a larger (10-mm) scope and allows for better visualization due to more illumination. The smaller (5-mm) trocar is used with a 4-mm scope; in the emergency room or intensive care unit this trocar is used for diagnostic purposes only. If the patient has had prior surgery, then the open laparoscopy technique may be selected with incision of the fascia and peritoneum under direct vision followed by placement of the Hasson 11-mm cannula, which is held in place by stay sutures.

If the closed method of creating pneumoperitoneum has been used, then careful primary trocar placement is vital. With proper patient positioning and use of a probe and suction/irrigator, most areas of the peritoneal cavity can be examined. Also, as described above, tilting allows areas of the abdomen to be seen and should be used in conjunction with dual bowel-grasping forceps to carefully examine the intestine from the ligament of Treitz all the way to the rectum.

The areas that are not well visualized are the bare area of the liver, the spleen (which is usually covered with omentum unless splenomegaly or a splenic hematoma is present), and the retroperitoneum. The pancreas can be visualized by either incising the avascular portion of the gastrocolic omentum to enter the lesser sac or through the foramen of Winslow where a flexible laparoscope may be helpful. However, these are time-consuming maneuvers and are rarely indicated in this situation.

Initially, in penetrating trauma the clinician should scrutinize the patient to ascertain if the peritoneum has been breached and if there is gross evidence of an injury. It is critical to remember the algorithm and the purpose of the laparoscopy (Fig. 10).

Using the suction/irrigator, probe areas of minimal or moderate hemoperitoneum can be irrigated and the source of bleeding investigated. Small liver lacerations can be coagulated or pressure applied. Laparoscopically applied hemostatic agents, such as thrombin gel film or argon beam coagulation, can also be utilized for small liver lacerations. New applications of fibrin glue to large liver lacerations are being investigated and appear promising (11).

Blunt Abdominal Trauma

Using the indications listed above, laparoscopy can be used most effectively in patients who have equivocal findings and can select out those who have stopped bleeding or who may be treated laparoscopically. Hemoperitoneum can be subdivided into four categories (9):

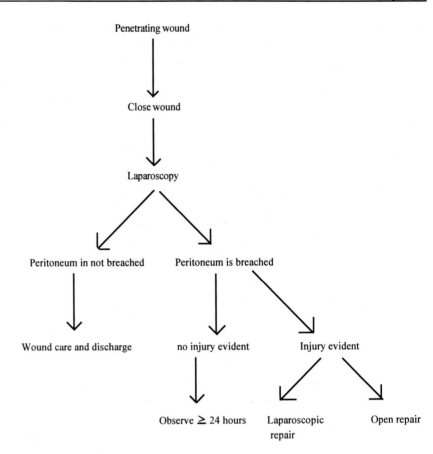

Figure 10. The algorithm for laparoscopy in penetrating trauma.

1. No hemoperitoneum: No blood is seen after thorough examination, and irrigation and suction produce a clear return.
2. Minimal hemoperitoneum: A small volume of blood is in the paracolic gutters or streaking on the loops of intestines. If no blood is seen after irrigation and aspiration, the patient may be observed and laparotomy avoided.
3. Moderate hemoperitoneum: A puddle of blood is in the paracolic gutters and when aspirated, returns. The source of bleeding can be localized laparoscopically and either coagulated if on the liver surface, or sutured if a mesenteric source is found. Brisk bleeding indicates immediate laparotomy.
4. Severe hemoperitoneum: When frank blood is aspirated from the Veress needle or the intestines are floating in a pool of blood, laparotomy is urgent.

Recently, more expanded applications of laparoscopy in blunt abdominal trauma have been reported. At the University of California at Davis, a patient who sustained a boxing injury to the lower left chest and had a class 2A splenic laceration with hemoperitoneum and falling hematocrit was examined laparoscopically. Hemoperitoneum was found and autotransfused back to the patient. There were no other injuries and the spleen was not bleeding, therefore, no laparotomy was done and the patient's blood was recovered laparoscopically and given back in a therapeutic manner (12). In the past, investigators who proposed laparoscopy had found similar uses—before the "laparoscopic revolution." In another study which compared diagnostic peritoneal lavage to diagnostic laparoscopy in 75 patients (13), it was found that laparoscopy had no advantage over diagnostic peritoneal lavage in blunt trauma but had an advantage in penetrating trauma, especially stab wounds. These investigators also found that laparoscopy is a safe procedure that can be performed under local anesthesia in the emergency department.

Penetrating Trauma

Laparoscopy may be useful in patients who are hemodynamically stable and where assessment of the abdomen may be difficult. This is most appropriate in patients sustaining stab wounds or in gunshot wounds where the entry and exit wounds seem compatible with an oblique, superficial trajectory across the abdomen.

The stab site should be sutured and examined laparoscopically to assess if there is any opening in the peritoneum. If there is no hole in the peritoneum, then no intraabdominal injury exists and the examination is complete. If there is an opening in the peritoneum, an additional trocar can be inserted and the abdominal contents examined for injury. If the injury is found, it can be repaired laparoscopically or by laparotomy; if no injury is found, then the patient should be observed for at least 24 hours. Occasionally, it is feasible to insert the cannula directly into the wound, although obviously there is the danger of introducing foreign matter.

Gunshot wounds diagnosed laparoscopically have been managed successfully, especially tangential wounds caused by small-caliber bullets and mostly in obese individuals (14). The entry and exit sites are closed, the peritoneal cavity is examined laparoscopically, and then the wound is debrided in routine fashion. Posterior penetrating wounds are difficult to evaluate and laparotomy should be strongly considered.

▲ COMPLICATIONS

Complications of the laparoscopic technique can be divided into four main areas: trocar and needle placement, energy source injury, dissection injury, and effects of pneumoperitoneum.

Incorrect Needle and Trocar Insertion

Insertion of the Veress needle and trocars can injure the small and large intestines, bladder, stomach, liver, omental vessels, major retroperitoneal vessels, or abdominal wall vessels. Most injuries occur with either the insufflation needle or the initial trocar due to the blind insertion of these instruments. Yuzpe (15) reported 274 needle and trocar injuries: 109 caused by the insufflator needle, 104 by the primary trocar, and 61 by the accessory trocar. Retroperitoneal vessel injury is the most serious and is potentially life-threatening. In a national survey of laparoscopic cholecystectomy by Deziel and colleagues (16), injury to the aorta, inferior vena cava, or iliac vessels occurred in 36 of 77,604 patients for a rate of 0.05%; of these 36 patients, 2 (9%) died from the injury. Early recognition and immediate repair are necessary to decrease morbidity and mortality from this complication. Hemodynamic instability, an expanding retroperitoneal hematoma, and obvious intraabdominal hemorrhage are indications for exploration of vessel injury.

The superior and inferior epigastric vessels may also be injured during insertion of the Veress needle or trocar; this injury is identified when blood is seen dripping along the cannula. The vessel can either be ligated or coagulated from within the peritoneal cavity or by direct suturing through a cutdown over the cannula site. In addition, a bolster-type through-and-through suture of the abdominal wall on either side of the cannula can be done (Fig. 11). To avoid injury, the abdominal wall vessels should be transilluminated before trocar placement and the trocar sites must be closely inspected when the trocars are removed.

Intestinal injury is reported to occur in 1 per 1,000 laparoscopic procedures. Often diagnosed late, this injury leads to peritonitis and sepsis and increased mor-

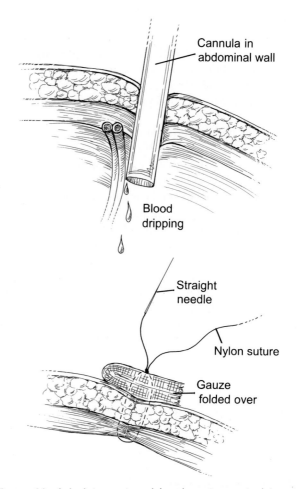

Cannula in
abdominal wall

Blood
dripping

Straight
needle

Nylon suture

Gauze
folded over

Figure 11. A bolster sutured in place to control trocar site hemorrhage.

bidity and mortality (17). Risk factors for intestinal perforation are previous abdominal operations, history of peritonitis, and bowel distention. Veress needle injury is usually apparent when intestinal contents are aspirated upon insertion. The open Hasson technique can then be performed or a new Veress needle inserted in a different location (i.e., right upper or other quadrant apart from adhesions). The perforation site should be examined and repaired if full-thickness laceration of the bowel wall is evident. In contrast to Veress needle injury, trocar intestinal injury is usually full-thickness and requires primary repair. The trocar should be left in the area of injury—to prevent spillage of the enteric content—until the site is identified and repaired.

Bladder injuries are rare and can be avoided by catheter drainage of the bladder intraoperatively. The stomach should be decompressed by orogastric or nasogastric suction to prevent perforation from needle or trocar placement.

In summary, by applying basic laparoscopic principles, needle and trocar injuries can be avoided, as follows:

1. Decompressing stomach and bladder by catheter drainage.
2. Placing the patient in reverse Trendelenburg position.
3. Using an alternative entrance site for the Veress needle or an open Hasson technique if there are incisions near the umbilicus (although the Hasson technique may be difficult if extensive adhesions are present).
4. Aspirating first from the Veress needle and confirming correct position before insufflation.

5. When the first trocar is placed, a careful examination of the needle and/or trocar site is required.
6. All subsequent trocars should be visualized during insertion, and transillumination of the abdominal wall to avoid vessels is important.
7. Examination of the trocar sites during the procedure and upon withdrawal of the cannulas will pick up any abdominal wall vessel bleeding that may need repair.

Cautery/Laser Injury

If unrecognized, thermal bowel injury that occurs during electrosurgery (monopolar and bipolar) or laser use can cause subsequent sepsis and death. Although the use of lasers for laparoscopic cholecystectomy was popular initially, increased expense, longer operative time, and less effective hemostasis have caused a decline in laser popularity. Thermal injuries can occur by direct contact of electrosurgical probes, a poorly insulated shaft to the bowel, or, indirectly, through current flowing through the path of least resistance (which may be adjacent bowel wall rather than the intended tissue), back to the ground electrode on the patient. To reduce thermal injury, the following precautions should be taken:

1. Use the lowest possible setting for coagulation.
2. Inspect probes and other instruments with cautery potential for intact insulation along the entire shaft.
3. Observe the cautery tip at all times during use.
4. Activate the cautery only when it is in contract with the target tissue.
5. Keep the cautery tip and shaft away from bowel during the procedure.

Dissection Injury

Mechanical perforation due to manipulation and dissection injury can occur with laparoscopic instruments if improperly applied with the wrong instrument for the job or with too much force on the tissue. A study by Levy and colleagues (18) of gross and histologic bowel injuries during laparoscopy revealed that many of the injuries that were thought to have occurred from cautery injury were actually mechanical perforations from laparoscopic instrumentation. These can be avoided if the instruments are introduced and used under full view and the correct instrument is used for retraction, dissection, or grasping without excessive force.

Effects of Pneumoperitoneum

The effects of pneumoperitoneum are usually well tolerated by most patients, but in the elderly or those with limited cardiopulmonary reserve, they can cause significant hemodynamic changes (10). Pneumoperitoneum causes an increase in carbon dioxide and a lowering of the pH, which may lead to cardiac dysrhythmias. It can also decrease total lung compliance and functional residual capacity. Areas of ventilation-perfusion mismatch can occur due to compression of the lung bases and when the Trendelenburg position is used for pelvic or lower abdominal laparoscopy (19,20). Cardiac output and central venous pressures decrease with a pneumoperitoneum greater than 20 mmHg (21), and can either increase or decrease based on whether or not the patient is hypovolemic or is in the Trendelenburg or reverse Trendelenburg position (22). In addition, venous stasis is enhanced by the reverse Trendelenburg position and increased intraabdominal pressure, resulting in a higher risk of deep venous thrombosis and pulmonary embolus. This risk can be decreased by the use of pneumatic compression devices to the lower extremities during all laparoscopic procedures.

SURGICAL PEARLS

The amount of intraabdominal bleeding should be carefully evaluated. Continued bleeding will most likely require a laparotomy.

Laparoscopy for stab wounds will help exclude patients with no intraabdominal damage.

Laparoscopy for gunshot wounds may similarly be valuable if the bullet is small caliber, the patient is obese, or the course of the wound suggests the abdominal cavity has been missed.

In blunt abdominal trauma, the main role of laparoscopy is to exclude or grade the hemoperitoneum.

Posterior penetrating injuries are difficult to evaluate laparoscopically, since injury to the small and large intestines may be inadvertently missed in over 50% of the cases.

The aims of the laparoscopy should be clearly defined before commencing—the emergency room is no place for a long and meaningless search.

Pneumothorax and pneumomediastium are also possible complications of pneumoperitoneum. This can occur by injury to the diaphragm or by dissection of carbon dioxide through the retroperitoneal tissues and mediastinum to the pleural and mediastinal space. If there is a sudden increase in ventilatory pressure or desaturation, then a pneumothorax should be suspected and placement of a thoracostomy tube is indicated to prevent tension pneumothorax and to reexpand the lung.

The effects of pneumoperitoneum can be reduced if the intraabdominal pressures are kept below 15 mmHG. In the elderly, who may have reduced compensatory mechanisms, and in patients with reduced cardiopulmonary reserves, pulmonary artery and arterial catheters should be used to monitor and direct treatment of the effects of pneumoperitoneum. Mechanical ventilation, end tidal carbon dioxide monitoring, oxygen saturation monitoring along with blood pressure, ECG, and temperature monitoring, should be standard, as the constant insufflation causes cooling.

☑ CONCLUSION

Diagnostic laparoscopy has been available for over 90 years as a direct view into the peritoneal cavity. Through recent advancements in the laparoscope, video imaging, and instrumentation, diagnostic and therapeutic maneuvers can be accomplished by "minimally invasive surgery." All specialties have seen increasing uses for laparoscopic surgery. The use of laparoscopy in trauma has been expanded from merely a diagnostic tool to a therapeutic modality in selected cases. This has resulted in a quicker and more specific diagnosis and avoidance of unnecessary laparotomies in many studies. Further prospective studies are needed that compare laparoscopy, CT imaging, diagnostic peritoneal lavage, ultrasound imaging, and other modalities. However, the technique (including methods of reducing the possible complications of the procedure itself) and interpretation of laparoscopic findings should be integrated in general surgery resident training and become a part of the trauma surgeon's skills in diagnosing and treating injured patients.

REFERENCES

1. Gazzaniga A, Stanton W, Bartlett R. Laparoscopy in the diagnosis of blunt and penetrating injuries to the abdomen. *Am J Surg* 1976;131:315–318.
2. Carnevale N, Baron N, Delany HM. Peritoneoscopy as an aid in the diagnosis of abdominal trauma: a preliminary report. *J Trauma* 1997;17:634–41.
3. Root HO, Hauser D, McKinley C, LaFave J, Mendiola R. Diagnostic peritoneal lavage. *Surgery* 1965;57:633–637.
4. Du Priest RW Jr, Rodriguez A, Khaneja SC, Soderstrom C, Maekawa K, Agella R, Cowley R. Open diagnostic peritoneal lavage in blunt abdominal trauma victims. *Surg Gynecol Obstet* 1979; 148:890.
5. Cox EF. Blunt abdominal trauma: a 5 year analysis of 870 patients requiring celiotomy. *Ann Surg* 1984;199:467.
6. Federele M, Crass A, Brooke J, Trunkey D. Computed tomography in blunt abdominal trauma. *Arch Surg* 1982;117:645.
7. Sherwood R, Berci G, Austin E, Morgenstern L. Minilaparoscopy for blunt abdominal trauma. *Arch Surg* 1980;115:672.
8. Sackier JM. Laparoscopy in the intensive care unit patient. In: Brooks D, ed. *Current techniques in laparoscopy*. Philadelphia: Current Medicine, 1994.
9. Berci G, Sackier JM, Paz-Partlow M. Emergency laparoscopy. *Am J Surg* 1991;161:332–335.
10. Paw P, Sackier JM. Complications of laparoscopy and thoracoscopy. *J Intern Care Med* 1994;9: 290–304.
11. Ishitani MB, McGahren ED, Sibley DA, Spotnitz WD, Rodgers BM. Laparoscopically applied fibrin glue in experimental liver trauma. *J Pediatr Surg* 1989;24:9:867–871.
12. Smith RS, Meister RK, Tsoi E, Bohman H. Laparoscopically guided blood salvage and autotransfusion in splenic trauma: a case report. *J Trauma* 1993;34:313–314.
13. Salvino C, Esposito T, Marshall W, Dries D, Morris R, Gamelli R. The role of diagnostic laparoscopy in the management of trauma patients: a preliminary assessment. *J Trauma* 1993;34:506–515.

14. Sosa J, Sims D, Martin L, Zeppa R. Laparoscopic evaluation of tangential abdominal gunshot wounds. *Arch Surg* 1992;127:109–110.
15. Yuzpe AA. Pneumoperitoneum needle and trocar injuries in laparoscopy: a survey on possible contributing factors and prevention. *J Reprod Med* 1990;35:485–490.
16. Deziel DJ, Millikan KW, Economou G, et al. Complications of laparoscopic cholecystectomy: results of a national survey of 4,292 hospitals and analysis of 77,604 cases. *Am J Surg* 1993;165: 9–14.
17. Wolfe BM, Gardiner BN, Leary BF, Frey CF. Endoscopic cholecystectomy: an analysis of complications. *Arch Surg* 191;126:1192–1198.
18. Levy BS, Soderstrom RM, Dail DH. Bowel injuries during laparoscopy: gross anatomy and histology. *J Reprod Med* 1985;30:168–172.
19. Wittgen CM, Andras CH, Fitzgerald SD, et al. Analysis of hemodynamic and ventilatory effects of laparoscopic cholecystectomy. *Arch Surg* 1991;126:997–1000.
20. Verischelen L, Serreyn R, Rolly G, et al. Physiopathologic changes during anesthesia administration during gynecological laparoscopy. *J Reprod Med* 1984;29:697–700.
21. Motew M, Ivanovich AD, Bieniarz J, et al. Cardiovascular effects and acid-base and blood gas changes during laparoscopy. *Am J Obstet Gynecol* 1973;115:1002–1012.
22. Sibbald WJ, Paterson NAM, Holliday RL, et al. The Trendelenburg position: hemodynamic effects in hypotensive and normotensive patients. *Crit Care Med* 1979;7:218–224.

GALLBLADDER

important for the
these alternatives,
garding these issue

A patient with t
with less specific s
evaluation for conf
documented acalcu
unless prohibitive
tion, selected patic
tomy in several clir
suppressive therap
a prolonged period
in this latter categ
solitary gallbladde
stones. Studies ha
stones will develo
small but not insig
disease as their in
elective cholecyste
candidates and hav
mellitus has histor
this setting, more
symptomatic chol
bid complications

Contraindicatio
have decreased in
contraindications
Patients with adv
general anesthesia
methods where ap
for cholecystecton
in this setting, th
complications, as
there are several i
tomy in the settin
data at this time t
pneumoperitoneu
obese patients ca
conferred benefit,
and placement, ai
omy. Prior abdom
indication, depenc
rience. Finally, in
accessible via lap
tings, the surgeon
assessment of his
tomic risks the la

▼ INTRAOPERA

Final preopera
antibiotic prophyl
and application ol
prophylaxis. In pa
laxis is added.

relatively normal a
may reveal gallsto
appropriate sympto
out undergoing pla
liver function stud
the above complair
cystitis will often
can help to define
hepatocellular dise

Other laborator
ate in excluding e
the nature of the p
intestinal contrast
lography, and car
classic clinical set
is less specific. Th
tomy, since this t
laparotomy in the

Another issue
acalculous cholec
symptoms of bilia
tions. In this settir
fraction (GBEF)
phy. When perfo
35% has been sh
This study is les
historical evaluati
distinguish betwe
ter of Oddi dysfu
der. Nevertheless
toms and an abn
preoperative sph
unlikely to respor
associated with a
In addition, the l
scopic sphincter
overlap in the in
significant numbe
try eventually rec
scopic sphincter
with typical sym
pathology and th
cholangiography
function, with th
may dictate fur
sphincterotomy.

A final point
ative endoscopic
siderable enthus
oscopic cholecy
fact that preope
possibility of co
was identified ir
gery by preope
carry less weigh
become a reality

in th
post
altho
ing i
divis
brar
"ca
and
on t
mult
surf
4).

sup

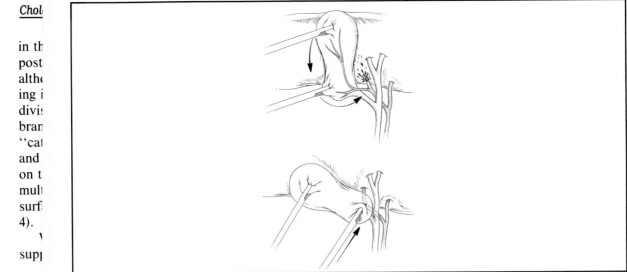

13

Cholecystectomy in Chronic Cholecystitis

John D. Mellinger
Department of Surgery,
St. Mary's Health Services
Grand Rapids, Michigan 49503

Operative Laparoscopy and Thoracoscopy, edited by B. V. MacFadyen, Jr. and J. L. Ponsky. Lippincott-Raven Publishers, Philadelphia © 1996.

Once the patient is in the operating room and anesthetized, a Foley catheter and oral-gastric tube are placed to decompress these structures before laparoscopic access. The patient should be well secured to the table, using footboards, shoulder braces, and safety straps as necessary, to allow changes in patient position that the operation may require. The patient is then antiseptically prepared from the nipples to the groin and from table to table. Towels are then positioned to allow wide exposure from the right midaxillary line to the left of the midline, and from the chest wall above the right costal margin to the right lower quadrant. Towel clips are avoided in the epigastric area to prevent interference with cholangiography. A Mayo stand is often placed over the patient's upper chest prior to placement of the laparotomy drape, and can serve as an area for the surgeon to keep the instruments he is using available on a rotating basis (e.g., suction-irrigator, scissors, clip applier, hook, or spatula).

I use the commonly employed operating room organization as depicted (Fig. 6). Important additional points with regard to operating room configuration and setup include the immediate availability of laparotomy instruments, and the use of an operating table equipped for static film cholangiography or, ideally, real time C-arm or overhead fluorocholangiography. Carts especially designed to house video monitors as well as ancillary equipment such as insufflators, suction-irrigation pumps, light source, camera, and electocautery apparatus are helpful in simplifying operating room organization. Other options to this configuration include placing the patient in a modified lithotomy position with the surgeon standing between the patient's legs, as has been popularized in Europe.

Specific instrumentation requirements for the procedure include high-resolution video monitors, carbon dioxide insufflators capable of delivering flow rates of at least 4 l per minute, and a high-intensity xenon light source. I also find a pressurized suction-irrigation apparatus highly valuable in certain circumstances, particularly if troublesome bleeding is encountered, although this is not necessary in most instances. It is also helpful to have a variety of cautery-adaptable dissecting

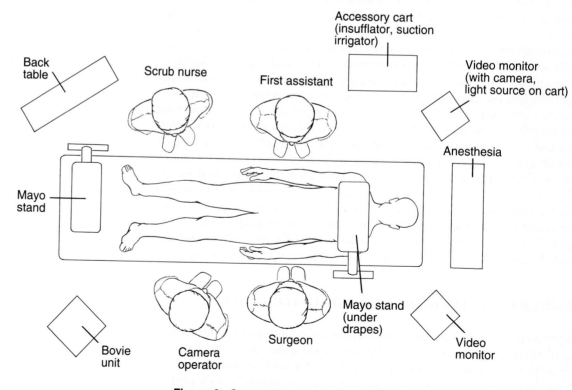

Figure 6. Operating room configuration.

tools, graspers, control devices such as clip applier and suture, trocars with adapters, and cholangiography equipment reviewed by the surgeon at the start of the case. This minimizes the frustration of the surgeon and operative team during the procedure if a particular device is needed but not already at hand. It is critically important for the surgeon to be proficient at "trouble-shooting" video, optic, insufflation, and thermal equipment malfunctions when they occur, and this is often best accomplished by a thorough inspection prior to the start of the procedure.

It is our preference to use the technique of open laparoscopy routinely. By using this approach, the surgeon can standardize his operative sequence whether in a virgin or reoperative setting, has complete assurance regarding safe peritoneal entry, and is almost always able to remove the gallbladder expeditiously through an appropriately sized fascial incision at the completion of the procedure. A 2-cm, transverse, or longitudinal skin incision is made at the infraumbilical margin and the subcutaneous tissues are developed bluntly at the cephalad extent of the incision to the point where the umbilical dermis is most closely approximated to the underlying linea alba. In morbidly obese patients, patients with prior lower abdominal surgery, or patients with an unusually long torso, it may be necessary to place this incision above the umbilicus. Once the fascia is visualized, it is grasped with a Kocher clamp and elevated into the wound. Using this method, subcutaneous retractors are rarely necessary. A second Kocher clamp is applied below the other and the fascia opened with Mayo scissors or a scalpel for a distance of approximately 2 cm between the two clamps. In thin patients, the peritoneum can be similarly opened in immediate sequence. In more obese patients, who often harbor a well-developed preperitoneal adipose layer, it may be necessary to reapply the Kocher clamps and delineate the peritoneum further before incising it. A Hasson-type trocar works nicely in this setting. Our own practice is to place two absorbable sutures in figure-of-eight fashion at the superior and inferior margins of the fascial incision, position a standard 10-mm trocar without its pointed internal obturator into the peritoneal cavity between these untied sutures, and then to tighten the sutures down onto the fascia using short segments of rubber tubing and a Rommel tourniquet technique. This facilitates opening of the incision for gallbladder removal and allows the preplaced sutures to be used for fascial closure at completion of the case. It is helpful to place the trocar in at the angle it will occupy for the majority of the case before tightening these sutures, in order to minimize leakage of pneumoperitoneum during the procedure.

The closed technique using a Veress needle is certainly an acceptable and time-attested alternative means of achieving peritoneal access for pneumoperitoneum. The needle is checked for a smoothly functioning spring mechanism and then introduced through the infraumbilical skin incision. At the fascial level, the tip of the needle is directed in a cephalad direction until the needle tip is felt to catch on the relatively thin subumbilical fascia. The needle is then maintained in this "engaged" position by gentle pressure and redirected toward the pelvis, away from the sacral promontory, and advanced with steady pressure. If in the true midline, the surgeon will often be able to sense two distinct "pops" as the needle traverses the fascia and peritoneum. If this technique is used in the reoperative setting, alternative sites of puncture away from prior surgical scars or a preoperative ultrasonic visceral slide test should be employed to minimize the risk of underlying visceral injury. Aspiration, flushing, and a saline drop test are routinely performed before attempting carbon dioxide insufflation through the needle.

Whatever the means of peritoneal access, carbon dioxide insufflation is commenced at a flow rate of not more than 2 l per minute. This helps to minimize the possibility of vasovagal reactions, which have been described with rapid peritoneal distention in the setting of high-flow initiation of pneumoperitoneum. This is especially important when the open technique is used, since high-flow rates are easily achieved through the larger caliber trocar. Initial low flow also minimizes the chance of overwhelming gas embolism if needle or trocar placement is faulty, and helps protect against large-volume insufflation into the preperitoneal space or other areas of aberrant placement. Careful monitoring of initial pressure readings is mandatory, and insufflation should be stopped immediately and placement checked if initial pressures >5 mmHg are noted. Pressure limits not exceeding 15 mmHg are employed throughout the procedure, with good exposure being possible in most instances with limits in the 10–12 mmHg range. Ongoing assessment of the distribution of pneumoperitoneum by observation and percussion is also important during the initial phases of insufflation. It is useful for the surgeon and anesthesiologist to communicate during this phase of the procedure to monitor hemodynamic responses to pneumoperitoneum. This communication should continue during the conduct of the operation, with particular reference to the patient's acid-base and carbon dioxide excretion status, especially in the setting of underlying cardiopulmonary disease. Typically, adequate pneumoperitoneum is achieved after 3–4 l of insufflation, with this being dependent on patient size and abdominal wall muscle tone. Again, we feel that many of the above concerns with safe initiation of pneumoperitoneum are well-addressed by routine use of the open technique, and this is our standard practice.

Once pneumoperitoneum is achieved, the laparoscope (10 mm) is introduced and a general abdominal visual inspection performed. If the Veress needle is utilized, the operator will, or course, have to first position an umbilical trocar, using similar anatomic precautions to those described above. It is our preference to use radiolucent disposable trocars, although well-maintained reusable trocars are equally acceptable and are adaptable to cholangiography by positional change or substitution of the trocar for a radiolucent obturator (prefabricated or made from available suction tubing) at the time of the cholangiogram. It is worth emphasizing that while the shield devices on many reusable trocars may help minimize the risk of trocar-induced visceral injury, there is a large historical volume of diagnostic and gynecologic laparoscopic experience, which attests to low rates of visceral injury using standard, reuseable trocars, and careful placement technique. The technique of careful placement under conditions of adequate pneumoperitoneum

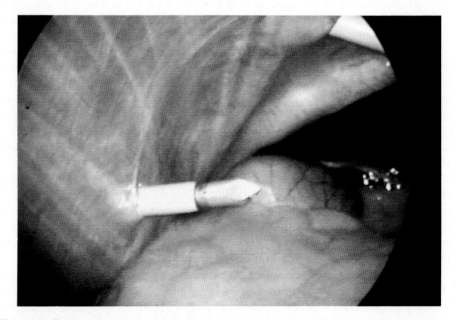

Figure 7. Trocar placement under laparoscopic visualization; note incomplete activation of safety shield.

and laparoscopic visualization of trocar peritoneal entry, rather than shield devices, is the key to safe placement (Fig. 7).

In this regard, further trocars are placed in the right paramedian epigastrium (10 mm), right midclavicular line just below the costal margin (5 mm), and right anterior axillary line between the umbilicus and right costal margin (5 mm) (Fig. 8). Each of these is placed under laparoscopic visualization after transillumination of the abdominal wall to identify and avoid injury to prominent subcutaneous or epigastric vessels in the respective areas of trocar placement. Skin incisions are made just large enough to allow facile trocar introduction, and mild subcutaneous bleeding is controlled either by trocar placement and tamponade or subcutaneous injection of epinephrine-containing local anesthetic. Placement is sometimes facilitated by blunt spreading of the subcutaneous tissues to the fascial level with a hemostat prior to trocar introduction, and this may also minimize the likelihood of subcutaneous vessel injury. The site of planned trocar penetration of the peritoneum in each of these locations must be cleared of any adhesions, even if nonvisceral in nature, before trocar introduction. In instances of extensive adhesion formation, this may require placement of initial trocars in other locations to allow adhesiolysis to be accomplished. The epigastric trocar is usually positioned just to the right of the falciform ligament, taking care not to directly penetrate this structure and increase the likelihood of vessel injury or subsequent internal hernia formation. If the falciform ligament is unusually large, placement of the epigastric trocar to the left of the ligament may be useful in allowing it to be elevated anteriorly and out of the laparoscope's area of domain during the subsequent conduct of the operation.

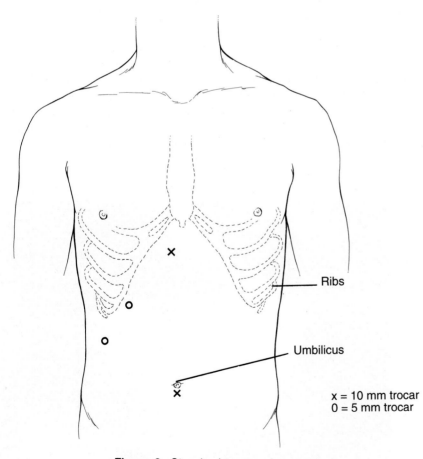

Figure 8. Standard trocar placement.

Following trocar placement, the fundus of the gallbladder is grasped by the surgeon and elevated via the epigastric trocar, and is then handed off to a grasper placed through the anterior axillary line trocar by the assistant (Fig. 9). The assistant then further elevates the fundus anteriorly and cephalad by advancing the grasper up toward the dome of the right hemidiaphragm. Optimal exposure, especially in overweight patients, is often facilitated by placing the patient in a slight reverse Trendelenburg position. All instrument introductions and withdrawals throughout the entire procedure are made under direct laparoscopic visualization, requiring continual vigilance on the part of the camera operator and appropriate communication and coordination on the part of surgeon and assistant. Adhesions to the inferior aspect of the gallbladder are not infrequently encountered, and if present are mobilized by the surgeon until the infundibulum of the gallbladder is clearly visualized. This dissection usually does not require cautery, although thermal energy may be used if the adhesions are vascular and are clear of surrounding visceral structures, notably the transverse colon and duodenum.

We employ a standard monopolar electrocautery unit rather than laser for the thermal aspects of the dissection. The latter can certainly be used, although it offers no significant advantages over standard electrocautery, as has been documented in prospective evaluations, and is much more expensive and space-consuming. For those portions of the procedure in which thermal energy is employed, it should be used for brief (1- to 2-second) pulses, utilizing the minimal power unit settings required to achieve tissue coagulation. All conductive parts of the coagulating instrument must be within the laparoscopic visual field, and the active point of the coagulating device must be in contact only with the tissue to be coagulated and away from any conductive objects, such as clips or metallic trocars. Inadvertent thermal injuries, including delayed ductal injuries and strictures, as well as inadvertent visceral injuries, will be avoided by following these precautions assiduously.

Once the infundibulum is clearly visualized, this is grasped and retracted laterally to open up the region of the hepatobiliary triangle. Hunter has appropriately emphasized that this right lateral retraction on the gallbladder infundibulum or neck may help minimize the potential for common duct injury, since cephalad retraction on this area tends to place the cystic duct and common duct in immediate and parallel proximity. The assistant generally performs this retraction using the midclavicular trocar, although it is acceptable and, in some cases, preferable for the surgeon to manipulate this area so as to have two-handed, coordinated control

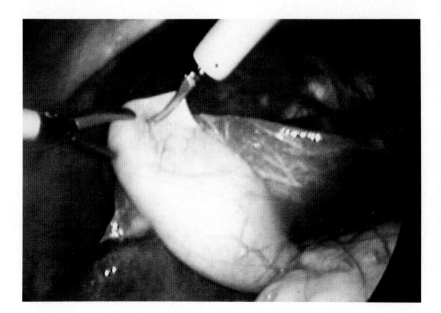

Figure 9. Handoff maneuver, allowing assistant to obtain wider purchase of fundic tissue for subsequent retraction.

of the dissection of the hepatoduodenal ligament. It is important not to place this grasper on the presumed area of the infundibulum if this is not clearly visible, since mistaken placement on more distal structures may mislead the surgeon into inadvertent dissection of the common duct and predispose to ductal injury. If the gallbladder is quite distended or the infundibulum large or redundant, several options may be helpful in ensuring adequate exposure. Use of a larger, atraumatic grasping forceps will often facilitate a more secure purchase of the enlarged organ and be sufficient (Fig. 10). Other options include applying the fundic retractor more distally on the body of the gallbladder, which may achieve a mechanical advantage in lifting the more distal gallbladder out of the hepatorenal fossa, placing a fifth trocar to allow simultaneous bimanual manipulation by the assistant and surgeon, or aspirating the gallbladder with a long spinal needle or laparoscopic aspiration needle. We have on rare occasion employed a "homemade" fixed infundibular elevator in such instances, made by passing a standard endoscopic polypectomy snare through a 12-gauge intravenous catheter positioned directly through the abdominal wall. The snare is tightened on the enlarged infundibulum and then placed under moderate anterior tension by placing a hemostat on the catheter-snare complex at the skin level, which keeps the infundibulum in an elevated position while freeing the distal grasper for more focal manipulation.

Once the gallbladder is so appropriately positioned for dissection of the hepatoduodenal ligament, the surgeon first inspects this area closely. It is often possible to identify the ductal and arterial anatomy by simple inspection in the thin patient. In the more obese or chronically inflamed situation, identification of more obvious anatomic landmarks such as Calot's node is often possible, and can help direct the surgeon as the dissection proceeds. Dissection of the hepatoduodenal ligament itself is commenced on the gallbladder by grasping the inferior margin of the ligament on the organ and stripping downward and medially in smooth, sweeping fashion. All dissection should initially be off the gallbladder neck toward the common duct and porta hepatis, so as to minimize undue trauma to the latter structures. Bites of tissue that do not easily sweep away should be reevaluated for structural content before being cauterized or more forcibly manipulated, and, in general, cautery use is avoided during this initial dissection, at least until the ductal and arterial anatomy becomes apparent. The hepatoduodenal ligament itself quickly defines into anterior and posterior peritoneal reflections following the initial dissection, and the dissection continues by limiting the bites of tissue grasped to these defined leaves of mesothelium and adherent fibroareolar tissue.

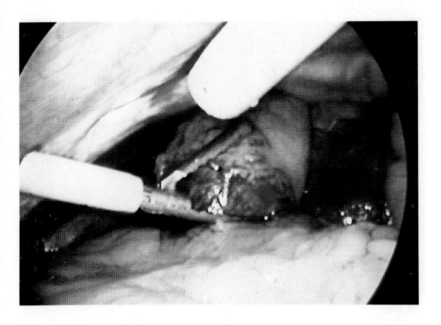

Figure 10. Wide-angled atraumatic grasper being positioned to control redundant and distended infundibulum.

Successive identification and dissection of these peritoneal investments is facilitated by alternating lateral (for the anterior leaf), and cephalad-medial (for the posterior leaf) retraction of the infundibulum by the assistant (Fig. 11). Use of a 30-degree laparoscope can also facilitate specific visualization of these anatomic areas, and should be employed routinely in situations where the anatomy is not clear, since simple rotation of the laparoscope can allow anteroposterior and mediolateral alterations in the field of view. This alternating, blunt, highly focal dissection is continued until the gallbladder neck and gallbladder-cystic duct junction are freely mobilized. In instances of dense fibrosis, the dissection may need to be carried up onto the gallbladder to achieve such mobility, and this can be done safely before arterial control if the dissection is kept at the peritoneal investment level. If peritoneal or fibrotic tethering of the infundibulum to the cystic duct or more medial structures is encountered, these attachments are similarly mobilized with facility after the gallbladder neck has been mobilized as described. If the attachments are unusually thick or tenacious and resist gentle, deliberate dissection, the surgeon may attempt transcystic cholangiography to further define the anatomy, or may choose to convert to an open procedure. The decision to so convert should never be viewed as a failure, but rather as mature judgment, appropriately utilized in the patient's best interests when operative findings preclude confident continuation of the laparoscopic approach. In general, if the surgeon finds himself tempted to use ablative cautery or forceful dissection to free tissue too resistant to respond to normal dissection during this early portion of the procedure, he should consider conversion before proceeding further.

Once the neck and cystic duct junction are so mobilized, with the infundibulum retracted laterally, the surgeon continues to dissect until the inferior margin of the proximal cystic duct is well visualized. If an arteriolar structure is encountered prior to clear identification of the cystic duct, it may be one of the cystic artery anatomic variants previously described, and if this can be clearly demonstrated, the structure may be controlled with clips and divided. Care should be taken, however, in this instance. A. M. Davidoff has identified a classic pattern of common bile duct injury, which includes early identification and division of an arterial structure, presumed by the surgeon to be the cystic artery, which appears to cross over a ductal structure presumed to be the cystic duct. In this instance, the vessel turns out to be supplying the common hepatic duct, which is subsequently divided as the surgeon proceeds in his mistaken medial plane of dissection. It is thus

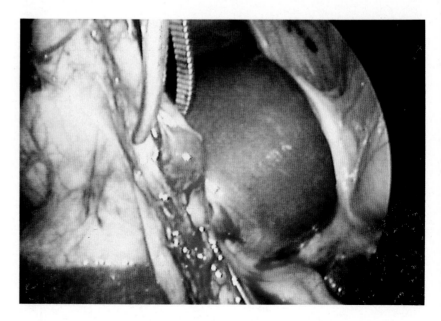

Figure 11. Both anterior and posterior leaves of the hepatoduodenal ligament are demonstrated in lower portion of visual field, with intervening fibroaerolar tissue between the two, as the gallbladder neck is retracted in a cephalad and medial direction. Note node of Calot near dissector.

prudent for the surgeon to carefully reassess if an artery is encountered early, and not to proceed laparoscopically if the anatomy appears confusing.

At this point, the dissecting instrument is insinuated with tips closed adjacent to the superior aspect of the gallbladder-cystic duct junction and "nuzzled" in a plane parallel to the cystic duct so as to open the plane around the duct (Fig. 12). The assistant again can be of help by alternating the direction of infundibular retraction as the surgeon proceeds so the dissector tip can be appreciated posteriorly as the dissection advances. An angled dissector may be of assistance if the hepatobiliary triangle does not open easily with retraction, and the 30-degree laparoscope may help considerably with visualization at this point. Once the dissector has fully circumvented the cystic duct, its tips are opened and the duct itself further dissected and cleaned until a segment suitable for cholangiography and subsequent clip or ligature control is developed. The duct is not cleared all the way to the common duct junction unless this is required to clarify confusing anatomy or the cystic duct is so short as to require such mobilization for adequate control. The surgeon must remain vigilant to avoid tenting the common duct into a "pseudocystic duct" as this is performed. Small, twiglike cystic duct arteries are often encountered in the course of this dissection, and are cleared to allow full duct exposure. Clips and cautery are avoided in most instances without undue difficulty because of the small size of these branches and the potential danger of cautery and encumberance of clips in this area. If obscuring bleeding from these vessels occurs, it is generally able to be observed and irrigated until spontaneous cessation occurs, typically in rapid fashion.

It is our practice to perform routine cholangiography. While studies are available that document the acceptability of selective cholangiography, we are impressed with the benefits of routine performance. These include ongoing facility with the technique for those instances where it is truly necessary, preparation of the surgeon-in-training for more advanced procedures such as transcystic common duct exploration, and protection against common bile duct injury. L. Way has appropriately emphasized that the vast majority of laparoscopic common duct injuries occur in the setting of either omitted or misinterpreted operative cholangiography. In our own experience, 10% of the cholangiograms reveal information not otherwise apparent that affects the patient's subsequent operative or postoperative management. The most frequent finding we have encountered is an otherwise unexpected, unusually short cystic duct, which can, if occult, easily be the beginning of a laparoscopic common duct misadventure.

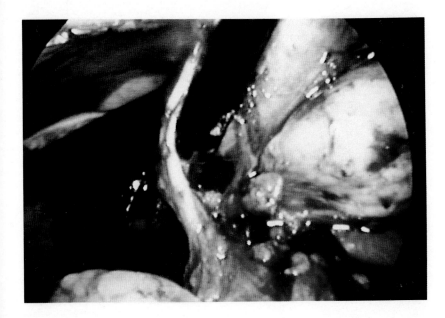

Figure 12. "Nuzzling" technique, with tips of dissector closed, in initial cystic duct circumvention.

The cholangiogram is obtained after first controlling the cystic duct proximally with a clip (Fig. 13). Clips should always be applied on well-defined tissue, taking care to visualize both tips of the clip applier before occlusion of the clip. Our typical practice is to pass the infundibulum to the epigastric port grasper and incise and intubate the cystic duct from the midclavicular port. Scissors are used to partially transect the duct, after which a cholangiogram clamp loaded with a pre-flushed 4 French ureteral catheter is advanced and the duct intubated (Fig. 14). It is frequently helpful to position the clamp immediately anterior to the ductotomy and push the clamp firmly onto the tissue just proximal to this site, as this provides mechanical advantage in introducing the catheter and allows the same to approach the duct at an appropriately tangential angle. Saline flushing of the catheter may facilitate advancement if it engages on valves of Heister. Once in the duct, the catheter is secured by closing the clamp while continuing to flush, closing only so tight as to prevent leakage while maintaining flow. Other techniques include a variety of commercially available balloon-tipped catheters and catheter-trocar systems that do not require use of one of the laparoscopic trocars. A detailed

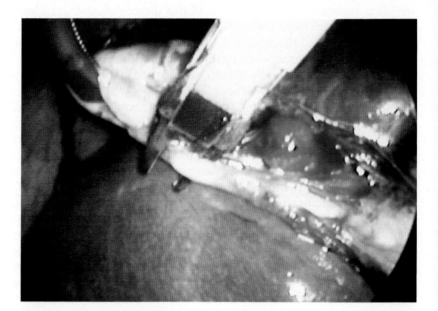

Figure 13. Control of cystic duct as gall-bladder neck with clip. Note lateral retraction of gallbladder neck opening hepato-biliary triangle and clear visualization of tips of clip applier.

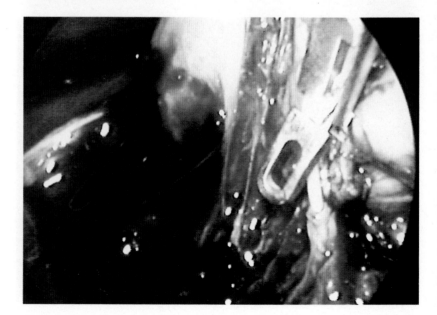

Figure 14. Introduction of cholangio-gram catheter by specially designed clamp.

discussion of cholangiography and its interpretation is in Chapter 18. I would only add that optimal filling of the hepatic radicles often requires placing the patient in Trendelenburg position and/or administration of 3 to 5 mg of intravenous morphine sulfate, which can increase sphincter of Oddi tone and diminish duodenal runoff. If poor duodenal runoff is noted, glucagon (1 mg intravenous) may be tried, especially if narcotics have been used as part of the anesthetic management. Incomplete biliary visualization on cholangiography dictates either further dissection to fully exclude any possibility of hepatic or common duct impingement, or conversion to an open procedure.

After review of the cholangiographic findings, the cholangiography setup is removed, two clips are placed via the epigastric trocar on the cystic duct distal to the ductotomy (Fig. 15), and the duct is divided at the ductotomy site, taking care to incorporate no extraneous or undeveloped tissue within the scissor blades (Fig. 16). The clips must completely incorporate the duct in order to provide reliable closure. If the duct is unusually large, laparoscopic ligatures may provide more secure duct closure on the distal (nonspecimen) side. Failure to visualize

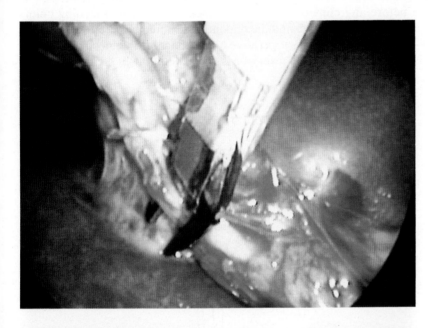

Figure 15. Control of cystic duct with clips distal to ductotomy site.

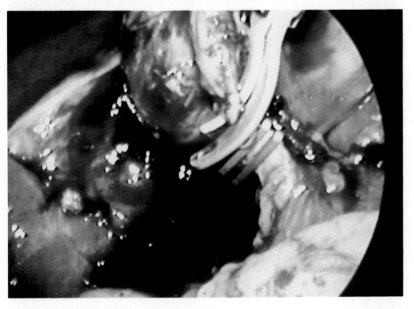

Figure 16. Division of cystic duct between clips; note clear visualization of tips on both scissors blades.

the tips of the scissor blades prior to closure, again using a 30-degree laparoscope if necessary, can lead to inadvertent injury to adjacent structures, including the cystic or right hepatic artery. After division of the duct, the cystic artery is similarly defined, clipped, and divided. It is helpful to watch for and appropriately control both anterior and posterior branches of the cystic artery in the course of this dissection, since failure to completely control the latter is the most frequent reason for troublesome or obscuring bleeding as the gallbladder is mobilized from its hepatic bed. If arterial bleeding is encountered at any time during the hepatoduodenal ligament phase of the dissection, we have found the following immediate sequence most helpful and uniformly successful in achieving rapid control. First, the assistant partially relaxes fundic elevation and simultaneously pushes the infundibular retractor and its incorporated tissue firmly against the area of bleeding (Fig. 17). This maneuver was initially described by S. Ko and M. Airan, and is efficacious. A fifth trocar is then immediately placed near the midline between the umbilicus and epigastric trocar. The surgeon then works bimanually with a dissector and suction-irrigator as the assistant slowly releases the compression. The bleeding point is grasped and elevated by the surgeon and fully delineated as to its source before any clips or ligatures are used to secure it. Bleeding points which appear brisk initially but cannot be reidentified should be carefully searched for, as they can be a source of postoperative hemorrhage. If the bleeding is found to originate from the right hepatic artery or is not expeditiously defined and con-

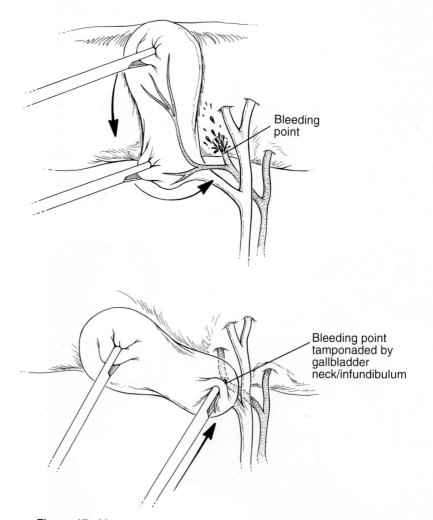

Figure 17. Maneuver to control bleeding in hepatobiliary triangle.

trolled, the procedure is immediately converted to open and formal exploration and repair performed.

The gallbladder can be mobilized from its bed using a variety of tools. Our preference is to use a cautery-adaptable, curved scissors. This allows spatulalike thermal dissection with tips closed or spreading and cutting as appropriate. The assistant changes his axis of retraction by elevating the gallbladder neck in alternating lateral and medial orientations to facilitate exposure of the opposing peritoneal investments of the organ. The surgeon first incises these structures and then dissects the plane of the hepatic bed, being ever-vigilant for nonfibroareolar structures in this plane, which may include the right hepatic artery or branches thereof supplying the gallbladder, accessory bile ducts, and cystic venous channels. Sizeable structures are best controlled with clips or ligatures rather than cautery. A very helpful maneuver for the surgeon in the course of this dissection is to gently push the liver bed tissue off the gallbladder; this often defines the appropriate plane of dissection prior to cautery application, which can obscure the same if applied to inadequately developed tissue. If the assistant maintains the gallbladder under optimal traction, this dissection proceeds expeditiously.

As the dissection approaches the fundus, the assistant may have to use other maneuvers to maintain optimal tension (Fig. 18). Such maneuvers may include "choking up" on the undersurface of the gallbladder by advancing the grasper on the neck up closer to the plane of dissection. The graspers on the gallbladder may also be simultaneously rotated in clockwise or counterclockwise fashion, or splayed in opposing medial and lateral directions, to maintain appropriate exposure and tension. It is occasionally at this point in the dissection that the gallbladder is inadvertently entered and bile spillage occurs. If stones are lost, attempts should be made to retrieve these, since delayed complications including stone migration, erosion, and abscess formation have been reported. Entry is prevented by continued traction by the assistant and patient dissection of the appropriate and precisely defined tissue plane by the surgeon. Laparoscopic retrieval bags or specially designed aspiration cannulas may be useful for stone retrieval if spillage occurs. If gallbladder entry occurs earlier in the dissection, attempts should be made to control the point of injury by occluding it with a grasper, if small and in a location suitable for ongoing retraction, or, more typically, by closing it with an endoscopic ligature.

Just before completing delivery of the gallbladder from its bed, a final inspection of the bed is made to ensure hemostasis is complete and no bile leakage

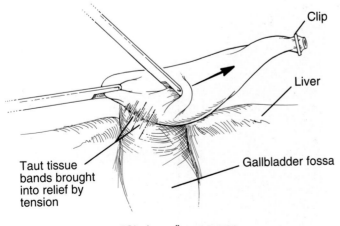

"Choke up" maneuver

Figure 18. "Choke up" and twisting maneuvers to facilitate fundic mobilization (see Fig. 21C).

apparent. The gallbladder is then delivered and placed up over the liver, maintaining the graspers' control of it. The laparoscope is then switched to the epigastric port and a toothed grasper passed via the umbilical port, up to the gallbladder, and used to grasp the gallbladder neck. The other graspers are then released and the gallbladder pulled up into the umbilical trocar as far as it comfortably advances. If the gallbladder is unusually thin, tense, or damaged, it may be placed into a specimen retrieval bag prior to removal to minimize the chance of rupture and spillage in removal. The Rommel tourniquets are then released, and the grasper, umbilical trocar, and gallbladder are removed as a unit under continuous laparoscopic visualization. Once the gallbladder is externally visible, it is grasped with a Kelly clamp and the laparoscopic apparati released from it. Because of the open laparoscopic entry method we employ, it is unusual to have difficulty in removing the gallbladder. If difficulty is encountered due to an unusually tense organ or numerous or large stones, this is most simply, expeditiously, and safely dealt with by enlarging the fascial incision with a scalpel or Mayo scissors applied to the margin of the fascial opening. A finger is inserted into the umbilical site to occlude it and it is inspected laparoscopically. Any remaining irrigation or spilled fluid in the perihepatic area is suctioned, and the 5-mm trocars are removed under laparoscopic visualization (Fig. 19). Significant bleeding is rarely encountered, but, if seen, can be dealt with by placement of a through-and-through suture under protective laparoscopic visualization, or by extension of the skin incision and external wound exploration. The laparoscope is then withdrawn into the epigastric trocar and removed while visualizing the tract during withdrawal. Forceful evacuation of pneumoperitoneum via the trocar sites is avoided by allowing this to occur at the reexplorable umbilical level, so as to minimize the chance of hernia formation at the trocar sites. The umbilical site is irrigated and the preplaced fascial sutures tied. The remaining sites are closed with subcuticular absorbable suture, as is the umbilical skin, and bandaid dressings applied.

In the rare instance where a drain is felt to be necessary, such as when poorly localized bilious drainage is noted from the hepatic bed or cystic duct control has been unusually challenging, this is easily placed by the following technique (Fig. 20). A grasper is advanced via the anterior axillary line trocar directly into the epigastric trocar and, in retrograde fashion, out the external orifice of the same after manual disarming of the valve as the grasper is advanced through it. The tubing end of a 10-mm Jackson-Pratt drain is advanced onto one flange of the grasper, the grasper jaws closed, and the grasper withdrawn all the way out the

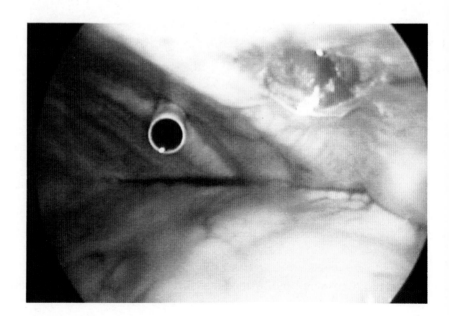

Figure 19. Trocar site inspection at time of trocar removal.

anterior axillary port with the trocar and drain in tow. A grasper through the midclavicular or epigastric ports may then be used to position the drain in the appropriate internal position in Morrison's pouch.

▲ COMPLICATIONS

The most important, specific, technical complications of laparoscopic cholecystectomy include common bile duct injury, hepatic arterial injury, visceral puncture or thermal injury, gallbladder rupture with stone loss and potential delayed complications secondary thereunto, and postoperative bile leak. Most of these are adequately discussed with regard to avoidance and management, should they occur, in the foregoing discussion. Common duct injury and postoperative bile leak are briefly elaborated upon in the comments that follow.

Common bile duct injury has clearly been the Achilles' heel of the laparoscopic method, both in a technical and political sense. To summarize what has been stated previously, this complication can be prevented by adherence to the following principles. The cystic duct must be dissected from the gallbladder neck downward and the gallbladder/cystic duct junction clearly delineated before any clips are applied. Infundibular retraction should be lateral, not cephalad. A 30-degree lapar-

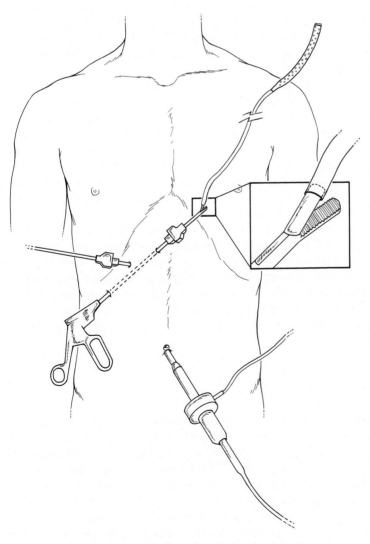

Figure 20. Technique for drain placement.

oscope should be liberally utilized, especially if confusing anatomy is noted. Thermal energy should not be used in proximity to the common bile duct or previously positioned metallic clips or graspers, and if the laser is used, the potential for "backstop" injury must be kept in mind. If bleeding develops, only clearly delineated and identified structures may be controlled with clip or cautery. If this is not possible in expeditious fashion, the case is converted to open before such control is attempted. Cholangiography is used routinely, and inadequate or incomplete cholangiograms dictate either repetition, more thorough dissection to document common duct integrity and safety, or conversion to an open procedure. Finally, if the surgeon is confused or unsure, laparotomy is performed.

If common duct injury does occur, the following points are worthy of emphasis. The problem is most easily dealt with at the time of injury. If the injury is missed and septic complications supervene, it is best to achieve drainage and control of the septic process and leave definitive reconstruction for the elective, prospectively planned setting. Definitive cholangiographic documentation of the injury by ERCP and/or percutaneous transhepatic cholangiography is required before reconstruction, and may allow for temporizing therapeutic stenting or decompression of many injuries. Durable reconstruction usually requires Roux-en-Y choledocho- or hepaticojejunostomy, especially where partial ductal excision or thermal injury has occurred, and the complexity and long-term failure rates are increased as the location of injury progresses proximally. Mucosa to mucosa anastomoses, using fine absorbable suture, are utilized, and the utility and duration of anastomotic stenting remain controversial. Subcutaneous Roux limb extensions are valuable in this setting for future access. Referral to more specialized biliary surgeons should be considered in many of these cases, particularly if the grasper is missed and the patient presents in complicated fashion.

Postoperative bile leak is a less catastrophic and more common complication. It should be suspected when relatively nonspecific complaints such as nausea, abdominal or shoulder discomfort, poor appetite, or abdominal distention alter the typically rapid early postoperative recovery. These symptoms may overlap with those secondary to more serious injuries, such as missed common duct or bowel injury, and the possibility of these problems must also be entertained when bile leak is suspected. The majority of such leaks arise from small sources in the gallbladder bed or from inadequate control of the cystic duct stump. Radionuclide scanning is a useful screening test, and can document the presence of bile leakage, as well as common duct patency. If a leak is evident, it is typically managed by ultrasound or CT scan-guided drainage. Once adequately externalized in this fashion, most such leaks will resolve spontaneously with continued observation. Should the leak be of higher output, a higher grade ductal injury should be suspected. In this setting, ERCP is helpful to delineate the anatomy of the leak, and endoscopically placed stents that obviate sphincter of Oddi resistance and bypass the area of leakage (e.g., cystic duct stump or sizable accessory duct) may accelerate closure.

☑ CONCLUSIONS

A thorough understanding of biliary anatomy and its laparoscopic appearance, fastidious adherence to safety principles, including careful use of thermal energy and continuous maintenance of laparoscopic visualization, routine use of operative cholangiography, and the presence of a premeditated algorithm for preventing and dealing with problems that may arise, including the judgment to know when to say "open," are all critical to the successful performance of laparoscopic cholecystectomy for chronic cholecystitis. Laparoscopic cholecystectomy for chronic gallbladder disease has not only been the midwife of the therapeutic laparoscopy revolution, but will likely remain its most widely applied constituent. What the

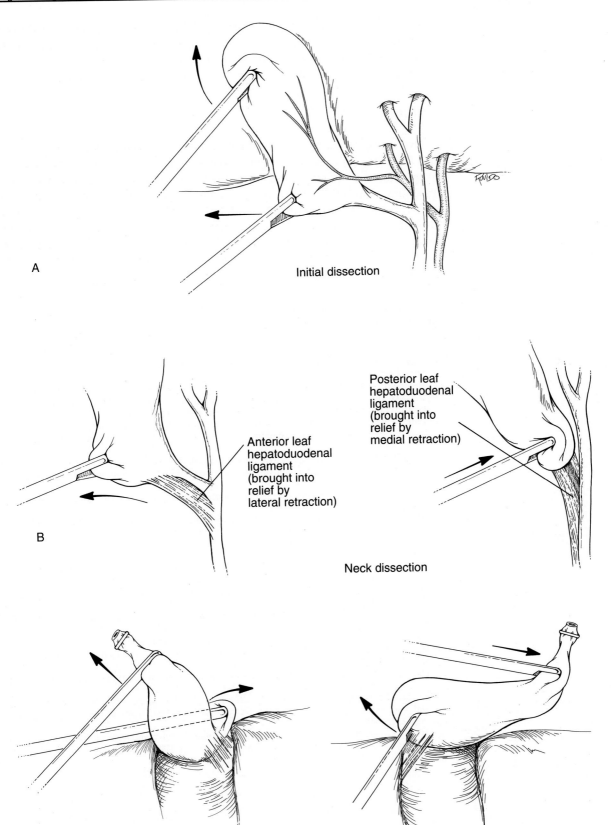

A Initial dissection

B Anterior leaf hepatoduodenal ligament (brought into relief by lateral retraction)

Posterior leaf hepatoduodenal ligament (brought into relief by medial retraction)

Neck dissection

C Opposing tensions

Figure 21. "Pearls" of exposure (initial lateral retraction of neck, followed by alternating medial and lateral retraction of same, followed by opposing tension maneuvers as in Fig. 18).

surgeon does often, he is required to do well. The precepts learned and patterns habitualized from this procedure will, for most general surgeons, form the basis of safety and judgment for all subsequent laparoscopic endeavors. The principles outlined above can serve the surgeon well in laying this foundation.

SURGICAL PEARL

One "surgical pearl" worthy of particular emphasis reiterates the surgical principle that "exposure is everything." Dynamic retraction, which continually seeks to optimize the surgeon's visualization of and mechanical advantage over the presenting anatomy, is the sine qua non of safe and expeditious laparoscopic cholecystectomy. The sequence of initial lateral retraction on the infundibulum, alternating medial and lateral retraction of the same as the gallbladder neck is dissected, and the use of twisting and other opposing means of bimanual retraction as the gallbladder bed dissection proceeds toward completion, will be valuable to the surgeon in this regard (Fig. 21).

RECOMMENDED READING

1. Scott-Conner CEH, Hall TJ. Variant arterial anatomy in laparoscopic cholecystectomy. *Am J Surg* 1992;163:590–592.
2. Hugh TB, Kelly MD. Laparoscopic anatomy of the cystic artery. *Am J Surg* 1992;163:593–595.
3. Berci G. Biliary ductal anatomy and anomalies: the role of intraoperative cholangiography during laparoscopic cholecystectomy. *Surg Clin North Am* 1992;72:1069–1075.
4. Fink-Bennett D, De Ridder P, Koloszi WZ, et al. Cholecystokinin cholescintigraphy: detection of abnormal motor function in patients with chronic acalculous gallbladder disease. *J Nucl Med* 1991;32:1695–1699.
5. Reed DN, Fernandez M, Hicks RD. Kinevac-assisted cholescintigraphy as an accurate predictor of chronic acalculous gallbladder disease and the likelihood of symptom relief with cholecystectomy. *Am Surg* 1993;59:273–277.
6. NIH Consensus Conference. Gallstones and laparoscopic cholecystectomy. *JAMA* 1993;269:1018–1024.
7. Sackier JM, Berci G. Phillips E, et al. The role of cholangiography in laparoscopic cholecystectomy. *Arch Surg* 1991;126:1021–1026.
8. Zucker KA, Bailey RW, Flowers J. Laparoscopic management of acute and chronic cholecystitis. *Surg Clin North Am* 1992;72:1045–1067.
9. Reddick EJ, Olsen D, Spaw A, et al. Safe performance of difficult laparoscopic cholecystectomies. *Am J Surg* 1991;161:377–381.
10. Schirmer BD, Dix J, Edge SB, et al. Laparoscopic cholecystectomy in the obese patient. *Ann Surg* 1992;216:146–152.
11. Soper N, Hunter JG, Petrie RH. Larpaoscopic cholecystectomy during pregnancy. *Surg Endosc* 1992;6:115–117.
12. Ponsky JL. Complications of laparoscopic cholecystectomy. *Am J Surg* 1991;161:393–395.
13. Hunter JG. Avoidance of bile duct injury during laparoscopic cholecystectomy. *Am J Surg* 1991;162:71–76.
14. Davidoff AM, Pappas TN, Murray EA, et al. Mechanisms of major biliary injury during laparoscopic cholecystectomy. *Ann Surg* 1992;215:196–202.
15. Kozarek R, Gannan R, Baerg R, et al. Bile leak after laparoscopic cholecystectomy: diagnostic and therapeutic applications of endoscopic retrograde cholangiopancreatography. *Arch Intern Med* 1992;152:1040–1043.
16. Trerotola SO, Savader SJ, Lund GB, et al. Biliary tract complications following laparoscopic cholecystectomy: imaging and intervention. *Radiology* 1992;184:195–200.

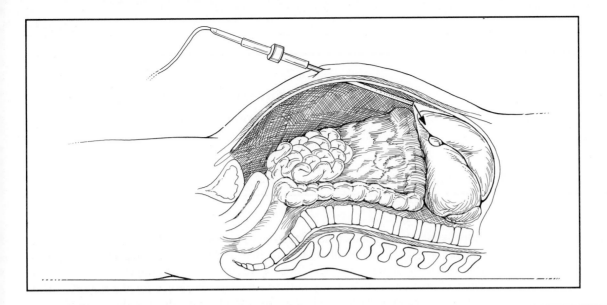

14

Cholecystectomy for Acute Cholecystitis

Douglas O. Olsen
Department of Surgery
Vanderbilt University
Baptist Hospital
Nashville, Tennessee 37203

Operative Laparoscopy and Thoracoscopy, edited by
B. V. MacFadyen, Jr. and
J. L. Ponsky. Published by
Lippincott-Raven
Publishers, Philadelphia, 1996

KEY WORDS

Gangrenous cholecystitis

Phlegmon

Gasless laparoscopy

Golden period

Gallbladder decompression

Sentinel lymph node

Acute hydrops

Infundibulum

Approximately 526,000 cholecystectomies are performed each year in the United States (1). Within this number, 10% to 30% of the patients will present with symptoms of acute cholecystitis (2). Since 1990, there has developed a consensus that laparoscopic cholecystectomy is the procedure of choice for the majority of patients who present with gallbladder disease (3). Yet, despite this general acceptance of laparoscopic cholecystectomy, some still question the application of this technique for the patient who presents with signs of acute inflammation of the gallbladder. This hesitation may be due to the literature reports that still consider acute cholecystitis to be a relative contraindication to laparoscopic cholecystectomy (4). These reports were based on the findings of early series that suggested there was a higher percentage of complications and conversions related to patients with acute cholecystitis (5–7). Therefore, many patients who present with symptoms of acute cholecystitis are denied the advantages of a laparoscopic cholecystectomy.

Patients with acute cholecystitis present certain challenges over those with routine gallbladder disease:

1. A debilitated systemic condition
2. Ileus
3. Inflammatory phlegmon surrounding the gallbladder
4. Distended gallbladder with thickened wall
5. Friable tissues, which bleed
6. Distorted anatomy

Except for the longer operative time that goes along with the increased-difficulty ratio, these problems can be overcome in the majority of cases, which will allow successful completion of the laparoscopic procedure.

Patients with acute cholecystitis can safely undergo laparoscopic cholecystectomy, providing that several criteria are met:

1. Achievement of safe access to the abdominal cavity
2. Maintenance of adequate exposure
3. Absolute identity of the anatomy

When a surgeon has adequate experience and uses good surgical judgment, even the most difficult case can be approached via a laparoscopic method. It is vital that the surgeon adhere to those basic surgical principles that dictate safe surgery, and that he use good judgment to convert to an open procedure when those specific conditions cannot be met.

ANATOMY

As mentioned above, absolute identification of the anatomy is crucial to performing a safe laparoscopic cholecystectomy. The challenges that an acutely inflamed gallbladder poses for the surgeon are perhaps most important in the proper identification of the anatomy. Due to the inflammation and scarring, the normal anatomic relationships can often be distorted, or impossible to recognize. Despite this difficulty, it is still imperative that the surgeon make an absolute identification of the anatomy before he proceeds with ligation and division of structures. Because the gallbladder is an end organ, the intense inflammation and necrosis is usually worst at the distal tip of the gallbladder. Even with an acute necrotizing cholecystitis, if the surgeon can work his way down the gallbladder to the more proximal portions of the organ, he can often find healthier tissues to grasp and work with. The inflammation and scarring can also cause the triangle of Calot to contract, bringing the common hepatic duct into close proximity to the cystic duct. For this reason, great care must be taken in the early dissection and identification of the portal structures. A key landmark that is often overlooked in the standard cholecystectomy is the "sentinel" lymph node that overlies the cystic artery (Fig. 1). This lymph node is very prominent in cases of acute inflammation and very easily identified. Dissection below this structure may lead to potential injury to the common bile duct or common hepatic duct. Keeping the dissection above this point and making an effort to clear the infundibulum of the gallbladder will often give sufficient length in the cystic duct to perform a cholangiogram. Since the pathophysiology of acute cholecystitis is cystic duct obstruction at the neck of the gallbladder, the usual clip that is placed on the neck of the gallbladder can be omitted, allowing the surgeon to perform his cholangiogram as close to the gallbladder as possible. This also minimizes any crush injury to the duct in the event that the common bile duct has been inadvertently cannulated. Because of the distortion of the anatomy with acute cholecystis, cholangiography plays a key role in verifying the anatomy prior to any ligation and division of structures.

▶ PREOPERATIVE PLANNING

Pneumoperitoneum

The indications for laparoscopic cholecystectomy are the same as that for an open cholecystectomy. The only exception might be pregnancy, which is more of a consideration from a medicolegal issue than a technical one. A pregnant

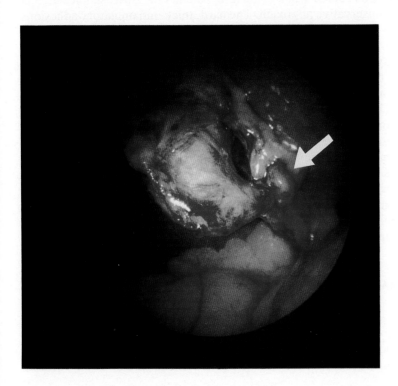

Figure 1. The sentinel lymph node is prominent in acute cholecystitis, and affords an important landmark during the dissection. The dissection should be at or above the level of this lymph node to prevent a possible bile duct injury.

patient presents the ideal situation for considering "gasless" laparoscopy, since the question regarding safety during pregnancy is related to the pneumoperitoneum. There are other rare patients who cannot tolerate a pneumoperitoneum because of underlying cardiopulmonary disease. In that case, the surgeon should carefully monitor the patient's cardiopulmonary parameters during the initial phase of establishing the pneumoperitoneum. If there is any instability in these parameters, the pneumoperitoneum should be vented immediately, and after the patient is stabilized, a second attempt at insufflation can be attempted with a lower pressure setting on the insufflator. If the second attempt fails, then either a "gasless" system can be utilized or a standard open approach be taken.

Preoperative Evaluations

Although there has been a considerable amount of literature addressing the issue of preoperative evaluation to determine which patients fall into the category of a "difficult" cholecystectomy, the preoperative workup and evaluation should be directed to analyzing the patient's systemic state and confirming the diagnosis of acute cholecystitis. This is especially true for the debilitated patient or patients who have comorbid conditions and for whom an operative procedure carries a significant risk. The inaccuracy rate of the preoperative diagnosis for acute cholecystitis can be as high as 25%, when comparing the preoperative diagnosis to interoperative findings and pathology (8). Although ultrasound will accurately confirm the diagnosis of cholelithiasis, it is not an accurate predictor of acute cholecystitis. A radionucleotide hepatobiliary scan is perhaps the most sensitive of studies available to confirm the diagnosis of acute cholecystitis. If the nuclear medicine study is negative, then the surgeon should entertain other explanations for the acute presentation of the patient.

Procedure of Choice

The "golden period" of 72 hours (9) that has been described in open cholecystectomy should be considered when evaluating patients for laparoscopic surgical therapy versus a conservative approach. The hard, thick, inflammatory adhesions characteristic in a patient with several days' history of symptoms, will present a challenge to even the most experienced laparoscopic surgeons. If a patient has a history of acute symptoms dating more than 5 to 7 days, then every attempt to treat the patient conservatively should be considered. This will maximize the chance of being able to undergo a successful laparoscopic operation after the inflammation has had a chance to subside in 4 to 6 weeks.

Criteria for conservative management hinges on the patient's responding to medical therapy and not progressing to a septic state. Fortunately, the majority of patients who have had symptoms for over a week will generally respond to intravenous fluids and antibiotics. The surgeon should not forget the alternatives, which include tube drainage of the gallbladder with interval cholecystectomy. This may be the ideal management strategy for the severely debilitated patient, or the patient who is found to have a significant degree of inflammatory changes that preclude a safe laparoscopic dissection.

▼ INTRAOPERATIVE MANAGEMENT/SURGICAL TECHNIQUE

Anesthesia

All patients should be adequately hydrated and on appropriate antibiotics prior to initiating the operative procedure. General anesthesia should be used in all cases except for the severely debilitated patient who will undergo a laparoscopically guided cholecystostomy. This procedure can be done very nicely under a local anesthetic and has been described elsewhere in detail (10).

Nasogastric suction is especially important in the patient with acute cholecystitis, since many of these patients have a certain degree of ileus due to the underlying inflammatory state, and every effort to enhance the exposure will benefit the patient. A Foley catheter should be considered, since there is often the issue of fluid hydration with the acutely ill patient. If a Foley catheter is not used, then it is imperative that the patient void on call to the operating room to decompress the bladder.

Trocar Placement

The surgical procedure is based on a four-puncture technique, with the primary trocar placed at the umbilicus and three accessory punctures in the right upper quadrant (Fig. 2). Since the acute gallbladder is usually thickened and difficult to extract at the end of the procedure, utilizing an open technique for trocar insertion will not only add to the safety of abdominal access, but will facilitate organ extraction at the end of the procedure. After completion of exploration of the abdominal cavity, the patient is placed in a steep reverse Trendelenburg position with a slight tilt to the left.

The placement of the accessory ports are tailored to the individual clinical situation. The placement of these trocars is more critical in the case of the acute gallbladder, however, since the liver is often edematous and does not retract as easily as a normal liver. In this case, the midclavicular trocar is placed directly

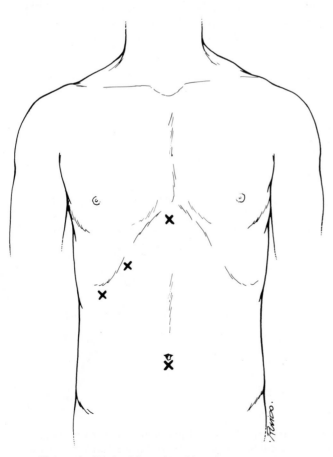

Figure 2. Typical locations for the trocar ports.

over the fundus of the gallbladder, and the lateral trocar is positioned to enter the abdominal cavity just at the lower edge of the liver. The epigastric trocar is positioned as high in the epigastrium as possible, without being above the liver edge, so as to maximize the angle between the telescope and the working instruments (Fig. 3). This will facilitate a clear view of the tips of the instruments and the clip applier when working within the porta hepatis.

Procedural Evaluation

The gallbladder is assessed for the likelihood of a laparoscopic dissection, and *it is at this point* that the surgeon needs to assess the likelihood of being able to carry out the dissection. If the inflammatory tissues have hardened, and will not easily peel off the gallbladder, then a decision needs to be made between proceeding with a cholecystectomy, which at this point will most likely require an open procedure, or performing instead a laparoscopic cholecystostomy. Once the dissection is carried farther than this point, the ability to end with a simple tube cholecystostomy becomes less likely.

Decompressing the gallbladder laparoscopically and allowing the inflammatory process to subside will allow the surgeon to perform an interval laparoscopic cholecystectomy with greater success.

Gaining Exposure

The gallbladder is exposed by bluntly peeling the inflammatory phlegmon off the fundus of the gallbladder (Fig. 4). The earlier in the presentation that the patient comes to the operating room, the easier the peeling of the phlegmon. With the fundus of the gallbladder exposed, the tense inflamed gallbladder is decompressed. This can be done in several ways, including the use of a cyst puncture needle (Fig. 5), a spinal needle inserted through the anterior abdominal wall, or

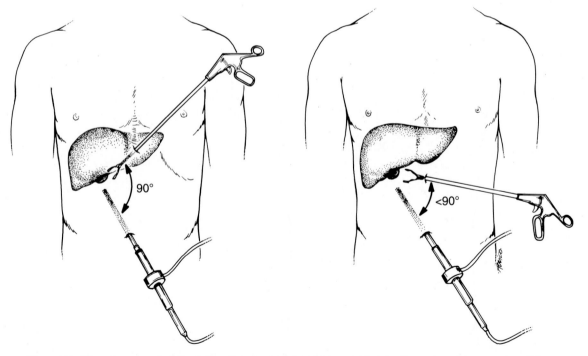

Figure 3. The placement of the epigastric trocar should be as high in the epigastrium as possible, to maximize the angle formed between the camera and the working instrument. This allows maximum visualization of the tip of the dissecting instrument.

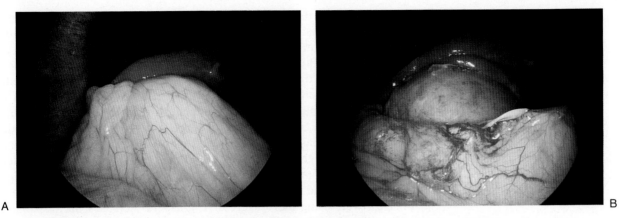

Figure 4. A: A dense omental pack is typically found covering the acute gallbladder, obscuring its view. **B:** The omental pack is gently peeled away from the fundus of the gallbladder.

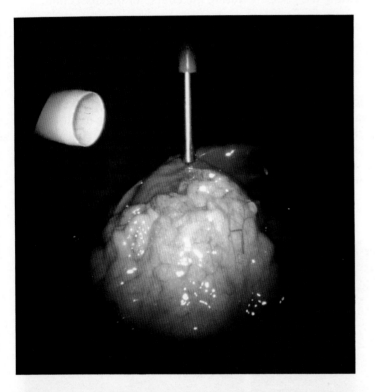

Figure 5. The gallbladder can be decompressed with a cyst aspiration needle. Because of the thickness of the gallbladder wall, the needle hole does not generally need to be closed. Decompression of the acute gallbladder is required to allow grasping and control of the gallbladder.

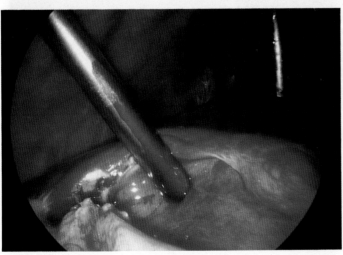

Figure 6. To allow drainage of thick bile and gravel, the midclavicular trocar can be inserted into the fundus of the gallbladder. This allows the insertion of a suction irrigation instrument into the gallbladder to drain and wash out the debris that is normally within an acutely inflamed gallbladder.

a direct puncture with a trocar (Fig. 6). I prefer to utilize the midclavicular trocar to puncture through the distended fundus and aspirate and flush out the gallbladder.

By inserting a suction irrigator through the trocar, the gallbladder can be completely emptied of all fluid and washed clean. This minimizes contamination to the abdominal cavity if the gallbladder is torn during the course of the procedure.

Using the trocar method to decompress the gallbladder does require a loop ligature closure of the puncture hole to eliminate any spillage of residual fluid or small stones during the course of the procedure (Fig. 7). When the gallbladder is decompressed, it can easily be grasped and elevated. Because of the thickened wall, a more aggressive grasper than what is normally used for a standard cholecystectomy is required. I prefer a 5-mm toothed grasper that can firmly hold the diseased gallbladder and allow the necessary traction to carry out the dissection (Fig. 8). However, using more aggressive graspers increases the possibility of tearing the gallbladder, but with the gallbladder decompressed, this is of less concern. To minimize tearing of the gallbladder with the toothed graspers, the surgeon should avoid repositioning the graspers during the course of the dissection.

Porta Hepatis

In a patient who demonstrates acute cholecystitis, exposure of the porta hepatis can be difficult. As discussed earlier, in acute cases the liver is often edematous and does not allow the same upward traction that opens up the porta hepatis in the noninflamed gallbladder patient. Therefore, instead of trying to lift the gallbladder up over the liver (Fig. 9), the surgeon should place the fundal retractor on the body of the gallbladder and lift the gallbladder straight up (Fig. 10). Also, any degree of ileus will minimize the open space created by the pneumoperitoneum, thereby creating an obstacle for a clear view of the porta hepatis (Fig. 11).

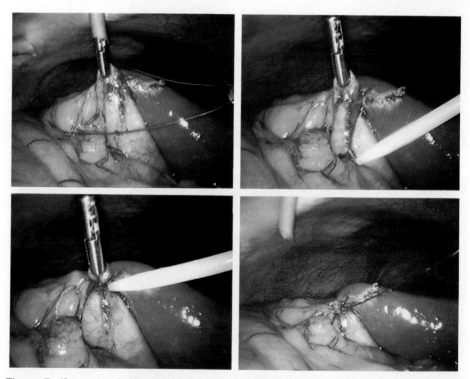

Figure 7. If a trocar is inserted into the gallbladder fundus to drain the gallbladder, then the hole created must be closed with a loop ligature to prevent spillage of debris and stones during the case.

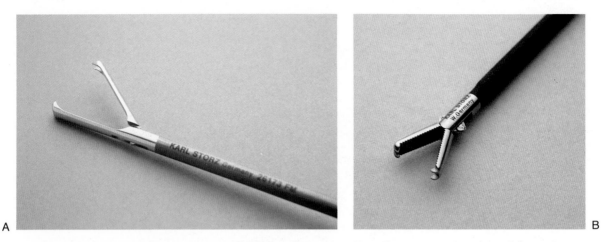

A   B

Figure 8. A,B: Toothed graspers are often required to allow the surgeon to adequately grasp and hold the thickened acute gallbladder.

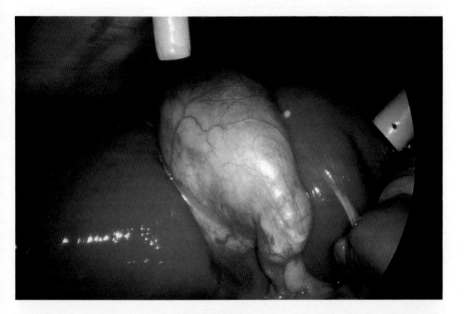

Figure 9. With a normal gallbladder, the fundus can be retracted over the edge of the liver, giving a wide open view of the portal structures. With an acute gallbladder, this cannot normally be accomplished because of the edema in the liver.

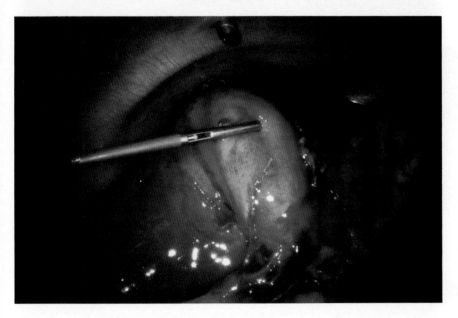

Figure 10. With the acute gallbladder, the retracting grasper is placed on the midbody of the gallbladder and lifted straight up to allow exposure of the portal structures.

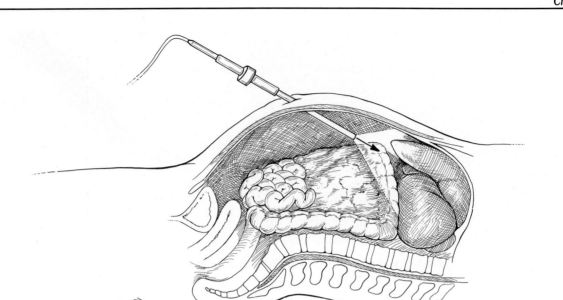

Figure 11. A thickened omental pack, along with a distended transverse colon, often blocks the view of a 0-degree telescope.

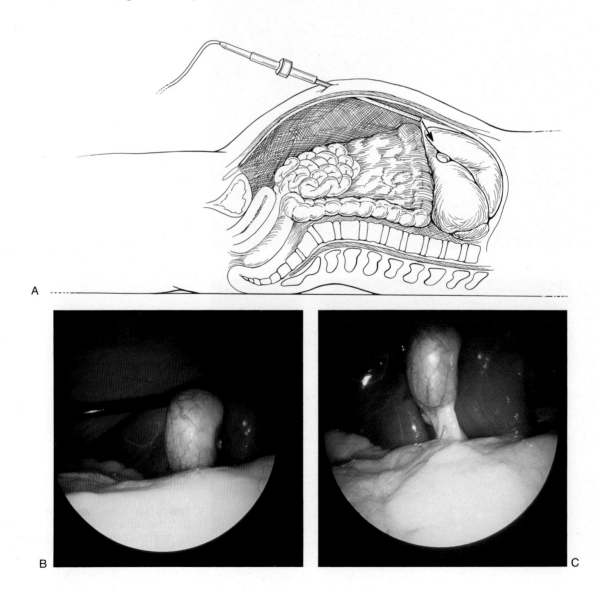

The surgeon should not proceed further until full visualization of the operative field is achieved. Using a 30-degree telescope to look over the "horizon" will often give the surgeon the open field he needs to proceed (Fig. 12). If this does not help achieve an open field, then a 5th puncture can be used to introduce a blunt retracting instrument to retract the transverse colon and omentum downward (Fig. 13). Only after the surgeon has obtained a good field of view of the porta hepatis should he or she proceed to dissection of the cystic duct.

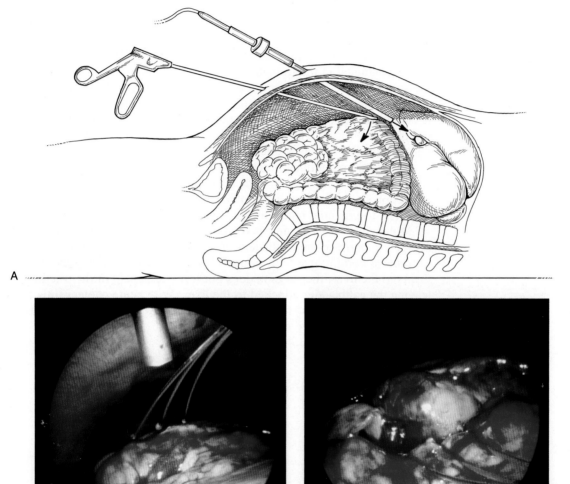

A

B

C

Figure 13. A: To further increase the exposure when there is thickening of the omentum and transverse colon, a 5th puncture can be placed to insert a retracting instrument to distract downward the transverse colon and omentum. **B,C:** The addition of a 5th puncture allows the placement of a retractor to distract downward the transverse colon and omentum and can increase the ability to open up the visual field.

Figure 12. A: The use of an angled telescope allows the surgeon to look over the structures that may be obscuring the view of a 0-degree telescope. **B,C:** These two pictures demonstrate the difference between a 0-degree telescope (Fig. 11B) and a 30-degree telescope (Fig. 11C). The "down" look that is achieved with the angled scope can greatly increase the surgeon's ability to visualize the portal structures.

The Cystic Duct

The dissection of the cystic duct is initiated high up on the gallbladder, actually mobilizing the neck and body of the gallbladder by opening up the lateral and medial peritoneal attachments (Fig. 14). The vast majority if not all of this dissection is performed bluntly. The only structures that should be divided by cautery or sharp dissection are structures that are *absolutely* identified before their division.

The use of aqua dissection with a blunt irrigation probe works very nicely in defining the tissue planes in the acute gallbladder.

Triangle of Calot

Early dissection of the triangle of Calot should be avoided. The only anatomy that is contained in the triangle of Calot is anatomy that will cause problems for the surgeon. The lateral margin of the triangle of Calot is defined by the cystic duct. Keeping the dissection confined to the lateral margin until the cystic duct is clearly identified will minimize potential injury to structures that might lie in the triangle of Calot, including a right hepatic artery, an aberrant right hepatic duct, or accessory biliary ducts.

As already mentioned, attention should be given to the sentinel lymph node, which is always very prominent in a case of acute cholecystitis (Fig. 1). The dissection should be at or above this landmark. Dissecting below the lymph node may lead to potential injury to the common bile duct or common hepatic duct.

Mobilizing the neck and body of the gallbladder as described, enables the surgeon to perform the equivalent of a "fundus" first dissection that we have all become so comfortable with in open surgery. By maintaining the fundal attachments to the liver, the surgeon does not lose the benefit of the traction gained by leaving the gallbladder attached to the liver. With acute cholecystitis this is even more important because the inflammatory changes that are present cause extreme difficulty with exposure of the porta hepatis.

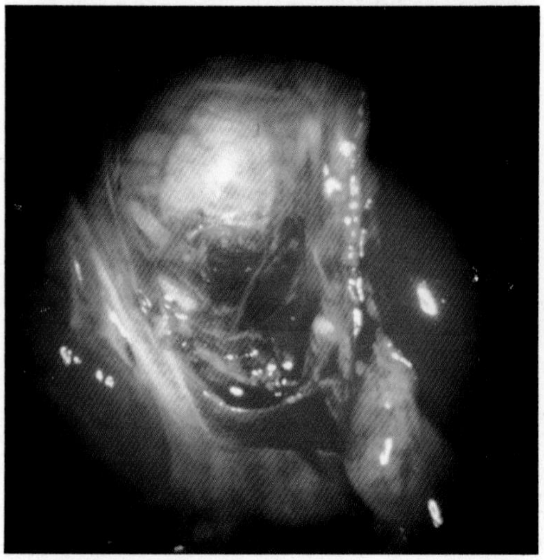

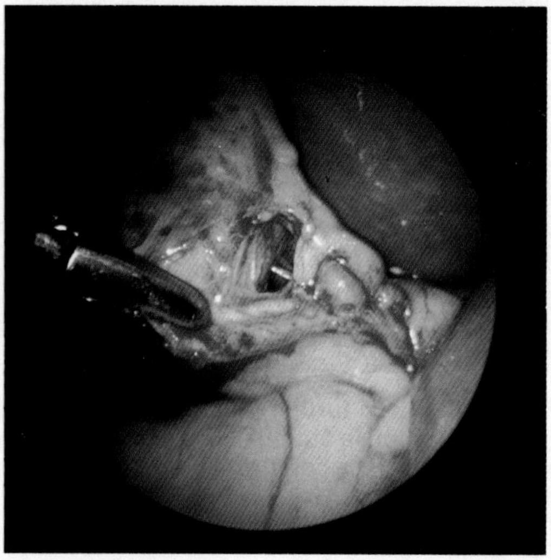

Figure 14. A: The peritoneum covering the cystic duct is best opened laterally at the neck of the gallbladder. This area is relatively avascular, and will avoid many of the bleeding problems that can occur if the dissection is initiated anteriorly. **B:** As the cystic duct and the neck of the gallbladder are exposed laterally, the dissection is carried anteriorly, bluntly pushing the cystic artery off of the cystic duct. This will expose the infundibulum of the gallbladder for positive identification of the cystic duct. The dissection must be circumferentially with no intervening tissue which could hide an aberrant duct.

Infundibulum

An especially difficult problem is the acute hydrops. Due to the impacted stone in the neck, the dissection is often difficult and the anatomy especially confusing. Hartmann's pouch tends to lie much lower in patients with acute cholecystitis, and can often adhere to the common bile duct. For this reason, it is extremely important to mobilize the neck and body of the gallbladder to clearly identify the infundibulum of the gallbladder. Some gallbladders do not have a true infundibulum and demonstrate nothing more than that of a long tapering body. If this is the case, and if there is any doubt, the dissection should be carried out higher up on the gallbladder.

Cholangiography

In the case of acute cholecystitis, the classic landmark of the cystic duct/common bile duct junction can rarely be demonstrated without a difficult and dangerous dissection. For this reason it is generally recommended that cholangiography be performed in all cases of acute cholecystitis. A cholangiogram not only confirms the anatomy (Fig. 15), but verifies the absence of any retained stones in the proximal cystic duct or common bile duct (Fig. 16). Cholangiography through the gallbladder is difficult in acute cholecystitis due to cystic duct obstruction at the neck. For this reason, that routine cystic duct cholangiography is recommended. A surgeon can obtain a cystic duct cholangiogram in nearly every case without undue risk to the common duct if a high dissection on the neck of the gallbladder is performed, exposing the most distal aspect of the cystic duct where

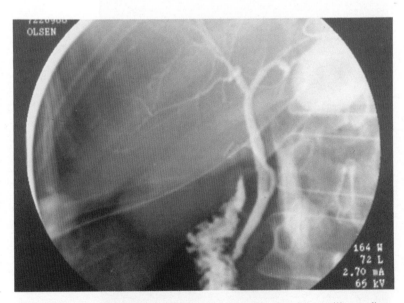

Figure 15. A cholangiogram through the cystic duct will confirm proper identification of the anatomy. This is especially important with acute cholecystitis because of the acute inflammatory changes making identification of the structures difficult.

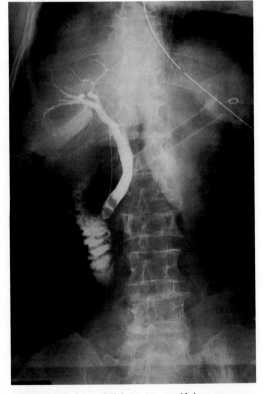

Figure 16. In addition to verifying proper identification of the anatomy, the cholangiogram will also help in diagnosing common bile duct stones.

it joins the neck of the gallbladder. An additional advantage of routine cholangiography in acute cases is that it will also identify any aberrant anatomy that may lie in the triangle of Calot (Fig. 17). This anatomy can be obscured by the inflammatory reaction and be at risk when the gallbladder is removed from the liver bed.

With the cystic duct positively identified and confirmed by cholangiography, the structure is ligated with clips and divided (Fig. 18). I recommend further securing the closure with a loop ligature because of the inflammatory nature of the tissues. Maintaining upward traction on the neck of the gallbladder, the dissection is carried out bluntly until the cystic artery is identified as it enters the gallbladder (Fig. 19). The cystic artery is clip ligated and divided with scissors. The gallbladder is dissected off the liver bed using either cautery, laser, or harmonic scalpel. The use of an energy source for dissection should be avoided until the cholecystohepatic ligament is bluntly dissected. This prevents a potential "burn" injury to a right hepatic duct that might be lying deep in the triangle of Calot.

Constant repositioning of the gallbladder, which exposes the lateral or medial serosal attachments, will help the surgeon stay in the proper plane of dissection. The dissection should be from the lateral or medial serosal attachments of the gallbladder toward the middle of the gallbladder bed. Dissection that is performed up the middle of the gallbladder bed will increase the risk of getting out of the plane of dissection, thereby either perforating the gallbladder or cutting into liver substance. Carefully examine the liver bed prior to dividing the last attachments of the gallbladder in order to take advantage of the exposure gained by upward retraction on the liver (Fig. 20).

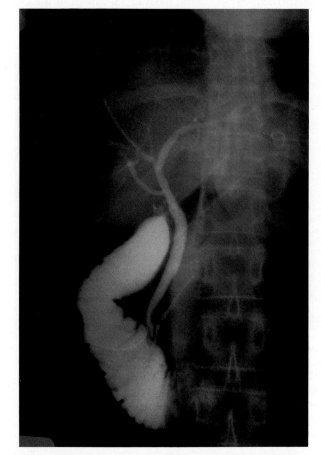

Figure 17. An additional benefit of the cholangiogram is to identify aberrant anatomy that can occur in as many as 7% of cases. This aberrant anatomy can be at risk of injury during the dissection and removal of the gallbladder.

Extraction

With the gallbladder off the liver, the camera is switched to the epigastric trocar so that the larger incision at the umbilicus resulting from the open technique can be used to extract the gallbladder. It is usually advisable to place the gallbladder into a specimen bag prior to extraction because of the inflammation and friability of the gallbladder (Fig. 21). This minimizes any risk of wound infection at the trocar site where the gallbladder is removed and also minimizes the risk of spilling material into the abdominal cavity if the gallbladder is torn while trying to remove it through the puncture site.

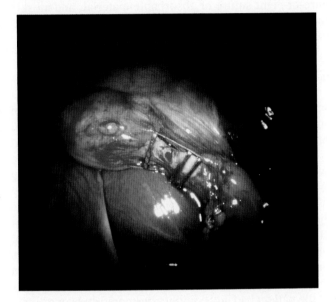

Figure 18. The cystic duct is ligated and divided only after it is *positively* identified.

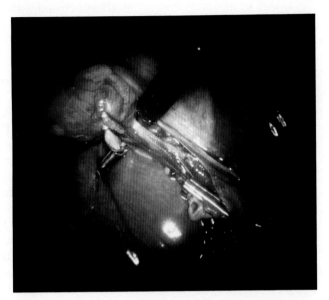

Figure 19. Once the cystic duct is identified, ligated, and divided, the cystic artery is easily found as it courses into the gallbladder. The dissection is kept right on the wall of the gallbladder to prevent an injury to an aberrant right hepatic artery.

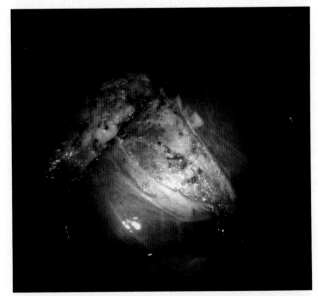

Figure 20. Prior to dividing the last attachments of the gallbladder to the liver bed, inspection of the bed is made to identify any bleeding sites.

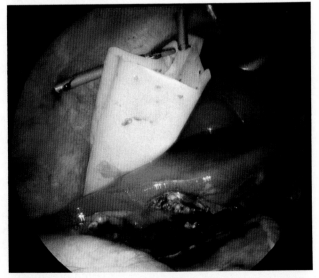

Figure 21. The inflamed, necrotic gallbladder is best extracted in a specimen bag. This will prevent spillage of material while removing the gallbladder through the umbilical puncture site and minimize possible wound infection at the extraction site.

Drains

If there is concern because of the acute inflammation, bile spillage, or other factors, then a drain can be placed in the liver bed for postoperative drainage. This is accomplished by placing a grasper through the lateral port and passing it through the umbilical puncture after the gallbladder has been removed. The free end of the drain is secured by the grasper and brought out through the lateral puncture site. After this procedure, the Hasson trocar is then reinserted in the umbilicus and the pneumoperitoneum is reestablished. The drain can then be manipulated into position to evacuate the gallbladder bed. The fascia at the umbilicus is always closed with a figure-of-eight suture of absorbable material, and all skin incisions closed with a subcuticular closure. The nasogastric tube is removed in the operating suite prior to waking the patient.

Postoperative Management

Postoperative antibiotics are generally continued due to the septic nature of the disease process. Because of the contamination that generally exists with an acute case, antibiotics minimize the risk of abscess and wound infection. An oral antibiotic will allow early discharge when the patient demonstrates an afebrile course and can tolerate oral intake without nausea or vomiting. Pain can generally be controlled with either an oral narcotic analgesic or a nonsteroidal antiinflammatory agent.

Hospital stay will be dictated by the overall degree of sepsis that the patient originally demonstrated. If the patient initially presented early in the course of the disease process, then he can generally be discharged within 24 to 36 hours after the operative procedure. If a drain has been placed, it can usually be removed within 24 hours unless there is a specific indication to leave it longer, such as heavy or bilious drainage. If the patient had any complicating comorbid conditions, or did not demonstrate an uncomplicated postoperative course, then the length of hospitalization is dictated by this concern. The patient should not have any significant complaints of nausea, vomiting, or pain after the first 24 hours. If these reactions are encountered, then the surgeon should be suspicious of complicating conditions. Any questions of bile leak should be investigated first with a nuclear medicine study and, if a leak is confirmed, followed by an endoscopic retrograde cholangiopancreatography.

▲ COMPLICATIONS

There have been a number of reports that demonstrate the effectiveness of laparoscopic cholecystectomy for the acute gallbladder (2,11,12). These studies show that acute cases do not demonstrate any increase in complications as a result of laparoscopic cholecystectomy when compared to other nonacute series. There are more postoperative complications but these are related to the septic nature of the disease process, rather than an increase due to a laparoscopic approach. If anything, complication rates may even be lower for acute cases performed laparoscopically. In these reports, a higher rate of conversion to open cholecystectomy was noted for acute gallbladders—in one series, as high as 10%. But in my experience, between 1990 and 1993, *no laparoscopic cholecystectomy procedures for acute gallbladder have been converted,* despite an overall conversion rate of 5% noted previously (2). This clearly indicates that *experience* is the issue in the success of completing the procedure laparoscopically. An inexperienced surgeon will demonstrate a slightly higher rate of conversion, but this is *not* an increase in technical complication! Conversion is not a complication when it is done electively before a complication occurs.

2. Olsen DO, Asbun HJ, et al. Laparoscopic ch
   1991;8:426–431.
3. Kalser SC, Bray EA, et al. National Institut
   ment on gallstone and laparoscopic cholecy
4. Soper N. Effect of nonbiliary problems on
   522–526.
5. Cameron JC, Gadaez TR. Laparoscopic ch
6. Soper N. Laparoscopic cholecystectomy. Ir
   Mosby-Year Book; 1991:583–655.
7. Baily R, Zucker K, et al. Laparoscopic cl
   tients. *Ann Surg* 1991;214:531–541.
8. Schofield PF, Nulton NR, Baildam AD. Is
   14.
9. Schwartz S. Gallbladder and extrahepatic
   gery. New York: McGraw-Hill; 1984:1307
10. Auguste LJ. Laparoscopic guided percuta
    58–60.
11. Unger S ,Edelman D, et al. Laparoscopic t
    1991;1:14–16.
12. Phillips E, Carroll B, et al. Laparoscopic
    58:273–276.
13. Welch N, Hinder RA, et al. Gallstones in
    Surg Laparosc Endosc 1991;1:246–247.
14. Fitzgibbons R, Annibali R, Litke B. Gallbl
    copy and pneumoperitoneum. *Am J Surg*

Complications that are more likely to occur with the acute gallbladder include:

1. Bowel perforation (duodenum)
2. Perforation of the gallbladder
3. Bile duct injury
4. Postoperative subhepatic hematoma or biloma
5. Wound infection

Perforation

The risk of perforation of the duodenum is a result of the inflammatory process and the fact that the duodenum adheres to the inflamed gallbladder. Care should be taken to divide these adhesions carefully and avoid cautery dissection. A cautery burn can seem benign until it dehisces 4 to 5 days postoperatively. Duodenal perforation should be considered if there is any evidence of increasing abdominal pain with bloating, elevated white blood cell count, temperature, elevated amylase, or fluid collection within the abdominal cavity detected by ultrasound or computed tomography scan. Diagnosis can be confirmed by a contrast study using a water-soluble agent.

Perforation of the gallbladder may be considered by some to be expected and not a complication. Due to the inflamed, friable nature of the tissues, perforation is common. The need to use aggressive graspers to control the gallbladder also increases the likelihood of perforation. To help minimize the consequences of perforation, the gallbladder should be decompressed in the early phase of the procedure. Any spilled stones should be retrieved. This is facilitated by the use of a spoon grasper (Fig. 22) or a specimen bag. Even though a retained stone usually causes few problems (13,14), there have been anecdotal reports of serious complications occurring due to stones that were left in the abdominal cavity, including infection, abscess, and even bowel perforation.

Duct Injuries

Bile duct injuries have always been recognized as a possible outcome in biliary tract surgery. With acute cholecystitis, the inflammatory process makes identification of the anatomy difficult and can increase the potential for injury. If the surgeon adheres to the basic principle of surgery, that no structure is ligated or divided until it is positively identified, then the serious injury of common bile duct ligation and division should never occur. If there is any question of the anatomy, the

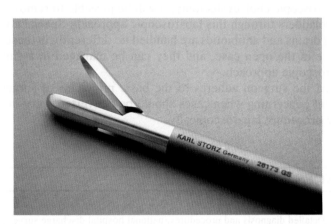

Figure 22. A 10-mm spoon grasper makes removal of spilled stones a simple matter.

246

SURGICAL PEARLS

Early decompression o
the gallbladder to allow th
gallbladder to be grasped an
elevated.

Use of toothed graspers t
allow an adequate hold on th
thickened gallbladder.

Liberal use of heparinize
irrigation solution to clear tl
dissection field of blood, ai
keep it free of clots for ease
aspiration.

Use of an angled sco
and/or a retractor insert
through a 5th puncture to c
tain adequate visualization
the portal structures. NO c
section of the triangle of Ca
should be attempted until v
ualization is achieved.

Avoid dissection in the
angle of Calot until the cy
duct has been identified. S
the dissection lateral to the
angle, and high on the ne
body of the gallbladder.

LIBERAL use of cho
giography to verify pro
identification of the anato
NO structure should be lig
and divided until the cy
duct has been identified.

Identification of the c
artery after the cystic duc
been identified, ligated,
divided.

If there are any ques
regarding the anatomy or
culty in exposing the s
tures, convert to an oper
cedure.

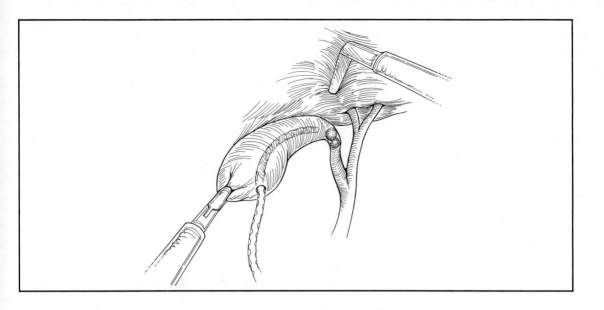

15

Cholecystotomy

Eckart Frimberger
Department of Gastroenterology
Medizinische Klinik
Munich, Germany

Operative Laparoscopy and Thoracoscopy, edited by
B. V. MacFadyen, Jr. and
J. L. Ponsky. Lippincott-Raven
Publishers, Philadelphia © 1996.

KEY WORDS

Cholecystoscopy	Litholysis
Extracorporeal Shock Wave Lithotripsy (ESWL)	Lithotripsy
Gallbladder Stone	Percutaneous Cholecystolithotomy (PCCL)
Laparoscopic Cholecystotomy (LCT)	Oral Bile Acid Therapy (BAT)

For decades, the only surgical option for a patient with gallbladder stones was a cholecystectomy, since other treatment modalities were not available. With the advent of alternative methods, such as litholysis as the sole treatment or in combination with extracorporeal shock wave lithotripsy (ESWL), percutaneous cholecystolithotomy (PCCL) and laparoscopic cholecystotomy (LCT) with primary closure of the gallbladder, there is now a wider array of options for treatment of gallbladder stones.

I introduced the laparoscopic technique for closing an incision in an intraabdominal hollow organ by suture and clips in 1979 and 1989. Later, laparoscopic cholecystotomy was introduced by E. Mühe in 1985, Mouret in 1987, and J. Perissat and Dubois in 1989.

● ANATOMY

The gallbladder is located on the inferior surface of the right lobe of the liver and drains through the cystic duct into the common hepatic duct, which then becomes the common bile duct. The primary blood supply is from the cystic artery, which is a branch of the right hepatic artery. The cystic artery divides into an anterior or superficial branch that lies on the anterior surface of the gallbladder, whereas the posterior branch of the cystic artery lies on the posterior surface of the gallbladder and is usually not visualized in laparoscopic cholecystotomy. Since neither the cystic artery (anterior or posterior) branches are ligated or cauterized during this procedure, bleeding on the anterior surface of the gallbladder may occur unless adequate cauterization of the gallbladder wall is performed. Figure 1 illustrates the anatomy of the gallbladder and its blood supply. The incision is made in the fundus or in the upper portion of the anterior surface of the gallbladder wall; this will minimize the potential of injury to the cystic, hepatic, or right hepatic ducts. For variations on the cystic duct, refer to Chapter 13.

▶ PREOPERATIVE PLANNING

Etiology of Gallbladder Stones

Gallbladder stones have long been thought to result from gallbladder disease. Today, a multifactorial concept has evolved for the formation of stones, including the secretion of lithogenic cholesterol-supersaturated bile by the liver, pronucleating and antinucleating factors, gallbladder motility, and gallbladder mucin. The lithogenic potential may not be constant during an individual's life, and it can be increased by pregnancy, obesity, rapid weight loss during weight reduction, and in the immediate postoperative period after abdominal surgery.

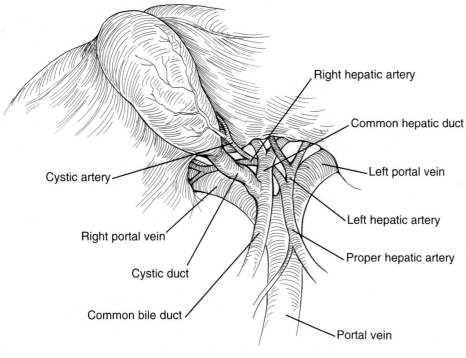

Figure 1. Blood supply of the gallbladder.

Clinical Presentation

The typical symptomatic patient with gallbladder stones presents with what is considered biliary pain—a steady, noncolicky, long lasting (>½ hour) pain in the right upper quadrant, or the epigastrium forcing the patient to stop what he is doing and take antispasmodics. This symptomatology is generally accepted as evolving from biliary origin, but the positive predictive value is not very high. Persistent symptoms after treatment, for instance after cholecystectomy, may indicate that the complaints had other causes, such as irritable bowel syndrome. Even right upper quadrant tenderness during palpation is not specific for gallbladder disease.

Special Tests

The gallbladder is primarily evaluated by ultrasonography. The function of the organ is verified by oral stimulation (fatty meal), and endoscopic retrograde cholangiography (ERC) is only carried out when suspicion of common bile duct stones are indicated by elevated liver function studies or enlarged caliber of the bile ducts detected by ultrasound. Proper contraction of the gallbladder (diminution of the resting volume by at least 30%) confirms a patient cystic duct and a gallbladder ejection rate of less than 30% indicates a poorly functioning gallbladder. Oral cholecystography should be carried out in cases that are not clear. Concomitant peptic ulcer disease is ruled out by an endoscopic examination of the upper gastrointestinal tract.

Patient Selection and Indications/Contraindications

The typical symptomatic patient selected for LCT wishes that the gallbladder and its function are preserved and that the operative trauma and risk are minimized. The gallbladder must be functioning as demonstrated by OCG, its wall not thickened, and there is no previous upper abdominal surgery preventing the laparoscopic access to the gallbladder due to adhesions. The ideal patient for LCT has a limited number of stones, not more than five, and has a relatively low risk of stone recurrence. Patients with stones having formed during phases of increased lithogenesis, such as pregnancy or prolonged parenteral nutrition, are ideal candidates for LCT because they may remain stone-free for the rest of their lives. Sometimes it may be difficult to convince a patient with a gallbladder containing numerous stones to undergo cholecystectomy when he or she insists on keeping the gallbladder and its function intact, despite traditional medical advice supporting its removal. Since the risk of stone recurrence in this subset of patients is high, cholecystotomy is not recommended. LCT is not indicated in patients with a nonfunctioning gallbladder, thickening of the gallbladder wall, obstruction of the cystic duct, or who have had upper abdominal surgery, or are unfit for general anesthesia.

Nonsurgical Options

Percutaneous cholecystolithotomy (PCCL) is a semiendoscopic method that is not restricted to cholesterol stones, such as with oral dissolution medication. All types of stones, regardless of number and diameter, may be treated. The gallbladder is punctured under ultrasonographic control after a fluoroscopically controlled guidewire is inserted. Access to the gallbladder is achieved by bouginage over the guidewire, after which a sheath is inserted into the gallbladder. Under the view of a rigid laparoscope, stones are grasped and extracted. After stone clearance, a Foley catheter is left in the gallbladder, which may be removed after formation of a stable fistulous tract. Disadvantages of this technique are that access to the gallbladder is gained only by fluoroscopic control transhepatically, and organs along the puncture line may be perforated. Another disadvantage is that the catheter must be left in place for 10 to 15 days and can cause patient discomfort. In addition, adhesions form between the gallbladder and the abdominal wall.

For patients with mild symptoms due to radiolucent gallbladder stones up to a diameter of 5 mm and a patent cystic duct, dissolution with oral bile acid therapy is a noninvasive treatment option. Urodeoxycholic acid (UDCA) 8–10 mg/day is given until the gallbladder is free of stones. In this group, comprising 3% of all patients with gallbladder stones, UDCA can be successful in more than 50%, but it requires at least 2 years of therapy.

Extracorporeal shock-wave lithotripsy (ESWL), in current use in Europe, has not been approved by the U.S. Food and Drug Administration; for this reason it is restricted to investigational programs. In combination with urodeoxycholic acid, ESWL may be offered to patients with a single radiolucent stone up to a diameter of 20 mm. In this setting, 84% of patients are free of stone fragments after 1 year. In larger solitary stones with a diameter between 20 and 30 mm and in patients with two or three gallbladder stones, primary efficacy is reduced to 57% and 51%, respectively. During the phase of stone clearance after ESWL up to one-third of patients suffer from biliary colic due to the passage of fragments.

▼ INTRAOPERATIVE MANAGEMENT/SURGICAL TECHNIQUE

The patient is placed on the operating table in the supine position and prepared as for laparoscopic cholecystectomy.

The Verres needle is introduced through a 1-cm umbilical incision and a CO_2 pneumoperitoneum is established with the pressure limit set at 15 mmHg. The risk of the insertion of the first (umbilical) cannula is reduced by initial insertion of a small-caliber cannula (6 mm), which is replaced later by an 11-mm trocar. The abdominal wall is pulled up with a forceps or by hand, and the cannula is inserted at the umbilicus. A 5-mm telescope is introduced and the insertion sites for the two additional cannulas are selected. Positioning of the following cannulas is carried out under endoscopic vision. The right-paraumbilical 6-mm cannula is inserted at the level of the umbilicus or a few centimeters caudally. The 13-mm operative cannula, mounted with a stopper, is inserted approximately 5 cm distal to the gallbladder and a few centimeters lateral to its fundus. The stopper is fixed in such a position so that the internal part of the cannula protrudes 2 to 3 cm into the abdominal cavity. The operative cannula and the paraumbilical cannula should not be located on the same craniocaudal line passing the gallbladder region: the operative cannula should be located approximately 2 cm laterally and the paraumbilical cannula 2 cm medially. The sites envisaged for cannula placement are indented with the finger from outside. The intraabdominally visible indentation corresponds to the chosen point. Finally, the 6-mm umbilical cannula is replaced by the 12-mm cannula using the same puncture channel. Again, the insertion is endoscopically controlled by the 5-mm telescope inserted through the operative cannula. Figure 2 shows the location of the three cannulas.

Exposure of the Gallbladder

The pivot arm laparoscope (Fig. 3) with the arm retracted is inserted through the umbilical cannula. Other instruments used in this technique are seen in Figure 4. After extension of the arm of the laparoscope to an angle adjusted to the individual anatomic situation, in the range of 120 to 150 degrees, the liver lobe is elevated with the arm placed medially to the gallbladder (Figure 4A). After elevation of

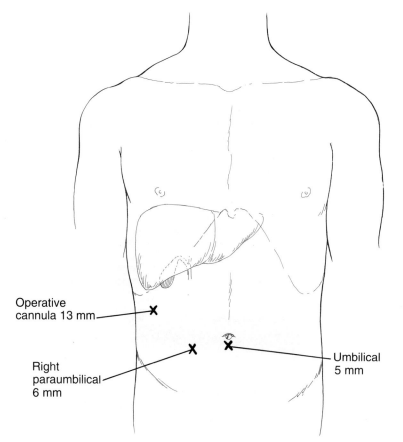

Operative
cannula 13 mm

Right
paraumbilical
6 mm

Umbilical
5 mm

Figure 2. Cannula puncture sites for LCT. Umbilical cannula (12 mm); access for the pivot arm laparoscope connected to the videocamera. Paraumbilical cannula (6 mm); access for the gallbladder grasping forceps, cholecystotome, coagulation forceps (in case of need), hook to narrow the incision margins, 12 F drain. Operative cannula (13 mm); access for the operative laparoscope, cholecystoscope, stone bag (in case of need).

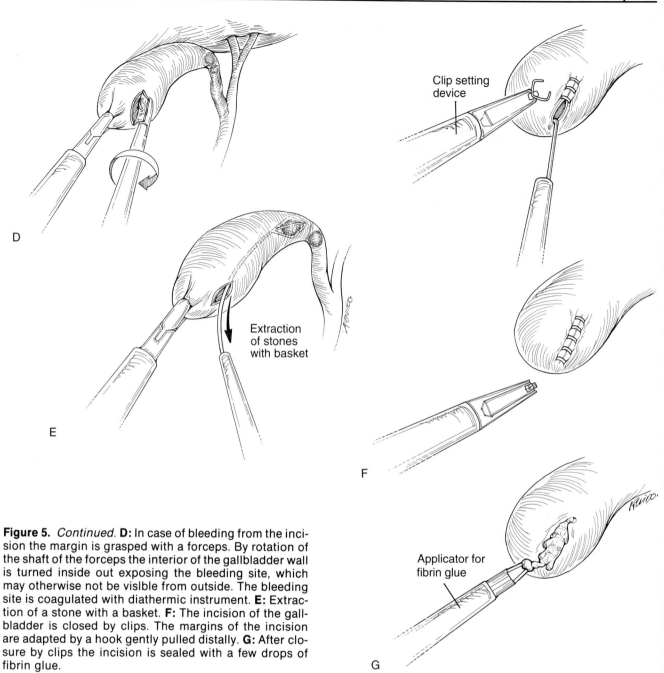

Figure 5. *Continued.* **D:** In case of bleeding from the incision the margin is grasped with a forceps. By rotation of the shaft of the forceps the interior of the gallbladder wall is turned inside out exposing the bleeding site, which may otherwise not be visible from outside. The bleeding site is coagulated with diathermic instrument. **E:** Extraction of a stone with a basket. **F:** The incision of the gallbladder is closed by clips. The margins of the incision are adapted by a hook gently pulled distally. **G:** After closure by clips the incision is sealed with a few drops of fibrin glue.

Incision of the Gallbladder

An adequate access to the gallbladder may be established with a diathermic needle knife or a papillotomelike cholecystotome with a rigid shaft (Fig. 4B). The cholecystotome is inserted into the puncture hole via the paraumbilical cannula (Fig. 5C); for the diathermic cut the instrument is moved slowly and gently both dorsally and caudally. The length of the incision is commensurate with the size of stones to be extracted.

Bleeding from the incision is never severe because of the small caliber of the blood vessels in the gallbladder wall. Nevertheless, measures to stop bleeding have to be carried out quickly and efficiently because even relatively small amounts of blood obscure the endoscopic view, rendering the manipulations more difficult. Hemostasis should be achieved by the least coagulation necessary because large coagulation zones may cause the closure of the gallbladder incision by clips to be less safe. In order to visualize the bleeding vessel, the incision margin is grasped with a forceps through the paraumbilical cannula. Forceps are used to grasp the undersurface of the gallbladder wall and by rotation of the shaft, the interior of the gallbladder wall is turned inside out (Fig. 5D) presenting the bleeding site, which usually retracts a little from the incision margin so that it may not be seen from outside. The exposed bleeding site is coagulated with a forceps with narrow jaws. If necessary a Verres needle is inserted through the abdominal wall close to the gallbladder for rinsing.

Cholecystoscopy

The operative laparoscope may be inserted into the gallbladder if the incision is long enough. With the rigid endoscope, complete inspection of the gallbladder up to the opening of the cystic duct may be difficult, depending on the individual anatomic situation. More suitable is a flexible cholecystoscope (4–6 mm diameter flexible endoscope, with a working length of 40 to 60 cm, and a working channel of 2 mm) inserted into a rigid shaft sparing the bending section of the instrument (Fig. 3). The cholecystoscope is inserted through the operative cannula. Saline is instilled through the endoscope into the gallbladder in order to distend the organ. In case the view is not entirely clear due to remaining bile, the liquid is aspirated and rinsed.

Stone Extraction

Stones are extracted with a basket (Fig. 5E) or a three-armed grasper. The endoscope should be retrieved with the deflection section straightened; otherwise the sharp edges of the cannula will damage the cover of the scope. The extraction of multiple stones and large stones may be cumbersome and time-consuming. In these cases a bag is introduced before stone extraction by the operative trocar and placed on the liver surface. The opening of the bag oriented in a caudal direction is kept in place with a forceps introduced through the paraumbilical cannula.

Closure of the Gallbladder

The gallbladder incision is closed with titanium clips and fibrin glue. With a small hook inserted through the paraumbilical trocar, the margins are adjusted by a gentle pull caudally. With the clip-setting device (Fig. 4D) introduced through the laparoscope clips are set one by one, usually beginning at the cranial part of the incision (Fig. 5F), at a distance of 4 mm between the clips. The clips are loaded excentrically on the tip of the clip-setting device. In order to visualize the open clip with the laparoscope, the clip has to be adjusted until it is in the field of vision of the laparoscope, that is, in the position closest to the lens of the laparoscope (Fig. 5G). The clipped incision is sealed with a few drops of fibrin glue applied with a two-channel applicator (Fig. 4E and 5H). The viscosity of the fibrin glue Beriplast can be adjusted to the appropriate honeylike thickness. The aspect of the gallbladder closed by clips and fibrin glue is shown in Fig. 6.

Insertion of a Balloon Catheter into the Gallbladder

Alternatively to the closure by the clip method, a balloon catheter may be inserted into the gallbladder. This technique is applied only if closure by clips is not feasible or if it is intended to use the fistulous tract created by the catheter

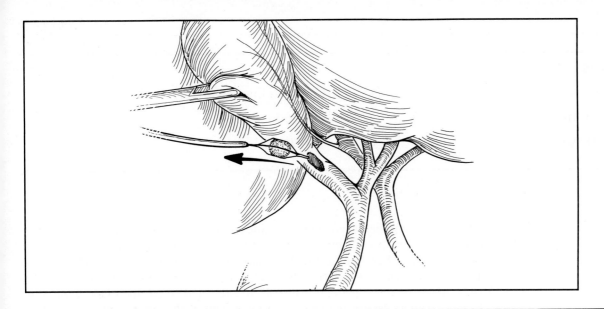

Transcystic Common Bile Duct Exploration

Karl A. Zucker
Department of Surgery
University of New Mexico
Albuquerque, New Mexico 87131

Robert K. Josloff
Temple University
Surgical Care Specialist, Inc.
Abington, Pennsylvania 19001

Operative Laparoscopy and Thoracoscopy, edited by B. V. MacFadyen, Jr. and J. L. Ponsky. Lippincott-Raven Publishers, Philadelphia © 1996.

KEY WORDS

Papillotomy   Common bile duct (CBD) exploration

Choledocholithiasis   Cystic duct

Choledochoscope   Antegrade

Although most patients with symptomatic cholelithiasis are now offered a laparoscopic approach to cholecystectomy, individuals with common bile duct stones often remain a challenge for the minimally invasive surgeon. An estimated 5% to 15% of all patients with cholelithiasis also have common bile duct (CBD) stones (1,2). Many of these patients will still be subjected to an open laparotomy and formal common bile duct exploration, especially if the stones are discovered at the time of laparoscopic surgery. In some cases the surgeon may elect to complete the cholecystectomy under laparoscopic guidance and recommend that the patient undergo postoperative endoscopic retrograde cholangiography (ERC) and sphincterotomy. Although usually successful, biliary endoscopy is an invasive procedure that is uncomfortable, relatively expensive, and associated with a 3% to 5% incidence of major complications (3,4). The benefits of laparoscopic versus traditional open surgery have persuaded many surgeons to attempt definitive therapy of common bile duct stones at the same time as laparoscopic cholecystectomy. Today laparoscopic surgeons are using techniques borrowed from both conventional methods of CBD exploration and flexible biliary endoscopy so that they may effectively manage choledocholithiasis without the need for an open laparotomy or postoperative endoscopic retrograde cholangiography and sphincterotomy.

Two methods of accessing the bile ducts during laparoscopic surgery have thus far been described. The same opening made in the cystic duct for introducing the cholangiogram catheter may be enlarged so that various endoscopic devices can be maneuvered into the main bile ducts or a separate incision can be made along the anterior surface of the common bile duct (choledochostomy) to allow for direct insertion of these same instruments. In keeping with the growing trend of "minimally invasive surgery" the most popular method of accessing the biliary system during laparoscopic surgery has been by way of the cystic duct. With this approach the surgeon can often avoid the need to tediously expose and manipulate the common bile duct and in most cases eliminate the need for postoperative biliary drainage (i.e., T-tube). Early attempts at laparoscopic transcystic common bile duct exploration were often frustrated by the inability to maneuver existing endoscopes and instruments through smaller ducts (5). In the past few years dramatic advances in fluoroscopic equipment, flexible choledochoscopes and endoscopic instrumentation have made it possible to accomplish transcystic bile duct exploration in the majority of patients with choledocholithiasis. In this chapter the various methods of transcystic duct exploration of the common bile duct and the equipment used are described.

■ ANATOMY

It is essential that any surgeon embarking on either a laparoscopic or conventional operation of the biliary tract be familiar not only with the normal anatomy of this region but also the many variations described in the literature (8). Fortunately, the anatomy of the cystic and common bile ducts is usually well delineated by the intraoperative cholangiogram obtained before attempting common bile duct exploration. Therefore it is important that this radiographic record of the juncture

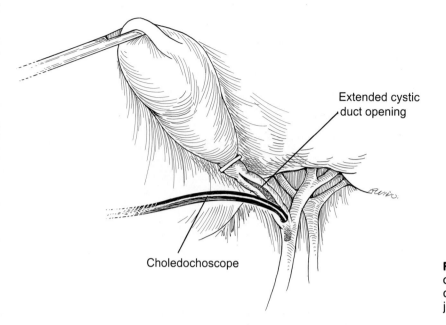

Extended cystic
duct opening

Choledochoscope

Figure 1. If the cystic duct is long, the opening made for the cholangiogram catheter may be extended closer to the juncture of the common bile duct.

of the cystic and common bile ducts, the entire extrahepatic biliary tree, and preferably some portion of the more proximal intrahepatic bile ducts be of sufficient quality that the surgeon can visualize the anatomy and adequately prepare for the subsequent exploration. Of particular importance are the length and luminal diameter of cystic duct, the location of the cystic-common bile duct junction, and the ampulla. In patients with very long cystic ducts, the opening created for inserting the cholangiogram catheter may be a considerable distance (>2.0 cm) from the common bile duct juncture. In this circumstance it may prove useful to extend the cystic duct opening distally toward the common bile juncture to allow for easier manipulation of the subsequent instruments into the main biliary tree (Fig. 1). Occasionally, the intraoperative cholangiogram will demonstrate one or more stones within the proximal cystic duct (Fig. 2). These should be removed first, as

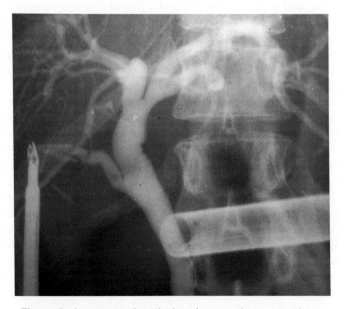

Figure 2. Intraoperative cholangiogram demonstrating a small stone within the cystic duct.

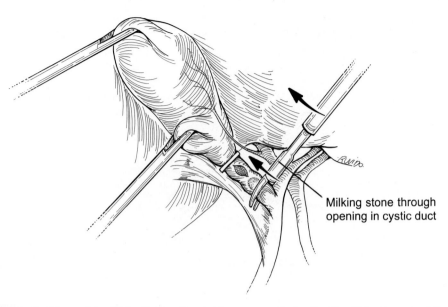

Milking stone through
opening in cystic duct

Figure 3. Stones(s) within the cystic duct can usually be "milked" back out of the opening made for the cholangiogram catheter.

they may later drop into the common bile duct and be more difficult to extract. Usually these stones can be "milked out" of the cystic duct opening with an atraumatic forceps (Fig. 3).

If the lumen of the cystic duct is small (<3.0 mm diameter) it will usually be necessary to dilate the duct before insertion of a choledochoscope (usually 3.0 mm or larger in diameter). Also, if any calculi visualized within the common hepatic or bile ducts are significantly larger than the cystic duct lumen it may be necessary to forego transcystic exploration and go immediately to a separate choledochostomy for access into the biliary tree and removal of calculi. The course of the cystic duct may also be important in determining the feasibility of transcystic exploration. Ideally, the cystic duct should be reasonably short and dilated to at least 4 to 5 mm, and it should insert directly into the lateral or anterior aspect of the midportion of the main bile duct. If the cystic duct has a long, tortuous course with insertion very distal on the common bile duct, it would probably be futile to attempt exploration through this route. As expected, most cystic ducts fall between these two extremes, and experience will dictate to surgeons what the limitations of their equipment and experience will allow.

One of the more common anomalies encountered by biliary tract surgeons is the aberrant right hepatic duct lying very close to the cystic duct. Another important variant is the situation where the cystic duct joins the right hepatic duct rather than the common bile duct. Knowledge of these and other anomalies is essential in diminishing the incidence of major bile duct injuries. Finally, the surgeon should not neglect a very careful inspection of the cholangiographic view of the distal common bile duct and ampulla. Occasionally, the intraoperative cholangiogram may demonstrate that the ampulla empties into a large duodenal diverticulum. Such a finding would imply that postoperative ERCP and sphincterotomy would be far less likely to be successful than the 90% to 95% success rate often quoted in the literature (3). This anatomic variation may persuade the surgeon to be more aggressive in completing intraoperative common bile duct exploration and even converting to open laparotomy if all laparoscopic attempts have been unsuccessful.

▶ PREOPERATIVE PLANNING

It is recommended that all patients undergo screening for choledocholithiasis before planned laparoscopic cholecystectomy. In our practice this usually entails obtaining a careful history that would reveal possible prior episodes of jaundice or pancreatitis, routine liver function tests, serum bilirubin levels, pancreatic amylase or lipase levels, and a careful examination of the preoperative ultrasound scans that would show signs of common bile duct dilation. In some cases, larger stones in the distal common bile duct may actually be visualized with a high-quality sonogram. If there is strong preoperative evidence of choledocholithiasis, this information may help the surgeon determine the most appropriate course of therapy for the patient. If the surgeon plans an exploratory common bile duct laparoscopy, then he or she can ensure that the necessary equipment is available, adequate time in the operating room has been planned for, and, if necessary, arrangements can be made to have an assistant available who is experienced in these techniques. In some cases the surgeon may decide that preoperative biliary endoscopy or an open laparotomy and formal common bile duct exploration is indicated. Unfortunately, many patients with choledocholithiasis will manifest no preoperative evidence of common bile duct stones; these stones can be discovered during the course of routine cholangiography (5,6). Therefore it is advisable for all surgeons performing laparoscopic biliary tract surgery to be comfortable with the various methods of common bile duct exploration.

Laparoscopic exploration of the bile ducts should be performed before removing the gallbladder from the liver bed. Cephalad and right lateral retraction of the gallbladder and liver is the easiest method of exposing the cystic and common bile ducts. In almost every patient an intraoperative cholangiogram is performed as a prelude to common bile duct exploration. The most popular technique employs a small catheter inserted into the biliary system through an opening made in the proximal cystic duct (7). In addition to determining the presence of one or more filling defects within the common or hepatic bile ducts, the intraoperative cholangiogram should also be examined in order to assess the feasibility of accessing the biliary tree via the cystic duct (Figs. 4 and 5). The caliber of the cystic duct lumen, as well as the length and site of insertion into the main bile duct, are all important features that can be used to predict the success of this approach.

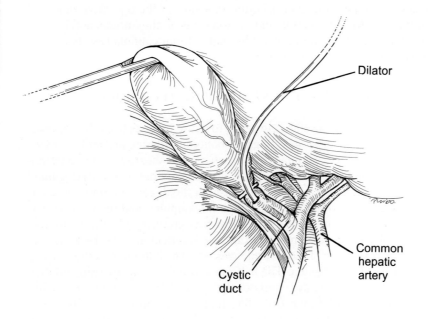

Figure 4. Sequential passage of flexible dilators of increasing diameter may be used until the lumen of the cystic duct is large enough to accommodate the choledochoscope.

if the ducts are normal or only slightly dilated. We have found it useful to remove the back wall of the T-tube and then trim one end shorter. The longer limb is first maneuvered into the main bile duct followed by the shorter end. The catheter can then be secured within the duct by placing one or more 3-0 or 4-0 absorbable sutures under laparoscopic guidance. Although extracorporeal knot-tying is currently very popular among most laparoscopic surgeons, the bile ducts are usually too friable to withstand the upward tension associated with this technique. Therefore, intracorporeal knot-tying with a 6- or 7-inch long suture must be used. After removing the gallbladder from the liver bed, the long end of the T-tube can then be pulled out through one of the lateral 5.0-mm port sites and sutured in place.

In most cases we also place a closed suction drainage catheter under the gallbladder fossa before completing the operative procedure. This is done in case of bile leakage around the T-tube insertion site. After the gallbladder has been extracted from the peritoneal cavity the abdomen is reinsufflated and the drain positioned under direct vision. The external tip of the catheter is then grasped and pulled out through the remaining lateral 5.0-mm port site. Usually this catheter can be removed 48 to 72 hours after surgery.

Transcystic Antegrade Sphincterotomy

DePaulo and his associates (14) in Brazil have recently described the technique of laparoscopic antegrade sphincterotomy, which has added a powerful new tool

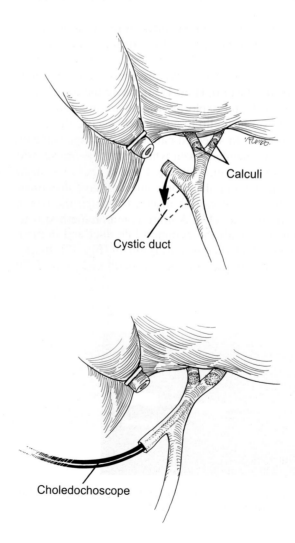

Figure 16. Dividing the cystic duct near the neck of the gallbladder will allow for easier passage of the choledochoscope into the proximal bile ducts.

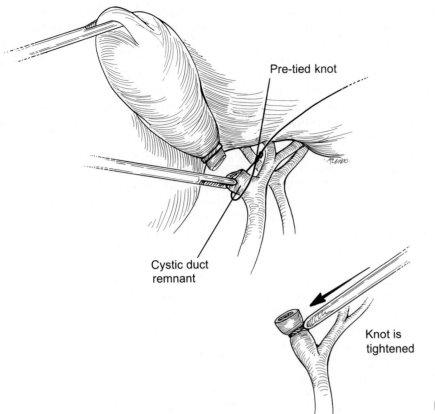

Pre-tied knot

Cystic duct
remnant

Knot is
tightened

Figure 17. Laparoscopic-guided ligature of the cystic duct remnant.

T-tube

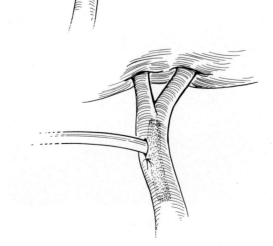

Figure 18. Insertion of a T-tube through a short cystic
duct remnant.

to the armentarium of the minimally invasive surgeon. With this procedure the surgeon can quickly and safely perform a sphincterotomy at the time of laparoscopic intervention and thus spare the patient the discomfort and possibly added morbidity of a later ERCP. Since this is a new technique, the indications for laparoscopic sphincterotomy are still being examined, but DePaulo has used it with great success in those patients with multiple large and small common bile duct stones, those with one or more stones impacted in the distal common bile duct, and in those with choledocholithiasis and very dilated ducts where there was evidence of abnormal biliary emptying or dyskinesia (14).

The technique of laparoscopic antegrade sphincterotomy is relatively straightforward and easy to perform (14,15). A standard endoscopic sphincterotome is inserted through the cystic duct opening and passed through the distal common bile duct and out through the ampulla. A side-viewing duodenoscope is introduced through the mouth and positioned in the second portion of the duodenum. Ideally a video duodenoscope is used so that the surgical team can manipulate the sphinctertome into the proper position under direct vision. The flexible endoscope is therefore used only to confirm that the cutting wire of the sphincterotome is at the 12 o'clock position (Fig. 19). This view is easily obtained with the duodenoscope, despite the fact that the patient is lying in the supine rather the prone position (which is the position used during traditional ERCP). After confirming the proper position of the sphincterotome, electrical current is applied and the papillotomy/ sphincterotomy is completed. The duodenum is then carefully observed for any signs of bleeding or other complications. DePaulo states that this laparoscopic antegrade technique of sphincterotomy should be associated with fewer complications than the traditional endoscopic retrograde method. This is because the sphincterotome is more easily maneuvered through the bile ducts and into the ampulla than the more traditional retrograde technique. Therefore, problems such as pancreatic duct cannulation, creation of false passages, and perforation should be far less common than with the retrograde approach. In DePaulo's preliminary experience with 21 patients the procedure took an average of 17 minutes to complete, and there were no complications associated with the antegrade approach

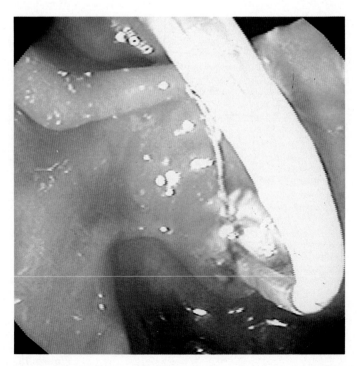

Figure 19. Endoscopic image confirms the cutting wire is at a 12 o'clock position.

(14). Our own early experience in New Mexico appears to confirm the findings of DePaulo (15). In the last two years we have been able to successfully clear the bile ducts in 12 of 15 patients with complicated choledocholithiasis (multiple large calculi, one or more stones impacted at the ampulla) after all the other methods described earlier in this chapter had failed. In one patient the sphincterotome was erroneously thought to have perforated the common bile duct. Subsequent open exploration revealed no such injury. In another patient with acute, necrotizing cholecystitis the cystic duct remnant proved to be too friable to allow passage of the sphincterotome. The only complication experienced in this group of difficult patients was a small duodenal mucosa tear resulting from passage and manipulation of the side-viewing duodenoscope. This was repaired after conversion to open laparotomy, and the patient experienced no other problems from this incident.

The only disadvantages of this technique are the prolonged anesthetic times and the need to have the endoscopic equipment available in the operating room. At our institution we now have a portable endoscopic cart with side-viewing video duodenoscope that can be brought to the operating room with a few minutes notice.

▲ COMPLICATIONS

In general, the same problems associated with conventional methods of common bile duct exploration can also occur when attempting laparoscopic transcystic exploration (Table 1).

Thus far the reported experience with laparoscopic transcystic common bile duct exploration has not been extensive enough to determine whether the incidence of retained stones is any greater or less than with conventional surgery. In one of the largest reported experiences of laparoscopic common bile duct exploration, Joseph Petelin (16) in Kansas reported an overall incidence of 2%. In the past, the diagnosis of persistent choledocholithiasis following open common bile duct exploration was easily made when the surgeon obtained a postoperative T-tube cholangiogram. However, as mentioned previously, many surgeons do not routinely use T-tubes, especially if the exploration has been successful and accomplished solely via the cystic duct. Therefore retained stones can now be confirmed only with the aid of a postoperative ERCP, transhepatic cholangiogram, or reexploration. Since common bile duct stones may remain asymptomatic for variable periods of time, it is probable that many surgeons will mistakenly underreport the true incidence of this problem.

Although false-positive cholangiograms were a recognized problem with conventional surgery, many surgeons now have the impression that they are seeing more such studies in this era of laparoscopic cholecystectomy. This impression is based on the number of negative common bile duct explorations (both laparoscopic and after conversion to open laparotomy) and normal ERCPs performed shortly after the laparoscopic cholangiography (usually the next day) (17,18). One

Table 1. *Complications associated with open and laparoscopic common bile duct exploration*

Retained bile duct (intra- or extrahepatic ducts) stones
False-positive cholangiogram
Bile duct injury (at or near junction of cystic duct)
Bile leak (from cystic or common bile duct)
Perforation/false channel of distal common bile duct
Trapped stone basket
Bleeding (hemobilia)
Bleeding (intraperitoneal)
Postoperative cholangitis
Postoperative pancreatitis

possible reason for this phenomenon may be that gas bubbles are more likely to enter the cystic duct opening in a patient with a pneumoperitoneum pressure of 15 mmHg. For this reason and others, some surgeons are taking a "wait and see" approach to those patients without any prior symptoms suggesting choledocholithiasis, who have normal-sized bile ducts on the cholangiogram and small defects that may be consistent with gas bubbles. If such patients later manifest symptoms consistent with retained common bile duct stones, an ERCP may be performed.

Fortunately, bile duct injuries related to transcystic exploration are exceedingly rare. Most often such injuries are related to avulsion of the cystic and common bile ducts associated with insertion of various devices into the biliary tree or removal of large stones through small orifices of the cystic and common bile ducts. In most cases these injuries are not circumferential and therefore are easy to repair and usually have very favorable outcomes. Interestingly, few data are available concerning this problem from either the conventional or laparoscopic surgical literature. It would seem likely that such injuries will become even less frequent as surgeons become more experienced in such techniques and as the instrumentation continues to improve.

In the past, perforation or the creation of false channels in the distal common bile duct was a serious problem in open bile duct exploration. Usually this was related to overly aggressive attempts to clear the distal common bile duct and ampulla with rigid dilators. This maneuver was largely abandoned by the mid-1980s and was replaced by rigid, and then flexible, choledochoscopy. Although it would seem likely that this problem might be more frequent with fluoroscopic methods of duct exploration as compared to choledochoscopy, this complication has not yet been reported by surgeons performing minimally invasive biliary tract surgery.

Bile leakage from the cystic or common bile duct may occur after either open or laparoscopic common bile duct exploration. No information is yet available as to whether there is a greater incidence of this problem in patients undergoing transcystic exploration without insertion of a T-tube or a similar bile duct drainage catheter. The most likely reason for such leaks is partial or complete obstruction of bile flow across the distal common bile duct from edema or a retained stone. Since the cystic duct remnant is usually traumatized during transcystic bile duct exploration, clips alone may not be adequate for a secure closure. Therefore, we routinely apply a pretied ligature after dividing the cystic duct. If there is any concern about the integrity of the bile duct closure or postoperative obstruction, we insert a T-tube.

Occasionally a stone forceps or a similar device may become trapped or frozen within the distal common bile duct or ampulla. This problem has long been described in the biliary endoscopy literature (i.e., ERCP/sphincterotomy) with most large series reporting a frequency of less than 1% (4). This problem usually occurs when attempting to retrieve one or more stones impacted at the ampulla.

Bleeding, either into the peritoneal cavity or lumen of the biliary tree (hemobilia), is usually the result of excessive force when manipulating instruments within the bile ducts. Postoperative pancreatitis has been described after both laparoscopic and open common bile duct exploration and even occasionally after simple cholangiography alone (from forceful pancreatic duct distention with contrast). Once again, the main culprit appears to be the use of excessive force at or near the ampulla, which may result in direct trauma to the pancreatic duct, edema at its orifice into the ampulla, or the creation of false channels into the pancreas or pancreatic duct.

✓ CONCLUSIONS

The management of patients with choledocholithiasis will present an exciting challenge for the minimally invasive surgeon over the next few years. It is likely

---

SURGICAL PEARLS

Key features of a choledochoscope are a working accessory channel and a deflectable tip greater than 120 degrees.

During exploration of the bile duct, it is important to keep the head elevated and to flush the bile duct with saline. This often pushes the CBD stones distally where they can be more easily grasped with a wire basket.

Dilation of the cystic duct to larger than 5 mm may tear the cystic duct-common duct junction.

Even with division of the cystic duct, advancement of the choledochoscope into the proximal bile duct can be difficult.

Caution must be used when extending the cystic duct incision, since it may extend into the common bile duct.

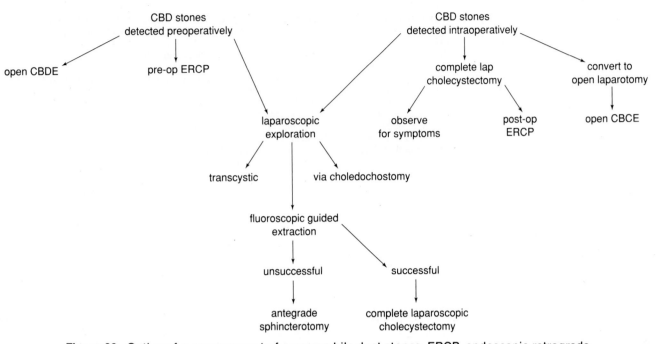

Figure 20. Options for management of common bile duct stones. ERCP, endoscopic retrograde cholangiopancreatography; CBDE, common bile duct exploration.

that no one method of management will be successful for all individuals with common bile duct stones. Therefore the overall management of such patients will continue to include such options as biliary endoscopy, conventional open exploration as well as the laparoscopic methods presented in this chapter. Our current algorithm for managing patients with suspected choledocholithiasis is described in Fig. 20. Although this aspect of laparoscopic surgery is still evolving, it seems clear that the trend will be for surgeons to manage more of these patients completely under laparoscopic guidance. As this occurs, our algorithm will undoubtedly be modified to expand the role of laparoscopic common bile duct exploration in the management of patients with choledocholithiasis.

REFERENCES

1. Gerber A, Apt MK. The case against routine operative cholangiography. *Am J Surg* 1982;143: 734–736.
2. Pangana TJ, Stahlgren LH. Indications and accuracy of operative cholangiography. *Arch Surg* 1980;115:1214–1215.
3. Reiter JJ, Bayer HP, Mennicken L. Results of endoscopic papillotomy: a collective experience from nine endoscopic centers in West Germany. *World J Surg* 1978;2:505–509.
4. Cotten PB, Lehman G, Vennes JA. Endoscopic sphincterotomy complications and their management: an attempt at consensus. *Gastrointest Endosc* 1991;37:383–390.
5. Narhwold DL. The biliary system. In: Sabiston DC, ed. *Textbook of surgery*. Philadelphia: WB Saunders; 1991:1042–1075.
6. Cuschieri A, Bouchier IAD. The biliary tract. In: Cuschieri A, Giles GR, Moossa AR, eds. *Essential surgical practice*. London: Wright; 1988:1021–1075.
7. Bailey RW, Zucker KA. Laparoscopic cholangiography and the management of choledocholithiasis. In: Zucker KA, ed. *Surgical laparoscopy*. St. Louis, MO: Quality Medical Publishing; 1991: 201–240.
8. Schwartz SI. Gallbladder and the extra-hepatic biliary system. In: Schwartz SI, ed. *Principles of surgery*. New York: McGraw-Hill; 1984:1308.
9. Petlin JB. Laparoscopic approach to common duct pathology. *Surg Laparos Endosc* 1991;1:33–41.
10. Hunter JG. Laparoscopic transcystic common bile duct exploration. *Am J Surg* 1992;163:53–57.
11. Hunter JG, Soper NJ. Laparoscopic management of bile duct stones. *Surg Clin North Am* 1992; 72:1077–1097.

12. Zucker KA, Bailey RW. Laparoscopic cholangiography and management of choledocholithiasis. In: Zucker KA, ed. *Surgical laparoscopy: update*. St. Louis, MO: Quality Medical Publishing; 1993:145–193.
13. Quatelbaum JK, Dorsey HD. Laparoscopic treatment of common bile duct stones. *Surg Laparosc Endosc* 1991;1:26–32.
14. DePaulo AL, Hashiba K, Bafutto M, Zago R, Machado MM. Laparoscopic antegrade sphincterotomy. *Surg Laparosc Endosc* 1993;3:157–160.
15. Curet MJ, Pitcher DE, Martin DT, Zucker KA, Laparoscopic antegrade sphincterotomy: a new technique for the management of complex choledocholithiasis. *Ann Surg* 1995;221:149–155.
16. Petelin J. Laparoscopic common bile duct exploration. *Am J Surg* 1992;161:77–83.
17. Flowers JL, Zucker KA, Graham SM, Scovill WA, Imbembo AL, Bailey RW. Laparoscopic cholangiography: results and indications. *Ann Surg* 1992;215:209–216.

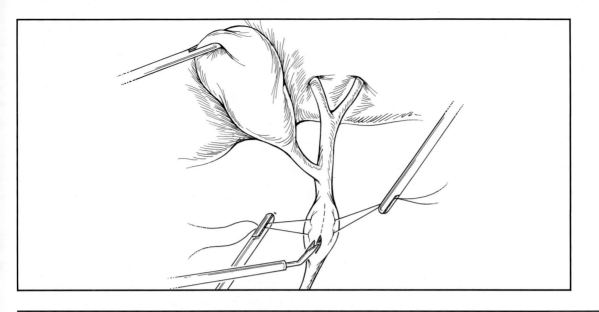

17

Choledochotomy in Laparoscopy

Edward H. Phillips
Department of Surgery
Cedars-Sinai Medical Center
University of Southern California
Los Angeles County Medical Center
Los Angeles, California 90048

Operative Laparoscopy and Thoracoscopy, edited by B. V. MacFadyen, Jr. and J. L. Ponsky. Lippincott-Raven Publishers, Philadelphia © 1996.

Laparoscopic cholecystectomy has become the standard surgical treatment for patients with symptomatic cholelithiasis, but the treatment of choledocholithiasis remains controversial. Because 10% to 15% of all patients undergoing cholecystectomy will have common bile duct (CBD) stones (1,2), it is important to have a strategy to treat them. Because their presence increases operative mortality 30-fold from 0.1% to 3%, the proper treatment of common duct calculi can be a matter of life and death.

Laparoscopic choledochotomy offers the ability to access both the proximal and distal bile duct, remove large stones, perform lithotripsy, lavage stone fragments, and use larger diameter flexible choledochoscopes than the transcystic duct approach, and allows for the placement of a T tube so that postoperative cholangiography can be obtained. If necessary, retained stones can be removed through the T-tube tract. Laparoscopic choledochotomy is applicable in most situations of choledocholithiasis, except when the diameter of the bile duct is small. In 5% to 10% of cases of common duct stones, the technique of choledochotomy is the only laparoscopic way of ridding the bile duct of multiple large calculi (2). Laparoscopic choledochotomy is also the basic technique of common duct exploration known to biliary surgeons, and only the skills of flexible choledochoscopy and laparoscopic suturing need to be acquired to apply the technique laparoscopically.

■ ANATOMY

The CBD lies within the porta hepatis. It is lateral to the hepatic artery and anterior to the portal vein. The right and left bile ducts carry bile from the liver into the common hepatic duct, and then into the CBD, which proceeds posteriorly on or through the head of the pancreas, into the duodenum via the papilla of Vater. The distal bile duct is partly covered by pancreatic tissue in 44% of people and is completely covered by the pancreas in 30% (Fig. 1) (3). The pancreatic duct enters the distal common duct near the papilla of Vater. A "common channel," where the pancreatic duct enters the distal bile duct within 1 cm of the papilla, is found in 75% of individuals; in 25%, the pancreatic duct enters separately on the papilla (Fig. 2) (4).

Anatomic variants in the extrahepatic biliary tree are almost the norm, but surgically significant anomalies occur in 10–15% of cases (5). The cystic duct can originate from the CBD at any location—lateral, medial, anterior. It can wrap around it or share a common wall for a variable distance. In other individuals the cystic duct originates from the right hepatic duct, but in 0.1% of cases it originates from the left hepatic duct (2).

The CBD receives its blood supply through the hepatic and gastroduodenal arteries. Two axial vessels form at approximately 3 and 9 o'clock in relation to the circumference of the CBD (Fig. 1). They originate in the retroduodenal portion, and run the length of the duct. Awareness of the location of these vessels is important when choosing a site for a choledochotomy or a biliary enteric anastomosis (Fig. 3).

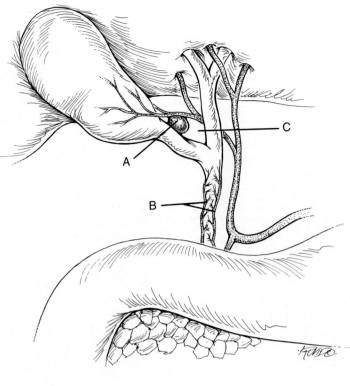

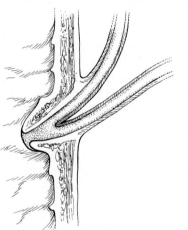

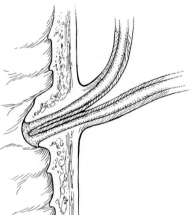

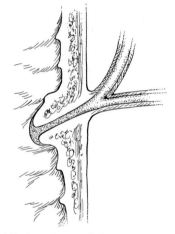

Figure 1. Anatomy of the common bile duct. **A:** Cystic duct lymph node. **B:** Common bile duct arteries. **C:** Calot's triangle (cystic duct, common bile duct, and liver edge).

Figure 2. Variable anatomy of the common bile duct and pancreatic duct at their entrance into the ampulla of Vater.

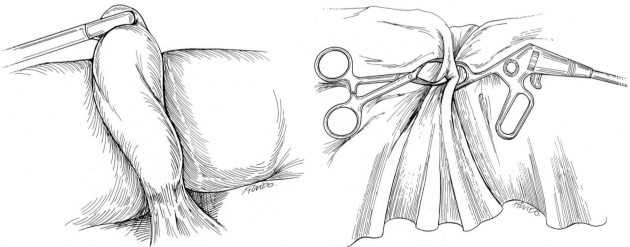

A

B

Figure 3. A: Stable retraction of the gallbladder during common bile duct exploration, provided by grasping the dome of the gallbladder, elevating it over the liver. **B:** Securing the handle of the laparoscopic grasper to the surgical drapes.

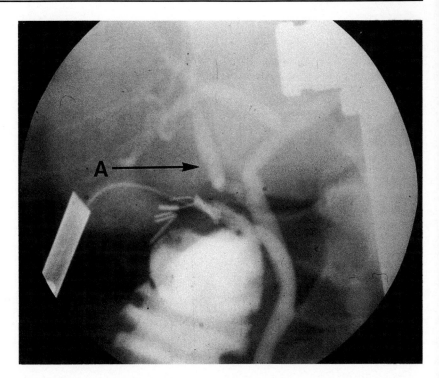

Figure 4. "Accessory" right hepatic duct.

The arterial blood of the gallbladder is supplied by the cystic artery, which is also variable in its origin and relationship to the cystic duct and common duct (6). It usually arises from the right hepatic duct and lies within Calot's triangle (Fig. 1). Often it can be found immediately deep to the cystic duct lymph node.

Calot's triangle is formed by the liver edge superiorly, the common hepatic duct medially, and the cystic duct inferolaterally. In 1% of cases an "accessory" right hepatic bile duct runs within Calot's triangle. This is really an anomalous course for the right anterior or posterior segmental bile duct of the liver. It is important to recognize this anomaly and avoid mistaking it for an artery, which would be clipped and transected distally and cut off flush with the liver; a bile leak from the liver bed will inevitably ensue (Fig. 4).

The lymphatics of the gallbladder drain from the body of the gallbladder toward the porta hepatis through the cystic duct lymph node, which often lies superficial to the cystic artery (Fig. 1). The venous blood drains into small veins, which drain into the portal vein. Occasionally, there is a vein large enough to be called a cystic duct vein.

▶ PREOPERATIVE PLANNING

All patients considered for laparoscopic cholecystectomy should have an ultrasound examination of the liver, gallbladder, CBD, and pancreas. The diameter of the bile duct should be noted, as well as echoes that might signify calculi within it. Changes in the diameter of different areas of the biliary system are also important to identify. Dilated intrahepatic bile ducts with a normal-sized distal bile duct would suggest a tumor at the bifurcation of the right and left bile ducts. Dilation of the extrahepatic bile ducts without a calculi would suggest either an ampullary or pancreatic tumor or a choledochal cyst. Careful analysis of the entire ultrasound examination can give needed information preoperatively and will indicate the need for further studies, such as endoscopic retrograde cholangiopancreatography (ERCP).

It is important to evaluate liver function; especially levels of serum alkaline phosphatase, transaminase, and bilirubin; prothrombin time and albumin level;

and, when abdominal pain and tenderness are present, serum amylase should be obtained. A baseline amylase level can be helpful when an ERCP or common duct exploration is anticipated.

Nuclear biliary studies are usually not helpful when evaluating the CBD for the presence of calculi. Currently, intravenous cholangiography is being reevaluated and may play a role in the preoperative assessment of patients suspected of having bile duct calculi (7). MRI has recently been shown to be useful in identifying CBDS.

These studies notwithstanding, the preoperative diagnosis of choledocholithiasis is imprecise. Only a portion of patients with common duct calculi have a dilated CBD on ultrasound or have abnormal liver function tests. In fact, 4% of patients undergoing cholecystectomy have unsuspected common duct stones (2). While approximately two-thirds of patients with common duct calculi have elevated liver function tests, only one-third of patients whose liver function tests are abnormal preoperatively harbor CBD stones at surgery (8).

Clinical presentations include epigastric pain that tightens around the waist like a vice and radiates through to the back, shoulder, or neck. This may be associated with nausea and/or vomiting, darkening of the urine, and lightening of the color of the stool (9). Jaundice follows, and occasionally shaking chills, fever, and tachycardia, as the gallstones are complicated by ascending infection. These patients are at high risk for renal failure as the result of bacterial endotoxin. Cahill and colleagues (10) have shown oral administration of sodium deoxycholate preoperatively prevents endotoxin absorption from the intestine and can prevent renal injury in these severely ill patients.

Often it is difficult to discriminate between obstructive cholecystitis with empyema of the gallbladder with or without common duct calculi and cholangitis associated with choledocholithiasis. In fact, in our experience, 18% of patients with acute cholecystitis had common duct stones at the time of surgery (11). Patients with empyema usually have a tender mass, but this finding may not be appreciated in obese or diabetic patients. Early surgical intervention is advisable.

Sometimes preoperative ERCP is needed for diagnostic reasons, but several prospective studies comparing preoperative ERCP, sphincterotomy and cholecystectomy versus cholecystectomy and "open" CBD exploration failed to show any advantage to ERCP or endoscopic sphincterotomy preceding surgery (12). Stain and coworkers (13) found preoperative ERCP and endoscopic sphincterotomy more morbid than open common duct exploration. Heinerman and associates (14) found preoperative ERCP to be less morbid than open surgery, but 72% of common duct explorations in his study were performed along with transduodenal sphincterotomy.

Shortly before the beginning of the laparoscopic era, Morgenstern and coworkers (15) reviewed 220 cases of open CBD exploration. Mortality was zero in patients under 60 and 4.3% in patients over 60, which suggests that preoperative sphincterotomy with 1% mortality (16) may be riskier than "open" duct exploration in younger patients, and endoscopic sphincterotomy may be safer in older patients. At the present time there are no comparable data on the risks of endoscopic sphincterotomy, or the long-term sequelae, in younger patients.

Several studies show that elderly patients suspected of having common duct calculi complicated by cholangitis or significant comorbid illness, or patients with worsening acute pancreatitis, are candidates for preoperative ERCP and possibly endoscopic sphincterotomy (17).

▼ INTRAOPERATIVE MANAGEMENT/SURGICAL TECHNIQUE

Surgery should be performed on patients with suspected choledocholithiasis only after appropriate intravenous hydration and antibiotic administration. Cefoperazone (Pfizer Canada, Inc.) as a single-drug therapy has been shown to be as

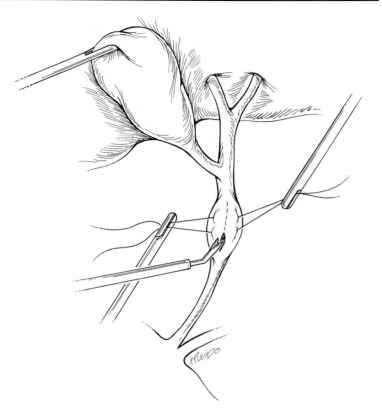

Figure 6. Elevation of stay sutures in the common duct to facilitate the safe performance of the choledochotomy.

injury to the portal vein. Electrocautery or laser energy is less controllable and should not be used to create the choledochotomy.

The length of the choledochotomy should be a few millimeters longer than the diameter of the largest CBD stone. Longer incisions require more suturing later when the choledochotomy is closed. The angle of the choledochotomy is based on the preexploration decision about the likelihood of a biliary bypass. If a biliary bypass is considered, the choledochotomy should be performed close to the duodenum. It should be performed in a horizontal or oblique orientation. If a biliary bypass is unlikely, a vertical choledochotomy affords easier suturing around the T tube when the choledochotomy is closed and greater ease of access to the proximal and distal bile ducts.

After the choledochotomy is performed, immediate insertion of a flexible choledochoscope through the subxiphoid trocar site allows for forceful irrigation of the CBD by means of the working channel of the endoscope and direct stone visualization (Fig. 7). This visualization allows for safer stone removal. Experience with rigid choledochoscopy in open common duct explorations conclusively shows that choledochoscopy decreases the incidence of retained stones (24,25). If a choledochoscope is available, there is no advantage in performing any "blind" manipulation. If a choledochoscope is not available, the patient's condition and the operator's experience in laparoscopically performing irrigation and balloon catheter trolling of the duct should be the determining factors when deciding to convert to "open" duct exploration or merely placing a T tube.

The choledochoscope should be bidirectional, and have a working channel of at least 1.2 mm (Fig. 8). Because the choledochotomy is usually at least 1 cm in length, and because the subxiphoid port is a 10-mm trocar, the standard 8-mm OD flexible choledochoscope can be used when performing laparoscopic choledochotomy. The larger diameter endoscopes allow for a large working channel, better light transmission, and improved optics. Of course, the 2.7- to 3.1-mm OD endoscopes used for transcystic duct exploration can be used, as long as they have a 1.2-mm working channel.

After the sutu
through the most
formed. The CBI
should be instilled
giogram shows tl
no calculi within
the gallbladder r
intravenously is
drainage into the
grasper pushing (
dye is injected v
drain should be [
choledochotomy

If a choledoc
common duct a
wire basket can
stones, and a bi
12-French or lai

Patients Requiri

Three types

1. With multip
   ration
2. With steno
   for reformi
3. With prima

In any categor
borderline case
the availability
Because endos
operative drair

The three l
choledochoje
formed either
tomy is slightl
limb. Howeve
jejunostomy i
should an ana

The chole
choledochodu
a "sump" sy
and literally b
However, if t
not occur. Se
of choledoch

Sphincter
technique for
been used fo
denal wall, it
suture line, t

The two l
and retrograc
the cystic d

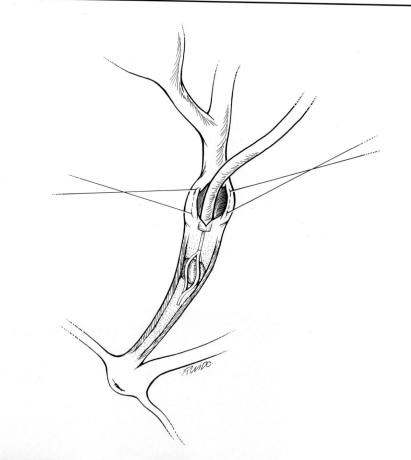

Figure 7. Choledochoscopy and stone removal with wire basket.

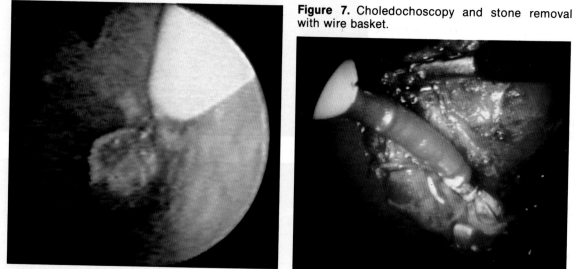

Irrigation solution is needed, and must be warmed to prevent hypothermia. Though direct visualization through the choledochoscope is possible, attaching a television camera to the choledochoscope for viewing on a television monitor facilitates the team approach for removal of bile duct calculi. The nurse or assistant can operate the stone-capturing basket in conjunction with the surgeon manipulating the endoscope (Fig. 9) (26). The shaft of the endoscope should be held in the surgeon's left hand, while the thumb of the right hand controls the deflection lever. While the right hand gently deflects the tip right and left or up and down, the left hand inserts or withdraws the endoscope while torquing the shaft to keep the lumen of the bile duct centered.

ACKNOWLEDGMENTS

I thank Raul Rosenthal, M.D., for his assistance with the preparation of this document; my partners, Brendan J. Carroll, M.D., F.A.C.S. and Moses J. Fallas, M.D., for their hard work; and Emma Matt and Lizabeth Knight for their help in its organization. Thank you to Morris Franklin, M.D., George Berci, M.D., and Gino Hasler for providing the figures.

REFERENCES

1. Way LW, Admirand WH, Dunphy JE. Management of choledocholithiasis. *Ann Surg* 1972;176: 347–359.
2. Phillips EH, Carroll BJ, Pearlstein AR, et al. Laparoscopic choledochoscopy and extraction of common bile duct stones. *World J Surg* 1993;17:22–28.
3. Skandalakis JE, Gray SW, et al. Biliary tract. In: Skandalakis JE, Gray SW, et al., eds. *Anatomical complications in general surgery*. New York: McGraw-Hill, 1983.
4. Ellis H. Choledocholithiasis. In: Schwartz SI, Ellis H, eds. *Maingot's abdominal operations*. 9th ed. E. Norwalk, CT: Appleton & Lange, 1989.
5. Phillips EH, Berci G, Carroll B, et al. The importance of intraoperative cholangiography during laparoscopic cholecystectomy. *Am Surg* 1990;56:792–795.
6. Schwartz SI. Anatomy of the extrahepatic biliary tract. In: Schwartz SI, Ellis H, eds. *Maingot's abdominal operations*. 9th ed. E. Norwalk, CT: Appleton & Lange, 1989.
7. Salky B. Personal communication. Mount Sinai Hospital, New York.
8. Cranley B, Logan H. Exploration of the common bile duct: the relevance of the clinical picture and the importance of preoperative cholangiography. *Br J Surg* 1980;67:869–872.
9. Diehl AK, Sugarpek NJ, Todd KH. Clinical evaluation for gallstone disease: usefulness of symptoms and signs in diagnosis. *Am J Med* 1990;89:29–33.
10. Cahill CJ, Pain JA, Bailey ME. Bile salts, endotoxin and renal function in obstructive jaundice. *Surg Gynecol Obstet* 1987;165:579.
11. Phillips EH, Carroll BJ, Fallas MJ. Laparoscopically guided cholecystectomy: a detailed report of 453 cases by one surgical team. *Am Surg* 1993;59:235–242.
12. Neoptolemos JP, Steigman G, Goff J, et al. Pre-cholecystectomy endoscopic cholangiography and stone removal is not superior to cholecystectomy, cholangiography, and common duct exploration. *Am J Surg* 1992;163:227–230.
13. Stain SC, Cohen H, Tsuishyosha M, Donovan AJ. Choledocholithiasis: endoscopic sphincterotomy or common bile duct exploration. *Ann Surg* 1991;213:6.
14. Heinerman PM, Boeckl O, Pimpl W, Selective ERCP and preoperative stone removal in bile duct surgery. *Ann Surg* 1989;209:267–272.
15. Morgenstern L, Wong L, Berci G. Twelve hundred open cholecystectomies before the laparoscopic era: a standard for comparison. *Arch Surg* 1992;127:400–403.
16. Cotton PB, Vennes J, Geenen JE, et al. Endoscopic sphincterotomy complications and their management: an attempt at consensus. *Gastrointest Endosc* 1991;37:383–386.
17. Mee AS, Vallon AG, Croker JD, et al. Nonoperative removal of bile duct stones by duodenoscopy sphincterotomy in the elderly. *Br Med J* 1981;3:521–523.
18. Bergeron MG, Mendelson J, Harding GK, et al. Cefoperazone compared to ampicillin plus tobramycin for severe biliary infections. *Antimicrob Agents Chemother* 1988;32:1231–1236.
19. Berci G, Hamlin J, Morgenstern L. Operative fluorocholangiography: utopia or overlooked entity. *Gastrointest Radiat* 1978;3:401–406.
20. Carroll BJ, Phillips EH, Daykhovsky L, et al. Laparoscopic choledochoscopy: an effective approach to the common duct. *J Laparoendosc Surg* 1992;2:15–21.
21. Hunter JG, Soper NJ. Laparoscopic management of bile duct stones. *Surg Clin North Am* 1992; 75:1077–1080.
22. Petelin JB. Laparoscopic approach to common duct pathology. *Surg Laparoendosc Endosc* 1991; 1:33–41.
23. Moosa AR, Easter DW, Van Sonnenberg E, et al. Laparoscopic injuries to the bile duct: a cause for concern. *Ann Surg* 1992;215:203–208.
24. Escat J, Fourtanier G, Maigne C, et al. Choledochoscopy in common bile duct surgery for choledocholithiasis: a must. *Gastrointest Endosc* 1991;37:166–167.
25. Shore JM, Shore E. Operative biliary endoscopy: experience with the flexible choledochoscope in 100 consecutive choledocholithotomies. *Ann Surg* 1970;171:269.
26. Ashby BS. Operative choledochoscopy in common bile duct surgery. *Ann R Coll Surg Engl* 1985; 67:279–283.
27. Carroll BJ, Phillips EH, Chandra M, Fallas M. Laparoscopic transcystic duct balloon dilatation of the sphincter of Oddi. *Surg Endosc* 1993;7:514–517.
28. Arregui ME, Davis CJ, Arkush AM, Nagan RF. Laparoscopic cholecystectomy combined with endoscopic sphincterotomy and stone extraction or laparoscopic choledochoscopy and electrohydraulic lithotripsy for management of cholelithiasis with choledocholithiasis. *Surg Endosc* 1992; 6:10–15.

29. Carroll B, Chandra M, Phillips E, et al. Biliary lithotripsy as an adjunct to laparoscopic common bile duct stone extraction. *Surg Endosc* 1993;7:356–359.
30. Berci G, Cuschieri A. *Practical laparoscopy.* London: Baillière Tindall, 1986.
31. Bean WJ, Mahorner HR. Removal of residual biliary stones through the T-tube tract. *South Med J* 1972;65:377.
32. Panis Y, Fagniez PL, Brisset D, et al. Long term result of choledochoduodenostomy versus choledochojejunostomy for choledocholithiasis: French association for surgical research. *Surg Gynecol Obstet* 1993;177:33–37.
33. DePaula A, Hashiba K, Bafutto M, Grecco E. Laparoscopic transcystic sphincterotomy in the management of 76 cases of choledocholithiasis. *SAGES Sci Session* 1993.
34. Franklin ME, Dorman JP. Laparoscopic common bile duct exploration. In: Braverman M, ed. *Surgical technology international,* Vol. 2. San Francisco, CA: Surgical Technology International, 1993.
35. Franklin ME. Laparoscopic choledochotomy for management of common bile duct stones and other common bile duct diseases. In: Arregui M, ed. *Principles of laparoscopic surgery.* St. Louis: Quality Medical Publishing, Inc., 1993.
36. Franklin ME, Pharand D, Rosenthal D. Laparoscopic common bile duct exploration. In: Zucker K, ed. *Surgical laparoscopy and endoscopy.* 1993.

KEY WORDS

Bile duct injury

Cholecystography

Choledocholithiasis

Fluoroscopy

Transcystic biliary access

● ANATOMY

Bile enters and exits the gallbladder via the cystic duct. While identification of the cystic duct-common bile duct junction is the most critical anatomic landmark during open cholecystectomy, the gallbladder-cystic duct junction is of much greater import during safe LC. The cystic duct-common bile duct junction is usually not identified during LC. Indeed, it can actually be difficult to visualize this area during LC, especially when using non-angled laparoscopes. Laparoscopic IOC remains the best technique for precise delineation of biliary tract anatomy, and is mandatory prior to applying occlusion devices when anatomy remains unclear.

While the cystic duct is classically portrayed as entering the right lateral aspect of the common bile duct at an acute angle, this anatomic configuration is not the most common. Berci and Hamlin (1981) found that the latter anatomic arrangement occurred in only 17% of patients, the most common situation being posterior entry of the cystic duct into the common bile duct (Fig. 1). Other variations are demonstrated in Fig. 1. A short cystic duct, entering the common hepatic or right hepatic ducts (Fig. 2) may occasionally be encountered, and is cause for concern and special care. Finally, accessory biliary ducts can occur, which may not only confuse anatomic interpretation but may also require clipping or ligation in order to avoid postoperative bile leak.

▶ PREOPERATIVE PLANNING

Following its introduction in 1937 by Mirizzi, intraoperative cholangiography (IOC) saw little use until technical improvements afforded better quality images. The increased popularity of IOC during open cholecystectomy was associated with a significant decrease in common bile duct exploration (CBDE) and increased incidence of positive explorations. The role of IOC continues to be discussed, especially since laparoscopic cholecystectomy (LC) has become the treatment of choice for symptomatic cholelithiasis. Without the ability to palpate the common duct, a positive IOC becomes the most reliable indicator for CBDE. Laparoscopic IOC is a valuable technique which can be performed in most cases. Failures are most often due to an unusually small cystic duct or stone impaction in the cystic duct stump.

When LC was introduced, endoscopic retrograde cholangiopancreatography (ERCP) was the favored treatment modality when choledocholithiasis was suspected. Thus, if signs or symptoms of a common duct stone were present preoperatively, the patient underwent ERCP and stone extraction was attempted prior to LC. If stone extraction was not possible, formal open cholecystectomy and CBDE were performed. With the advent of laparoscopic common duct exploration and stone extraction, laparoscopic surgeons now have a new set of options allowing the treatment of both cholelithiasis and choledocholithiasis with a single, minimally invasive procedure. Clearly, the latter approach mandates use of laparoscopic IOC.

Routine IOC is also proposed to prevent certain types of iatrogenic biliary injuries. Since retraction techniques used in LC may distort normal anatomy, IOC can provide vital anatomic information, especially in the presence of inflammation or unclear anatomy. Besides providing an anatomic "road map" to aid in safe dissection, IOC allows early detection of iatrogenic injury. Indeed, if the right hepatic or common ducts are misidentified as the cystic duct, IOC may reveal this injury. Early identification may allow one to repair an incision, in lieu of excision, of a common duct segment.

As with IOC during open cholecystectomy, many have espoused selective use of laparoscopic IOC. Proponents of selective laparoscopic IOC cite increased operative time and cost, false-positive or equivocal studies, and reports of injury

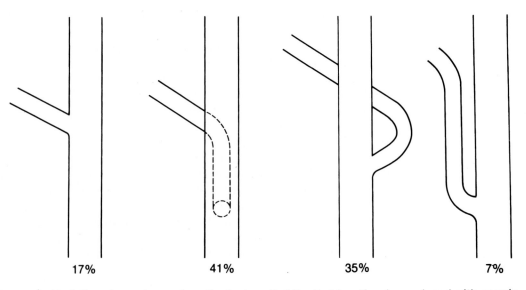

17%   41%   35%   7%

Figure 1. Variations in anatomy of cystic duct-cystic bile duct junction (reproduced with permission from Cuschieri A, Berci G: Laparoscopic Biliary Surgery, Second edition, Boston, 1992, Blackwell Scientific Publications, p. 126).

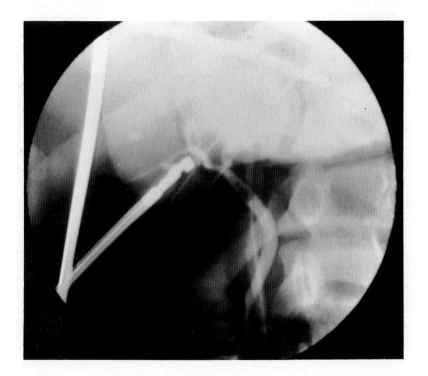

Figure 2. Laparoscopic cholangiogram demonstrating aberrant short cystic duct entering right hepatic duct. The filling defects are air bubbles.

secondary to cholangiography as arguments against routine IOC. Indications utilized for selective cholangiography include evidence of choledocholithiasis or dilated intra- or extrahepatic ducts on preoperative sonogram, elevated serum bilirubin or liver function tests, history of jaundice or gallstone pancreatitis, multiple small gallstones, enlarged cystic duct, or unclear anatomy at the time of cholecystectomy. If a policy of selective cholangiography is adopted, it is imperative that laparoscopic surgeons have the expertise and experience to avail themselves of IOC when it is most needed. For this reason, several authors advocate routine IOC to gain proficiency in techniques and confidence in the ability to obtain a cholangiogram in cases where it is most needed: when the anatomy is distorted, in the presence of inflammation, or in cases of unusually small caliber cystic ducts.

▼ INTRAOPERATIVE MANAGEMENT/SURGICAL TECHNIQUES

There are several techniques for performing LC, most of which involve alternative methods of cannulating the cystic duct or using different radiologic modalities. Adequate radiologic support is a critical component of any technique. Quality equipment, a trained technician, and a staff radiologist experienced in reading intraoperative biliary studies are vital needs. Although conventional portable x-ray equipment is sufficient to perform IOC, many currently favor digital cinefluoroscopy (Fig. 3). This method requires less contrast agent and allows clear demonstration of early biliary filling. Indeed, small stones may be obscured by the larger amount of contrast used in conventional studies, and may only be seen early in fluoroscopic studies. Similarly, if dye extravasation occurs, fluoroscopy facilitates identification of the anatomic site of extravasation, be it a pericatheter leak or a ductal injury. Hard copies can be made from the study for review by a radiologist or inclusion with the patient's radiologic file. In rare cases, such as extremely obese patients, fluoroscopic images may not be adequate, and conventional radiographs are then required.

Transcystic Cholangiography

As with open cholecystectomy, LC is most commonly obtained via the cystic duct. In this technique, exposure and dissection of the cystic duct-gallbladder junction gives circumferential access to the cystic duct. A clip applier is inserted

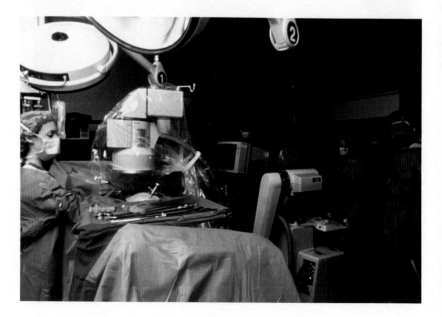

Figure 3. Digital cinefluoroscopy equipment which facilitates laparoscopic cholangiography, and is essential for more sophisticated procedures (e.g., common duct exploration).

via the subxiphoid port, and is used to place a clip as high as possible on the cystic duct-gallbladder junction. Care should be taken to ensure that gallbladder contents or any other structures are completely excluded. If the clip applicator is maintained in the closed position and not released, the grasp of the proximal cystic duct can be used to place it on tension, facilitating catheter insertion. Since the midclavicular port is frequently utilized for transcystic biliary access, optimal placement of this trocar is critical. For this reason, the midclavicular trocar is usually placed last. Placing the trocar after elevating the gallbladder allows for placement based on the resultant position of Calot's triangle (Fig. 4A). Ideally, the midclavicular trocar should be placed in the same plane as the cystic and common ducts, and should allow nearly perpendicular access to the cystic duct.

Microscissors are introduced through the midclavicular port and used to make a small incision in the cystic duct, just distal to the clip (Fig. 4B). This crucial step should be performed with great caution. While the incision must be large enough to accept the catheter, it should not transect the duct or injure posterior structures. If the duct is transected, it becomes extremely difficult to maintain tension on the cystic duct stump and cholangiography may become impossible. Transection also causes collapse of the cystic duct lumen, adding to the challenge. Should the duct be inadvertently divided, the best course is often simply to regain control of the stump and ligate it with an endoloop or two clips. The former is favored with short cystic duct stumps. If clips are used, they should be placed carefully and deliberately in order to avoid common duct injury.

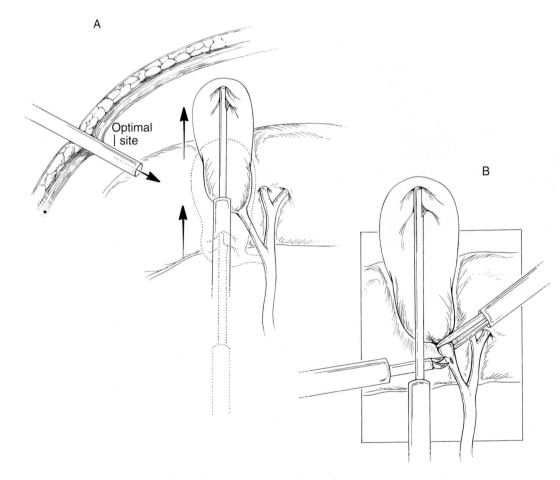

Figure 4. A: Elevating the gallbladder with graspers inserted via the right inferior trocar prior to insertion of the right superior trocar allows the latter trocar to be inserted at an optimal site, based on the final location of Calot's triangle. **B:** Optimal location of the right superior trocar provides perpendicular access to Calot's triangle.

After making an adequate incision, the catheter is introduced into the abdomen through a lateral abdominal port (Fig. 5) or a separate puncture site (Fig. 6). If one of the exiting ports is used, it should be selected based upon which offers the best approach to the ductal incision. This is usually the right midclavicular port (see above). The catheter is then guided into the cystic duct with graspers and carefully clipped in place with a single clip. This clip must be applied so as to prevent extravasation while not occluding the catheter. This method of cholangiography leaves only a single port for retraction and exposure. If exposure is inadequate, a separate puncture site should be used to insert the catheter. This alternative method permits selection of the angle and location of insertion based upon ductal anatomy, and does not require the use of an existing port which might be utilized to maximize exposure.

When the catheter is secured, the graspers are removed from the field; any metal trocars should be replaced with radiolucent plastic rods. Most disposable plastic trocars will not interfere with the study and may be left in place. The catheter is then connected to a syringe of sterile saline previously rid of air bubbles. Bile is aspirated, and the ductal system is irrigated with sterile saline to ensure easy flow and no leakage. If using conventional films, two radiographs are usually obtained: the first after injecting 5-10 cc bolus of water-soluble contrast, the second after injecting 15-20 cc. If using digital fluoroscopy, contrast is injected under direct vision until the entire biliary tree is visualized (Fig. 7) and contrast is seen to flow freely into the duodenum (Fig. 8). Intermittent exposures should be taken for review and documentation.

Another method of cystic duct cannulation uses one of several available clamps specifically designed for cystic duct cannulation and occlusion (Fig. 9). The cathe-

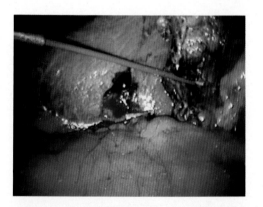

Figure 5. Cholangiography catheter inserted through the right superior trocar. (Courtesy of Dr. E. H. Phillips.)

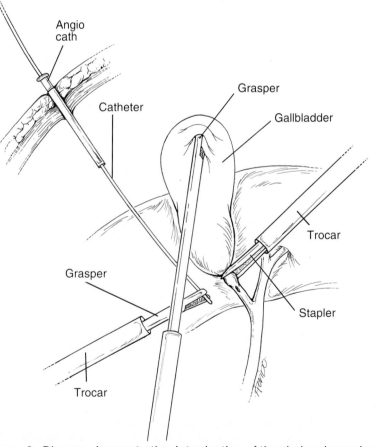

Figure 6. Diagram demonstrating introduction of the cholangiography catheter via an angiocatheter inserted at a separate puncture site.

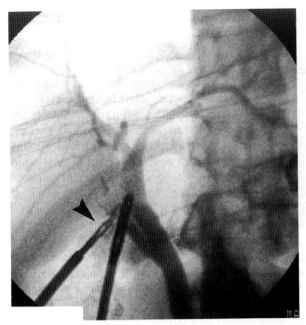

Figure 7. Laparoscopic cholangiogram demonstrating complete filling of the biliary tree. Note the cholangiogram catheter clamp *(arrow)*.

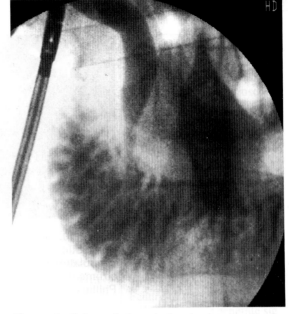

Figure 8. Enlarged view during laparoscopic cholangiography demonstrating the biliary sphincter zone, as well as flow of contrast into the duodenum.

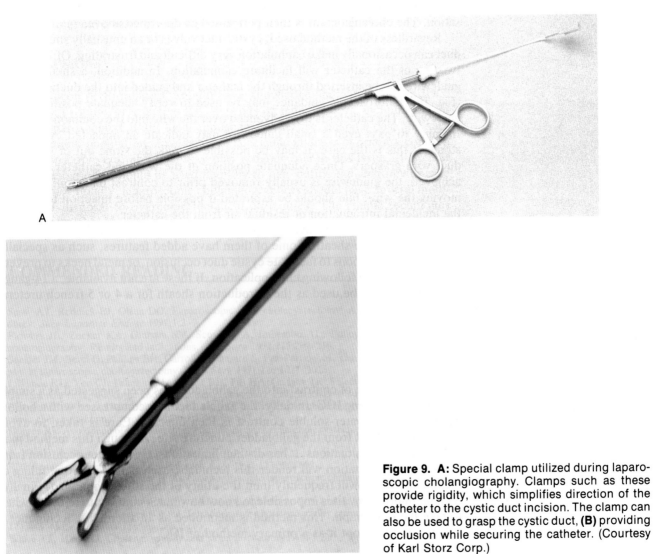

Figure 9. **A:** Special clamp utilized during laparoscopic cholangiography. Clamps such as these provide rigidity, which simplifies direction of the catheter to the cystic duct incision. The clamp can also be used to grasp the cystic duct, **(B)** providing occlusion while securing the catheter. (Courtesy of Karl Storz Corp.)

19

Transhepatic Biliary Laser Lithotripsy

Desmond H. Birkett
Department of Surgery
Boston University School of Medicine
Boston, Massachusetts 02118

Operative Laparoscopy and Thoracoscopy, edited by
B. V. MacFadyen, Jr. and
J. L. Ponsky. Lippincott-Raven
Publishers, Philadelphia © 1996.

KEY WORDS

Cholangiogram   Laser

Choledocholithiasis   Lithotripsy

Choledochoscopy   Transhepatic

The management of retained or recurrent bile duct stones by open operation has been replaced largely by endoscopic retrograde cholangiography and papillotomy, a procedure first described by Classen and Demling (1). This minimal access method of treating choledocholithiasis carries a lower incidence of morbidity and mortality than in an open operation. However, in 5% to 10% of patients, papillotomy cannot be performed because of inexperience of the endoscopist, a difficult papilla, or anatomic reasons, the most common of which are a periampullary diverticulum, which heightens the risk of duodenal perforation, and the altered anatomy of a previous Bilroth II gastrectomy, particularly with an anticolic hookup. In these circumstances, the alternative is to resort to an open operation, which carries a significant morbidity and mortality rate in elderly patients with comorbidities. In this group of patients the treatment of choice for choledocholithiasis is by way of a transhepatic route to the biliary tree.

The transhepatic approach is an extension of transhepatic drainage of the biliary tree for biliary decompression and transhepatic stent placement for the relief of biliary obstruction. To treat stones by way of the transhepatic route the track must be enlarged to permit endoscopic access to the stone. At times this requires a track of some considerable size for the larger stones. With the introduction of lithotripsy, biliary stones can be removed in small fragments through percutaneous tracts that are considerably smaller than the stone to be removed. The less dilatation of the transhepatic tract, the less likelihood of complications such as biliary leak or bleeding from the erosion of intrahepatic veins or arteries.

Chen and Jan (2) were the first to describe transhepatic laser lithotripsy using the Nd:YAG laser in 2 of 14 patients with intrahepatic and common duct stones; the remaining patients were treated with electrohydraulic lithotripsy. Orii and colleagues (3) found from their experience with Nd:YAG laser lithotripsy through the T-tube tract that at a wavelength of 1,064 nm only pigment stones were fragmented.

Nishioka and coworkers (4) investigated a variety of wavelengths from 450 to 700 nm and found that 504 nm was the wavelength that gave the most effective stone fragmentation with the best combination of low energy requirements and the fewest pulses. Fragmentation at this wavelength was achieved by an acoustic effect brought about by the conversion of light energy to mechanical energy, forming a plasma at the surface of the stone, which, on contraction, generated a shockwave that fragmented the stone. This theory was supported by the work of Teng and colleagues (5).

The 504-nm coumarin pulsed dye laser became the laser of choice for the treatment of both renal and biliary stones and was found to be more effective in fragmenting pigment than cholesterol stones. Josephs and Birkett (6) reported the use of the coumarin pulsed dye laser in the treatment of retained common duct and intrahepatic stones and found that stones could be fragmented to a size that washed through the sphincter of Oddi into the duodenum. They also point out it is not the size of the stone to be removed that is the dominant factor, but rather it is the size of the endoscope that has to be passed to the site of the stone.

The use of laser lithotripsy in combination with small-instrument transhepatic endoscopy makes this technology useful for the treatment of common duct stones that cannot be treated by retrograde papillotomy with stone extraction.

● ANATOMY

The radiologist must know the anatomy of the intrahepatic bile ducts to aid in locating them with the needle. The right hepatic duct has a main anterior and a main posterior branch, with segmental branches off these. It is in the anterior branch of the right hepatic duct that is chosen for needling.

The common hepatic duct starts at the junction of the right and the left hepatic duct, a junction that is just intrahepatic in most patients, but in a minority of patients the right and left hepatic ducts join outside the substance of the liver. The right hepatic duct is formed by the union of an anterior branch and a posterior branch, a junction that is within the substance of the liver, but they may join quite distally to form a very short right hepatic duct. It is in the anterior hepatic duct or the junction of the right hepatic duct that the radiologist aims to place the needle so that he is well within the substance of the liver. The right lobe of the liver is situated under the costal margin and the superior surface is in direct contact with the undersurface of the diaphragm as it passes down and is inserted into the edge of the rib cage. The pleura of the right pleural cavity may extend deep down between the lower rib cage and diaphragm such that a percutaneous needle directed at the right hepatic duct within the substance of the liver will pass across the pleural space, thereby running the risk of a pneumothorax.

The anatomy of the biliary tree from the endoscopist's point of view is very straightforward. The endoscope is introduced initially into the right hepatic duct and on advancing the endoscope the orifice of the hepatic duct will be noted on the right side. The distance that the right duct must be traversed endoscopically to find the left duct orifice depends on the point of entry into the ductal system. A good cholangiogram performed after access has been achieved is a great help to the endoscopist. As the endoscope is passed into the common hepatic duct the endoscopist must be prepared for some significant angulations, usually to the right, due to postoperative changes brought about by scarring. The upper biliary sphincter can be seen opening and closing and can be traversed easily with small endoscopes. The distal sphincter can then be seen in the distance and tends not to open and close quite as much. The distal sphincter can also be crossed easily into the duodenum.

▶ PREOPERATIVE PLANNING

Transhepatic endoscopic laser lithotripsy is an excellent minimal access method of treating common duct and intrahepatic stones, but should not be used as the first treatment option unless other minimally invasive techniques are not possible.

Endoscopic retrograde papillotomy with stone removal is the first choice for the nonoperative treatment of common duct or intrahepatic stones, provided there is not an already established percutaneous access, such as the presence of a T-tube tract. In patients with a T tube in place, access through the T-tube tract is considered the best route for the treatment of retained common duct stones, particularly for common hepatic or intrahepatic stones. In those patients who have no potential for T-tube tract access or who cannot have a successful endoscopic retrograde papillotomy performed, then transhepatic endoscopy, lithotripsy, and stone removal is the most appropriate method of treatment.

There are several reasons why an endoscopic retrograde papillotomy may fail or may not be possible:

1. A previous Bilroth II gastrectomy, particularly when the anastomosis was constructed in an anticolic manner and results in an afferent limb that is usually too long to allow the duodenoscope to reach the ampulla

2. The stone is too large to be pulled through the papillotomy and is easily fragmented
3. Periampullary duodenum diverticula
4. Impossible to intubate the sphincter of Oddi
5. Comorbidities in the patient, such as being unable to lie prone or being unable
   to undergo the necessary sedation

A transhepatic approach should be undertaken in patients who fit in the above
categories.

▼ INTRAOPERATIVE MANAGEMENT/SURGICAL TECHNIQUE

There are two methods of performing transhepatic endoscopy and laser lithotripsy: first, a staged procedure through a chronically established track between
the skin of the lower right rib cage or upper abdomen and the right hepatic duct,
and second, a one-stage procedure through a sheath placed from the skin of the
lower right rib cage into the right hepatic duct at the time of the initial transhepatic
cholangiogram. Through this sheath an endoscope is passed to enable laser lithotripsy to be performed under direct vision.

Staged Procedure

The procedure is performed in the radiology department using fluoroscopy.
Under sterile conditions, antibiotic coverage, and intravenous sedation a radiolo-
gist performs a skinny Chiba needle cholangiogram to visualize the biliary tree
(Fig. 1). With the biliary tree well opacified and the presence of stones confirmed,

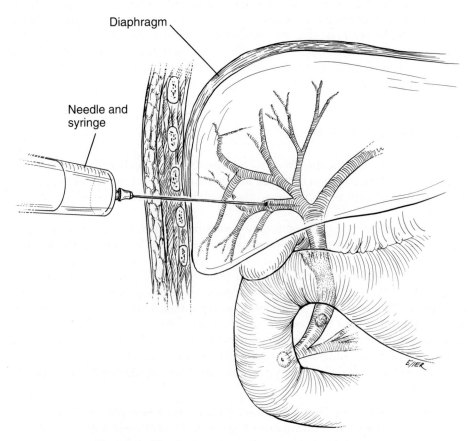

Figure 1. Needle location of the right hepatic duct.

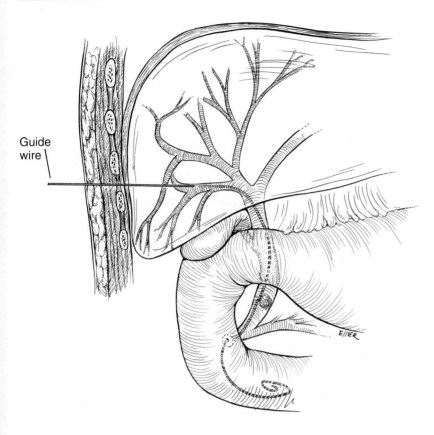

Figure 2. Percutaneous placement of a guidewire across the lower rib cage and the liver into the right hepatic duct.

the radiologist removes the Chiba needle and introduces a larger needle and introducer into the right hepatic duct at an angle to the right duct that will permit easy passage of an endoscope into the right duct and on into the distal biliary tree. An 0.038-in. guidewire is then fed through the introducer into the right hepatic duct and on down the common duct, through the sphincter of Oddi, and on into the duodenum (Fig. 2). With the wire in place, the introducer is removed and an 8.3 F transhepatic pigtail catheter is passed over the wire into the right hepatic duct, advanced into the common hepatic duct, and anchored in place. The extracorporal portion is fastened securely to the skin.

Over the next 10 to 14 days the track is serially dilated up to either size 11 F or size 16 F to permit passage of either the 3.2-mm ureteroscope URF P2 (Olympus Corporation, Inc., Lake Success, NY) or the 4.9-mm flexible choledochoscope CHF B3 (Olympus Corporation, Inc., Lake Success, NY), respectively, depending on which endoscope is to be used for the lithotripsy and stone removal (Fig. 3).

Once the track is mature and dilated to the correct size, the second stage of the procedure is performed. This is also performed in the radiology department on a fluoroscopy table or in the operating room with good C-arm fluoroscopy. The procedure is performed under intravenous antibiotic coverage and sedation, and sterile conditions. First a transhepatic cholangiogram is performed to again document the presence of the stones and to show their current position. The transhepatic catheter is removed from the transhepatic tract and a flexible endoscope, with saline running through the instrument channel, is passed into the track and advanced under direct vision into the biliary tree and down to the site of the stone. Saline irrigation is necessary to distend the biliary tree to permit good visualization and to wash away any debris that might be present. A liter bag of normal saline attached to a standard intravenous giving set and hung 3–4 ft above the patient is connected to the instrument channel of the endoscope through a "Sure-Seal" valve (Applied Urology, Inc., Laguna Hills, CA) which gives an

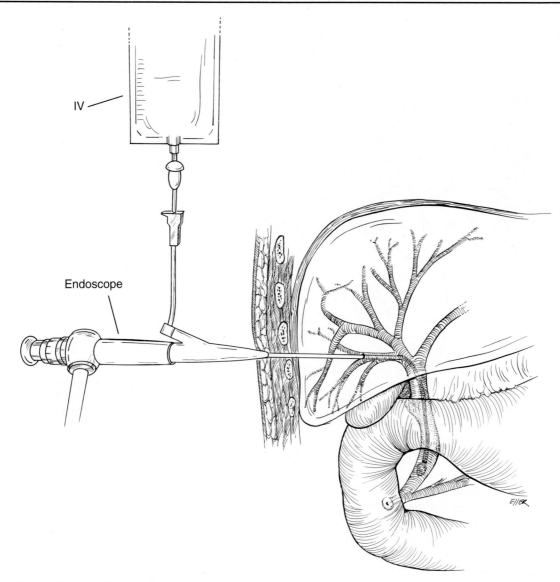

IV

Endoscope

Figure 3. Choledochoscope passed through the mature transhepatic duct into the biliary tree.

excellent seal around the laser fiber and other accessories without leakage of saline. When using the smaller 3.2-mm endoscope it is often necessary to use a pressure bag on the liter bag of saline to keep the irrigation flowing when the laser fiber or other instruments are partially occluding the instrument channel of the endoscope. If the stone is in the left hepatic duct or a branch of either major intrahepatic duct, fluoroscopy may be helpful in directing the endoscope into the correct position to reach the stone. Once the stone is visualized, a highly flexible 200-μm quartz fiber attached to a 504-nm coumarin pulsed dye laser, such as the Pulsolith (Technomed International, Inc., Danvers, MA) is passed through the "Sure-Seal" valve and the instrument channel of the endoscope and placed in direct contact with the surface of the stone. The laser set at 80–100 mJ and 5 Hz is discharged by foot pedal control onto the stone surface while the laser discharge is carefully monitored under direct vision to prevent ductal damage. If the laser is discharged at a rate faster than 5 Hz, the fast flashing blends into one bright light, preventing visualization of the fiber tip, the stone, and its fragmentation. It is very important to watch the tip of the fiber at all times to ensure a good fiber stone contact for effective rapid fragmentation and to avoid accidental discharge of the laser on the wall of the bile duct, reducing the chance of ductal perforation by the laser. Fragmentation is often more rapid if the laser is fired at the edge of the stone as this breaks off fragments that are small enough to be washed away through the sphincter of Oddi by the flow of saline. Stones often fragment easily and more rapidly by chipping fragments off the edge of the stone rather than by placing the fiber in the center of the stone, which often takes many pulses to fragment into large pieces. Cholesterol stones do not fragment as easily as pigment stones, but once the white cholesterol shell has been cracked more rapid progress can be achieved by firing at the pigment center. It may be necessary to turn the stone or fragment to expose a pigmented surface. As the stone is fragmented into small pieces they can be fragmented into even smaller pieces until they can be washed into the duodenum or removed by basket extraction.

There are two types of baskets that are used, a spiral wire basket and a hexagonal wire basket. The former is easier to use in ducts that are curved, since the wires of a hexagonal basket are spread out by the curve and a stone will not engage in the basket. The size of the basket to be used depends on the size of the endoscope being passed. The small 3.2-mm ureteroscope will take a 3 F basket, while the channel of the larger 4.9-mm choledochoscope will accommodate a 5 F basket. The basket is passed through the instrument channel of the endoscope, advanced beyond the fragment, opened, and pulled back to engage the fragment. Once the fragment is seen to be between the wires of the basket, the basket is closed to secure the fragment and, once secure, the basket, endoscope, and fragment are pulled out of the transhepatic track. The endoscope is passed back through the transhepatic track to ensnare further fragments, to perform further lithotripsy, or to inspect the biliary tree for completeness of stone removal.

Once the biliary tree is cleared of stones, and this is confirmed by good visualization or by cholangiography, the track is not reintubated and the skin site is dressed with gauze and allowed to close. If it is necessary to perform another endoscopy and possible lithotripsy at a later date, a catheter is placed into the tract to preserve its patency and secured in place ready for the next session, which can be performed at any time convenient to the patient and surgeon.

One-Stage Procedure

Transhepatic lithotripsy can be performed as a one-stage procedure, an alternative that has distinct advantages for the patient, but this may make it more difficult and lengthy for the surgeon and radiologist.

The procedure is performed in the radiology department with fluoroscopy, under antibiotic coverage, intravenous sedation, and sterile conditions. The radiologist performs a Chiba needle transhepatic cholangiogram to opacify the biliary tree (Fig. 1). A larger needle and introducer are passed into the main right hepatic duct through which an 0.038-in. guidewire is introduced into the biliary tree and advanced through the sphincter of Oddi into the duodenum (Fig. 2). It is important for the angle of entry into the right hepatic duct to permit easy entry of a sheath and endoscope. The tract is then acutely dilated over the wire up to 11 F. After dilatation, an 11 F Cath Seal sheath and introducer (UMI, Inc., Ballston Spa, NY) are passed over the guidewire into the right hepatic duct, and the wire and introducer are removed (Fig. 4).

Once the access has been established, the 3.2-mm ureteroscope is passed through the sheath into the right hepatic duct and advanced down the biliary tree under direct vision to the site of the stone (Fig. 5). A 200-μm quartz fiber attached to a 504-nm coumarin pulsed dye laser, such as the Pulsolith, is passed through the instrument channel of the endoscope and placed in contact with the stone and the laser activated. For effective fragmentation the procedure must be performed under direct vision, washing the fragments away with the flow of saline, which is pressurized by a pressure cuff on the bag of saline. When using the small endo-

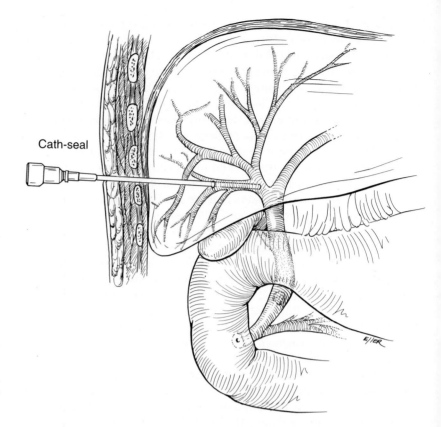

Cath-seal

Figure 4. Cath-seal sheath placed across the rib cage and liver into the right hepatic duct.

scope it is necessary to fragment the stone into pieces that can be washed through the sphincter into the duodenum. As mentioned in the previous section, cholesterol stones fragment slowly as the laser light is not absorbed as well by the white color of the stone and the tricks mentioned previously help considerably. To speed up fragmentation of these stones it is important to focus either on cracks in the stone or at the edge of the stone to remove part of the cholesterol shell and expose the underlying pigment. When the laser can be aimed at pigment, the light energy is better absorbed, and fragmentation proceeds at a faster rate. It is not possible to basket extract fragments through the sheath as it is too small and rigid and may be dislodged from the right hepatic duct if a fragment gets caught on its edge.

Once it is felt that the biliary tree is free of stones and fragments by direct visualization, a cholangiogram should be performed through the sheath. This can be performed through the arm of the sheath or by passing a radiologic catheter through the valve of the sheath into the biliary system. If the biliary tree is determined to be free of stones, the sheath is removed over a Gelfoam plug. Bleeding is not usually a problem. This is probably due to a combination of the compression of vessels by the sheath and the length of the procedure, which results in the clotting of any vessel in the path of the track. Despite this we place a Gelfoam plug to reduce the chances of bleeding. If the biliary tree needs to be reexamined at a later date for further stone fragmentation or clearance of remaining fragments, then a 10 F transhepatic catheter is placed through the transhepatic sheath and into the right hepatic duct before removing the sheath. The sheath is removed over the catheter. This tube should be clamped off for two reasons, to reduce the chance of biliary infection and also to permit the flow of bile to wash remaining fragments out of the biliary tree into the duodenum. Before performing further endoscopy and lithotripsy a cholangiogram should be performed to confirm the presence of stones, since the flow of bile may have washed the biliary tree free of stones and fragments.

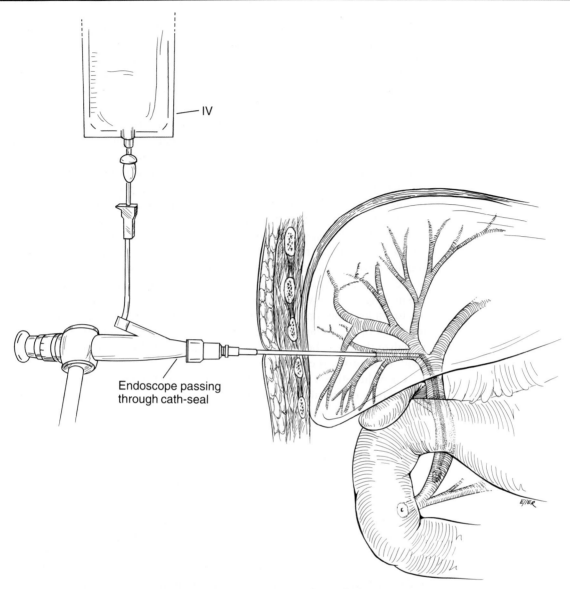

Figure 5. Choledochoscope passed through the cath-seal sheath.

The one-stage procedure is preferable because of the shorter time and fewer procedures required to treat the stone burden. However, if access is difficult to establish or takes a long time, then it is better to stage the procedure. Clearly the ability of the patient to tolerate a long procedure will necessitate a staged technique. The chance of losing access to the biliary tree is lower with a staged technique because of an established and mature transhepatic tract. Should there be any doubt about the ability to perform a one-stage procedure, then it should be staged.

▲ COMPLICATIONS

The complications of this minimal access procedure can be divided into two groups: those related to the stage of radiologic access and those related to the stage of the biliary endoscopy and lithotripsy.

A percutaneous needle puncture through the lower right rib cage aimed at the main right hepatic duct may violate the pleural space and cause a pneumothorax,

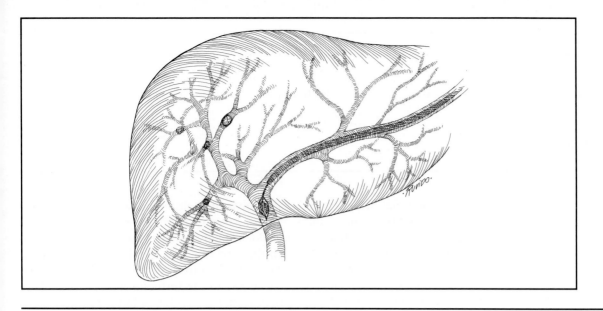

20

Choledochoscopy

Jeffrey L. Ponsky
Department of Surgery
Case Western Reserve University
School of Medicine
Cleveland, Ohio 44016

Operative Laparoscopy and Thoracoscopy, edited by
B. V. MacFadyen, Jr. and
J. L. Ponsky. Lippincott-Raven
Publishers, Philadelphia © 1996.

Endoscopic examination of the biliary tree is not a new technique, yet the importance and sophistication of the method have grown with the emergence of minimally invasive surgery. Initially, choledochoscopy was performed with rigid endoscopes through a choledochotomy at the time of common bile duct exploration. More recently, most practitioners have switched to flexible fiberoptic (or video) choledochoscopes to achieve greater access to the tortuous areas of the biliary tree (Fig. 1). The method has benefited from the revolution in video technology, enabling all members of the operative team to visualize the interior of the duct and participate in the diagnostic and therapeutic dimensions of the procedure (Fig. 2). The technology has been adapted for peroral use via ampullary cannulation, allowing direct examination of the bile ducts at the time of endoscopic retrograde cholangiopancreatography (ERCP). The choledochoscope may also be introduced through a T-tube tract in the postoperative period in order to deal with retained stones after surgery. Most recently, choledochoscopy has become important in the examination of the biliary tree at the time of laparoscopic cholecystectomy, passing the instrument(s) via the cystic duct or through a laparoscopic choledochotomy. These advancements have permitted the biliary surgeon to diagnose and treat maladies of the bile ducts in a minimally invasive fashion.

◉ ANATOMY

The classical anatomy of the biliary tree is well known to all surgeons. The structure of the system is characterized by its simplicity and variability. The right and left hepatic ducts converge to form the common hepatic duct. The gallbladder empties via the cystic duct into the common hepatic duct to begin the common bile duct (CBD). The distal CBD is surrounded by a muscular sphincter and traverses the duodenal wall prior to opening into the intestinal lumen. The pancreatic duct joins the system proximal to the ampulla of Vater. A common channel of variable length is present in most individuals (Fig. 3).

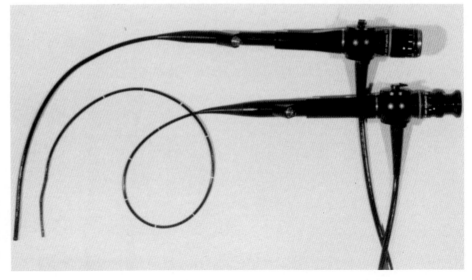

Figure 1. The standard flexible choledochoscope *(top)* has a diameter of approximately 5 mm, while the ureteroscopes used for transcystic choledochoscopy are about 3 mm in diameter.

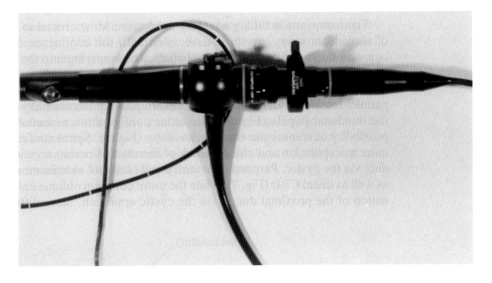

Figure 2. Video cameras can be easily attached to the eyepiece of the choledochoscope.

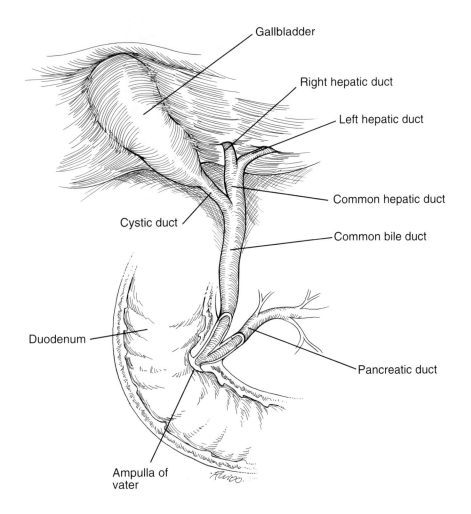

Figure 3. The normal anatomy of the biliary system.

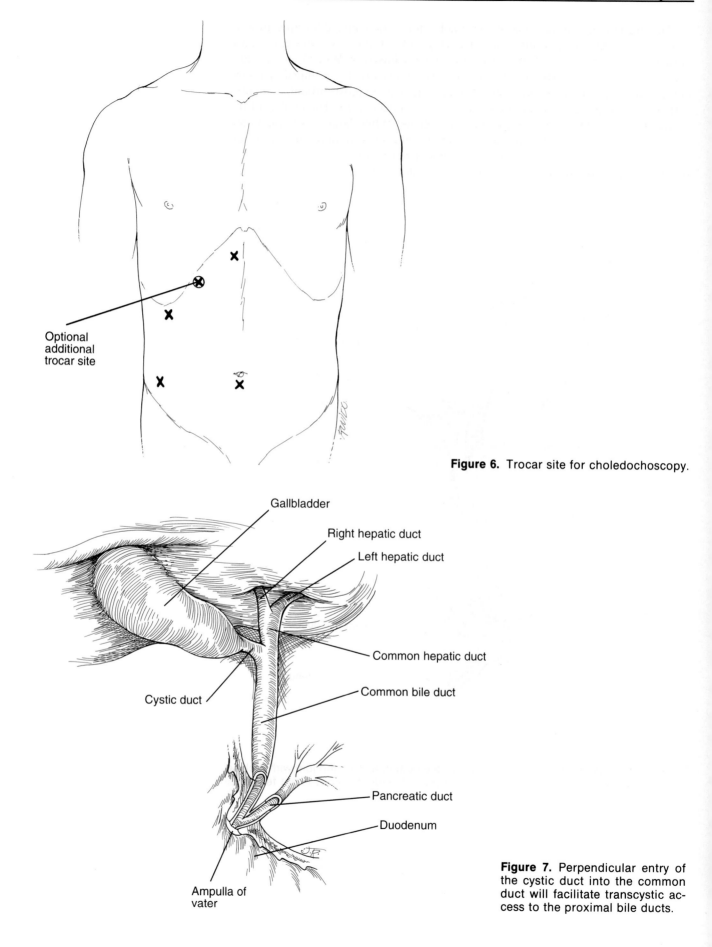

Figure 6. Trocar site for choledochoscopy.

Optional additional trocar site

Gallbladder

Right hepatic duct

Left hepatic duct

Common hepatic duct

Common bile duct

Cystic duct

Pancreatic duct

Duodenum

Ampulla of vater

Figure 7. Perpendicular entry of the cystic duct into the common duct will facilitate transcystic access to the proximal bile ducts.

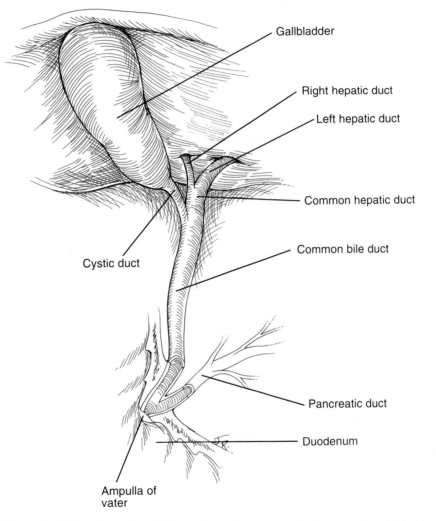

Gallbladder

Right hepatic duct

Left hepatic duct

Common hepatic duct

Cystic duct

Common bile duct

Pancreatic duct

Duodenum

Ampulla of vater

Figure 8. Oblique junction of the cystic and common ducts is most common. Transcystic choledochoscopy is usually easy to perform but often is limited to the distal common duct.

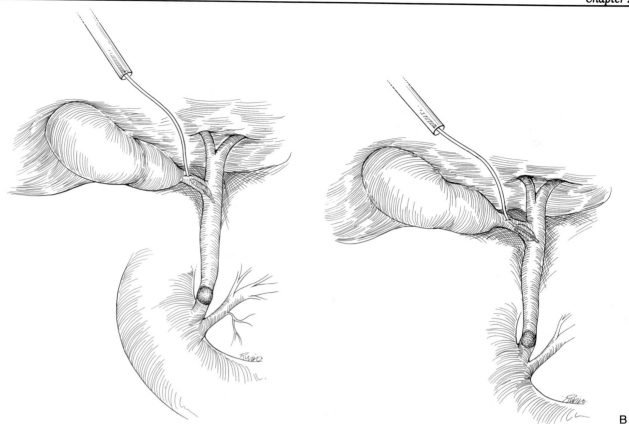

A

B

Figure 12. A: Hydrostatic balloon dilaters are inserted into the cystic duct. **B:** The hydrostatic balloon dilator is slowly inflated in the cystic duct. Close observation is necessary to look for evidence of tearing of the duct wall or the common duct junction.

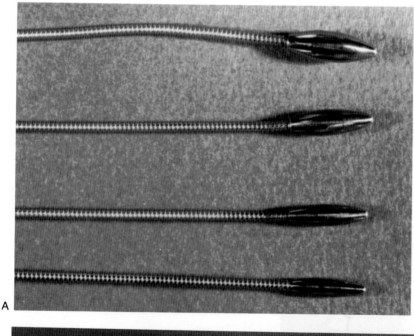

A

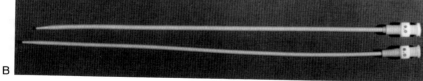

B

Figure 13. A: Metal-tipped graded ureteral dilators may be used over a wire to dilate the cystic duct. **B:** Plastic ureteral dilators can be used for cystic duct dilation. The course of the tip of the dilator should be noted to prevent inadvertent common duct injury.

Once the scope is within the common bile duct lumen, it is necessary to infuse saline solution through the scope's channel in order to distend the duct and achieve optimal visualization. This can be done by the simple attachment of intravenous tubing, from a bag of saline, to the channel of the scope. In most cases, the endoscope will proceed distally in the common duct, toward the duodenum. Visualization of the ductal interior is usually best upon withdrawal of the scope, so the scope should be passed as far distally as it will go easily. If resistance is met, force should be avoided and observation of the duct commenced. Because the presently available endoscopes employ only two-directional tip control, it is necessary to twist the shaft of the instrument a bit as it is withdrawn. This, in combination with two-way tip deflection, will provide a complete view of the ductal interior. Inspection of the proximal ductal system may be difficult owing to the obliquity, which generally characterizes the cystic duct-common bile duct junction. In some cases, however, with slight traction applied to the cystic duct, the obliquity can be straightened and the scope advanced into the proximal system.

With saline infusion, stones may be seen to "float" within the duct. Small stones frequently can be flushed or pushed distally to exit into the duodenum. Larger stones will require lithotripsy or extraction techniques. A wire stone basket, much the same as used by urologists, is a valuable tool in manipulating ductal calculi. The basket may have three or four wires and passed through the working channel of the scope. Once the stone is observed, the basket is used to surround the stone. It is useful to pass the basket beyond the stone, opening it prior to pulling it back. Once the basket is in proximity to the stone, capture may be facilitated by back-and-forth movements or twist of the basket (Fig. 14). Closing

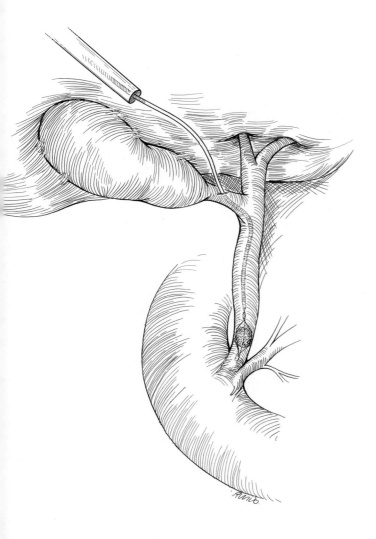

Figure 14. To-and-fro motion of the basket will often facilitate capture of the stone.

the basket once the stone is engaged may result in morselization of the stone. Although this may be desirable for larger stones, the many fragments resulting may themselves require extraction or flushing. It may be preferable to attempt only partial closure of the basket and to coax the intact stone backward through the cystic duct orifice where it can be removed. A stone may also be extracted by trapping it between a balloon and the scope's tip, securing it as it is pulled out of the ductal system (Fig. 15). When multiple passes of the scope and basket are required, as when stone fragments are being retrieved, the use of an introducer sheath passed through the opening in the cystic duct can facilitate multiple entries of the endoscope. The sheath is the same as is used for introduction of central venous lines. It is advanced into the cystic duct over a wire after the duct is dilated.

When stones are very large or impacted, lithotripsy may be accomplished under direct vision using electrohydraulic devices or pulse dye laser energy. The probe or fiber for the device is passed into the duct via the channel of the endoscope. Each device must be applied directly to the surface of the stone. The electrohydraulic lithotripter can produce ductal perforation if incorrectly aimed. While the pulse dye laser carries less risk of perforation, it can also injure the ductal wall, and great care must be taken with either instrument to apply energy only to the surface of the stone.

Following completion of the examination, the cystic duct must be adequately closed. While metal clips are satisfactory in routine cholecystectomy, the tissue

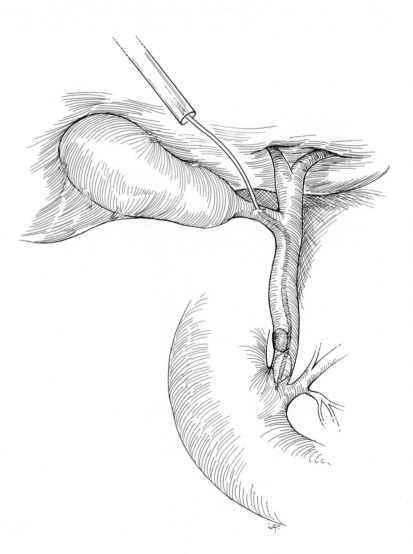

Figure 15. A stone can be trapped between the inflated balloon and the scope's tip and held there as the scope is removed.

edema resulting from ductal dilation and manipulation can predispose to clip dislodgment. Therefore, it is advisable to use a suture ligature, usually a pretied loop ligature, alone or in combination with a clip to seal the duct.

Choledochoscopy via a Choledochotomy

Direct choledochoscopy has become an integral part of laparoscopic choledochotomy. It is perhaps more important than in traditional open choledochotomy because, in the laparoscopic procedure, the surgeon must use his eyes to supplant tactile sensation. The standard flexible choledochoscope, approximately 5 mm in diameter, can be used for the procedure (Fig. 16). It can be introduced through a 5-mm trocar and inserted directly into the choledochotomy. Saline irrigation should be carried out to distend the duct. The scope is directed proximally and distally to completely examine all areas of the extrahepatic system. Inspection is usually best upon withdrawal of the scope after complete insertion. When stones are encountered, they may be dislodged and removed using balloons or wire baskets passed through the scope's channel. Lithotripsy can be used when necessary using the electrohydraulic lithotripter or pulse dye laser. Again, these endoscopes have only two-directional tip control and torsion must be applied to the shaft as the scope is withdrawn in order to view all of the ductal interior.

Choledochoscopy via the Transhepatic Route

When biliary stones are suspected or demonstrated within the intrahepatic ducts, extraction may be attempted by the transhepatic route. The first step in this approach must be a transhepatic cholangiogram. When successful access is obtained a catheter is left in place to establish a tract. Bilateral access is optimal. The catheters are exchanged over guidewires periodically and progressively larger catheters are introduced until the tracts are approximately 10 French in size and of adequate caliber to permit entry of a 3-mm endoscope.

After the tracts are mature, the catheters are removed and a small-caliber endoscope is inserted (Fig. 17). Fluoroscopic guidance is useful to guide the extraction. Balloons, baskets, and lithotripsy devices may be employed. Multiple interventions may be required and catheters should be replaced into the tracts following the procedure and left in place until the tracts are no longer required.

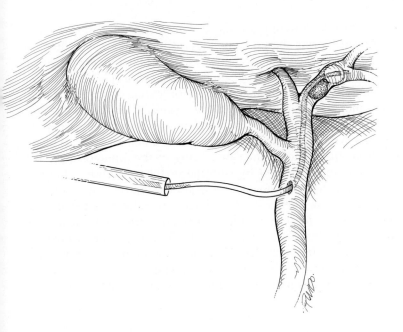

Figure 16. A standard flexible choledochoscope, with a diameter of approximately 5 mm, is invaluable in the performance of common bile duct exploration at the time of laparoscopic choledochotomy.

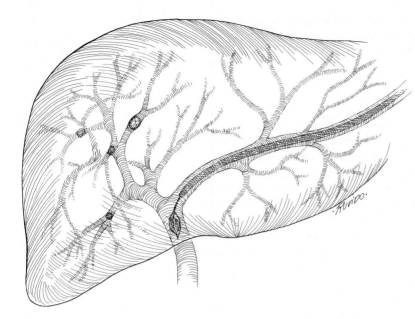

Fig. 17. Transhepatic cholangioscopy can be performed using the small-caliber choledochoscope (3 mm) after transhepatic tracts are mature.

Choledochoscopy via the Postoperative T-Tube Tract

Following choledochotomy, postoperative T-tube cholangiography is generally performed prior to removal of the T-tube. When stones are identified they are most often removed by radiographic or endoscopic intervention. In some cases, choledochoscopy via the mature T-tube tract can permit manipulation and removal of stones under direct vision. The T-tube tract is generally allowed to mature for 6 weeks. The T-tube is removed and, under fluoroscopic guidance, the choledochoscope is inserted into the tract to observe and attack any retained stones. Baskets, balloons, or lithotripsy devices can be used to facilitate stone extraction. Following stone extraction, a tube should be placed into the duct through the tract to effect temporary ductal drainage until edema has resolved and a final normal cholangiogram has been obtained.

▲ **Complications**

Complications of choledochoscopy are unusual, and not often severe. Yet, some problems can occur during the procedure. Avulsion of the cystic duct, or worse, tearing of the common duct, can occur as cystic duct dilation is performed. This risk may be minimized by very slow, gradual, dilation with close observation of the ducts as the dilation proceeds. Should thinning or tearing of the ductal walls appear, the dilation should be rapidly terminated. Avulsion of the cystic duct from the gallbladder is of little concern. The more proximal cystic duct may be regrasped, secured in a clamp, and used for access to the common duct. Avulsion of the cystic duct from the common duct or tearing of the common duct will require careful attention and treatment by suturing or tube insertion. Often, at this juncture, open choledochotomy should be considered. Injury to the duct, with avulsion or tearing, may occur when a stone is pulled forcefully back through the cystic duct. When excessive force is required to remove the stone, it may be better to fragment the stone before removal to avoid this complication. Injury of the bile duct wall may occur during choledochoscopy when power sources, such as the electrohydraulic lithotripter, are used to fragment stones. If inadvertent bursts of energy from the instrument hit the bile duct wall instead of the stone,

SURGICAL PEARLS
Working over a guidewire in the common bile duct provides easy repeated access.

Withdrawal of the stone basket, with the entrapped stone, may sometimes be facilitated by leaving the basket in the open position rather than trying to fully tighten it.

Lithotripsy devices such as the electrohydraulic probe or pulse dye laser should be in direct contact with the stone prior to application of power.

they may damage the tissue, occasionally causing perforation of the duct. This may be avoided by ensuring that the probe is firmly and unequivocally in contact with the stone when power is applied.

☑ CONCLUSIONS

Endoscopic examination of the common duct has become an important component of the complete assessment and treatment of choledocholithiasis. Improvements in fiberoptic and video technology have permitted excellent visualization through progressively smaller caliber endoscopes and enabled direct examination of the common bile duct via multiple routes. The modern biliary surgeon should be familiar with the endoscopic options available for diagnosis and therapy of common duct pathology and adept at their performance. Each adds an expanded dimension to the comprehensive treatment of biliary pathology.

RECOMMENDED READINGS

1. Apelgren KN, Zambos JM, Vargish T. Intraoperative flexible videocholedochoscopy: an improved technique for evaluating the common duct. *Am Surg* 1990;56:178–181.
2. Berci G. Intraoperative and postoperative biliary endoscopy (choledochoscopy). *Surg Clin North Am* 1989;69:1275–1286.
3. Carroll B, Phillips E. Laparoscopic removal of common duct stones. *Surg Clin North Am* 1993;3:239–246.
4. Dennis MJ, James MJ, Wherry D, et al. Choledoschoscopy via the cystic duct: evaluation of a new ultrathin disposable choledochoscope. *Ann R Coll Surg Engl* 1990;72:147–148.

PANCREAS, LIVER, AND SPLEEN

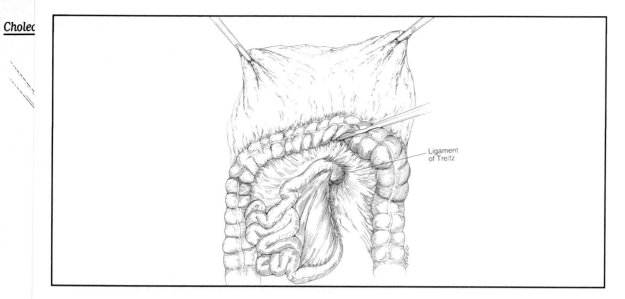

Ligament
of Treitz

21

Cholecystojejunostomy

Douglas B. Evans and Jeffrey E. Lee
Department of Surgical Oncology
The University of Texas M. D. Anderson Cancer Center
Houston, Texas 77030

David J. Winchester
Department of Surgery
Evanston Hospital
Northwestern University Medical School
Evanston, Illinois 60201

*Operative Laparoscopy and
Thoracoscopy,* edited by
B. V. MacFadyen, Jr. and
J. L. Ponsky. Lippincott-Raven
Publishers, Philadelphia © 1996.

Ga

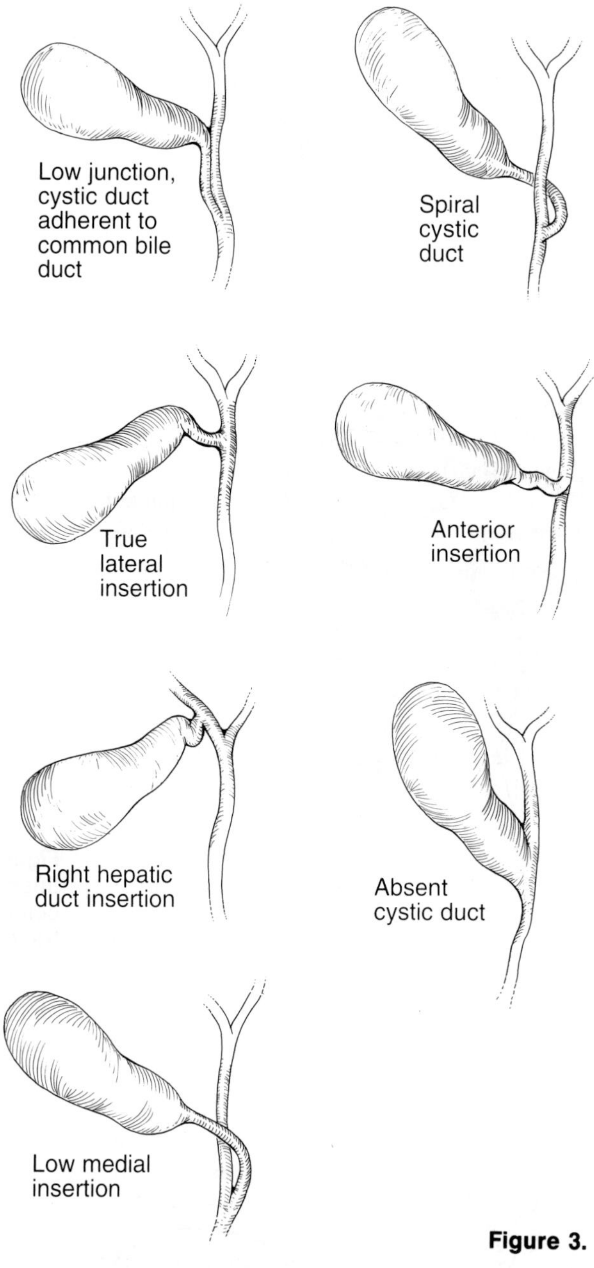

Figure 3. Anomalies of the cystic duct.

2. Positive margin resections (due to retroperitoneal tumor extension) offer no survival benefit compared with palliative chemoradiation, and no data exist to support "palliative" pancreaticoduodenectomy.
3. Biliary decompression can be achieved by less invasive methods, thereby avoiding the complications (mortality, morbidity, and recovery time) of open laparotomy and allowing the patient's rapid entry into investigational treatment programs.

Advocates of surgical exploration in all patients presumed to have resectable pancreatic cancer (i.e., no evidence of lung or liver metastases) base their argument on one or more of the following reasons:

1. The cancer's resectability is best determined at the time of open laparotomy; further sophisticated testing is not cost effective (1).
2. If the cancer is found to be unresectable, operative biliary decompression is superior to endoscopic, percutaneous, or laparoscopic biliary drainage (2).

3. Prophylactic gastrojejunomy should be performed at the time of biliary-enteric bypass in patients with unresectable cancers (1,3).

4. Laparotomy provides an opportunity to perform sphlanchniectomy to improve pain control in patients with locally advanced, unresectable disease (4).

5. As there is no effective nonsurgical treatment for patients with adenocarcinoma of the pancreas, a delay in patient recovery following palliative biliary bypass or gastric bypass or both is of little consequence.

Data from the University of Texas M. D. Anderson Cancer Center have clearly demonstrated that the resectability of malignant tumors of the pancreatic head and periampullary region is best determined by thin-section computed tomography (CT) scans (5). Direct intraoperative assessment of the degree of retroperitoneal tumor extension in relation to the superior mesenteric artery origin is not completed until the final step of tumor resection, after gastric and pancreatic transection, when the surgeon is committed to resection even if all tumor cannot be safely removed. In contrast, as illustrated in Figs. 4 through 6, the relationship of the

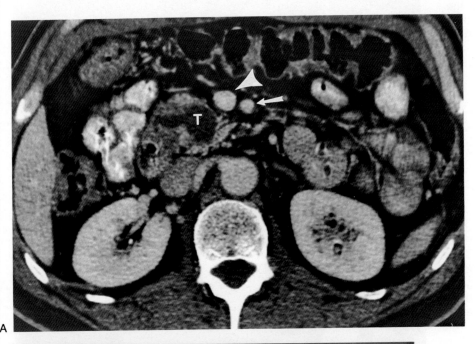

A

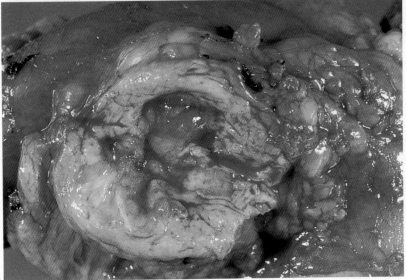

B

Figure 4. A: Thin-section, contrast-enhanced CT scan **(A)** specimen photograph **(B)** of a resectable adenocarcinoma of the pancreas. Carefully examine the normal fat plane between the tumor *(T)* and the superior mesenteric vein *(arrowhead)* and the superior mesenteric artery *(arrow)*. Note the cystic change within the tumor.

tumor to the mesenteric vessels is accurately assessed during the bolus phase of a contrast-enhanced thin-section CT scan. Excision of all retroperitoneal tissue lateral to the superior mesenteric artery at the time of pancreaticoduodenectomy (Fig. 7) is necessary to ensure a negative margin of excision and to prevent iatrogenic arterial injury (5–7). Palliative or margin-positive resection offers no significant survival benefit when compared to palliative chemotherapy and external-beam radiation therapy (chemoradiation) (5,8). The cost of a more extensive preoperative evaluation is insignificant compared with the cost of unnecessary laparot-

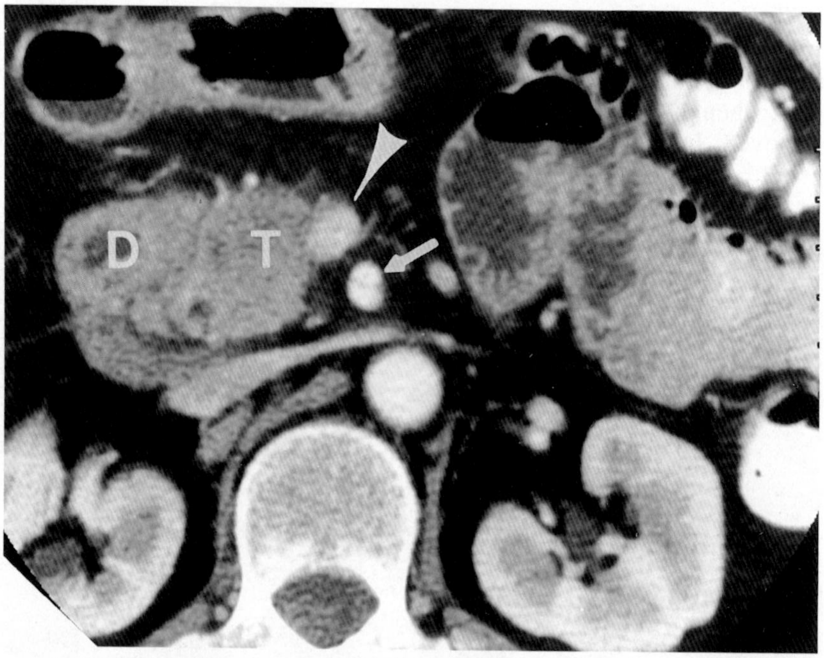

Figure 5. Thin-section, contrast-enhanced CT scan demonstrating probable tumor *(T)* adherence to the lateral wall of the superior mesenteric vein *(arrowhead)*. Note the normal fat plane between the tumor and the superior mesenteric artery *(arrow)*. This patient required segmental resection of the superior mesenteric vein at the time of pancreaticoduodenectomy. D, duodenum.

Figure 6. Thin-section contrast enhanced CT scan demonstrating an unresectable adenocarcinoma of the head of the pancreas. Note the absence of a fat plane between the tumor *(T)* and both the superior mesenteric vein *(arrowhead)* and the superior mesenteric artery *(arrow)*. Successful margin-negative resection would require en-bloc resection of both the superior mesenteric vein and the superior mesenteric artery. We currently do not perform arterial resection in patients with adenocarcinoma of the pancreas. The value of good quality CT is underscored when one realizes that at surgery, direct extension of tumor to involve the superior mesenteric artery can be appreciated only after gastric and pancreatic transection, a point in the procedure at which the surgeon has committed to resection. Therefore, locally advanced, unresectable disease is most accurately determined by CT, preventing needless laparotomy in the majority of patients with pancreatic cancer.

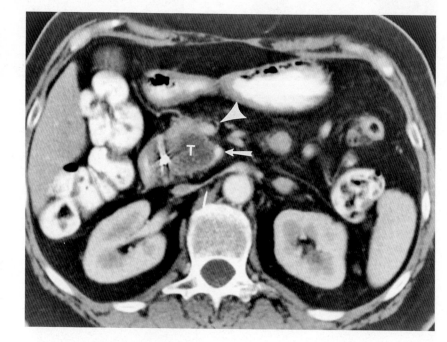

omy. Our diagnostic schema for the patient presumed to have adenocarcinoma of the pancreatic head is presented in Fig. 8.

Studies comparing the complications and efficacy associated with operative versus endoscopic biliary decompression have demonstrated that operative biliary-enteric bypass offers little advantage (9–12). Initial procedure-related incidences of mortality, morbidity, and hospital stay are fewer with endoscopic stent placement than with operative biliary bypass. Late complications (recurrent jaundice, cholangitis) occur more frequently with stent placement than with operative

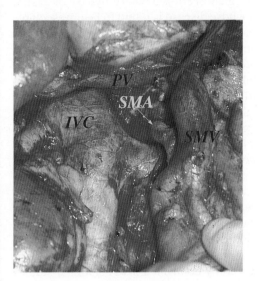

Figure 7. Intraoperative photograph following pancreaticoduodenectomy. The retroperitoneal dissection results in complete visualization of the inferior vena cava *(IVC)*. The superior mesenteric vein *(SMV)* and portal vein *(PV)* are retracted medially exposing the superior mesenteric artery *(SMA)*, the lateral border of which marks the retroperitoneal margin of excision.

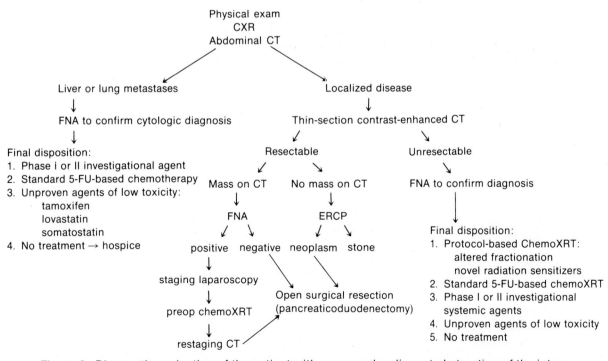

Figure 8. Diagnostic evaluation of the patient with presumed malignant obstruction of the intrapancreatic portion of the common bile duct. Open surgical bypass procedures are performed only on patients whose cancer is found to be unresectable at the time of planned pancreaticoduodenectomy. CT, computed tomography; CXR, chest radiograph; FNA, fine needle aspirate performed under CT guidance; ERCP, endoscopic retrograde cholangiopancreatography; chemoXRT, chemoradiation; 5-FU, 5-fluorouracil.

bypass, yet overall survival rates associated with the two procedures are similar. Of importance, survival is short (3–8 months) in patients with unresectable adenocarcinoma of the pancreas. If patients were appropriately selected for operative or endoscopic biliary decompression, all retrospective studies would demonstrate lower mortality and morbidity rates and longer durations of survival in patients treated with operative palliative bypass due to the obvious bias involving patient selection; patients having a good performance status and no apparent metastatic disease would be selected for surgery. Patients having advanced disease and a short life expectancy would be managed by endoscopic or percutaneous biliary stent decompression. At our institution, open operative biliary bypass or gastric bypass or both are reserved for patients whose disease is found to be unresectable at the time of laparotomy for planned pancreaticoduodenectomy. We do not perform prophylactic gastrojejunostomy and agree with other authors that gastric outlet obstruction is most often a manifestation of end-stage disease (13–15).

While injection of alcohol into the celiac ganglia has been reported to be effective in the palliation of pain resulting from unresectable adenocarcinoma of the pancreas, laparotomy for this purpose alone is not justified (4). Further, accurate intraoperative injection into the celiac ganglion is not an easy procedure, and it requires some degree of operator experience. The same procedure can be performed percutaneously under CT guidance (16), and many patients achieve improved pain control following palliative external-beam irradiation, usually delivered with a radiosensitizing dose of chemotherapy (17–19).

Adenocarcinoma of the pancreas remains relatively insensitive to currently available systemic chemotherapeutic agents, as assessed by response and survival rates (20). However, few patients are willing to accept no treatment for an aggressive and often newly diagnosed disease. We maintain a major institutional commitment to enter all eligible patients into carefully controlled investigational studies exploring the potential benefits of innovative treatment strategies. While patients need to be honestly counseled regarding the aggressive nature of their disease, treatment options do exist for those with an acceptable performance status. These patients require a safe, rapid, and durable method of biliary decompression to allow rapid entry into Phase II investigational studies.

In summary, we perform laparotomy only in patients with tumors of the pancreatic head determined to be resectable by radiologic studies. Resectability is

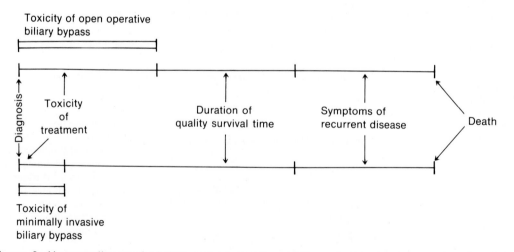

Figure 9. How quality survival time can be lengthened by reducing treatment-related toxicity even when overall survival time remains unchanged, using the TWiST index (*Time Without Symptoms of disease or Toxicity of treatment*). For example, open surgical biliary or gastric bypass or both are associated with a 2-week hospitalization and a 3- to 4-week recovery period. Laparoscopically assisted cholecystojejunostomy is performed with a 2-night hospital stay and a 7- to 10-day recovery period.

Table 1. *Indications for the three most common types of biliary decompressive procedures in patients with malignant obstruction of the intrapancreatic portion of the common bile duct*

Biliary decompressive technique	Operative indications
Open cholecystojejunostomy or choledochlojejunostomy[a]	Procedure of choice in patients taken to surgery for a potentially curative pancreaticoduodenectomy and found to be unresectable
Endoscopic stent or transhepatic biliary catheter	Favored procedure in patients with symptomatic jaundice and advanced disease when a stent is needed prior to hospice care
	Also applicable in patients with unresectable disease who have good performance status and ready access to an interventional gastroenterologist or radiologist in the event of stent occlusion
Laparoscopic or laparoscopically assisted cholecystojejunostomy	Our preferred method of biliary decompression in patients with potentially resectable disease who undergo a diagnostic laparoscopy before preoperative chemoradiation
	Also a good alternative to stent placement in unresectable patients who do not have ready access to specialists required for stent change

[a] We prefer Roux-en-Y choledochojejunostomy.

defined by a patent superior mesenteric-portal venous confluence, no encasement of the celiac axis or superior mesenteric artery, and no extrapancreatic metastatic disease. Patients with locally advanced or metastatic disease can achieve a longer period of good-quality survival simply by avoiding the complications (mortality, morbidity, recovery time) that attend a major palliative abdominal operation (Fig. 9). Laparoscopic cholecystojejunostomy has been included in our surgical options for biliary decompression, as illustrated in Table 1. Similar to open cholecystojejunostomy or choledochojejunostomy, laparoscopic cholecystojejunostomy avoids the use of a stent and, therefore, the potential late complications of recurrent jaundice and cholangitis. Laparoscopic cholecystojejunostomy has the additional advantage, as a minimally invasive technique, of allowing rapid patient recovery.

Laparoscopically assisted cholecystojejunostomy is dependent on a patient cystic duct. Therefore, patients with large tumors that extend to the cystic duct-common duct junction are not candidates for this technique. Likewise, patients with extensive portal adenopathy or carcinomatosis are best treated by endoscopic or percutaneous stent placement. The patient with symptomatic jaundice and ascites presents a unique technical challenge. Clearly, a subset of these patients will have such advanced disease (and poor performance status) that pain control and hospice care are all that is indicated. For the occasional patient who presents with the rapid onset of jaundice and ascites and requires palliative treatment, we prefer endoscopic stent placement followed by early peritoneovenous shunting [double-valve, high-flow Denver shunt (Denver Biomaterials, Inc., Evergreen, Colorado)] if an initial attempt at diuretic therapy is unsuccessful. If endoscopic stenting is not technically possible, we prefer to proceed with laparoscopic cholecystojejunostomy in the absence of high-volume carcinomatosis. Transhepatic biliary drainage with an internal-external catheter is not advised in patients with ascites, as the ascitic fluid will leak around the catheter at the skin entrance site. In patients with malignant ascites, the surgeon should avoid using transabdominal catheters and making large abdominal incisions because of the risk of ascitic leak. Although we have limited experience with laparoscopically assisted cholecystojejunostomy followed by peritoneovenous shunt, we have been pleased with the quality of palliation provided the patient.

Technique No. 1

After the establishment of pneumoperitoneum, a 30-degree telescope is placed at the umbilical incision. Port positioning is indicated in Fig. 5. The stomach is visualized, and the bulging pseudocyst may often be seen pushing the stomach forward. A 4-cm longitudinal incision is made in the anterior wall of the stomach over the most prominent portion of the pseudocyst, which is usually in the midgastric or central region (Fig. 6). The pseudocyst is nonlocalized again by insertion of a needle and aspirating cyst contents. This incision is performed with either electrocautery scissors or the L hook. Generally the pseudocyst is seen bulging through the posterior wall and a 1-cm window is created through the posterior wall of the stomach into the pseudocyst cavity using electrocautery attached to either the scissors or L hook (Fig. 7). This window needs to be large enough to accommodate the EndoGia stapler. At this time, a biopsy of the cyst wall is performed and then the 30-mm EndoGia (U.S. Surgical, Norwalk, CT) stapler is introduced into the stomach, and one arm of the instrument is advanced into the pseudocyst and the second arm is positioned on the gastric lumen side (Fig. 8).

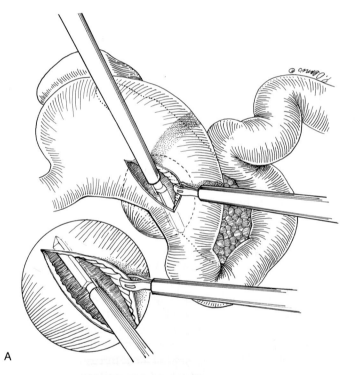

A

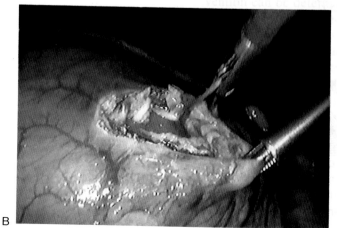

B

Figure 6. A: The stapler is inserted into the stomach with one arm of the stapler in the gastric side and the other on the pancreatic cyst side. **B:** The anterior wall of the stomach is opened overtop the most prominant part of the pseudocyst.

The instrument is closed and fired and a second firing of the EndoGia may be carried out if a larger opening is necessary (Fig. 9). An alternative to stapling is performed by creating a 3- to 6-cm cystgastrostomy with electrocautery scissors and suturing this opening with a running locking 2-cm suture. At this point, a large communication is created between the pseudocyst and the stomach, and hemostasis is excellent. If bleeding should occur, interrupted 2-0 silk can be used to stop the bleeding. The gastrostomy is closed with either sutures or staples, and the operation is completed (Fig. 10).

Technique No. 2

A nasogastric tube is inserted into the stomach and pneumoperitoneum is established. A 10-mm trocar is inserted at the umbilicus and the 30-degree telescope is placed through this trocar. The stomach is visualized and insufflated with CO_2 via a standard CO_2 insufflator with a pressure limit of 8–10 mmHg. When the

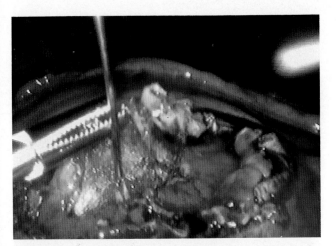

Figure 7. An incision with electrocautery on the posterior wall of the stomach is made. Aspiration with a spinal needle through the fibrous capsule of the pseudocyst is carried out to confirm the presence of cyst contents.

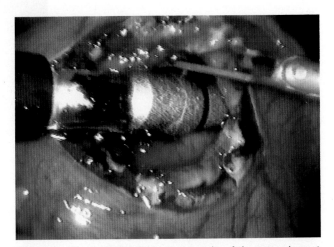

Figure 8. The anterior fibrous capsule of the pseudocyst is entered, and an opening is created large enough to place one arm of the EndoGIA.

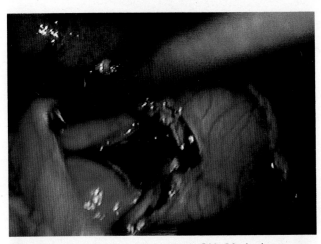

Figure 9. Two firings of the EndoGIA 30 device are required to create an opening of adequate size. Superb hemostasis is mandatory.

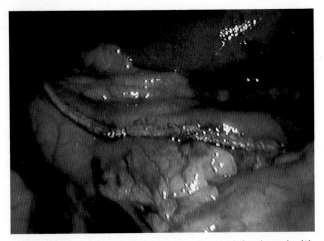

Figure 10. The anterior wall of the stomach is closed with the EndoGIA.

stomach is inflated (Fig. 11), two 5-mm radially expanding trocars (RED: Inner-dyne, Mountain View, CA) are placed into the stomach (Fig. 12 and 13). These are used to obtain access into the stomach and will subsequently be used as the operating chambers. The position of the inflated stomach is variable, but one trocar is placed through the midline and another in the left upper quadrant (Fig. 14). The inflated stomach is then utilized as the operating chamber and a 5-mm telescope is introduced into the stomach through the RED device. Because of the gastric insufflation, the pseudocyst may not be obvious. A needle is introduced through the second RED port to aspirate pseudocyst contents and confirm the position of the pseudocyst if it is not evident (Fig. 15). Once the position of the pseudocyst is verified, an opening is developed between the pseudocyst and the posterior wall of the stomach (Fig. 16). A 3- to 5-cm opening is created using

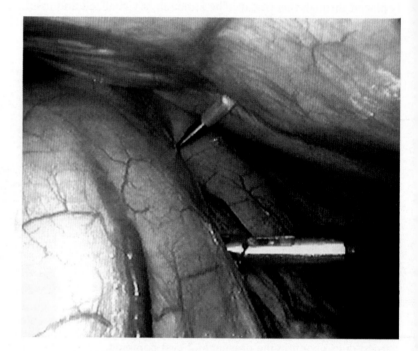

Figure 11. After inflating the stomach through the nasogastric tube, the RED trocar is passed through the anterior abdominal wall into the stomach.

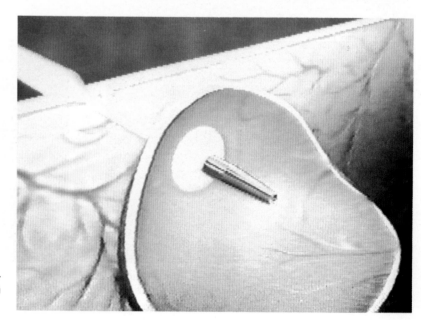

Figure 12. This depiction illustrates the balloon on the RED device which will hold it in place.

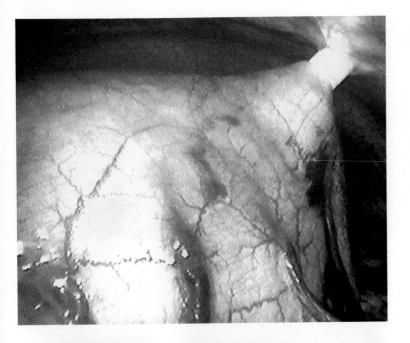

Figure 13. The placement of the RED trocar along the greater curve with the balloon inflated is depicted.

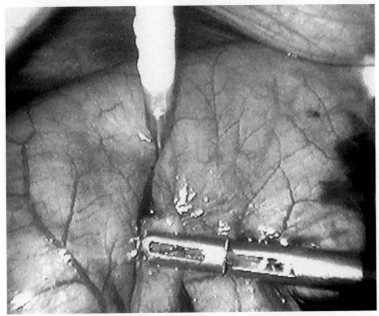

Figure 14. Placement of a second RED trocar on the anterior wall of the stomach to allow entry of a 5-mm telescope into the stomach is demonstrated.

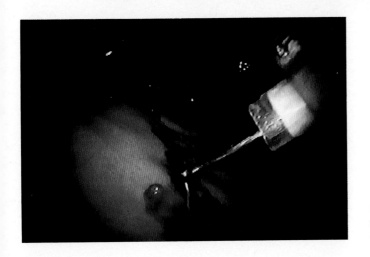

Figure 15. With the 5-mm telescope in the inflated stomach, needle aspiration of the pseudocyst is depicted to confirm position.

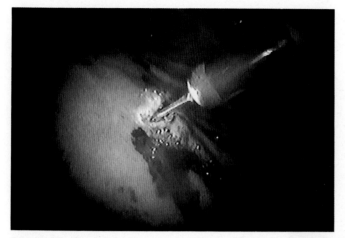

Figure 16. The hook electrode is used to create an opening into the pseudocyst.

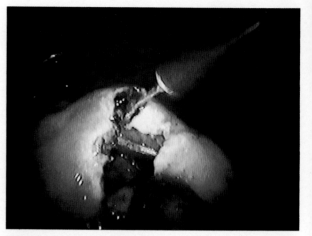

Figure 17. An opening of suitable size is created. Superb hemostasis is mandatory.

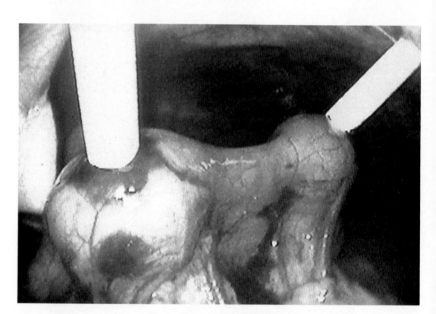

Figure 18. After deflation of the stomach and reinsufflation of the abdomen the RED devices may be seen in the appropriate position.

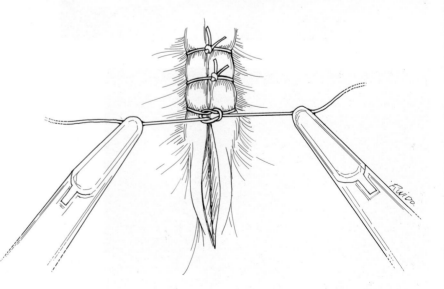

Figure 19. The small incisions are closed with interrupted figure-of-eight absorbable sutures.

electrocautery scissors or a hook, the cyst contents are evacuated, and a biopsy is taken of the pseudocyst wall (Fig. 17). Any bleeding from the cystgastrostomy site should be ligated or cauterized. Thus far in our experience, it has not been necessary to perform intraluminal suturing. Pneumoperitoneum is reestablished and the stomach is deflated (Fig. 18). The intragastric trocars are removed after their balloons are deflated. After the trocars are removed, the small holes in the stomach are sutured with intracorporeal knots (Fig. 19). It appears that postoperatively, patients have less pain, shorter length of stay, and less disability when compared to open surgery.

▲ COMPLICATIONS

When approaching any operation by means of the laparoscope, conversion to open surgery may be necessary if the pseudocyst cannot be localized. If the pseudocyst is not in firm apposition to the posterior gastric wall then these relatively simple methods of pseudocyst drainage cannot be considered and a more complex Roux-en-Y drainage procedure may be necessary. The first case in which we attempted the endoluminal approach (technique no. 2) failed because of nonapposition of the pseudocyst to the posterior wall of the stomach. This occurred despite preoperative CT scanning, which suggested strong fibrous adherence to the stomach wall. In one patient, the creation of the pneumoperitoneum visibly caused separation between the stomach wall and the pseudocyst. The patient developed significant fever postoperatively, suggesting the development of a leak. However, this problem resolved on intravenous antibiotic therapy. Because of this complication, we feel that it is important to suture or staple the pseudocyst wall to the stomach. We now prefer technique no. 1.

Stapling will minimize the risk of bleeding or pseudocyst/stomach separation. Although we have treated only two patients in this fashion, there were no postoperative complications and early discharge occurred. There has been no pseudocyst recurrence with a follow-up of 6–18 months in these patients. The possibility that the cyst might recur is often related to inadequate drainage between the cyst and the stomach. It is important to create a large communication between the cyst and the stomach and the application of two 30-mm EndoGIA staples will ensure this large communication. Bleeding and leakage from the anterior gastric wall incision can be minimized by meticulous attention to surgical technique.

Complications associated with internal drainage of pseudocysts include bleeding, particularly from the pseudocyst-gastric wall margin, sepsis, and pancreatic fistula. The possibility of any of these is quite small but can cause significant morbidity.

☑ CONCLUSIONS

Many therapeutic modes of treatment have been suggested for pancreatic pseudocysts, but the vast majority spontaneously will resolve and require no definitive treatment. Persistent large (>6 cm) or symptomatic pseudocysts should be treated and the most reliable is surgical drainage. It is likely that the results of open surgical drainage in terms of pseudocyst recurrence will be achieved by the laparoscopic approach with the added benefit of small incisions, less pain, and earlier return to work. It is our belief that a stapled communication is preferable to a nonstapled, nonsutured approach. For the laparoscopic surgeon, these two approaches are relatively straightforward, and if the technique fails, conversion to open surgery is mandatory. It is imperative for the operating surgeon to understand the natural history of pancreatic pseudocysts so that surgery is offered in a timely fashion when necessary.

SURGICAL PEARLS

A recent CT scan (within 1 week) should be available in the operating room before surgery to assess pseudocyst size, location, thickness of cyst wall, and adherence to gastric wall.

Intraoperative ultrasound may be helpful to localize the pseudocyst during surgery.

It is imperative to establish total hemostasis of the anastomosis.

An adequate communication measuring 4–6 cm is required.

Trocar positioning is essential to facilitate access to the stomach, stapling of the anastomosis, and to allow easy suturing of the gastric wall.

REFERENCES

1. Rosai J. Pancreas and periampullary region. In: *Ackerman's Surgical Pathology*. St. Louis, MO: CV Mosby; 1989:757–789.
2. Adams DB, Anderson MC. Changing concepts in the surgical management of pancreatic pseudocysts. *Ann Surg* 1992;58:173–180.
3. Anderson R, Janzon M, Sundberg I, Bengmark S. Management of pancreatic pseudocysts. *Br J Surg* 1989;76:550–552.
4. Mullins RJ, Malagoni MA, Bergamini TM, Casey JM, Richardson JD. Controversies in the management of pancreatic pseudocysts. *Am J Surg* 1988;155:165–172.
5. O'Malley VP, Cannon JP, Postier RG. Pancreatic pseudocysts: cause, therapy and results. *Am J Surg* 1985;150:680–682.
6. Sankaran S, Walt AJ. The natural and unnatural history of pancreatic pseudocysts. *Br J Surg* 1975;62:37–44.
7. Grace PA, Williamson RCN. Modern management of pancreatic pseudocysts. *Br J Surg* 1993;80:573–581.
8. Yeo CJ, Sarr MG Cystic and pseudocystic diseases of the pancreas. *Curr Prob Surg* 1994;431:165–252.
9. Neoptolemos JP, London NJM, Carr-Locke DL. Assessment of main pancreatic duct integrity by endoscopic retrograde pancreatography in patients with acute pancreatitis. *Br J Surg* 1993;80:94–99.
10. Bradley EL, Clements JL, Gonzalez AC. The natural history of pancreatic pseudocysts: a unified concept of management. *Am J Surg* 1979;137:135–141.
11. Yeo CJ, Bastidas JA, Lynch-Nyham A, Fishman EK, Zimmer MJ, Cameron JL. The natural history of pancreatic pseudocysts documented by computed tomography. *Surg Gynecol Obstet* 1990;170:411–417.
12. Kourtesis GK, Wilson SE, Williams RA. The clinical significance of fluid collections in acute pancreatitis. *Am Surg* 1990;56:796–799.
13. Vitas GJ, Sarr MG. Selected management of pancareatic pseudocysts: operative versus expectant management. *Surgery* 1992;111:123–130.
14. Williams KJ, Fabian TC. Pancreatic pseudocyst: recommendations for operative and non-operative management. *Am Surg* 1992;58:199–205.
15. Watt AJ, Bouwman DL, Weaver DW, Sachs RJ. The impact of technology on the management of pancreatic pseudocysts. *Arch Surg* 1990;125:759–763.
16. Becker JM. Pancreatic pseuodycsts. In: Cameron JL, ed., *Current surgical therapy*. 4th ed. BC Decker; 1992:426.
17. Johnson LB, Rattner DW, Warshaw AL. The effect of size of giant pancreatic pseudocysts on the outcome of internal drainage procedures. *Surg Gynecol Obstet* 1991;173:171–174.
18. Newell KA, Liu T, Aranha GV, Prinz RA. Are cystgastrostomy and cystjejunostomy equivalent operations for pancreatic pseudocysts? *Surgery* 1990;108:635–640.

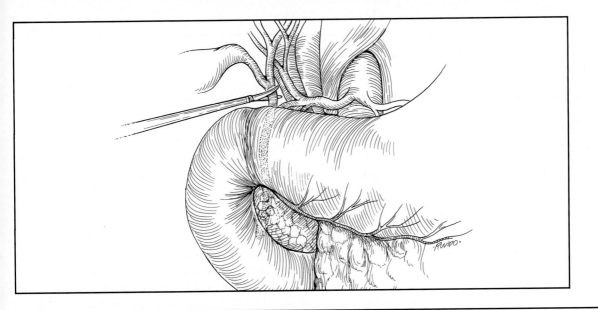

23

Pancreatoduodenectomy

Michel Gagner
Department of General Surgery
The Cleveland Clinic Foundation
Cleveland, Ohio 44195

Operative Laparoscopy and Thoracoscopy, edited by
B. V. MacFadyen, Jr. and
J. L. Ponsky. Lippincott-Raven
Publishers, Philadelphia © 1996.

KEY WORDS

Ampullary tumors

Hepaticojejunostomy

Pancreaticojejunostomy

Percutaneous fine needle aspiration

Pylorojejunostomy

Whipple procedure

● ANATOMY

The pancreas is a soft pink retroperitoneal gland that is approximately 15 cm long that extends from the second portion of the duodenum to the spleen hilum posterior to the stomach. The head of the pancreas is located from the duodenum to the superior mesenteric vessels, and the body consists of the middle one-third and the tail the distal one-third. Relations to the head of the pancreas are important for dissection in the Whipple procedure. The inferior part of the head has a posterior projection, call the uncinate process, that surrounds the mesenteric vessels. A groove between the neck of the gland and the head permits the location of the gastroduodenal artery. The upper border of the head of the pancreas is delineated by the first portion of the duodenum, and extended laterally to the pylorus of the stomach. Inferiorly and to the right of the mesenteric vessels, the third and fourth portion of the duodenum also come in contact with the transverse colon. Posteriorly, the head overlies the inferior vena cava, and the uncinate process lies in front of the aorta (Fig. 1). The common bile duct lies posterior to the pancreatic

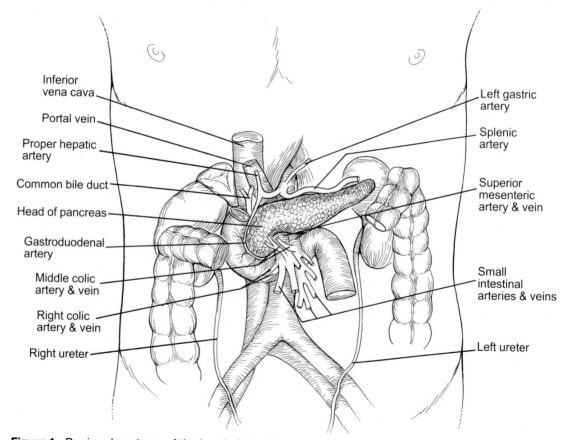

Figure 1. Regional anatomy of the head of the pancreas, with relations to the mesenteric vessels, common bile duct, pancreatic duct, gastroduodenal artery, pylorus, and vena cavae.

head and traverses the pancreatic tissue for a short distance close to the second portion of the duodenum.

The dorsal or main pancreatic duct runs the length of the pancreas and empties into the bile duct above the papilla. An accessory pancreatic duct (ventral duct) joins the dorsal duct at the head-body junction and variations. The portal vein lies posterior to the pancreas and is located at the division of the head and body of the pancreas. The tributaries of this vein include the splenic, superior, and inferior mesenteric veins, and as it travels to the liver it becomes part of the portal triad, which also includes the hepatic artery and common bile duct. The location of the stomach and pylorus in relation to the pancreas is important, since part of this organ is removed during the operation.

▶ PREOPERATIVE PLANNING

Pancreatic adenocarcinoma accounts for 90% of pancreatic tumors, and distant metastases are often found at the time of diagnosis. The most common clinical presentation is a mixture of weight loss, anorexia, jaundice, and sometimes pain and pruritus. Less frequently, a tumor of the periampullary region may invade the duodenum and produce mucosal ulceration with bleeding or an obstruction with vomiting. The jaundice is often progressive and profound and results from tumor obstruction or invasion of the common bile duct. Besides ampullary and islets cell tumors of the pancreas, other indications for a laparoscopic pancreatoduodenectomy include ampullary tumors, distal bile duct tumors, duodenal tumors, cystadenomas/cystadenocarcinomas of the pancreas, and chronic pancreatitis localized to the pancreatic head. Contraindications to this procedure include liver or peritoneal metastases and/or positive regional lymph nodes containing cancer. Other reasons not to perform this operation include an inability to localize the tumor, portal hypertension, portal vein invasion by a tumor, a large pancreatic mass, morbid obesity, coagulopathy, and previous extensive abdominal surgery.

On physical examination, jaundice and weight loss can be noted, and a palpable gallbladder in the right upper quadrant can sometimes be palpated. Hepatomegaly, ascites, and palpable nodes are rarely noted on physical examination, but when observed, they are signs of unresectability. Apart from the biochemical profiles, which may reveal an elevated bilirubin, serum and alkaline phosphatase, and liver enzymes, anemia may be present on the complete blood count. A chest radiograph should be performed to rule out pulmonary metastases. Often an initial ultrasound is performed by the referral physician and will reveal some degree of bile duct distension with or without a periampullary mass. I personally prefer to obtain a computed tomography (CT) scan of the upper abdomen to delineate the parapancreatic mass extension, to look for metastatic process in the liver or peritoneal cavity and, if portoScan is performed (intravenous contrast into the mesenteric artery), with 1- to 2-mm cuts of the CT scan or an angiogram, one can determine if the portal vein is involved with tumor. Magnetic resonance imaging (MRI) may show approximately the same information and may not give additional information over the CT scan. The biliary tree should be delineated preoperatively to plan the operation. This may be achieved by an endoscopic retrograde cholangiopancreatography (ERCP) or a percutaneous transhepatic cholangiogram (PTC). However, ERCP is the method of choice, since endoscopy may reveal a duodenal or ampullary tumor, and biopsy can be performed at the time of the procedure. Cytology brushings of the lower common bile duct may be obtained as well. A cholangiogram and pancreatogram may also be obtained for anatomic purposes. During the bile duct imaging a stent may be inserted, and resectability or unresectability can be considered. Percutaneous biopsy of the pancreatic mass is extremely important to obtain a diagnosis. A negative result, however, should not prevent further studies or diagnostic or therapeutic laparoscopy. If the patient is felt to be an operative candidate, a mesenteric angiogram should be performed preoperatively, since mesenteric artery or vein or portal involvement means incurability (not necessarily unresectability).

In deeply jaundiced and malnourished patients, preoperative bile duct decompression permits improvement of the hepatic, renal, and immunologic functions before surgery. The bilirubin response may be a prognostic factor. If the bilirubin level returns to normal or near-normal, the mortality rate is less than 10%; however, if the bilirubin level does not decrease after decompression, the 30-day mortality rate may be above 80%. Some surgeons may prefer to perform a diagnostic laparoscopy and do peritoneal washing for cytology. This may be followed by a second procedure such as choledochojejunostomy and/or gastric jejunostomy or possibly a Whipple procedure. It is my policy to perform a diagnostic laparoscopy first and then to continue the procedure if the tumor is resectable during the same anesthesia. Warshaw and Castillo, at the Massachusetts General Hospital, have found in a series of 72 patients that if CT scan, angiography, and laparoscopy are negative for tumor, resectability is 78%.

Laparoscopic staging of periampullary tumors is a different technique that involves biopsy of the pancreatic lesion and inspection of the body and tail of the pancreas by using cautery and endoscopic clips to create a window between the traverse colon and the greater curvature of the stomach. A laparoscopic Kocher maneuver is important to evaluate the first and second portion of the duodenum, the head of the pancreas, and the vena cava. The ligament of Treitz is also inspected for mesojejunal involvement, and regional lymph nodes in the periduodenal and pericholedochal areas are also sampled along with lymph nodes around the hepatic artery. Finally, one can follow a branch of the middle colic vein superior to the mesenteric vein with the blunt irrigation-suction probe to eliminate portamesenteric vein involvement. If available, laparoscopic ultrasonography with or without Doppler can be used to evaluate vessel involvement. After all these maneuvers, it is possible to determine resectability in more than 90% of unresectable lesions.

Preoperatively, the bowel is prepared with 4 L of GoLitely, and a broad-spectrum cephalosporin is given on call to the operating room. Heparin is administered subcutaneously the day before the operation and 4 units of blood are crossmatched.

▼ INTRAOPERATIVE MANAGEMENT/SURGICAL TECHNIQUE

Pancreatoduodenectomy is performed in three parts: first, the staging procedure; second, resection, and third, reconstruction. The technique used is the same as in open surgery with the modification of Longmire and Traverso, which is a pylorus-preserving pancreatoduodenectomy.

Part One: Staging

The patient is placed in the supine position with slight reverse Trendelenburg positioning, and both legs are abducted. The surgeon will be at ease when standing between the legs of the patient so he can suture in front of him, and assistants are standing on both sides of the patient. An indwelling Foley catheter, a nasogastric tube, a central venous line, and an arterial line for monitoring should be inserted in the patient. A Veress needle is first inserted at the umbilicus, and CO_2 insufflation of the abdomen to 15 mmHg pressure is performed. A 10-mm trocar is then inserted at the umbilicus and a 30-degree 10-mm laparoscope is inserted for the diagnostic laparoscopy.

If no obvious peritoneal or liver metastases are seen, a second 10-mm epigastric trocar and right and left paramedian trocars are inserted under the laparoscopic

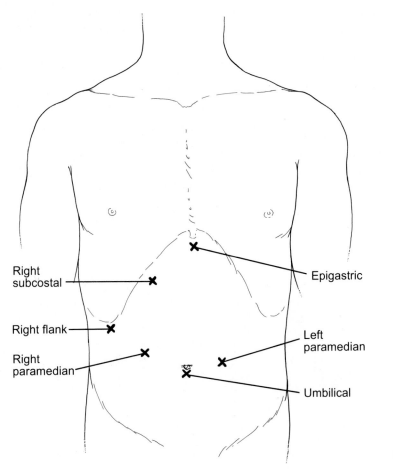

Right
subcostal

Epigastric

Right flank

Left
paramedian

Right
paramedian

Umbilical

Figure 2. Positions of trocars.

vision (Fig. 2). These trocars will permit a full evaluation of the tumor extension and the possibility of resection. Through the epigastric port a laparoscopic Babcock forceps is used to grasp the greater curvature of the stomach. The position of the camera at this point is changed to the right paramedian trocar, and the surgeon works with both hands using the umbilical and paramedian left trocar. Both instruments are used to dissect the gastrocolic ligament below the gastroepiploic vessels, so as to enter into the lesser sac. Transverse branches from the gastroepiploic arcades are clipped, but the arcade itself is preserved, since this will provide the blood supply to the pylorus and antrum. After a 10-cm window is created, the body and tail of the pancreas are inspected for possible seeding.

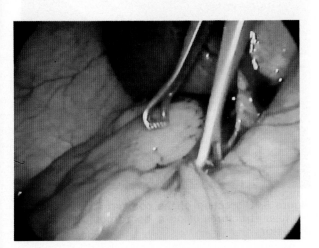

Figure 3. Laparoscopic Babcock forceps positioned on the second portion of the duodenum for a Kocher maneuver.

It is also possible to inspect the upper part of the lesser sac by creating a window in the gastrohepatic ligament below the left caudate lobe so as to assess local invasion.

A laparoscopic Kocher maneuver is conducted by positioning the Babcock forceps on the second portion of the duodenum and lifting anteriorly and superiorly (Fig. 3). The dissection will then be made between the lateral border of the second and third portion of the duodenum from the transverse colon and vena cava (Fig. 4). This will free the entire duodenal arcade and the posterior aspect of the head of the pancreas and uncinate process (Fig. 5), and any suspicious nodes should be biopsied. When the dilated common bile duct and common hepatic duct are identified (Fig. 6), a cholangiogram can be performed directly through the anterior aspect of the duct, using a percutaneously placed 22-gauge metallic spinal needle. Rarely, choledocholithiasis or localized tumor extension are found on the proximal

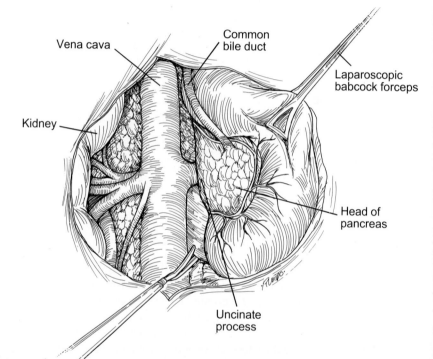

Figure 4. Laparoscopic Kocher maneuver. Exposure of the vena cava.

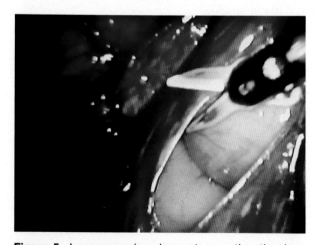

Figure 5. Laparoscopic scissors transecting the duodenojejunal junction after full mobilization of the duodenum and pancreas superiorly.

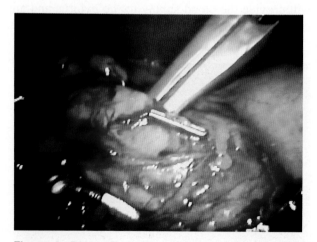

Figure 6. Dissection of the common bile duct from the hilar structures using a laparoscopic right-angle dissector.

bile duct. If the gallbladder is present it should be used for liver retraction to expose the liver hilum, and later in the procedure the gallbladder is resected.

If a diagnosis for malignancy has not been confirmed, it is our policy to perform a fine-needle aspiration, inserting a 22-gauge needle directly into the palpable mass in the anterior head of the pancreas. This is facilitated with a Franzen aspirating syringe apparatus for cytology, and multiple aspirations are layered on the glass for microscopic examination. Finally, to complete the workup, a branch of the middle colic vein is identified and followed until it reaches the anteroinferior aspect of the superior mesenteric vein (Fig. 7). An irrigation-suction probe is used for gentle blunt dissection, and sterile saline is injected in the proper plane between the pancreatic neck and superior mesenteric and portal veins (Fig. 8).

Part Two: Resection

The peritoneum covering the common bile duct is opened anteriorly and laterally so that it can be dissected free posteromedially from the portal vein and the right hepatic artery. Using a large curved needle, a No. 2 nylon suture is passed through the abdominal wall in the right subcostal area and passed under the bile duct to create a suspension with minimum retraction. The bile duct is transected with scissors at least 2 cm above the pancreatic border, preferably above the cystic common bile duct junction, and the suspension suture is removed (Figs. 9 and 10). Bile under pressure is aspirated, and a specimen is sent for

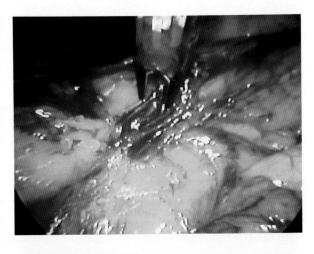

Figure 7. Dissection of the middle colic vein to the superior mesenteric vein.

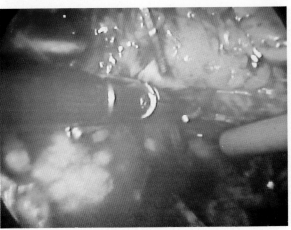

Figure 8. Blunt dissection of the superior mesenteric vein inferiorly from the pancreatic neck superiorly using an irrigation-suction probe.

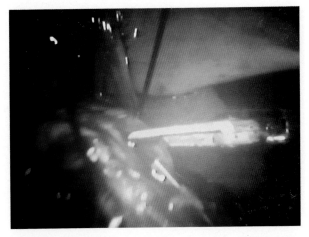

Figure 9. Complete transection of the common bile duct using laparoscopic scissors, after a bile duct suspension using nylon sutures.

culture. The next structure to be divided is the first portion of the duodenum, approximately 1 cm distal to the pylorus, which can be easily identified by looking interiorly for the veins of Mayo and by palpating a slight firmness in the area. If there is any doubt, a preoperative gastroscopy could be performed and the pylorus identified by transillumination. The dissection of the gastrocolic ligament is completed, and the gastroepiploic vessels originating from the gastroduodenal vessels are double-clipped with titanium clips (Fig. 11). Then a right-angle dissector is more easily passed under the pylorus to create a 1-cm window (Fig. 11), which allows the passage of an endoscopic linear stapler (Fig. 12). Since a 60-mm stapler is used (Fig. 13), the umbilical trocar is changed to an 18-mm trocar by using a 10-mm plastic rod for dilation and maintenance of the tract. Reducers from 18 mm to 10 mm or to 5 mm must be used throughout the procedure.

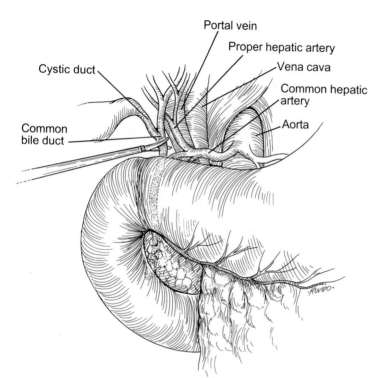

Figure 10. Transection of common bile duct.

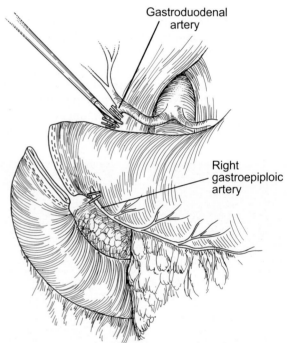

Figure 11. Line of transection on the duodenum, 1 cm from the pylorus. The gastroduodenal vessels are double-clipped with titanium clips.

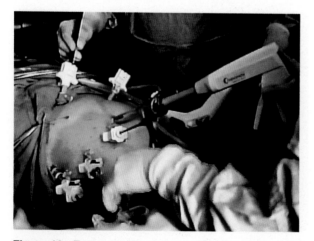

Figure 12. External view of the six trocars position and insertion of the endoscopic linear stapler for duodenal and jejunal transection.

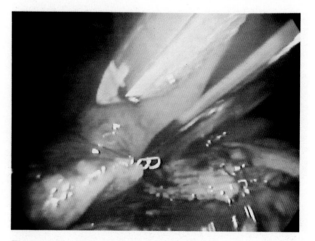

Figure 13. Endoscopic linear stapler removal after complete transection of the first portion of duodenum, 1 cm distal to the pylorus.

Similarly, the duodenojejunal junction is transected as close to the ligament of Treitz as possible with the same stapler just to the right of the mesenteric vessels (Fig. 14). The proximal jejunum will retract in the retroperitoneum and will be freed at the ligament of Treitz. After proximal duodenal transection, the gastroduodenal artery is exposed as the antrum of the stomach is pushed toward the upper left quadrant. The artery is dissected from the pancreatic neck and more so superiorly near its origin from the hepatic artery. It is double-clipped and divided with titanium clips (Fig. 15), and a 30-mm endoscopic linear stapler with vascular staples can be used. The pancreas that is anterior to the superior mesenteric vein and portal veins is transected by scissors (Fig. 16), starting on the inferior

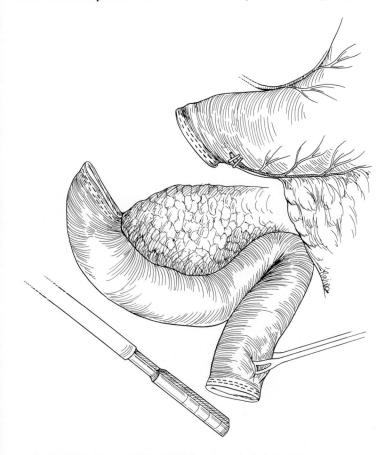

Figure 14. Duodenojejunal transection plane.

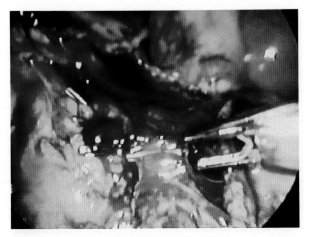

Figure 15. Double ligature with titanium clips of the gastroduodenal artery.

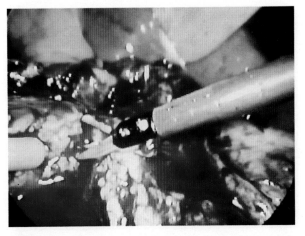

Figure 16. Transection of the pancreatic neck using straight endoscopic scissors over the mesenteric vein.

aspect and going superiorly. This sections the inferior and superior pancreatic vessel arcades, which is controlled with a combination of metallic clips and cautery. The pancreatic duct is easily seen because of magnification, and it is often left open or cannulated with a 5 F pediatric feeding tube. Once hemostasis is achieved on the transected pancreas, the uncinate process is resected from the superior mesenteric vessels, approximately 1 cm distal to them, using two cartridges of a 60-mm endoscopic linear stapler (Figs. 17 and 18). The resected specimen is then inserted into a large plastic endoscopic bag with a purse string to position it in the lower quadrant of the abdomen for later extraction. Three forceps are needed to perform this task: one forceps is placed on the lower lip of the bag, another on the superior lip, and finally one Babcock is used to push the specimen into the bag. The purse string is pulled tight and the bag is closed, which helps to maintain all contents (potentially malignant cells or gastrointestinal secretions) in the bag.

Part Three: Reconstruction

Three anastomoses need to be created, and therefore a good two-hand technique with fast intracorporeal knot-tying is necessary. The proximal jejunal loop is prepared for this task, by further mobilization at the ligament of Treitz, and

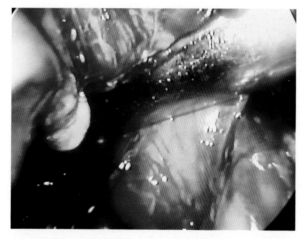

Figure 17. Uncinate process transection and stapling, using a 60-mm endoscopic linear stapler.

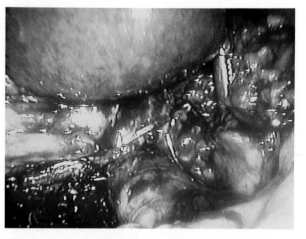

Figure 18. Endoscopic view after pancreatoduodenal resection before reconstruction.

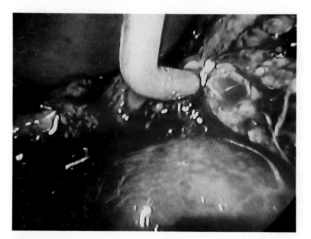

Figure 19. Inspection of the pancreatic duct for size and consistency.

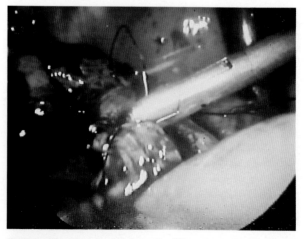

Figure 20. First anastomosis. The pancreaticojejunal anastomosis (end-to-side) is created with intracorporeal interrupted absorbable sutures.

several vessels are taken with the hook cautery and metallic clips. The loop is placed in a retrocolic fashion and a window is created in the transverse mesocolon for passage of the jejunum using soft-bowel forceps. The reconstruction recreates a duodenum by performance of end-to-end pylorojejunostomy, an end-to-side pancreaticojejunostomy, and an end-to-side choledochojejunostomy. The first anastomosis is the pancreaticojejunostomy, which is placed 10 cm distal to the proximal jejunal end (Fig. 19). It is easier to perform with the free jejunal loop. I have used in one instance a 5 F pediatric feeding stent into the pancreatic anastomosis which exited outside the jejunal loop through the right side of the abdomen. The anastomosis is created using 4-0 absorbable monofilament sutures with a semicurved needle, anastomosing the duct to the antimesenteric side of the jejunum, through the whole wall (Fig. 20). Four to six interrupted sutures are first positioned posteriorly. I have sealed the pancreatic and the biliary anastomosis with fibrin glue after suturing (Fig. 21), which is delivered by a catheter passed through the abdominal wall. Next, the choledochojejunostomy is placed 10 cm distally and is created in a similar fashion with intracorporeal sutures placed posteriorly, and no stent or T tubes are necessary (Fig. 22). Between 6 and 10 sutures are placed. The distance between all of these anastomoses is approximately 10 cm. Excess proximal jejunum and staple lines are excised, and the pylorojejunostomy is created using a 3-0 absorbable monofilament suture with a curved needle. Starting superi-

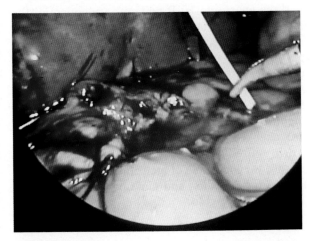

Figure 21. Both anastomoses are sealed using fibrin glue delivered through a percutaneous catheter.

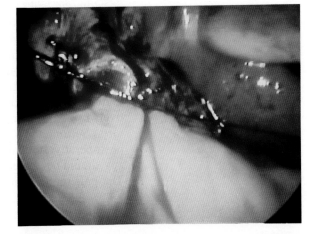

Figure 22. Second anastomosis. The hepaticojejunal anastomosis (end-to-side) is created with intracorporeal interrupted absorbable sutures.

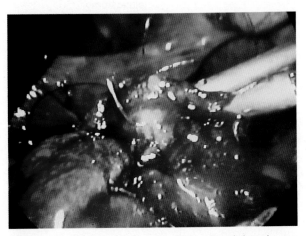

Figure 23. Third anastomosis. The pylorojejunal anastomosis (end-to-end) is created with intracorporeal running posterior and anterior absorbable sutures.

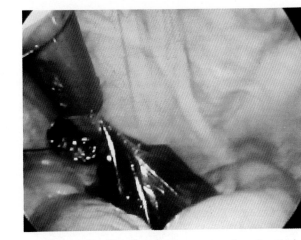

Figure 24. The duodenopancreas is extracted.

orly, a running posterior suture is followed by a running anterior suture (Fig. 23). The gallbladder can be removed after the specimen is extracted by means of the largest trocar—18 mm—in the umbilicus (Fig. 24). The specimen is turned longitudinally and extracted. Two Jackson-Pratt drains are positioned below and above the anastomosis and passed through the trocar sites in the right subcostal and right paramedian area (Fig. 25). A feeding jejunostomy is inserted approximately 30 cm distal to the hepaticojejunostomy on the antimesenteric side of the jejunal loop via the left paramedian trocar site. The nasogastric tube is left in place, and all fascial wounds are closed with 2-0 absorbable sutures.

Postoperative Care

This operation results in major gastrointestinal trauma to the patient and the postoperative morbidity rate is high (from 40% to 60%); the postoperative care is extremely important. I routinely use somatostatin analogs (octreotide), 50 μg subcutaneously every 8 hours, to decrease the likelihood of pancreatic fistulas for a minimum of 7 days. Similarly, the Jackson-Pratt drains are maintained for 7 days or longer if pancreatic juice continues to drain with an amylase content five times greater than normal. The nasogastric tube is also maintained for 7 days, at which time a gastrograffin swallow is performed to identify potential existence of anastomotic leaks at any of the three anastomosis. If no leaks are apparent, the nasogastric tube is removed and a liquid diet is started; the feeding jejunostomy is started on day 3 or 4 at half strength and increased progressively. Total parenteral nutrition has been administered to the first patient because I omitted placing a jejunostomy. Antibiotics are used for 5 to 7 days (cephalosporin). H2-blockers are administered intravenously postoperatively to decrease the likelihood of anastomotic jejunal ulcers. Prophylaxis for deep-vein thrombosis is initiated preoperatively by using heparin subcutaneously and is used until the patient is fully ambulatory. Serum glucose levels are checked every 6 hours intraoperatively and postoperatively, and an insulin drip is used as necessary. Pulmonary physiotherapy should be aggressive to decrease the incidence of atelectasis and pneumonia. The pancreatic stent is left in place for 6 weeks, and most patients are able to

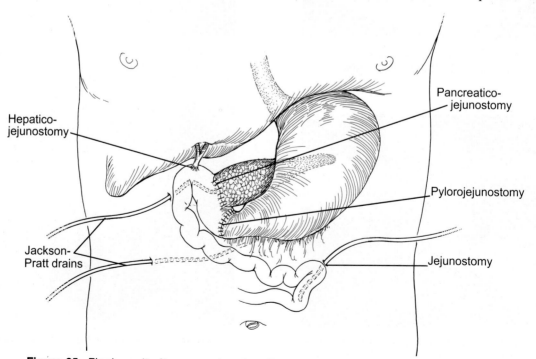

Figure 25. Final result after reconstruction. Drain placement and feeding jejunostomy.

manage this on an outpatient basis. In open surgery, the average hospital stay is 20 days with a 30-day mortality rate of 5%.

▲ COMPLICATIONS

The complications encountered are essentially the same as seen in open pylorus-preserving pancreatoduodenectomy. Delay in gastric emptying is the most frequent complication and occurs in 20% to 35% according to different series. Suturing between the pylorus and the jejunum should not be too tight, and the antrum-pylorus area should also not be devascularized. The most fearsome complication is the pancreatic leak, which often is due to the lack of a tight pancreaticojejunostomy. It is preferable to perform a mucosa-to-mucosa anastomosis than a dunking procedure that invaginates the pancreas transected plane into a loop of jejunum. Therefore laparoscopic suturing must be meticulous. Alternatively, a drain or stent through the anastomosis could be positioned to drain the pancreatic juice and decrease the incidence of a pancreatic fistula. It is more difficult to perform laparoscopically because the 5 F stent has to be inserted into the jejunal loop into the anastomosis and sutured at the anastomosis to prevent slippage. Hemorrhage is another complication that can be avoided by meticulous hemostasis during the procedure and corrections of possible coagulopathy. Biliary stenosis is prevented by meticulous suturing between the common hepatic duct and the antimesenteric side of the jejunal loop. Separate sutures of absorbable material should be used. Most complications in the postoperative period are related to advanced age, prolonged operative time, and increased operative blood loss. Intraabdominal sepsis is seen in fewer than 10% of patients and can be managed by antibiotics with or without the combination of percutaneous drainage of abscesses. Biliary leaks are often associated with a pancreatic leak and can be managed conservatively.

☑ CONCLUSION

An obvious selection of patients is necessary in order to decrease the likelihood of complications and to have a successful operation. It should be performed by an experienced team of surgeons in both advance laparoscopy and hepatopancreaticobiliary surgery. This should be evident if the 30-day mortality rate of open Whipple operation is below 5%. Since our policy is to perform a laparoscopic staging procedure on all potential candidates for a Whipple operation (after clearance with CT scan and angiogram), laparoscopic mobilization will usually provide gradual experience to the laparoscopic surgeon so that eventually he will be able to perform the operation with confidence. Now that we have shown that it is technically feasible in several patients, is this desirable and is it oncologically correct? More data must be collected and a larger series of patients is necessary to answer these questions. It may be that this intervention will evolve, the technique may improve with new instrumentation, and the indications may become more precise. It may also show in the future that extensive gastrointestinal reconstruction may give internal trauma and stress to such a degree that it will overcome the benefit of laparoscopy itself. At this stage of development, this operation should only be performed in selected institutions by highly trained surgeons. Data should be collected by following strict protocols of patient management and data collection.

RECOMMENDED READINGS

1. Braasch JW, Gagner M. Pylorus-preserving pancreatoduodenectomy: technical aspects. *Langenbecks Arch Chir* 1991;376:50–58.

SURGICAL PEARLS

The dissection between the anterior portion of the portal vein and the dorsal aspect of the pancreas should be done with an irrigation-suction cannula, using hydrodissection to provide a gentle dissection and prevent a portal vein rupture.

An 30- or 45-degree angulated laparoscope is best to provide a maximal view of the surgical field at different angles in order to perform the Kocher maneuver, transections, and anastomoses.

The hepaticojejunostomy and pancreaticojejunostomy anastomoses are best performed with a curved needle similar to the one used in open surgery. Interrupted intracorporeal sutures have to be placed meticulously to prevent an anastomotic leakage.

Transection of the pancreas is done with scissors only, so one can clearly identify the pancreatic duct and measure its diameter. Other structures can be transected with an endoscopic linear stapler to prevent intraperitoneal spillage of digestive secretions.

Extraction of the specimen is performed last, since it may require an enlargement of the incision. Therefore, during the reconstruction phase, the specimen is deposited in a sterile plastic bag toward the pelvis.

Extreme patience and a skillful assistant (four experienced hands) is the key to success for complicated laparoscopic digestive procedures.

2. Gagner M. Laparoscopic duodenopancreatectomy. In: Steichen F, Welter R, eds. *Minimally invasive surgery and technology*. St. Louis, MO: Quality Medical Publishing; 1994:192–199.
3. Gagner M, Pomp A. Laparoscopic pylorus-preserving pancreatoduodenectomy. *Surg Endosc* 1994; 8:408–410.
4. Miedema BW, Sarr MG, Van Heerden JA, Nagorney DM, McIlrath DC, Ilstrup D. Complications following pancreaticoduodenectomy: current management. *Arch Surg* 1992;127:945–949.
5. Warshaw AL, Fernandez del Castillo C. Laparoscopy in preoperative diagnosis and staging for gastrointestinal cancers. In: Zucker K, ed. *Surgical laparoscopy*. St. Louis, MO: Quality Medical Publishing; 1991:101–104.

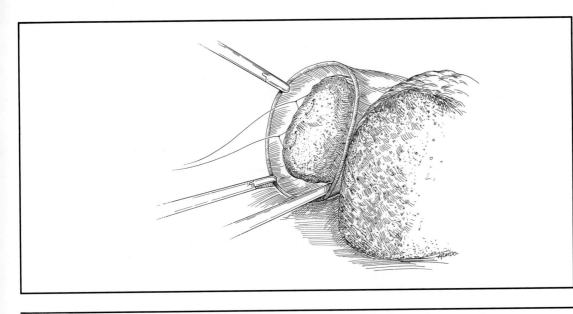

24

Hepatectomy

Makoto Hashizume, Kenji Takenaka,
and Keizo Sugimachi
Department of Surgery II
Faculty of Medicine, Kyushu University
Fukuoka 812, Japan

*Operative Laparoscopy and
Thoracoscopy,* edited by
B. V. MacFadyen, Jr. and
J. L. Ponsky. Lippincott-Raven
Publishers, Philadelphia © 1996.

KEY WORDS

Gas embolism   Liver cirrhosis

Hepatic resection   Microwave coagulator

Hepatocellular carcinoma   Ultrasonic dissector

Both cancer registry data and autopsy records show that the incidence of primary hepatocellular carcinoma has doubled in Japan in the last 10 years (1) although this incidence has not been observed in other countries. Despite recent progress in diagnostics, the rate of resectability remains low, and most patients are merely prescribed chemotherapy, mainly because of the advancement of the underlying liver disease. Unfortunately, not all such patients benefit from the anticancer drugs.

Laparoscopic surgery is steadily gaining in popularity as a minimally invasive procedure in almost all fields of general surgery since laparoscopic cholecystectomy was first reported in 1987 (2). In November 1994, in our hospital, laparoscopic hepatic resection was successfully performed for a hepatocellular carcinoma in a cirrhotic patient with poor liver function. This procedure is expected to provide a new choice of treatment for hepatic surgery and result in a better prognosis for those patients with advanced underlying liver disease.

◨ ANATOMY

Liver resections are performed based on a precise knowledge of the natural lines of division of the liver, which define the anatomic surgery of the liver (Fig. 1).

The liver appears to be divided into two livers by the main hepatic scissura through which the middle hepatic vein runs (3). The right liver is divided into two sectors by the right portal scissura through which the right hepatic vein runs. Each of these two sectors is further divided into two segments: the anteromedial sector, composed of segment V (S5) inferiorly and segment VIII (S8) superiorly, and the posterolateral sector, composed of segment VI (S6) inferiorly and segment VII (S7) superiorly. The left liver is also divided into two sectors by the left portal scissura through which the left hepatic vein runs. The anterior sector is divided by the umbilical fissure into two segments: segment IV (S4), the anterior part of which is the quadrate lobe, and segment III (S3), which is the anterior part of the left lobe. The posterior sector is composed of only one segment, segment II (S2), which is the posterior part of the left lobe. The Spiegel lobe, segment I (S1) is independent of the portal division and of the three main hepatic veins. It receives its vessels from the left, and also from the right, branches of the portal vein and hepatic artery; the hepatic veins are independent and end directly in the inferior vena cava. There are a total of eight segments in all.

The key anatomic consideration is a precise knowledge of the location of the portal and hepatic veins and the hepatic duct. The four sectors individualized by the three hepatic veins are called portal sectors, for these portions of the parenchyma are supplied by independent portal pedicles. The right and left sections of the liver are each divided into two parts by two other portal scissurae. These four subdivisions are usually called "segments" in the Anglo-Saxon nomenclature (4). According to Couinaud's nomenclature (3) they are called "sectors." A segment is the smallest anatomic unit of the liver. A thorough knowledge of the anatomic structure of the liver is thus an essential prerequisite to performing laparoscopic hepatic resection.

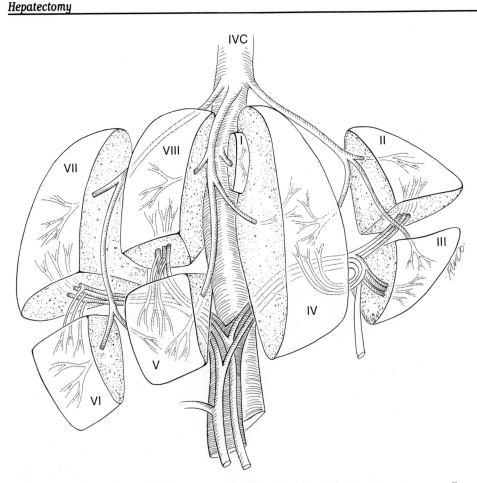

Figure 1. Anatomy of the liver. The liver is classified into eight segments according to Couinaud's nomenclature. Accurate and precise knowledge of the vascular structure is a prerequisite for hepatic surgery.

▶ PREOPERATIVE PLANNING

Diagnosis

Diagnostic studies on patients suspected of harboring hepatocellular cancer should be used to differentiate between progressive cirrhosis and the onset of cancer, by means of enzyme abnormalities, the presence of an elevated alpha-fetoprotein, and anatomic studies that display the presence of a mass. Many patients with hepatocellular carcinoma have a negative or normal alpha-fetoprotein; thus a negative test is no assurance that hepatocellular carcinoma does not exist.

Anatomic studies of the liver include initial echograms as the least invasive and most cost-effective procedures. Computed tomography scans of the liver are moderately accurate but not invariably so. The availability of noninvasive diagnostic techniques such as ultrasonography and computed tomography have greatly enhanced the possibility of detecting malignant growths in the liver at an early stage. Computed tomography scans should always be done with contrast agents, which help to greatly improve their accuracy (Figure 2). Computed tomographic imaging during arterial portography (CTAP) is the most sensitive modality for detecting and defining small liver nodules. Magnetic resonance imaging is useful in the detection and evaluation of large hepatocellular carcinomas.

Hepatic angiography is highly reliable (Fig. 3). Angiographically, only hepatocellular carcinoma, cancers of the pancreatic islet cells, and carcinoid tumors present as hypervascular relative to the surrounding liver. Rarely will other cancers produce a liver metastasis that is similarly hypervascular. Thus, an angiographic hypervascular mass in the liver tends to be almost diagnostic of a hepatocellular carcinoma, if islet cell cancers and carcinoid are excluded.

A percutaneous transhepatic biopsy of suspected hepatocellular carcinomas should be avoided if the patient is a potential candidate because of the extremely vascular nature of these cancers, which can bleed massively and often require emergency surgical control. If percutaneous transhepatic ethanol injection therapy is proposed for patients with a small tumor instead of an operation, biopsy is useful for an evaluation of the treatment.

One of the greatest concerns for the liver surgeon is in reducing the intrahepatic recurrence rate after a curative resection for hepatocellular carcinoma. Therefore, a more accurate preoperative assessment of the number and sites of intrahepatic metastatic nodules is essential, as is the development of a better method of preventing intrahepatic recurrence.

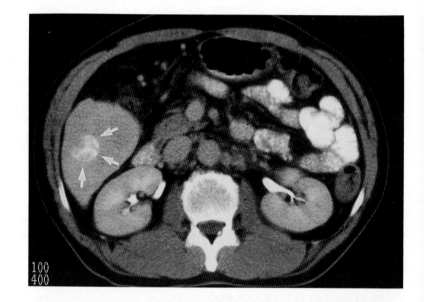

Figure 2. Computed tomography shows a 2-cm coin lesion with high density due to a selective injection of Lipiodol in segment 5 of the liver. The proposed volume of the hepatic tissue to be removed can be calculated by computed tomography.

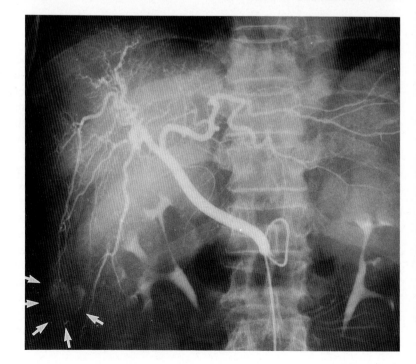

Figure 3. A selective hepatic arteriogram shows tumor staining in segment 5 of the liver, which helps to differentiate between a malignant tumor and hemangioma and also provides an image of the vascular structure of the resection line.

Special Tests

Hematologic changes are mostly related to cirrhosis and accompanying spleno-megaly, while other haematologic syndromes rarely occur. Biochemical investigations can show abnormal levels of bilirubin, alkaline phosphatase, transaminases, and serum proteins in both cirrhosis and hepatocellular carcinoma but do not distinguish between these conditions. In a patient known to have cirrhosis, an abrupt change in these values suggests a complicating hepatocellular carcinoma, particularly if there is an unexplained elevation in the alkaline phosphatase level.

The alpha-fetoprotein (AFP) level was first reported to be elevated in the blood of mice with hepatomas by Abelev and coworkers (5). The diagnostic usefulness of raised AFP levels was soon established; although raised AFP levels are also found in acute and chronic liver disease and in other malignancies, very high levels are suggestive of hepatocellular carcinoma. High AFP levels are associated with rapid tumor growth and tumor anaplasia. Other special tests, such as indocyanine green retention rate at 15 minutes, prothrombin time and the hepaplastine test are also reliable for determining the patient's hepatic function reserve.

Surgical and Nonsurgical Options

There are several choices in the treatment of hepatic tumors: systemic chemotherapy, selective transarterial chemotherapy (Lipiodolization), transarterial embolization (TAE), percutaneous ethanol injection therapy (PEIT), and hepatic resection. To improve the prognosis after a hepatectomy for hepatocellular carcinoma, adjuvant therapy and extended hepatectomy appear to be necessary when the functional capacity of the remaining liver permits.

Since 1982, we mainly prescribed ADM (Adriamycin; Kyowa Hakko Co. Ltd., Tokyo) mixed with an oily contrast medium (Lipiodol), which acts as a carrier of the drugs for tumor selectively (6). This mode of therapy, termed Lipiodolization, significantly prolongs survival, compared to the results achieved by hepatic artery ligation or the intraarterial administration of 5-fluorouracil (5-FU). Lipiodol accumulates in the vascular-rich masses, and a close relationship was also observed between the grades of deposits of Lipiodol in hepatocellular carcinoma on the plain abdominal radiograph and the antitumor effect. The hypovascular masses are not responsive to ADM, presumably because of the low concentration of antitumor agents as well as the insensitivity to ADM. With regard to pathologic factors, poorly differentiated hepatocellular carcinoma shows a high susceptibility to ADM, while resistance is noted in well-differentiated tumors. Hypovascular hepatocellular carcinomas respond poorly to ADM. Therefore, when hypovascular masses are clinically detected, MMC (mitomycin; Kyowa Hakko Co. Ltd., Tokyo) will probably be more effective than ADM. Otherwise, other types of treatment, such as percutaneous alcohol injection into the hepatocellular carcinoma nodules, can be tried (7). The succinate dehydrogenase inhibition (SDI) test is useful for determining when drugs will be most effective for a particular tumor.

The diagnosis of hepatocellular carcinoma at the time of Lipiodolization is based on the findings of an elevated alpha-fetoprotein (AFP) level, hepatic imaging, including CT and ultrasound, and/or biopsy. Indications for each treatment are as follows: when the hepatocellular carcinoma is local and resectable, and the clinical status and liver function of the patients are deemed adequate, a hepatic resection can be performed; when the hepatocellular carcinoma is not resectable, Lipiodolization is prescribed. The dose is determined with reference to the clinical status and biochemical parameters such as those based on the total bilirubin and indocyanine green test. In cases, in which the bilirubin exceeds 3 mg/dl and/or the indocyanine green test at 15 minutes is greater than 60%, Lipiodolization is contraindicated. When Lipiodolization is prescribed, a catheter is inserted percutaneously into the hepatic artery using Seldinger's technique. The patients undergo hepatic imaging at 3-month intervals. The serum AFP levels are regularly measured every month, and when the tumor appears to be growing, Lipiodolization is applied repeatedly.

Clinical Presentation

The clinical presentation of liver cancer is frequently masked by the underlying cirrhosis. Usually some uncharacteristic and vague symptoms bring the patient to the doctor. The onset of symptoms in cases with hepatocellular carcinoma may be insidious or sudden. Usually years of ill health, attributable to chronic liver disease, precede more acute symptoms, such as abdominal pain or jaundice.

Patients with underlying cirrhosis who are in a relatively steady state may clinically and biochemically deteriorate with the appearance of esophageal bleeding, liver failure, ascites, or pain (8). A majority of hepatocellular carcinoma patients experience abdominal discomfort or pain, and malaise, anorexia, weight loss, nausea, fever, and jaundice may also be observed. Clinical signs are most often those of tender hepatomegaly, often with a palpable hepatic mass, ascites, jaundice, vascular nevi, and distended abdominal surface veins. Less constant signs are splenomegaly, pyrexia, palmar erythema, gynecomastia, and increased skin pigmentation. Many of these features are due to concomitant cirrhosis, but hepatic pain is characteristic of an enlarging hepatic lesion. Such a sudden worsening of a stable clinical condition may be the result of the progressive growth of hepatocellular carcinoma with the destruction of an already compromised hepatic mass or the sudden worsening of the already established portal hypertension. Esophageal bleeding occurs in liver cancer to a large degree in those patients with intraluminal portal venous extension (9).

Patients without any underlying cirrhosis may also present with a palpable mass, pain, symptoms from a displacement of surrounding organs, ascites, bleeding, and evidence of portal hypertension. More subtle indications of hepatic dysfunction may also appear, such as weight loss and anorexia.

Hepatocellular carcinomas may occasionally first present with metastatic disease in bone or lung, but this is relatively uncommon. Spontaneous rupture of hepatic cell carcinoma occurs with some regularity and presents a dramatic picture of intraperitoneal hemorrhage and shock.

Patient Selection

Patients with multiple hepatocellular carcinoma are not candidates for curative resection. Large anatomic resections in cirrhotic livers lead to postoperative mortality and liver failure in a high percentage of cases (10). Peripheral wedge resections of small superficial hepatocellular carcinomas may be carried out on patients with cirrhosis with relative safety. In general, the presence of cirrhosis, even of relatively minor physiologic impact, precludes surgical resections of any significant size because of the incapability of hepatic regeneration or hypertrophy. Furthermore, most cancers arising with a background of cirrhosis are multiple, advanced, and demonstrate an extremely poor prognosis. Patients with underlying cirrhosis are thus not candidates for a resection of hepatocellular carcinoma because of poor results, high complication rates, increased blood loss, and a high incidence of multifocal disease.

The usual candidates for a resection of hepatocellular carcinoma are those patients with solitary lesions arising with the background of mild cirrhosis or chronic hepatitis. Cirrhosis is considered to be a limiting factor to massive excision, and extensive surgery may be unduly hazardous and life-threatening in such patients. Recent studies have paved the way for the development of techniques and indications for liver resection for hepatocellular carcinoma-associated cirrhosis (11).

The particular surgical resection is less important if the criterion of a margin of the liver of at least 1 cm is achieved. In cirrhotic patients with a tumor less than 4 cm in diameter, the extent of the margin from the cut surface to hepatocellular carcinoma (TW) is not linked to an early recurrence (12). However, when the tumor size exceeds 4 cm, 10 mm of TW is inadequate to achieve curability. When a wide resection is not feasible, then adjuvant therapy should be aggressive. Hepatocellular carcinomas that are small, focal, and lateral in the liver tissue can be easily removed with a wedge resection, as long as the criterion of reasonable local margins is achieved.

The other primary malignant tumors arising in the liver include cholangiocarcinoma, angiosarcoma, and primary lymphoma. These are rarely seen and thus provide few opportunities for surgical resection.

Metastatic carcinoma of the liver is a common cause of death from cancer. Unfortunately, liver metastases are usually but one manifestation of disseminated disease from cancers arising in the portal venous drainage area as well as in other parts of the body. Metastases to the liver are extremely common in carcinomas of the lung, breast, esophagus, stomach, pancreas, upper aerodigestive tract, and melanoma. Of the cancers listed, only carcinoma of the colon and rectum presents frequently with solitary or few metastases only in the liver. Most liver resections for metastatic cancer relate to carcinomas of the large bowel. Studies indicate that patients suitable for resection of metastatic colorectal cancer with curative intent usually have only one, two, or three tumor nodules in the liver, and no other extrahepatic metastatic disease. The particular biologic features that are associated with a higher long-term, disease-free survival rate include a primary colon cancer that was staged as Dukes B rather than Dukes C, a disease-free interval longer than 1 year, few hepatic metastases, confined to one lobe, and a surgical resection margin of more than 1 cm. Patients with a normal or low-serum carcinoembryonic antigen (CEA) level have a higher cure rate than those with a high value. In patients who display all these criteria, the disease-free survival rate at 5 years may approach 50%.

Indications and Contraindications

Hepatocellular carcinomas that are small, focal, and lateral are well indicated for a laparoscopic hepatic resection. At present, laparoscopic hepatic resection seems to be more appropriate for a partial resection of the lateral segment, S4, S5, or S6. It is also recommended for small tumors because the removal of the resected liver tissue is so limited through small incisions, and skin incisions have to be extended at the final-stage surgery to avoid any intraperitoneal dissemination of the tumor.

In cirrhotic patients, the balance between postoperative hepatocellular reserve and surgical curability will greatly influence the prognosis. Although the most widely accepted and standardized resectional procedures for hepatic carcinoma are either a formal lobar or a segmental resection, the indications for these techniques are limited when a primary carcinoma arises in the cirrhotic liver. In cirrhotic patients with a poor hepatocellular reserve, resection of small liver cancer, with limited procedure, enhances the possibility of cure. Provided that the patients for elective surgery are carefully screened, the life span can probably be extended with a limited hepatic resection (13). The limited hepatic resection assisted with laparoscopy therefore appears to be the procedure of choice, especially when there is a well-demarcated liver cancer nodule. A wide excision should be done for a noncapsulated mass.

In general, patients with an indocyanine green (ICG) test over 40%, prothrom-

Table 1. *Indications for a laparoscopic hepatic resection*

Hepatic tumor
    A small, focal, or lateral hepatic tumor
    A well-demarcated nodule
    A peripheral hepatic lesion: left lateral segment, S4, S5, S6
    Tumors which are well indicated for a wedge resection, or a partial, limited hepatic
      resection
Hepatocellular function
    Serum albumin over 3.5 mg/dl
    Total bilirubin below 1.5 mg/dl
    Indocyanine green retention rate at 15 minutes below 40%
    Prothrombin time activity over 60%

bin activity test less than 60%, serum albumin below 3.5 g/dl, and total bilirubin over 1.5 mg/dl, are considered poor risks for major hepatic resection (Table 1). In these patients with severely impaired liver function, limited hepatic resection is appraised, with reference to the degree of hepatocellular reserve. Independent of hepatocellular function, small peripheral cancer nodules are also removed in some patients (Fig. 4), and those patients are well indicated for laparoscopic hepatic resection. After surgery, the choice of adjuvant chemotherapy depends on the clinical status.

▼ INTRAOPERATIVE MANAGEMENT/SURGICAL TECHNIQUE

Positioning and Skin Incisions

When hepatic resection is performed on the left lateral segment (S2 or S3) the patient is operated on in a supine position and the surgeon stands on the right side of the patient. A minimal open laparotomy is performed 10 mm in length to insert a 10-mm trocar and an oblique type of laparoscope below the umbilicus. In order to minimize the intraoperative complications regarding the trocars, we prefer

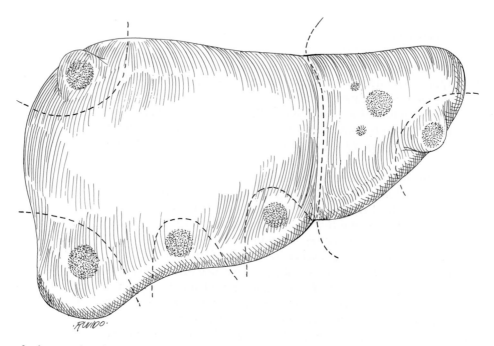

Figure 4. Appropriate location of hepatic tumors and resection lines for a laparoscopic hepatic resection.

a minimal open laparotomy to the use of an injection needle for making a pneumo-peritoneum. After the pneumoperitoneum is achieved by the infusion of carbon dioxide, three more trocars are inserted at the epigastrium and the left subcostal line for dissection. When a hepatic resection is performed on the medial segment (S4), the three other trocars are inserted at the epigastrium and bilateral subcostal line.

When hepatic resection is performed on the anteroinferior segment (S5) or posteroinferior segment (S6), the patient is operated on in a left-side semidecubitus position (Fig. 5). The surgeon stands on the left side of the patient (Fig. 6). A minimal open laparotomy is performed 10 mm in length for laparoscopy at the site 10 mm right of the umbilicus. After a pneumoperitoneum is made by the infusion of carbon dioxide, three more 10-mm trocars are inserted at the right subcostal line on the posterior axilar line, the anterior axilar line, and midclavicular line (Fig. 7).

When the posterior segment is resected, the site of insertion of the laparoscope is better moved toward the right lateral abdomen in order to obtain a better visual-

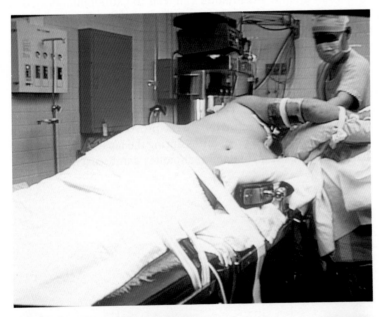

Figure 5. Position of the patient: Based on the location of the tumor either a supine position or semidecubitus position is alternatively chosen.

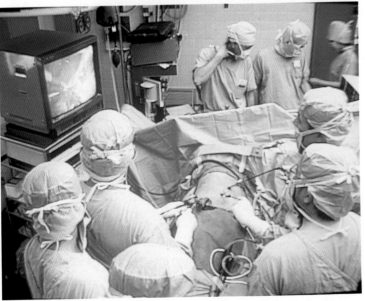

Figure 6. The operator stands on the left side of the patient when a hepatic resection is performed on the right lobe, while he stands on the right side when the operation is done on the left lateral segment.

ization. For a resection of the superior or posterior segment of the right hepatic lobe, either a lateral approach or thoracoabdominal approach is considered to be more appropriate.

Pneumoperitoneum or Airless Lifting System

The most critical complication is an air embolism through the injured hepatic vein. Pneumoperitoneum is necessary until all trocars have been inserted. If a moderate-size or larger hepatic vein is included in the hepatic tissue dissection plane, an airless lifting system may be an alternative way to prevent air embolism, rather than the use of a pneumoperitoneum. After all trocars have been inserted a U-shaped retractor is inserted into the peritoneal cavity or subcutaneously between the left and right subcostal region so as to elevate the abdominal wall along the falciform ligament. Then after the insertion of the U-shaped retractor the injection of carbon dioxide into the peritoneal cavity is stopped.

The intraperitoneal high pressure and possible rise in blood carbon dioxide content induced by carbon dioxide insufflation can lead to cardiopulmonary distress in patients with cardiovascular or pulmonary dysfunctions. It is also time-consuming to change the long forceps and to dissect inflamed tissue with a limited number of laparoscopic instruments. This is not the case when ordinary surgical instruments are used. The U-shaped retractor, which can elevate the abdominal wall, provides a clear operative field of vision without infusing gas into the abdominal cavity and enables the use of the ordinary surgical instruments through a skin incision made for the trocar; the intra- and extraperitoneal pressure are equal (14). The main advantages of this U-shaped retractor are the prevention of air embolism and a clear field of vision and operative procedures during the laparoscopic hepatic resection. The usual surgical instruments and techniques can be used.

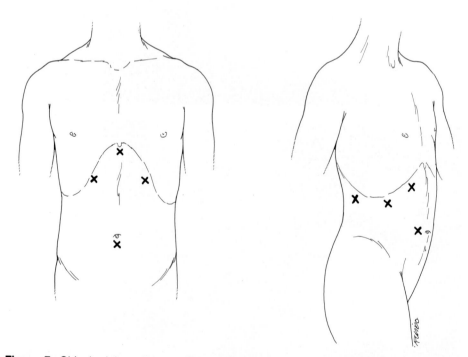

Figure 7. Skin incision: A laparoscope is inserted either 10 mm beneath or to the right of the umbilicus. The other three trocars are then inserted along the left subcostal line to the right subcostal line.

Intraoperative Final Examination

On entering the intraperitoneal cavity, the existence or absence of ascites, or metastatic lesions and the appearance of the liver surface, are examined by using a laparoscopic ultrasound (PEF-704LA; Toshiba, Tokyo *or* UST-5522-7.5; Aloka, Tokyo, Japan) (Fig. 8). After diagnostic intraoperative ultrasonography has been performed, it must be decided if hepatic resection is indicated and what procedures will be used. If intrametastasis or tumor thrombus has spread beyond the area that is considered for resection in light of the results of the patient's liver function tests, then a hepatectomy must be ruled out. Thus laparoscopic ultrasonography confirms the location of the tumor and decides the line where the liver should be resected; the resection line on the liver surface is marked with electrocautery (Fig. 9).

Intraoperative ultrasonography can be used as a direct guide for the division of the liver parenchyma (11). Every attempt to achieve a 2-cm margin around the hepatic mass should be made in order to ultimately achieve at least a 1-cm disease-free margin in the final specimen. With the aid of intraoperative ultrasound, the extent, number, and nature of the hepatic nodules or metastases can be detected, as well as their relationship to major venous structures and other aspects of the

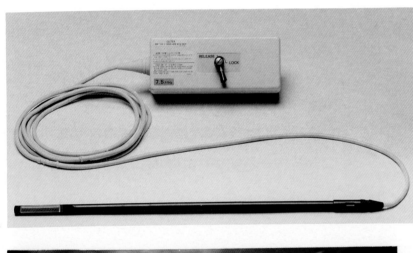

A

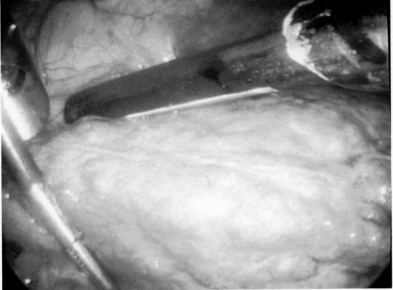

B

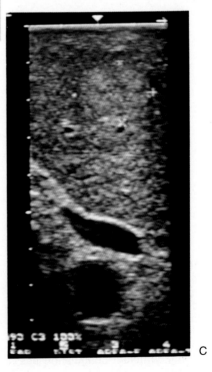

C

Figure 8. A: An ultrasonography probe. **B:** Intraoperative ultrasonography provides final decisions of the operative indication, procedures and resection line. **C:** The tumor is found on the video monitor and a marginal line is decided.

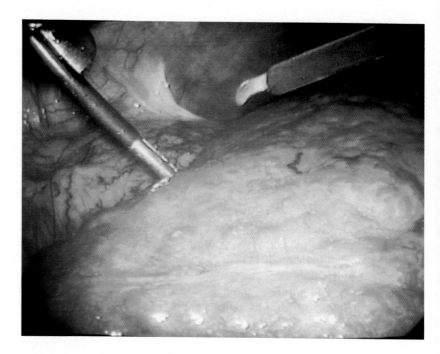

Figure 9. The marking of the resection line on the liver surface with electro-cautery.

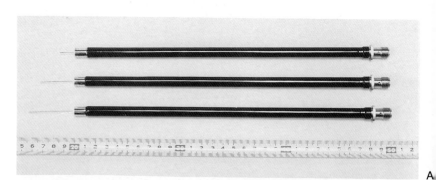

A

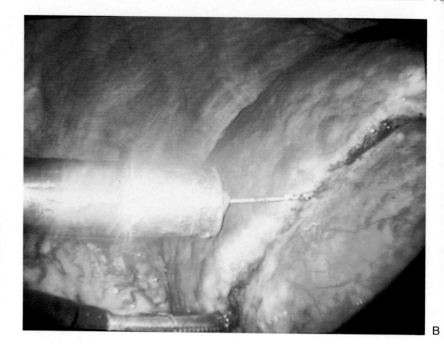

Figure 10. A: A microwave coagulator with different length tips. **B:** A microwave coagulator is useful for coagulating the surrounding parenchymal liver tissue and preventing unnecessary bleeding from the hepatic tissue. Puncture the needle of the microwave coagulator onto the resection line until sufficient coagulation has been obtained.

B

detailed anatomy of the liver. Ultrasonography is useful in determining the exact location of the cutting line and allowing a limited hepatic resection with an adequate resection margin in patients with a poor liver function.

Although this information may be obtained by preoperative ultrasonography, intraoperative sonography will provide much more information. The area of the lesion to be resected should be decided on the basis of the interrelationship between the tumor and blood vessels. When small partial resection of the liver is performed, when there is no landmark of suitable vessels near the tumor, and when an unknown vessel is encountered during division of the parenchyma, ultrasonic guidance is indicated. Of the hepatocellular carcinomas smaller than 5 cm in diameter, 61% (70/115) were invisible and nonpalpable (15). The detection of invisible and nonpalpable hepatocellular carcinoma is thus a simple and a primitive use of intraoperative ultrasonography. There are two methods for orienting the direction of division of the parenchyma. The first is to scan the liver only after the divided surfaces of the liver have been placed in the natural position. Because only a very small amount of the air gets into the divided surfaces of the liver, the transecting plane is demonstrated as a glittering line on the sonogram. When this echogenic line is not delineated, a sonolucent layer, due to the presence of blood, can be seen between the raw surfaces of the liver.

Resection of the Liver

After the resection line has been decided, a microwave coagulator (Microtaze; Nippon Shoji-Kaisha, Ltd., Osaka) is then used along the resection line to prevent any unnecessary bleeding from the surrounding parenchymal hepatic tissue (Fig. 10). An ultrasonic dissection (Olympus USU; Tokyo *or* Harmonic Scalpel; Ultra Cision, Rhode Island, USA) can also be used (16) (Fig. 11). The combination of a microwave coagulator and an ultrasonic dissector is considered to help minimize

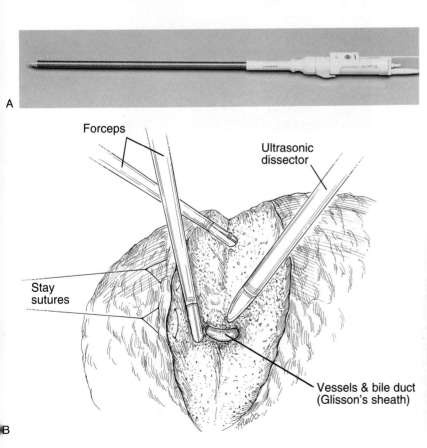

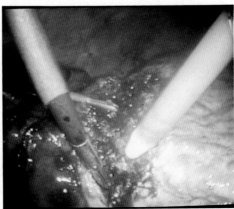

Figure 11. A: An ultrasonic dissector probe. **B:** An ultrasonic dissector is used to fragment the coagulated parenchymal tissue and to remove any fragments while irrigating with saline.

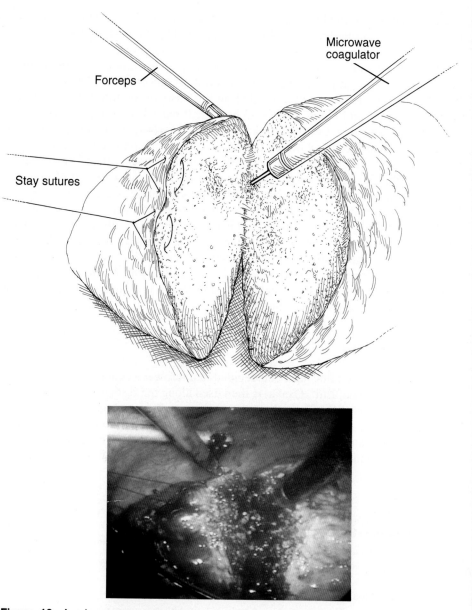

Figure 12. A microwave coagulator and ultrasonic dissector are alternatively used until the hepatic tissue has been completely separated.

intraoperative blood loss and prevent any resultant hepatic failure. They are alternatively used until the resecting plane has been completely dissected (Fig. 12). The small vessels and ducts encountered are coagulated. The moderate-sized hepatic vein or portal vein and bile duct in the Glisson's sheath are all clamped with a clip (Fig. 13) or extracorporeally ligated with a 75-cm length 3-0 silk, if necessary, and severed.

Partial resection of the peripheral liver or a left lateral segment resection may not require portal hepatis dissection or isolation and control of the central vascular structures, since the periphery of the liver is devoid of large venous structures, and bleeding can be controlled readily with local clamps, coagulation, and ligature. Such hepatic resections as either a required portal hepatis dissection or isolation are indicated for open hepatic surgery at this moment.

In order to keep a better operative field during surgery, stay sutures with 2-0 Prolene or 2-0 silk are placed on the resecting liver edge and pulled out through a trocar (Fig. 14). The bar of any forceps can be used for pushing the opposite site of the hepatic tissue up along the transecting line in order to maintain a sufficiently wide operative field.

Removal of the Tumor

The resected specimen is placed in a nylon bag (Fig. 15-A). The incision is extended a few centimeters at the subcostal line, and the bag, including the resected liver tissue, is then delivered out of the peritoneal cavity. When the tumor is suspected of malignancy, it is mandatory to avoid dissemination of the tumor or skin metastasis. Therefore, the size of the tumor is a limited factor for indication of the laparoscopic surgery in the malignant tumor. It is very important to select a sturdy bag and to make a sufficiently large skin incision, normally measuring up to 4 to 5 cm (Fig. 15B).

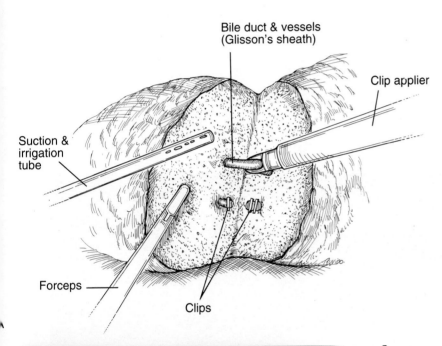

Bile duct & vessels
(Glisson's sheath)

Clip applier

Suction &
irrigation
tube

Forceps

Clips

Figure 13. A, B: The remnant vessels in Glisson's sheath after dissection with an ultrasonic dissector are clamped with clips and cut.

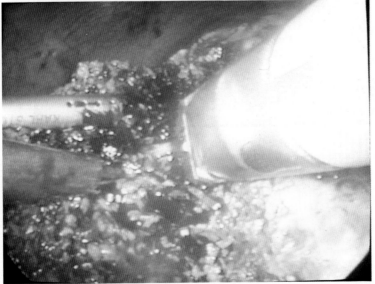

B

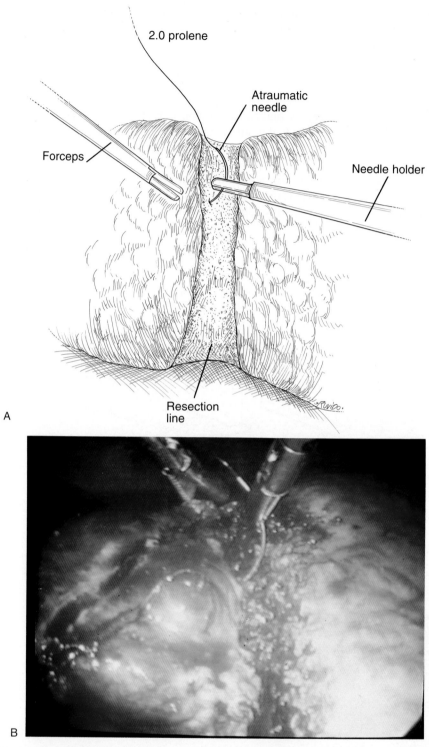

Figure 14. A,B: Stay sutures with 2-0 Prolene or 2-0 silk are placed on the edge of the resected tissue to maintain a good operative field.

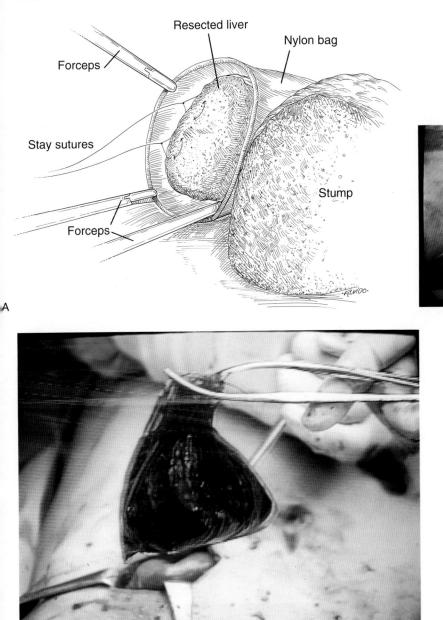

Figure 15. A: The resected hepatic tissue is put into a nylon bag and **B:** delivered from the peritoneal cavity through an extended skin incision by 4 cm.

Hemostasis

After sufficient hemostasis either with electrocautery or an argon beam coagulator (Fig. 16) and irrigation with warm saline, fibrin glue (Fig. 17) is applied for hemostasis on the cut surface of the remnant liver. Oxicell cotton (Fig. 18) is used for the hemostasis of an oozing from the injured branches of the hepatic veins or portal veins with compression for a short time by a forceps. A small piece of gauze tamponade is also useful for hemostasis of bleeding from the venous vessels. If the argon beam coagulator is used under pneumoperitoneum, the valves of the

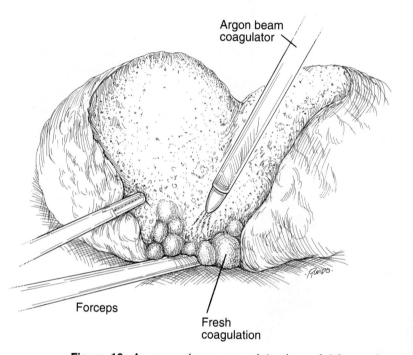

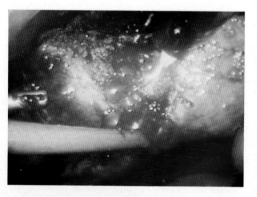

Figure 16. An argon beam coagulator is useful for performing hemostasis on any oozing that escapes from the dissection plane. Remember that all valves of the trocars should be open under the pneumoperitoneum, otherwise the intraperitoneal pressure will increase to extremely dangerous levels.

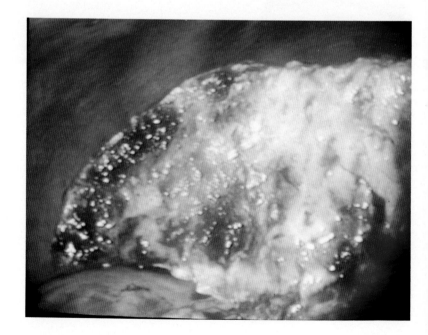

Figure 17. A fibrin glue is useful for performing hemostasis on the resecting plane.

trocars have to be open in order to avoid a rapid increase in the intraperitoneal pressure and air embolism, and more attention should be paid to the monitoring system.

Drainage

Two Penrose drains are placed: one in the right subdiaphragmatic space and the other on the cut surface of the liver. The ends of both drains are withdrawn through the incision at the most lateral subcostal line. Thereafter, the skin incisions are closed (Fig. 19).

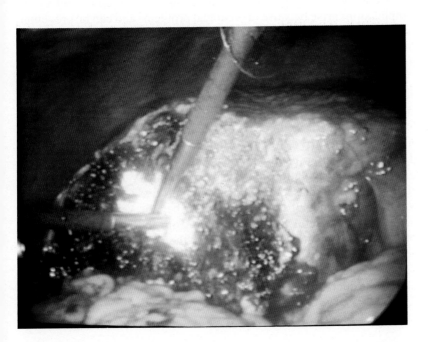

Figure 18. Oxicell cotton is also useful for hemostasis, especially when bleeding originates from the branches of the hepatic veins.

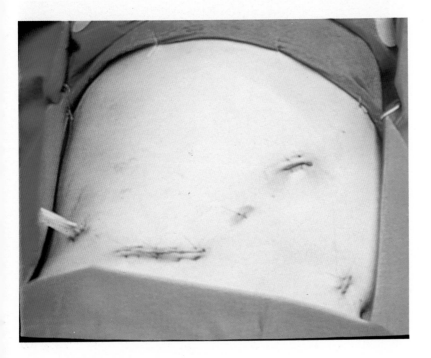

Figure 19. Postoperative abdominal wall. Two Penrose drains which are placed in the right subphrenic space and in the resected space are pulled out through a lateral abdominal skin incision.

Postoperative Management

Postoperative management is almost the same as that for conventional open surgery. Oral intake is permitted from the second day after operation, by which time the patient is free to move about. No pain medication is normally required. The patient is discharged after the seventh postoperative day when the postoperative course is essentially uneventful.

▲ COMPLICATIONS

The major complications encountered in laparoscopic hepatic resection are bleeding, bile leakage, gas embolism, intestinal damage, hypercapnia and so on. Most such complications arise because of technical problems and can be prevented by improvement in the techniques and instruments.

1. *Bleeding.* Oozing is easily controlled with either electrocautery or an argon beam coagulator. However, the argon beam coagulator should be carefully used if it is under pneumoperitoneum because the intraperitoneal pressure extensively increases and might cause hypercapnia, cardiopulmonary distress, or air embolism. Arterial bleeding is stopped with the use of a clip. Bleeding from larger vessels is also controlled with a clip or by extracorporeal ligation with 3-0 or 2-0 silk. Once bleeding has occurred it is important to catch the bleeding point with a device and to coagulate after a sufficient dissection of the vessel with the other device, otherwise blind coagulation may lead to secondary bleeding. A gentle dissection with an ultrasonic dissector will prevent unnecessary bleeding and provide the skeletalized branches of the portal vein or hepatic vein to be ligated or clipped. Oxicell cotton is useful to stop bleeding from the hepatic vein. Fibrin glue also works for the hemostasis of oozing from the small vessels.

2. *Bile leakage.* Small bile ducts at the periphery of the liver are well coagulated and no bile leakage occurs. When the hepatic dissection plate contains moderate-size to large bile ducts, careless operation might cause duct injuries, resulting

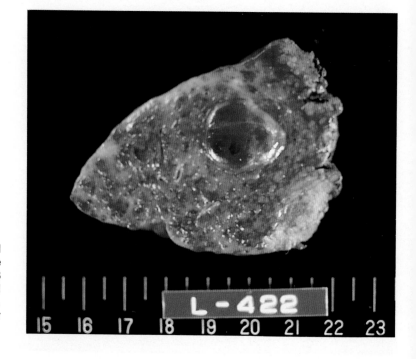

Figure 20. The cut surface of the resected specimen with liver cirrhosis. The size of the resected liver tissue measures 7.0 × 6.5 × 5.3 cm and weighs 115 g. The tumor size measured 1.8 × 1.6 cm with a resection margin of 13 mm. The operation was considered to be absolutely curative.

in bile leakage. While dissecting the hepatic parenchymal tissue the Glission sheath, including the bile duct, portal vein, and hepatic artery, should be carefully dissected. Biloma may be well drained using a drainage tube inserted under ultrasonography. A gram-negative infection may be complicated with the biloma, and antibiotics should be administered when the patient has a fever of unknown origin.

3. *Gas embolism.* Gas embolism is a serious complication (17). It occurs when carbon dioxide enters into any vessel that is punctured with a needle for pneumoperitoneum or into venous vessels that are severed or injured during surgery. During the operation a serial gas analysis should be taken; a decrease in the endotidal CO_2, an increase in $Paco_2$, and a reduction of Pao_2 suggests gas embolism. When massive gas embolism occurs, a decrease in venous return by a gas lock formed in the heart results in a decrease in the cardiac output. Then bubbles of carbon dioxide enter the pulmonary circulation and lead to pulmonary hypertension and heart failure. It is important to look for gas embolism and detect it early. Any bubble sound on auscultation is a useful tool for an early diagnosis to detect gas embolism. As soon as gas embolism is suspected, an injection of carbon dioxide should be stopped and all instruments that would cause an increase in the intraperitoneal pressure, such as an argon beam coagulator, should be stopped. Carbon dioxide should be deflated out of the peritoneal cavity. The patient should be in a head-down left lateral position. A catheter for intravenous hyperalimentation is also useful for removing air bubbles out of the heart. In addition, the site of venous injuries should be repaired as soon as possible. If the larger hepatic vein is contained in the dissection plane, then an airless lifting system would likely prevent gas embolism.

4. *Intestinal damage.* In the laparoscopic hepatic resection it is not necessary to touch the small or large intestine. The intestinal damage occurs when a trocar or needle is being inserted or when a dissecting device accidentally touches the intestine with the coagulating system switched on (18). Dissection should be carefully accomplished whenever there is any adhesion of the intestine with the liver surface. When the intestine is damaged, it should be repaired as soon as possible with interrupted suture of 3-0 silk, otherwise the site of the intestinal damage is often lost. If the intestinal contents spill over, sufficient irrigation with warm saline is mandatory. Thus, to prevent intestinal damage, the position of the patient and clear operative field are important factors. The assistants should do their best to obtain a wide operative field by mobilizing the small and large intestines.

5. *Hypercapnia.* Hypercapnia occurs when intraperitoneal pressure is extensively increased or the operation time is lengthened. The carbon dioxide used for pneumoperitoneum is easily absorbed through the peritoneum or the damaged tissue involving the capillaries or venules and enters into the systemic circulation, resulting in hypercapnia. It causes hypertension, tachycardia, or arrhythmia. It is easily detected during the operation by a gas analysis. The hypercapnia is corrected or prevented by hyperventilation because carbon dioxide is easily expired from the lung. If the patient has a poor pulmonary function or is elderly, then hypercapnia may occur easily and can continue for some time even after the cessation of carbon dioxide or the operation is finished. As a result, respiratory distress can occur. If the patient has a risk of hypercapnia, then the use of an airless lifting system is recommended.

☑ CONCLUSIONS

Laparoscopic hepatic resection is feasible with the help of an ultrasonic dissector and a microwave coagulator without any major complications. The indications for hepatic resection can be extended to patients with advanced underlying liver disease with the use of an assisted laparoscopy (Fig. 20).

SURGICAL PEARLS

In patients with severely impaired liver function, a limited hepatic resection is appraised, with reference to the degree of hepatocellular reserve. At present laparoscopic hepatic resection seems to be more appropriate for a wedge resection or a partial resection of the lateral segment, S4, S5, or S6.

Intraoperative ultrasonography is useful in determining the exact location of the cutting line and allows a limited hepatic resection with an adequate resection margin. Combination of a microwave coagulator and an ultrasonic dissector can help minimize intraoperative blood loss. It is mandatory to avoid dissemination of the tumor or skin metastasis.

Gas embolism is a serious complication. During the operation a serial gas analysis should be taken. An airless lifting system is an alternative way to prevent air embolism rather than use of a pneumoperitoneum. The argon beam coagulator should be carefully used if it is under pneumoperitoneum.

REFERENCES

1. Okuda K, Fujimoto I, Hanai A, Urano Y. Changing incidence of hepatocellular carcinoma. *Cancer Res* 1987;47:4967.
2. Reddick EJ, Olsen DO. Laparoscopic laser cholecystectomy: a comparison with mini-lap cholecystectomy. *Surg Endosc* 1989;3:131–133.
3. Couinaud C. *Le foie: etudes anatomiques et chirurgicales.* Paris: Masson, 1957.
4. Bismuth H. Surgical anatomy and anatomical surgery of the liver. *World J Surg* 1982;6:3–9.
5. Abelev GI, Perova SP, Khramkova NI, Postnikova ZA, Irlin IS. Production of embryonal alphaglobulin by transplantable mouse hepatomas. *Transplantation* 1963;1:174–180.
6. Kanematsu T, Furuta T, Takenaka K, Matsumata T, Yoshida Y, Nishizaki T, Hasuo K, Sugimachi K. A 5-year experience of Lipiodolization: selective regional chemotherapy for 200 patients with hepatocellular carcinoma. *Hepatology* 1989;10:98–102.
7. Livraghi T, Salmi A, Bolondo L, Marin G, Arienti V, Monti F, Vettori C. Small hepatocellular carcinoma: percutaneous alcohol injection: results in 23 patients. *Radiology* 1988;168:313.
8. Cady B. Hepatic tumors. In: McDermott WV Jr, ed. *Surgery of the liver.* Boston: Blackwell Scientific Publications; 1989:433–449.
9. Hashizume M, Kitano S, Koyanagi N, et al. Endoscopic injection sclerotherapy for 1,000 patients with esophageal varices: a nine-year prospective study. *Hepatology* 1992;15:69–75.
10. Takenaka K, Kanematsu T, Fukuzawa K, Sugimachi K. Can hepatic failure after surgery for hepatocellular carcinoma in cirrhotic patients be prevented? *World J Surg* 1990;14:123–127.
11. Makuuchi M, Hasegawa H, Yamazaki S. Ultrasonically guided subsegmentectomy. *Surg Gynecol Obstet* 1985;161:346–350.
12. Kanematsu T, Shirabe K, Sugimachi K. Surgical strategy for primary hepatocellular carcinoma associated with cirrhosis. *Semin Surg Oncol* 1990;6:36–41.
13. Kanematsu T, Takenaka K, Matsumata T, Furuta T, Sugimachi K, Inokuchi K. Limited hepatic resection effective for selected cirrhotic patients with primary liver cancer. *Ann Surg* 1984;199:51–56.
14. Kitano S, Iso S, Tomikawa M, Moriyama M, and Sugimachi K: A prospective randomized trial comparing pneumoperitoneum and U-shaped retractor elevation for laparoscopic cholecystectomy. *Surg Endosc* 1993;7:311–314.
15. Makuuchi M. Application of intraoperative ultrasonography of hepatectomy. In: Makuuchi M, ed. *Abdominal intraoperative ultrasonography.* Tokyo: Igaku-shoin; 1987:89–123.
16. Hashizume M, Sugimachi K, Kitano S, et al. Laparoscopic splenectomy. *Am J Surg* 1994;167:611–614.
17. Wittgen CM, Andrus CH, et al. Analysis of the hemodynamic and ventilatory effects of laparoscopic cholecystectomy. *Arch Surg* 1991;126:997–1001.
18. Deziel DJ, Millikan KW, Economou SG, et al. Complications of laparoscopic cholecystectomy: a national survey of 4,292 hospitals and an analysis of 77,604 cases. *Am J Surg* 1993;165:9–14.

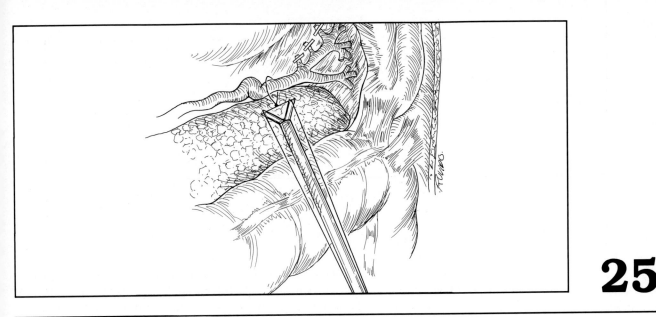

25

Splenectomy

M. M. Gazayerli and Tom Legge
Laparoscopic Laser Surge-on Institute
Troy, Michigan 48084–3525

Mary Lou Spitz
Department of General Surgery
St. Joseph Mercy Hospital
Pontiac, Michigan 48341–2985

Hosam S. Helmy
Department of Surgery
Cairo University
Cairo, Egypt

Mohamed Hakky
Department of General Surgery and Laparoscopy
Egypt Air Hospital
Cairo, Egypt

Operative Laparoscopy and Thoracoscopy, edited by B. V. MacFadyen, Jr. and J. L. Ponsky. Lippincott-Raven Publishers, Philadelphia © 1996.

● ANATOMY

The spleen invites laparoscopic removal because it is essentially intraperitoneal, its hilum is easy to dissect, it lies against the parietal peritoneum thus allowing lateral traction to expose the hilum, and steps can be taken to ensure the safety of its removal.

The spleen lies along the long axis of the left ninth rib close to the diaphragm. The pathologic spleen may be as small as the palm of the hand, or it may completely fill the abdomen, extending from the left upper quadrant to the right lower quadrant. There are certain advantages to dissecting a moderately enlarged spleen because the hilar vessels curve forward, being displaced anteriorly by the spleen. This advantage, however, is far outweighed by the difficulty of bagging the enlarged spleen; thus, extreme splenomegaly is a relative contraindication to a laparoscopic approach.

One can view the spleen as an outgrowth of the spine of a binder or book, with the anterior cover of the book being the gastrosplenic ligament containing the short gastric vessels and the posterior cover being the splenorenal ligament containing the splenic artery and vein. The upper pole of the spleen is attached to the diaphragm by the splenophrenic ligament, while the lower pole is attached to the colon by the splenocolic ligament. These two ligaments have no named vessels and are usually relatively avascular. However, in cases of hypersplenism they can become highly vascularized, containing large collateral vessels. Adhesions between the diaphragm and the lateral surface of the spleen can also develop to further challenge the surgeon. The inferior boundary of the splenic fossa is formed by the phrenocolic ligament, which is not attached to the spleen itself but cradles the lower pole of the spleen (Fig. 1).

In order to avoid complications during dissection of the hilum, there are three significant anatomic facts that must be kept in mind: the branching pattern of the splenic artery, the relationship of the splenic vein to the splenic artery, and the relationship of the tail of the pancreas to the spleen.

The most common type of branching of the splenic artery, called the *distributed* type, occurring in 70% of people, is that of a short splenic artery sending numerous long terminal branches to the splenic hilum. Since the arterial branching occurs from 3.5 to 12 cm proximal to the hilum, there are many more arteries entering over three-quarters of the hilar surface (Fig. 2A). With this type of vascular pattern care must be taken during dissection of the hilum. The less common branching pattern, called the *magistral* type, in 30% of people, occurs when a long splenic artery branches very close to the hilum, sending its short terminal branches directly into the midportion of the hilum (Fig. 2B). This type of splenic artery is, as expected, much easier to dissect and ligate.

The second relationship to be aware of is that of the splenic vein to the splenic artery. Most often, in 54% of individuals, it is located posterior and inferior to the artery. In the second most common pattern, in 44%, the vein is wrapped around the artery; however, distally it usually lies posterior to the artery. In the rarest pattern, occurring in only 2%, the vein is anterior to the artery.

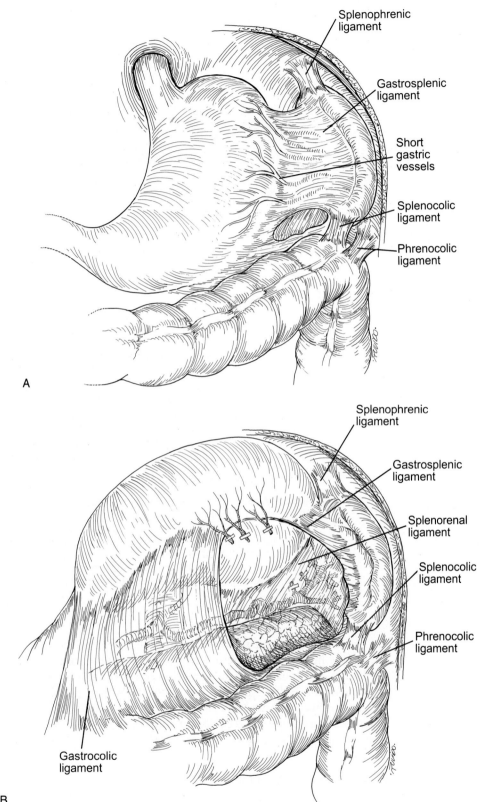

Splenophrenic ligament

Gastrosplenic ligament

Short gastric vessels

Splenocolic ligament

Phrenocolic ligament

A

Splenophrenic ligament

Gastrosplenic ligament

Splenorenal ligament

Splenocolic ligament

Phrenocolic ligament

Gastrocolic ligament

B

Figure 1. A, B: The splenophrenic ligament attaches the upper pole of the spleen to the diaphragm. The gastrosplenic ligament is the anterior leaf of the splenic hilum and contains the short gastric vessels. The splenocolic ligament attaches the lower pole of the spleen to the splenic flexure of the colon. The phrenocolic ligament supports the lower pole of the spleen if the spleen is not too enlarged. It forms the lower boundary of the splenic fossa. The splenorenal ligament is the posterior leaf of the splenic hilum and contains the splenic vessels as they run from the tail of the pancreas to the spleen.

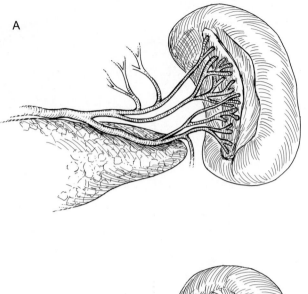

Figure 2. Branching patterns of the splenic artery. **A:** The distributed type. Note the short splenic trunk with its early proximal branching, the long multiple branches, and the large surface area of the hilum to which they branch. **B:** The magistral type. Note the long splenic trunk, the branching of the trunk very close to the hilum and many fewer branches going to a smaller surface area of the hilum.

The final significant relationship to note is that of the tail of the pancreas to the splenic hilum, both its actual location and whether or not it physically touches the hilum. The most common scenerio seen is the tail of the pancreas located at the midportion of the spleen at the hilum (in 50% of people), within 1 cm of the splenic surface (also in 50%) or actually lying against the spleen (in 33%). The other locations of the tail are near the inferior pole of the spleen (in 42%) or rarely near the superior pole of the spleen (in 8%).

▶ PREOPERATIVE PLANNING

Patients usually present to the surgeon with a diagnosis already made after having been worked up by their primary physician. A determination must then be made as to who is a surgical candidate and what further workup needs to be done; this is discussed at the end of this section. In selecting the patient for a laparoscopic approach, the surgeon must consider whether or not the patient falls into the appropriate category indicating surgery and whether or not the procedure can be safely accomplished. The three factors that make a laparoscopic approach hazardous and can be considered contraindicative are extreme splenomegaly, marked vascular adhesions to the parietal paritoneum, and a calcified splenic artery found on radiograph. These patients are much better served by an open splenectomy.

Any discussion of the indications for splenectomy apply to both open as well as laparoscopic splenectomy. The easiest way to discuss these indications is to break them down into three major categories: absolute indications, which are diseases that when diagnosed are best treated by surgical means as the first course of action; relative indications, which are disease conditions that become surgical candidates only when medical treatment fails or the physiologic stresses are such that surgery is indicated; and, finally, contraindications, which pertain to certain disease states that will not benefit from surgical intervention.

Absolute indications for splenectomy are few in number and can be categorized as traumatic splenic injuries, tumors, and abscesses of the spleen, and one specific hematologic disease, hereditary spherocytosis, which does not respond to medical therapy.

Relative indications are those conditions that cause symptomatic splenomegaly and can be broken down into two broad categories, primary hypersplenism and secondary hypersplenism. Hematologic diseases are the causes of primary hypersplenism, which is characterized by enlargement of the spleen due to sequestration of one or more blood cell types within the spleen, resulting in either destruction or a deficiency of that particular blood cell type. Secondary hypersplenism is caused by all disease processes, except those mentioned above, that cause severe physiologic consequences as a result of the splenomegaly induced by these diseases.

Primary hypersplenism is due to three categories of hematologic diseases: congenital hemolytic anemias, acquired hemolytic anemias, and thrombocytopenias. Congenital hemolytic anemias, which are autosomal dominant, result in early red blood cell (RBC) destruction due to a defective RBC membrane, an enzyme deficiency, or abnormal hemoglobin within the RBC. Gallstone formation induced by hemolysis of the RBC and formation of bilirubin stones within the gallbladder are accelerated by these diseases, and a preoperative ultrasound should always be done with a concomitant cholecystectomy scheduled at the time of splenectomy.

The hemolytic anemias that have defective RBC membranes are hereditary elliptocytosis (ovalocytosis) and hereditary stomatocytosis. The anemia due to a deficiency is pyruvate kinase deficiency and the anemias due to abnormal hemoglobins (Hb) are sickle cell anemia and thalassemia major (Cooley's anemia). In sickle cell anemia the normal HbA is replaced by HbS, which undergoes crystallization when subjected to decreased oxygen tension. In this disease, splenectomy is indicated only for sequestration crisis occurring in infants and small children. It is important to avoid splenectomy in children under 5 years old whenever possible, since over time repeated stasis will eventually cause splenic infarction leading to autosplenectomy. Thalassemia major is the persistence of fetal hemoglobin (HbF), with a concomitant reduction of the HbA levels, resulting in severe hemolytic anemia.

The acquired hemolytic anemias that may necessitate splenectomy are idiopathic autoimmune hemolytic anemia, which occurs when antibody and/or complement fix to the RBC membrane causing a decreased RBC survival, and Evans syndrome, which occurs when a hemolytic anemia is combined with either a thrombocytopenia or neutropenia.

Acquired thrombocytopenias that necessitate a splenectomy when medical treatment fails are idiopathic thrombocytopenic purpura (ITP), a variant of ITP seen in AIDS patients, and thrombotic thrombocytopenic purpura (TTP).

ITP occurs when antiplatelet antibodies, specifically immunoglobulin G (IgG), produced by the spleen results in splenic sequestration and destruction of platelets.

The two forms of ITP are acute and chronic. Acute ITP has a rapid, fulminant onset and occurs in children 2–5 years old. It is usually a self-limiting disease with spontaneous remission occurring in 90% of children within 6 months. Intravenous gamma-globulin is the treatment of choice for acute ITP, and steroids, the treatment of choice for chronic ITP, are ineffective when used for the acute form. Plasma exchange is much more effective for acute ITP than for the chronic form. Emergency splenectomy is indicated only for life-threatening hemorrhage.

Chronic ITP differs from acute ITP in that it occurs in an older age range, 20–40 years, spontaneous remission is rare, it is two or three times more common in women, and it is the most common cause of isolated thrombocytopenia. The management protocol involves three sequential lines of treatment. Steroids are the first and primary form of treatment and are very effective in inducing remission of bleeding and raising the platelet count. Splenectomy is the second treatment used and is indicated only if the steroids fail to produce a remission, if the patient relapses while on steroids or if high doses of steroids are required to maintain the platelet count. The relapse rate after a splenectomy is 10% and is often due to accessory spleens, which may be found in 30% of the cases. Thus it is important to look for and remove any accessory spleens during the initial splenectomy. The third line of treatment is immunosuppressive agents, which is indicated if a splenectomy is contraindicated or the patient fails to respond to a splenectomy. In this group, vincristine is the most effective drug. Other immunosuppressive drugs that can be used are azathioprine, cyclophosphamide, and danazol.

Mention should be made of AIDS patients who can present with chronic ITP. It is considered a variant of chronic ITP, since 90% of patients fail to respond to steroids, which means that 90% of these patients are candidates for the second line of treatment, splenectomy. There has been controversy about subjecting these immunocompromised patients to a procedure that theoretically can induce further immunocompromise.

TTP is a subendothelial hyalinization of arterioles with platelet trapping that causes occlusion of the arteriole as well as thrombocytopenia. Patients present with a classic pentad that includes fever, thrombocytopenic purpura, hemolytic anemia, neurologic disturbances, and renal failure. The initial therapy is plasmapheresis with fresh frozen plasma to remove von Willebrand factor, which is considered to be the causative agent inducing platelet aggregation. The majority of clinicians will also add steroids and dextran 70 as part of the treatment protocol. Splenectomy is indicated if the patient fails to respond to these treatments.

Secondary hypersplenism is the second major category of relative indications for splenectomy. The physiologic sequelae induced by the hypersplenism cause a domino effect, resulting in a vicious cycle such that one problem induces a second compensatory physiologic sequence that results in a third response that reinforces and further induces the first response. The result is hypermetabolism, increased cardiac output leading to high-output cardiac failure, portal hypertension, dilutional anemia, and decreased renal perfusion causing renal failure. The indications for splenectomy in this situation are fourfold:

1. Anemia, thrombocytopenia, or granulocytopenia supervene.
2. Physiologic mechanisms cause severe hypermetabolism or high-output cardiac failure.
3. The grossly enlarged spleen causes mechanical compression of the stomach or induces recurrent painful splenic infarcts.
4. Bleeding esophageal or gastric varices secondary to splenic vein thrombosis intervene.

The disease categories that result in secondary hypersplenism are also fourfold: splenic vein thrombosis, most commonly due to pancreatitis, may present with (i) bleeding esophageal varices, (ii) neoplasms, (iii) splenic cysts, and (iv) a miscellaneous category.

Neoplastic diseases that involve the spleen and require a splenectomy if the above indications are met include hairy cell leukemia, chronic lymphocytic leukemia (CLL), non-Hodgkin's lymphoma, Hodgkin's lymphoma, and agnogenic myeloid metaplasia. In the management of Hodgkin's lymphoma, a staging laparotomy may be necessary. This includes not only a splenectomy but also a 2-cm wedge biopsy of the left lobe of the liver with needle biopsies of both liver lobes and lymph node sampling at the following locations: splenic and liver hila, including cystic duct and common bile duct nodes; celiac axis; and paraaortic, mesenteric, mesocolic, and iliac lymph nodes. The procedure is completed with an iliac crest biopsy and oophoropexy in premenopausal women. In agnogenic myeloid metaplasia, progressive fibrosis and sclerosis of the bone marrow and extramedullary hematopoiesis cause splenomegaly.

Splenic cysts larger than 10 cm in diameter are at high risk for rupturing and resultant massive bleeding. The most common type of cyst is the pseudocyst, comprising 50–70% of splenic cysts. These occur as a response to prior splenic injury. The other two types of cysts are parasitic, most commonly echinococcal, and nonparasitic cysts.

Miscellaneous diseases that may induce splenomegaly include Felty syndrome, which is composed of a triad of rheumatoid arthritis, splenomegaly, and neutropenia. The three indications for splenectomy in this disease are serious or refractory infections despite the white cell count, intractable leg ulcers, and hemolytic anemia that is refractory to transfusions. Infiltrative diseases that fall into this category are amyloidosis, sarcoidosis, and Gaucher's disease. The final miscellaneous disease is porphyria erythropoietica, which is a congenital disorder of RBC pyrrole metabolism, resulting in premature destruction of the RBC in the spleen. Once again, these diseases are relative indications for splenectomy if they induce secondary hypersplenism.

Splenectomy is contraindicated if this surgery is not necessary to control the primary disease or, if done, will not result in cure or improvement of the disease process. This category includes glucose 6-phosphate dehydrogenase deficiency, thalassemia minor, chronic myelogenous leukemia (CML), chronic granulocytic leukemia (CGL), and portal hypertension.

Once it has been decided to do an elective splenectomy, special preoperative measures should include intramuscular pneumovacuum for all patients as well as having adequate amounts of platelets and blood components available for surgery. Preoperative workup varies based on the presenting diagnosis. CT scan of the abdomen is useful for evaluating splenic cysts, tumors, or abscesses; in determining the extent of splenic trauma; and in delineating accessory spleens. An ultrasound can be done to rule out cholelithiasis when indicated. Finally, as discussed later, an aortogram with selective splenic artery embolization immediately before surgery can also be done.

▼ INTRAOPERATIVE MANAGEMENT/SURGICAL TECHNIQUE

Three special instruments are required for the operation: an extracorporeal knotting device, such as the Gazayerli Knot Pusher (V. Mueller Inc., Chicago, IL) (Fig. 3); a linear vascular stapler; and, lastly, a 30- to 45-degree or full-flexing laparoscope, which, though not essential, greatly facilitates the procedure. The different angle of viewing provided by a 45-degree scope allows for excellent visualization of the hilum, the upper and lower poles of the spleen, and any attachments to them.

Also not essential, but adding to the safety of the procedure and level of the surgeon's comfort during the procedure, is a radiology department capable of selective embolization of the splenic artery. The help of the radiology department has been sought in the preoperative embolization of the splenic artery in 6 of our

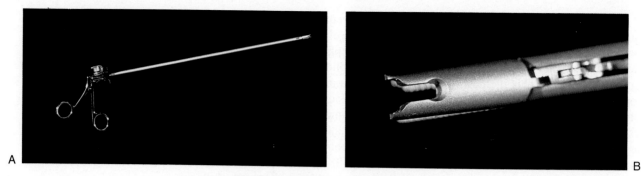

Figure 3. A, B: Gazayerli Knot Pusher.

42 splenectomies to date. This was carried out by means of coils (Figs. 4 and 5) in five cases and by a detachable balloon in one case. Such a measure eliminates the need to open the lesser sac and ligate the splenic artery in continuity as an early step of the operation. It has been criticized as an added expense but is well worth it in that patient safety is maintained, especially during the early learning curve of the surgeon as he or she gains experience with the procedure. Our recommendation is that, while the surgeon is learning the procedure, for the first few cases, preoperative embolization be performed. It is also a useful adjunct for the more experienced surgeon in dealing with a grossly enlarged spleen to both ensure patient safety and to allow the patient to become a candidate for a laparoscopic approach.

If splenic artery embolization is done, it is essential to take the patient directly from the radiology department to the operating room. When the splenic artery is embolized, the spleen is infarcted and must be removed as soon as possible. Although it sounds superfluous to stress that, it has come to our attention that in at least one patient the splenectomy was carried out the day following radiographic embolization. The patient was highly uncomfortable during this time delay, and at surgery it was reported that the spleen was dusky and friable.

The patient is positioned supine with the option of tilting the patient's left side partially; however, Delaitre, who described the first splenectomy in the French literature, has published a report on a modified position wherein the patient is placed in a right lateral position by means of an inflatable bean bag placed under the patient's left side. He calls this the hanged spleen position, and it is similar

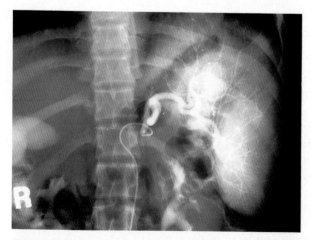

Figure 4. Splenic artery embolization. Selective arteriogram showing coils and thrombosed contrast material in the splenic artery. Note the compressed gastric air bubble.

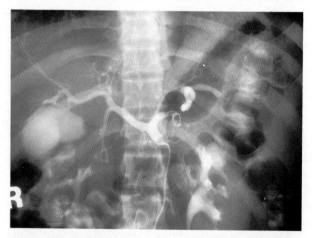

Figure 5. A second injection showing no flow through the thrombosed splenic artery. Note that the gastric air bubble has now expanded as the spleen begins to shrink in size.

to the position adopted for a nephrectomy. This may be helpful in a small spleen, but it is not recommended for enlarged spleens. Also, we have attempted three cases with the patient placed laterally in "the posterior approach" of Michel Gagner but do not feel that it is as comfortable as the traditional approach we are describing.

As far as port placement is concerned, if only a splenectomy is to be done, four or five ports are usually used. For clarity, these ports can be named epigastric, umbilical, pararectus, anterior axillary, and subcostal. Three 10- to 11-mm ports and one 11- to 12-mm port are placed, as much as possible, forming an arc, with the center of the arc located at the splenic hilum. Flexibility is essential, so the site of the three 10- to 11-mm ports varies slightly, depending on the body habitus. If the distance between the xiphoid and the umbilicus allows a port to be placed between them without hampering instrument movement, then the configuration in Fig. 6 would be used and can be referred to as the standard port placements. As seen in the illustration, the first port (epigastric) is placed just below the xiphoid, the second port (umbilical) at the level of the umbilicus, either above or below depending on the body habitus, and the third (pararectus) midway between them but positioned laterally just to the right of the right rectus muscle. An alternate placement pattern that deviates from the standard port placements is a variation in the placement of the pararectus port. Instead of placing it laterally to the right of the right rectus muscle, it may be placed in the linea alba midway between the epigastric and umbilical ports. The fourth port (anterior axillary), which is usually 12 mm, completes the arc and is placed in the left anterior axillary line. If further assistance is needed during the dissection, a fifth port (subcostal), often 5 mm, can be placed at the left costal margin and used for retraction instruments.

If a cholecystectomy is to be done simultaneously, it should be carried out first utilizing the traditional cholescystectomy port locations. Both the epigastric and umbilical ports placed for the cholecystectomy will be in the necessary operating arc for the splenectomy. The midclavicular port that has already been placed can be used for either posterior traction on the hilar structures by means of a fan retractor or for inferomedial traction on the greater curvature of the stomach by

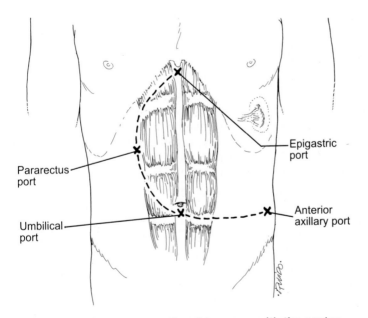

Figure 6. The ports are placed in an arc with the center of the arc at the splenic hilum. The minimum distance between each port should be the width of a hand.

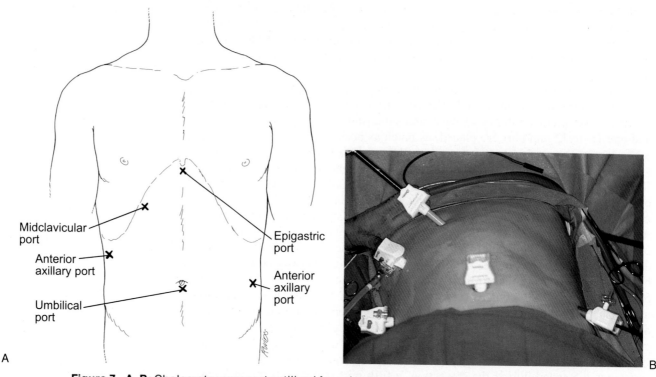

A   B

Figure 7. A, B: Cholecystecomy ports utilized for splenectomy. If a concomitant cholecystectomy is performed, an attempt is made to use the right midclavicular port for retraction. If a 5-mm port has been inserted initially, it will have to be replaced by a 10-mm port. A 12-mm right anterior axillary port is inserted after the cholecystectomy is completed. Ports from right to left: epigastric, midclavicular (pararectus), right anterior axillary, umbilical, and left anterior axillary.

means of a Babcock clamp. The fourth port, a 12-mm right anterior axillary port, is inserted after the cholecystectomy is completed (Fig. 7).

Through experience in using the ports with different instruments we offer the following port assignments as being the most comfortable way for the surgeon to do the necessary manipulations during the operation. However, flexibility is essential to meet the anatomic variations and respond to exposure needs such that, often during the procedure, the port usage will need to be changed around from the following suggestions.

The surgeon stands on the right side of the patient and uses the epigastric and umbilical ports for the left and right hands, respectively. The 45-degree laparoscope is introduced through the pararectus port. The camera operator stands preferably next to the surgeon, on the right side of the patient, to the right of the surgeon. The assistant, who stands on the patient's left side, will manipulate instruments through the left anterior axillary port and the optional subcostal port. The anterior axillary port will be used for lateral traction on the spleen during hilar dissection, by means of either an instrument or a fan retractor to provide countertraction, as well as passage of the linear vascular stapler to transect the hilar vessels. If extra traction is needed, such as in obese patients, a second pararectus port, as discussed above, can be placed and is handled by the camera person.

Before beginning the dissection an abdominal exploration is carried out, to inspect the abdominal contents and to look for accessory spleens that might or might not have been indicated by the preoperative computed tomography (CT) scan. Since 30% of patients will have accessory spleens, this step is critical to ensuring a successful outcome for the patient. If no preoperative embolization of the splenic artery has been done, the first step would be to enter the lesser sac and ligate the splenic artery in continuity at the upper border of the pancreas. It

reser (Figs. 11 and 12
these dividing the liga
incisi In our fourth st
tion above (Fig. 13).
incid relatively avascu
pleur need to be divid
be ur is to see the sple
ment task of removing
bord Placing the s
B it is not easy. S
tions enlarging one of
this t is needed—and s
unde is needed for a p
vein, spherocytosis po
causi suction tip into t
tion spillage. The suc
rectl it into the sac. O
instr out from a port s
T spleen is carried
impa and extraction is
large irrigation is carri
defec
be ha
near
last,
that t
can l
eithe
retra
T
in pa

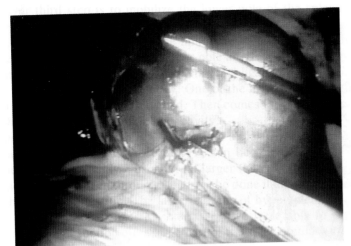

Figure 8. Dissection of short gastric vessels. An instrument or retractor is used to retract the spleen laterally. The short gastrics are being clipped then will be transected.

is advisable, for the first few cases of a surgeon's experience and when dealing with large spleens, to embolize the splenic artery and eliminate this step.

Our routine for the hilar dissection begins with exposing the hilum by first tackling the short gastric vessels below the hilum. The assistant starts by using the left anterior axillary port to retract the spleen laterally. The surgeon then dissects these vessels out, ligates or clips them individually, and finally transects the vessels (Fig. 8). This step results in good hilar exposure (Fig. 9). Our second step is to dissect the hilum. If a preoperative embolization has been carried out, the arteriogram will indicate the number of splenic vessels and their anatomic pattern, which is of great help in this part of the dissection. Once these vessels are dissected out they are ligated, preferably by extracorporeal knots (Fig. 10). The use of clips alone on the splenic vessels is hazardous because they can be easily dislodged during subsequent manipulation in the area. If preoperative embolization has been done, the splenic artery and vein can be ligated together. If embolization has not been done, the vessels must be ligated individually to prevent arteriovenous fistula formation. After ligation, the vessels are transected by a linear vascular stapling device introduced through the left anterior axillary port

The
arter
of th
disse
avoi

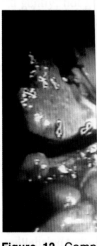

T
can l
vigo
avoi
clips
vide
may
irriga
be ca
stapl
is or

T
mal
sutu
splei

A
to th
men
but a
inju

Figure 12. Compl
splenic vessels are

Figure 13. Division
tric vessels above t

A

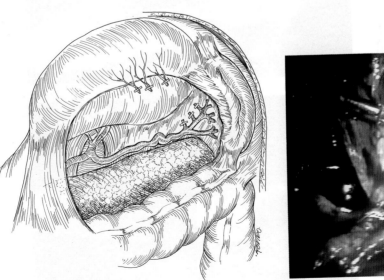

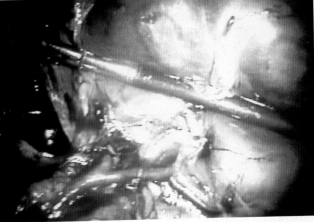

B

Figure 9. A, B: Splenic hilum. The splenic hilum is nicely exposed once the short gastrics are divided. The splenic artery is shown bifurcating into the substance of the spleen.

SURGICAL PEARLS

Do not attempt this procedure until you are comfortable with laparoscopic tying techniques learned via other laparoscopic procedures.

Preoperative embolization or early ligation in continuity of the splenic artery facilitates and increases the margin of safety of this procedure.

Preoperative embolization is recommended for the first few cases a surgeon does while on the learning curve and as an adjunct for grossly enlarged spleens.

If you embolize the splenic artery preoperatively take the patient to surgery immediately. You will have infarcted the spleen.

Utilization of surgical clips on the splenic artery is hazardous since they can be easily dislodged. Linear staplers or ligation is the preferred technique.

the clip or knot when the vessel retracts after it is divided. Similarly, dissection should be near but not on the colon wall.

Pancreatic injury remains a real potential complication with the laparoscopic approach as with any open approach. Once again, firm knowledge of the relationship of the tail of the pancreas to the spleen is essential. Direct visualization of the tail of the pancreas is often easier with the laparoscopic camera and aids in avoiding an injury. Most important of all is care during dissection of the splenic heilum. Structures located within the hilum and posterior to the hilum must be delineated before any use of cutting instruments, vascular staplers, cautery, and so on. Avoiding inserting instrument tips so that the tips cannot be seen at all times is a basic principle of any surgical procedure.

Splenosis from dissemination of fragments of spleen during extraction of the spleen can be avoided by placing the spleen within a sac and doing any further manipulations of the spleen, which may result in its disruption, within the sac.

Subphrenic abscess can be a real problem with the open approach. The literature is full of numerous articles discussing this complication, in particular the role of a drain placed in the splenic bed and its contribution to infection. However, the most important point is that fluid can collect from disrupted lymphatics due to blunt dissection of the tissues around the spleen. Once this fluid has collected it can then become infected. Short-term drainage (e.g., 24 hours) with a closed drainage system such as a Jackson-Pratt drain does not appear to increase the risk of infection and can be utilized if the surgeon has any concerns. In the laparoscopic approach the more precise dissection of pertinent structures under direct visualization and lack of widespread blunt posterior dissection should decrease the potential for fluid collections and their possible conversion to an abscess.

Wound problems that may occur include seroma, hematoma, infection, and herniation with or without small bowel obstruction. Since the incisions are small and the risk of gastrointestinal bacterial contamination is low there should be a much lower incidence of complications if adequate hemostasis within the port sites is obtained and if the fascia is closed appropriately. In obese patients or when exposure of the port site is difficult, the skin incision may be enlarged slightly to obtain hemostasis or to visualize the fascia better for its closure. Doing so will not increase the postoperative pain.

☑ CONCLUSIONS

Laparoscopic splenectomy provides several advantages over the open procedure. The dangers of subphrenic fluid collections that plague open splenectomy are eliminated. Recovery from surgery occurs more rapidly with less postoperative pain, a shorter hospital stay, and a quicker return to work.

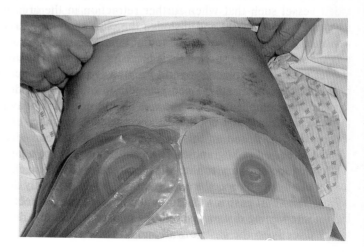

Figure 15. Patient with ileostomy (*right*) and colostomy (*left*) bags 36 hours after undergoing a laparoscopic splenectomy for idiopathic thrombocytopenic purpura.

Forty-two cases have been attempted. One case was converted to an open splenectomy because of bleeding from a calcified aneurysmal splenic artery as described above. Of the remaining 41 cases, 17 were familial spherocytosis, 21 were ITP, and 3 were schistosomiasis with hypersplenism. Splenic artery embolization was done in six cases, five with coils and one with a detachable balloon. These cases of embolization represent our learning curve.

One of the ITP patients posed a particular challenge. She had a total pelvic exenteration with a colostomy and ileal loop diversion. Her presenting platelet count was 26,000 while on steroid therapy. The splenectomy was successful despite the problems of a restricted abdominal cavity. She was discharged 36 hours after the surgery with a platelet count of 96,000 (Fig. 15).

RECOMMENDED READING

1. Akle CA, Wickham JEA, Gravett P, Dick R. Laparoscopic splenectomy [Correspondance]. *Br J Surg* 1993;80:126.
2. Cadiere GB, Delaitre B, Tulman S. Laparoscopic splenectomy: fifteen cases. *First European Congress of the European Association for Endoscopic Surgery.* Cologne, June 3, 1993;48 (abst).
3. Delaitre B, Maignien B. Splenectomie par voie coelioscopique: une observation. *Presse Med* 1991; 44:2263.
4. Delaitre B. Laparoscopic splenectomy: the "hanged spleen" technique. *Ann Chirurg* [*In press*].
5. Ferzoco SJ, Modlin IM. Splenic surgery. In: Ballantyne GH, Leahy PF, Modlin IM, eds. *Laparoscopic surgery.* Philadelphia: WB Saunders; 1994:154–164.
6. Flowers JL. Miscellaneous complications of laparoscopic surgery. In: Bailey RW, Flowers JL, eds. *Complications of laparoscopic surgery.* St Louis, MO: Quality Medical Publishing; 1995: 292–301.
7. Flowers JL. Laparoscopic splenectomy. In: Zucker KA, ed. *Surgical laparoscopy update.* St Louis, MO: Quality Medical Publishing; 1993:357–371.
8. Gazayerli MM, Hasan S, Richardson R. Laparoscopic splenectomy. *Gen Surg News* 1991;11:5.
9. Gazayerli MM. Splenectomy. *Laparosc Focus* 1991;1:2 p 1.
10. Gazayerli MM, Helmy HS, Hakki M, Spitz ML. Laparoscopic splenectomy. In: Rosen D, ed. *Minimal access general surgery.* Oxford, UK: Radcliff Medical Press; 1994:202–212.
11. Gazayerli MM, Spitz ML, Silbergleit A, Helmy HS. The spleen. In: Savalgi, Ellis, Rosser, eds. *Clinical anatomy for laparoscopic and thoracoscopic surgery.* Oxford, UK: Radcliff Medical Press, 1995.
12. Phillips EH. Laparoscopic Splenectomy. In: Hunter JG, Sackier JM, eds. *Minimally invasive surgery.* New York: McGraw-Hill; 1993:309–313.
13. Thibault C, Mamazza J, Letourneau R, Poulin E. Laparoscopic splenectomy. *Surg Laparosc Endosc* 1992;2:257–261.
14. Unger SW, Rosenbaum GJ. Laparoscopic splenectomy. In: Arregui MA, Fitzgibbons RJ, Katkhouda N, McKernan JB, Reich H, eds. *Principles of laparoscopic surgery basic and advanced techniques.* New York: Springer-Verlag; 1995:356–365.

SECTION VI

VERTEBRAL COLUMN

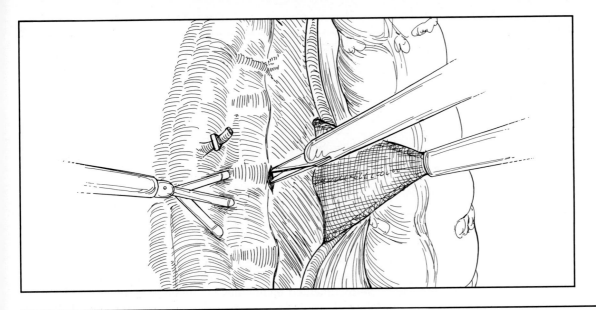

26

Spine Access Surgery

Lee L. Swanström
Department of Minimally Invasive Surgery
Oregon Health Sciences University
Portland, Oregon 97227

Operative Laparoscopy and Thoracoscopy, edited by B. V. MacFadyen, Jr. and J. L. Ponsky. Lippincott-Raven Publishers, Philadelphia © 1996.

KEY WORDS

Access

Fan retractors

Fixation plate

Fluoroscopy

Fusion

Gasless technique

Nucleatome

Scoliosis

Spinal foramina

General surgeons and spine surgeons have a long history of collaboration on the surgical treatment of diseases of the lumbar spine. While spine surgery is a very broad field with well-documented techniques involving percutaneous, posterior, anterior, and anterolateral procedures, many diseases of the spine and disk space lend themselves particularly well to anterior exposures (1). It was in the role of providing such exposure to spine surgeons that general surgeons have traditionally been involved (2). A great drawback to utilizing the anterior approach was the morbidity of the incisions required which delayed return to physical therapy, return to work, and had long-term complications of their own (3). This led to the avoidance of the anterior approach in all but highly selected cases and resulted in more difficult and sometimes less reliable posterior and percutaneous approaches being substituted for anterior surgery simply to avoid the morbidity of the access. The advent of minimally invasive surgery has caused a paradigm shift in the thinking of spine surgeons. With the avoidance of both wound morbidity and delayed recovery, spine surgeons are once again looking closely at which procedures are most efficacious when performed by an anterior approach. Because this field is new, long-term outcome studies are not available, and both the spine surgeon and the general surgeon providing access are feeling their way through uncharted territory. Indications for application, designs of new instruments, safety of exposure techniques, and the techniques themselves all remain to be worked out. Early experiences show that at least many traditional spine surgeries can be performed through minimal access, with only slight variation from the corresponding open procedure (4–7).

● ANATOMY

Diseases of the spine can be broadly categorized as follows:

1. Diseases of the spinal foramina, often due to either disk protuberance or hyperossification
2. Diseases of the vertebral body, which can be secondary to trauma, degenerative diseases, or tumors
3. Diseases of the disk space, which are either from disk rupture and protuberance or the poorly understood and extensive field of internal disk derangement
4. Problems with vertebral body alignment, which involve multiple segments often of both the thoracic and lumbar spine and are best characterized by childhood scoliosis

As may be expected, the treatment of each of these disease categories is radically different, but, generally, each involves disk removal, distraction of disk space, and often fusion or fixation. Some of these problems are best approached from the posterior direction, such as decompressing the nerve root foramina in foraminal stenosis or removal of posterior extruded solid disk fragments. Other problems require a combination of anterior and posterior exposure, such as scoliosis surgery and some complicated spinal fusion procedures. Still others can be approached either posteriorly or anteriorly, including routine disk surgery and fusions. Anterior exposures are complicated by the fact that the spine is a retroperitoneal structure in close proximity to important and easily traumatized structures such as the ureter, the aorta and its major branches, the vena cava, and the sympathetic nerve chain. Awareness of the location of and safe retraction of all these structures is a major element in safe laparoscopic exposure of the spine. Figure 1 illustrates the major vascular structures that the laparoscopic spine surgeon must identify, mobilize, and retract for exposure of the lumbar spine. Of particular concern is the infrarenal aorta and its lumbar segmental branches, which further branches into the left and right common iliac arteries. The L5, S1 exposures frequently require division or retraction of the median sacral vein and artery. The first branch of the common iliac vein, the iliolumbar vein, and the ascending lumbar vein are probably the most frequent cause of bleeding in lower lumbar exposures. These tether the common iliac vein, are often hidden by retroperitoneal fat, and are easily torn. For dissections of L4 and L5 in particular the iliolumbar vein should be identified early and securely controlled. Because of the anatomic position of the segmental lumbar veins, these vessels seldom need to be divided except for multilevel radical exposures. The lumbar vein and arteries cross the midbody of each vertebral segment and therefore are away from the disk, which is the area of dissection. Adequate aortic mobilization, on the other hand, frequently requires division of its lumbar branches. The aorta, which frequently lies directly over or slightly to the left of the vertebral column must be mobilized and retracted to the patient's right for all procedures other than L5, S1 diskectomies, which lie well below the bifurcation of the aorta. The left iliac artery is retracted for exposure of L4, S5 and several small unnamed branches exit from the posterior surface. The ileal lumbar artery is sometimes necessary to divide to allow full retraction of

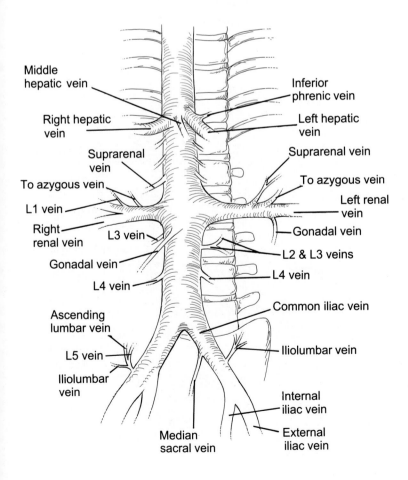

Figure 1. Relationship of major vascular structures to the lumbar spine.

the iliac artery. Other important retroperitoneal structures include the sympathetic trunk (Fig. 2), which lies atop the psoas muscle adjacent to the vertebral column, the gonadal vessels and ureter, which also lie atop the psoas muscle slightly further lateral. The left kidney, pancreas, and spleen lie immediately adjacent to T12, L1, and L2, and for access to this portion of the lumbar spine, these organs must be

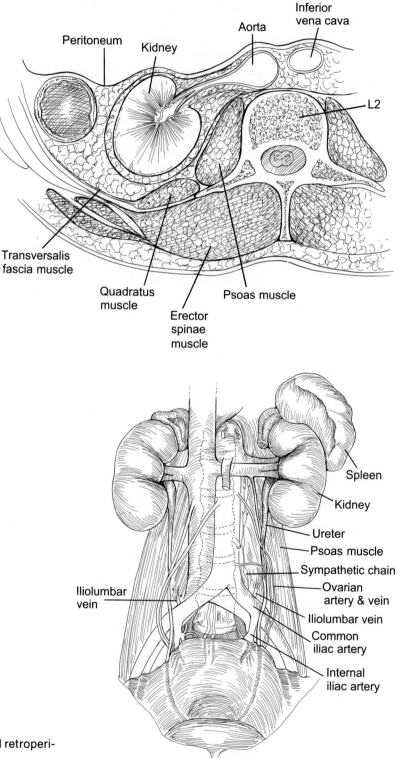

Figure 2. Retroperitoneal anatomy demonstrating the relative position of the iliac, aorta and lumbar arteries, the vena cava and its major and minor tributaries, and the psoas muscle.

Figure 3. Anterior view of the lumbar spine and retroperitoneal and vascular structures.

reflected anteriorly and medially (Fig. 3). The anatomy of the anterior lumbar spine itself includes somewhat depressed vertebral bodies, lateral spinous processes, and an intravertebral disk. The disk usually protrudes anteriorly compared to the vertebral bodies. The tough, shiny anterior spinous ligament overlies the anterior portion of the lumbar spine and is easily identified laparoscopically, while the ileal psoas and obturator muscles attach to the lumbar spinous processes. The spinal canal lies directly behind the bony vertebral column, and care should be taken to avoid breaking through the posterior disk annulus and into the spinal canal.

▶ PREOPERATIVE PLANNING

Proper patient selection for laparoscopic spine surgery presents a dilemma. The average spine surgeon is not well acquainted with the indications, restrictions, or contraindications of laparoscopic surgery. Conversely, the laparoscopic surgeon is, for the most part, unfamiliar with the proper indications, patient selection criteria, or the appropriate technique of spine surgery required. This creates a situation where the two surgeons must truly act as a team, not only during the surgery, but during the patient selection process and postoperative care as well. There are three main issues to consider with regard to appropriate patient selection. (1) Is the patient an appropriate spine surgery candidate and, if so, what is the appropriate technique? (2) Is the patient an appropriate laparoscopy candidate? (3) What is the appropriate laparoscopic access (e.g., transabdominal supine, medial visceral rotation, retroperitoneal, or lateral decubitus)? Obviously, the type of spine surgery will determine the type of access that is needed, and the laparoscopic surgeon's selection of patient position and access mode will influence the ability of the spine surgeon to do his part of the procedure. These patients must be thoroughly evaluated for their spine disease, which usually includes imaging studies—plain radiographs, computed tomography scans, or magnetic resonance imaging—and mylograms or provocative testing such as a diskogram. In addition, the laparoscopic surgeon must know his spine surgery partner well, as he relies on his knowledge to be sure that this patient needs spine surgery in the first place, anterior spine surgery in the second place, and exactly which spine procedure is necessary. The ultimate goal should be to perform the same surgery laparoscopically that would have been done in open surgery. Any obvious variations from this pattern, whether from patient positioning, angle of access, or different spine technique, should be performed under controlled, rigorous conditions, preferably with an IRB approval and a structured patient consent form. It must also be taken into account that this is a new and evolving field with no definitive answers.

In general, the anterior approach to the spine is indicated for the following surgical procedures: a thorough, complete diskectomy (e.g., ''internal disk derangements''), a fusion where the posterior elements are stable, severe traumatic fractures with resulting spinal cord compromise, reconstruction after vertebral corpectomy—as in tumor resections for partial diskectomies, central disk protrusions, as a last resort for multiple failed posterior fusions, and to mobilize and straighten the spine in scoliosis. Contraindications to the anterior approach are spinal cord compromise secondary to large extruded disk or vertebral fragments and dorsal nerve root compression secondary to foraminal stenoses. The contraindications for the laparoscopic part of the operation are standard for laparoscopy and include pregnancy, multiple adhesions (unless performing retroperitoneal laparoscopy), previous retroperitoneal spine surgery, and contraindications to general anesthesia. Our current treatment strategies and laparoscopic approaches for various diseases are listed in Table 1.

Table 1. *Treatment and laparoscopic techniques in lumbar spine disorder*

Diagnosis	Procedure	Laparoscopic approach
Isolated disk disease with central disk herniation (no fragments)	Nucleatome diskectomy	Transabdominal anterior
Internal disk derangement	Total diskectomy and fusion	Transabdominal anterior (L4/5, L5, S1) or lateral decubitus retroperitoneal (L1/2 to L4/5)
Vertebral instability secondary to degenerative disk disease	Fusion with interbody cages or bone graft and plating (Z plates)	Transabdominal anterior or lateral decubitus retroperitoneal
Traumatic vertebral fractures	Corpectomy and bone graft and anterolateral plating (Z plates)	Lateral decubitus retroperitoneal or medial visceral rotation
Scoliosis	Multidisk excision and bone grafting	Medial visceral rotation

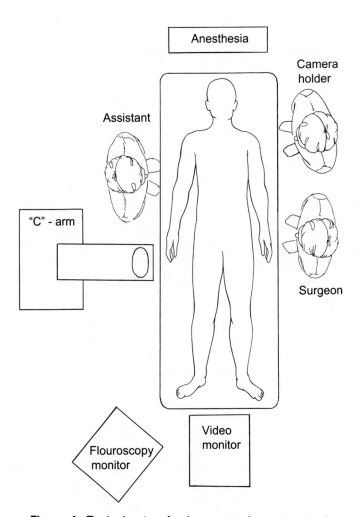

Figure 4. Typical setup for laparoscopic access to the mid and lower lumber spine.

▼ INTRAOPERATIVE MANAGEMENT/SURGICAL TECHNIQUE

Supine/Transabdominal Access

The supine/transabdominal access is indicated for simple nucleatome diskectomies at all levels, is required for placement of titanium cages at any level, and is the best access for any procedure on L5, S1. This approach can also be used for total diskectomies and fusions, although we find this to be less useful because of the need to continuously reflect the bowel out of the way and the need to retract the great vessels further to provide access.

Room Setup

The room setup for transabdominal access of the mid to lower lumbar spine is illustrated in Fig. 4. A single monitor is placed directly at the end of the bed. The patient is placed carefully in a true supine position with no rotation. The fluoroscopy monitor is placed at the end of the table where it is easily visible by both the neurosurgeon and laparoscopist. It is important to place the patient on an operating table that is fluoroscopy compatible; this often requires turning the standard operating table end for end. Typically five trocars are used (Fig. 5). The camera is placed in the subxiphoid midline position. After standard insufflation and introduction of the first trocar, the patient is placed in the Trendelenburg position to allow the small bowel to shift out of the way. Additional trocars are placed, including one in the right midquadrant and one in the left midquadrant. With sufficient Trendelenburg in the majority of cases, gravity will retract the small bowel out of the field. The right-sided port can then be used to retract the

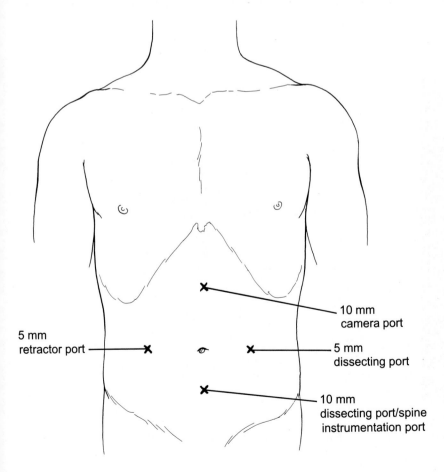

5 mm
retractor port

10 mm
camera port

5 mm
dissecting port

10 mm
dissecting port/spine
instrumentation port

Figure 5. Trocar position for lower lumbar access.

sigmoid colon laterally, exposing the root of the sigmoid mesentery. An additional trocar is inserted in the midline lower abdomen in the position directly over the disk to be operated on. The surgeon then looks for the appropriate landmarks and uses fluoroscopy to identify the area of peritoneum overlying the appropriate disk space (Fig. 6). Once this is confirmed an incision is made in the retroperitoneum ranging from 6 cm for a total diskectomy and fusion procedure to 1.5 to 2 cm for a partial diskectomy or nucleatome diskectomy. Dissection is initiated to the left of the major vessels, which is a relatively safe area (Fig. 7). Usually the psoas muscle is encountered first, and dissection can then be shifted medially until the anterior lateral portion of the spine is found. Meticulous hemostasis is necessary in this vascular tissue to keep the field clear. Dissection is best performed with a combination of blunt and sharp dissection. The surgeon usually holds a suction irrigator in the left hand to bluntly dissect the tissues and aspirate blood and lymph from the field. In the right hand, either a bipolar coagulating scissor (Everest Medical, Minneapolis, MN) or ultrasonic coagulating shear is used. Either ultrasonic coagulator or bipolar energy is safest in this area to prevent inadvertent burns to the aorta, stimulation of the psoas muscle, or injury to the sympathetic nerve chain. At this time fluoroscopy is often helpful to determine the direction of further dissection. Disk spaces tend to protrude above the level of the vertebral body, and it is wise to confine the dissection to the disk space if at all possible, as this is relatively avascular. Lumbar veins and arteries cross over the midportion of the vertebral bodies as illustrated in Fig. 8. For single level exposures not requiring total diskectomies, it is usually unnecessary to divide lumbar vessels. At L5, S1 the middle sacral artery frequently crosses the midportion of the disk space and must be sacrificed. If the sacral artery or lumbar are to be sacrificed, vessels, they should be securely hemoclipped before division or divided with ultrasonic coagulating shears (LCS™, Ultracision, Smithfield, RI) to ensure that they will not bleed and obscure the field. Once the confirmed disk space is identified,

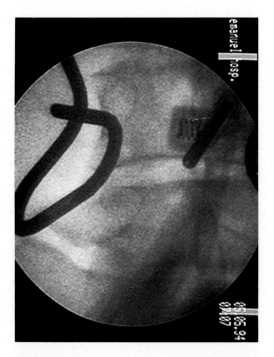

Figure 6. Fluoroscopy should be used liberally to maintain orientation in the retroperitoneum.

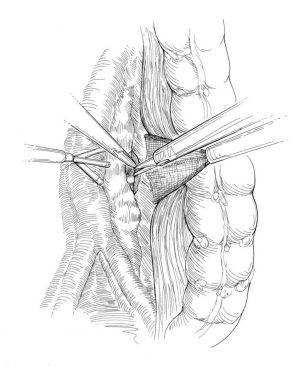

Figure 7. Blunt and sharp dissection is initiated to the left of the major vessels.

the vessels and areolar lymphatic tissue can be swept off the spine from left to right, staying in the prevertebral fascia plane (Fig. 9). Gradually the aorta, iliac artery, and iliac vein are gently swept past the midline of the spine, creating an exposure that is adequate for simple diskectomies (Fig. 10). Full exposure of the anterior spine for spinal fusion procedures will require further mobilization of the vessels, including dissection of the iliac artery and vein down to the level of the ureter. Early division of the iliolumbar vein, which is frequently torn by overvigorous retraction should be considered. A variable number of lumbar veins and arter-

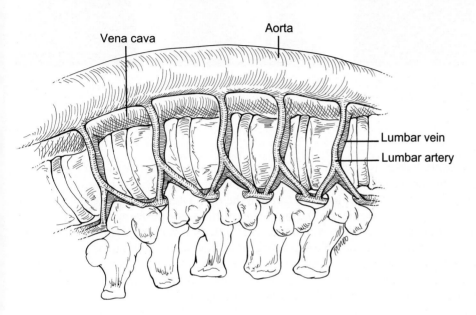

Figure 8. Segmental lumbar vessels cross the midportion of each vertebral body.

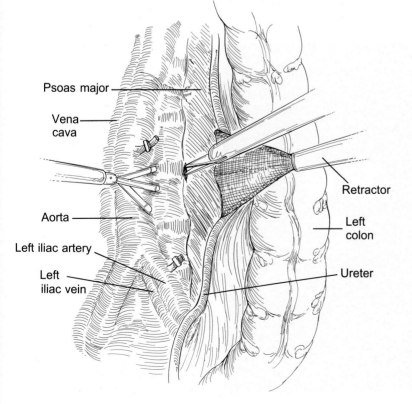

Figure 9. The aorta is progressively retracted to the right, often requiring division of several aortic branches. This exposes the anterior lumbar spine.

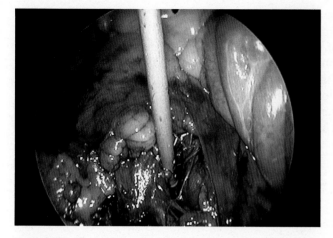

Figure 10. The retroperitoneal incision allows the left anterolateral spine to be exposed by retracting the aorta to the right.

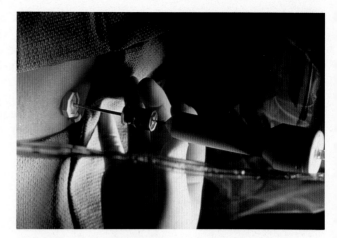

Figure 11. Automated nucleatome during activation after laparoscopic placement in the lumbar disk space.

ies can be taken as well to provide full mobilization of the vena cava and aorta. To maintain vessel retraction and disk exposure, we use a fan-type retractor (U.S. Surgical, Norwalk, CT) inserted through the right lateral port, placed beneath the great vessels and locked on the right side of the spine allowing the vessels to be rolled fully across the anterior spine. This retractor must be as broad as possible and very atraumatic to avoid lacerating or traumatically kinking the aorta or iliac vessels. The use of Steinmann pins is to be avoided, as these create a kinking of the vessels, which can lead to thrombosis. Diskectomy can then be performed by either placing a nucleatome trephine (Surgical Dynamics) through the anterior annulus or by incising a window in the anterior annulus with specially designed spine surgery instruments (Sofamor Danek, Memphis, TN) that can fit through a trocar placed exactly over the indicated disk space (Fig. 11). Careful laparoscopic

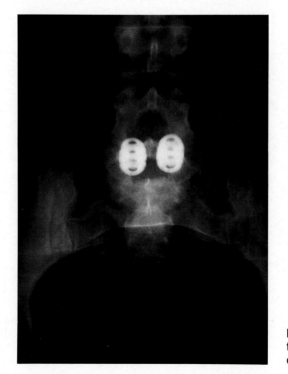

Figure 12. Anterior radiograph of titanium fusion cages placed laparoscopically at L5, S1.

visualization must be maintained at all times to prevent veins or arteries from slipping into the path of incoming diskectomy instruments. For this reason the laparoscopic surgeon should remain present in the operating room to ensure appropriate protection and retraction of the vessels. Once the diskectomy is complete and fusion devices (Fig. 12) or bone have been placed to the spine surgeon's satisfaction, the vessels can be allowed to relax back to their normal anatomic position. The incised retroperitoneum can be checked for hemostasis and irrigated as needed. The retroperitoneum is allowed to fall back closed without formal closure unless oozing is noted from the edges, in which case a simple running Vicryl suture can be used for hemostasis. The 10-mm trocar sites should be closed with full-thickness fascial closures to prevent postoperative herniation.

Anterior/Lateral Exposure

Anterior/lateral exposure by way of medial visceral rotation is indicated for multilevel disk procedures and exposure of the upper lumbar disk spaces from T12/L1–L2–3. Even with medial visceral rotation access to the upper lumbar spine is occasionally difficult. These cases are often better approached through a retroperitoneal approach. Patients are placed once again on a fluoroscopy table in full supine position. Five trocars are used. With this procedure, a dual laparoscopic monitor should be used at the head of the table and a fluoroscopy monitor placed so the surgeon can easily see it (Fig. 13). After insufflation of the abdomen with

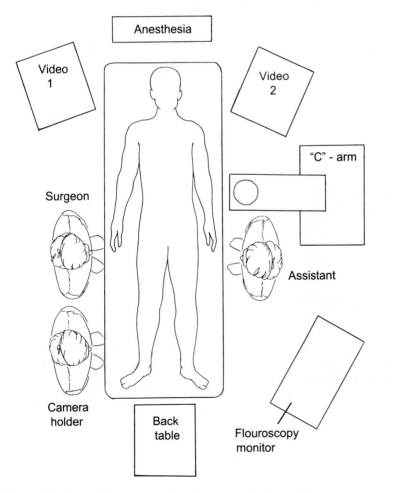

Figure 13. Operating room setup for upper lumbar spine exposures.

Medsystems, Menlo Park, CA) is placed through the left upper quadrant trocar site, and a small transverse muscle splitting incision is made in the left midquadrant to allow fracture reduction and insertion of anterior/lateral spine fixation plates (Z plate, Danek) (Fig. 18). One of the drawbacks to this approach is the difficulty in maintaining exposure by reflection of the large and small bowel. This is especially difficult in obese people. In these instances, it is often preferable to use a total extra peritoneal/retroperitoneal access approach.

Retroperitoneal Access

For multiple disk spaces, treatment of scoliosis, or vertebral body plating, the retroperitoneal approach is often preferable because it provides reliable, safe access to the anterior/lateral spine. Since these patients are positioned in the lateral decubitus position, this technique provides some restriction on the access for the spine surgeons and should only be undertaken with their awareness and consent. The patient is positioned on the operating table on a bean bag support in the right lateral decubitus position. The left arm should be placed on a support and positioned similar to a thoracotomy (Fig. 19). Arms and legs and axilla should be appropriately cushioned to prevent pressure injury or neuropraxia. It is very helpful to place the patient over the break in the table and before deflating the bean bag to break the table to open up the area between the rib cage and iliac crest. We start in the midposterior axillary line with a Visyport trocar (U.S. Surgical, Norwalk, CT) to permit access into the retroperitoneal fat. Once the fat has been identified, a retroperitoneal expansion balloon (Origin Medsystems, Menlo Park, CA) is then inserted and, under direct vision, insufflated for 1.2 L. Often during this balloon expansion the lateral spine can be identified. The balloon is then withdrawn and a Hasson trocar placed in its place, and insufflation of the retroperitoneum with a maximum pressure of 12 mmHg is instituted. Additional trocars, as illustrated in Fig. 20, can then be placed under direct vision and further dissection of the retroperitoneum can be performed as needed. Usual identification of the psoas muscle is noted first. Care must be taken not to disrupt the sympathetic chain, which lies along the medial aspect of the psoas muscle. The lateral vertebral body is identified and, using lateral fluoroscopy, the appropriate disk space is identified as well.

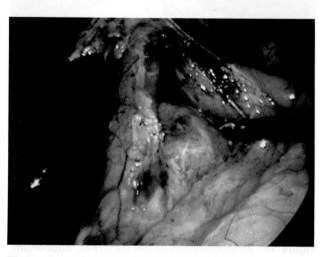

Figure 17. Access to T12, L1 is obtained by opening the esophageal hiatus to the right of the gastroesophageal junction, exposing the anterior spine for a nucleatome diskectomy.

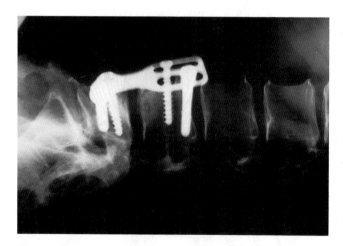

Figure 18. Laparoscopically placed spinal fixation plate between L4 and L5.

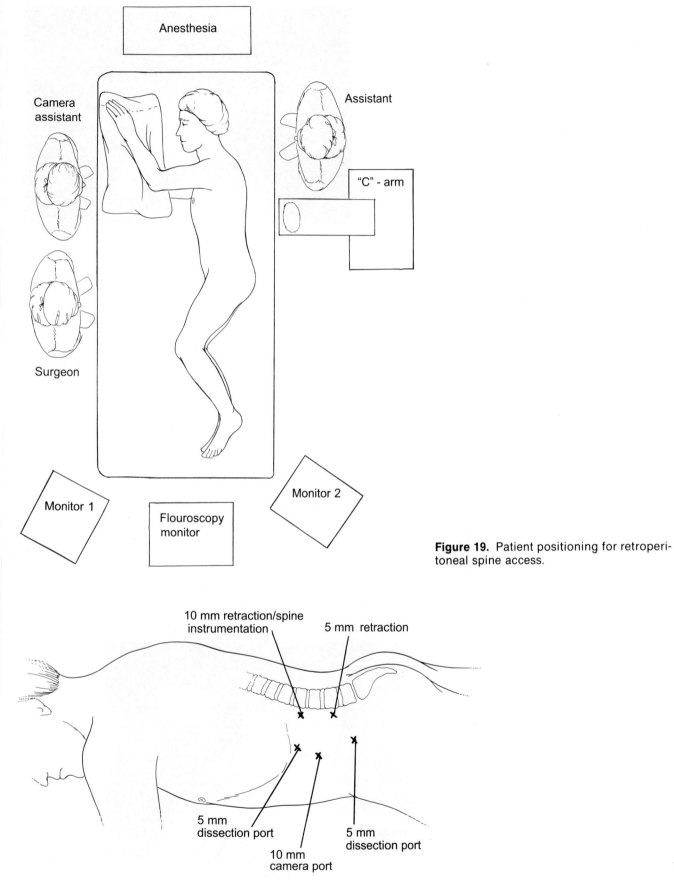

Figure 19. Patient positioning for retroperitoneal spine access.

Figure 20. Trocar placement.

superiorly, the lumbodorsal fascia laterally, and the internal oblique muscle inferiorly; the tip of the 12th rib lies at the apex of the triangle (Fig. 2). The inferior lumbar triangle is bounded by the latissimus dorsi muscle posteriorly, the external oblique muscle anteriorly, and the iliac crest inferiorly (Fig. 3); the floor of the triangle is formed by the internal oblique muscle.

The anatomic relations of the right kidney include the liver overlying the superior aspect of the anterior surface and the duodenum lying anteromedially, adja-

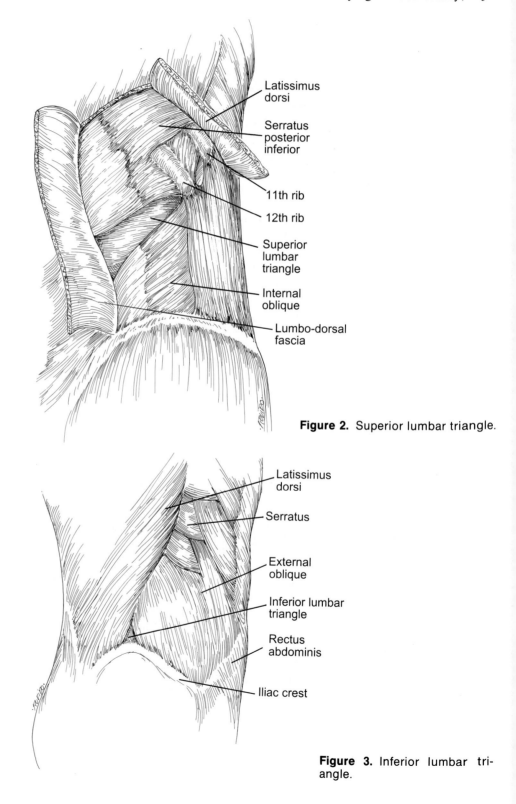

Latissimus
dorsi

Serratus
posterior
inferior

11th rib

12th rib

Superior
lumbar
triangle

Internal
oblique

Lumbo-dorsal
fascia

Figure 2. Superior lumbar triangle.

Latissimus
dorsi

Serratus

External
oblique

Inferior lumbar
triangle

Rectus
abdominis

Iliac crest

Figure 3. Inferior lumbar triangle.

cent to the renal hilum. The adrenal gland lies on the medial aspect of the upper pole of the right kidney. The posterior coronary ligament of the liver is reflected onto the right kidney and adrenal gland; as such, the triangular ligament of the liver, where the anterior and posterior layers of the coronary ligament meet, must be incised to the level of the diaphragm in order to reflect the liver medially and expose the superior border of Gerota'a fascia within which lies the adrenal gland. The hepatic flexure of the colon crosses anterior to the lower half of the kidney.

On the left, the spleen overlies the lateral aspect of the upper pole of the kidney; the adrenal gland lies directly on the anterior, medial area of the upper pole of the left kidney. The splenic flexure of the colon overlies the anterior lateral surface of the lower pole of the kidney. From a transperitoneal approach to the left kidney, the attachments of the spleen to the kidney (i.e., lienorenal ligament) and of the colon to the sidewall (phrenicolic ligament) must be incised in order to safely reflect the colon medially, thereby exposing the kidney. The body of the stomach lies anterior to the kidney; the body and tail of the pancreas sit anterior and medial to the upper pole of the kidney.

The vascular supply of the kidney is via a single renal artery originating from the lateral aspect of the aorta below the superior mesenteric artery. Multiple renal arteries are present in approximately 20% of the population. On the right, the renal artery passes behind the vena cava before entering the renal hilum where it branches to supply the five vascular segments of the kidney; on the left, the renal artery exits the aorta laterally and enters directly into the renal hilum. The right and left renal vein enter the vena cava laterally. The left renal vein is longer than the right and passes anterior to the aorta en route to the vena cava. The adrenal, gonadal, and ascending lumbar veins enter the left renal vein superiorly, inferiorly, and posteriorly, respectively. The right renal vein usually has no tributaries; likewise, the short right adrenal and gonadal veins enter the vena cava directly, posteriorly, and anteriorly, respectively.

Ureter

The upper ureter lies within the perirenal space, overlying the medial border of the psoas major muscle. As it courses toward the bladder, it passes under the gonadal vessels then over the distal half of the common iliac vessels. In the pelvis, the ureter dives medially, passing under the ductus deferens or round ligament and just medial to the medial umbilical ligament before entering the bladder wall.

Adrenal Gland

The right adrenal gland is triangular in shape and lies immediately lateral to the vena cava and posterior to the liver. The single right adrenal vein is short and empties directly into the posterior aspect of the vena cava. The left adrenal gland is flatter and lies on the anteromedial surface of the kidney, with the stomach located anteriorly and the spleen superiorly and laterally. The left adrenal vein is longer than the right and runs vertically to drain into the left renal vein. On either side, the arterial supply of the adrenal gland arises from branches of the inferior phrenic artery (superior adrenal artery), aorta (middle adrenal artery), and renal artery (inferior adrenal artery).

▶ PREOPERATIVE PLANNING

Patient Selection

As the instrumentation and experience of laparoscopic surgeons improve, the indications for a laparoscopic approach to kidney removal in the adult are rapidly

Table 2. *Laparoscopic nephrectomy*

Author (Ref.)	Attempted	Completed	Age (y)	OR time (h)	EBL (ml)
Rassweilwer (19)	6 (36)[a]	—	—	3–4	—
Coptcoat (27)	5 (27)[a]	—	—	4.5	—
Terachi (20)	5 (13)[a]	—	—	7.4	243
Kato (21)	5	5	—	6.4	430
Clayman	9	9	71 (29–90)	7.7 (7–9)	229 (50–600)
Total:	30	91%	—	Average: 6.1	286

[a] Number in parentheses indicates total number of nephrectomies in series and includes those performed for both benign and malignant disease. Values in table are tabulated for *all* patients in the series.

OR, operating room; EBL, estimated blood loss; MS, morphine sulfate; RCCa, renal cell carcinoma.

Nephroureterectomy

The development of a 12-mm laparoscopic GIA tissue stapling device provided the technology needed to extend the indications for laparoscopic nephrectomy to include transitional cell carcinoma of the upper urinary tract. Because of the high incidence of downstream tumors after resection of upper tract transitional cell tumors, the kidney, ureter, and cuff of bladder are routinely excised en bloc. With the laparoscopic GIA tissue stapler, a cuff of bladder is excised leaving a watertight bladder closure.

Procedure

The procedure begins in the cystoscopy suite with placement of a 0.035-in. Terumo guidewire (i.e., plastic, nonconducting) into the appropriate ureter. A 7 F 5-mm dilating balloon catheter is passed over the guidewire and positioned such that it straddles the ureteral orifice. After inflating the ballon enough to visibly open the ureteral orifice, the orifice and intramural tunnel are incised at the 12 o'clock position until fat is visible, which confirms extension of the incision up to and just through the vesical junction. This is accomplished with a 24 F resectoscope equipped with an Orandi knife. The dilating balloon is removed, and the entire inner surface of the now opened ureteral tunnel is electrocoagulated with a roller ball electrode. A retrograde 7 F 11.5-mm occlusion balloon catheter is placed in the renal pelvis over an Amplatz superstiff guidewire as previously described.

The patient is then moved to the open surgical suite, and the procedure is initiated in the supine position. The pneumoperitoneum is established as previously described and a 12-mm port is placed at the umbilicus. Under direct vision three more ports are placed: a 12-mm port in the midline between the umbilicus and symphysis pubis, a 12-mm port in the midclavicular line just below the costal margin, and a 5-mm port in the midclavicular line at the level of the anterior superior iliac spine (Fig. 16). Attention is directed initially to the distal ureter and ureterovesical junction. The peritoneum is incised *medial* to the medial umbilical ligament; the incision is continued cephalad along the colonic-peritoneal reflection (line of Toldt) (Fig. 17). The ductus (ras) deferens is identified, occluded with 9-mm clips, and divided. The ureter is identified and is dissected distally to the ureteral hiatus. A 9-mm clip is placed across the lower ureter. The medial umbilical ligament is secured with two pairs of 9-mm clips and divided. Traction on the

for renal tumors

Analgesics (MS) (mg)	Oral intake (days)	Hospital (days)	Compli-cations	Adrenal-ectomy	Pathology
—	—	—	—	5	RCCa
—	—	4.8	—	—	RCCa
—	—	—	—	—	—
—	—	10	—	5	RCCa
48	1	5.9	4 (44%)	7	7 RCCa 1 oncocyt., 1 multilocular cyst
48	1	6.7	—	57%	—

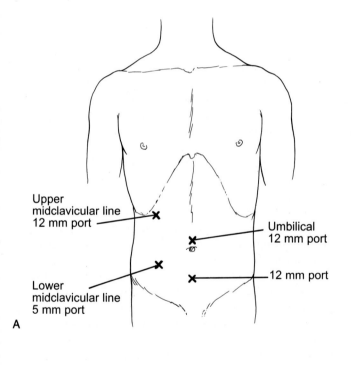

Upper midclavicular line 12 mm port

Umbilical 12 mm port

12 mm port

Lower midclavicular line 5 mm port

A

Lower midclavicular 5 mm port

Lower anterior axillary line 5 mm port

Upper anterior axillary line 5 mm port

Upper midclavicular line 12 mm port

12 mm port

Umbilical 12 mm port

B

Figure 16. A: Initial port placement with patient in the supine position to secure the distal ureter and cuff of bladder during nephroureterectomy. **B:** Remaining ports are placed once the patient is turned to the lateral decubitus position.

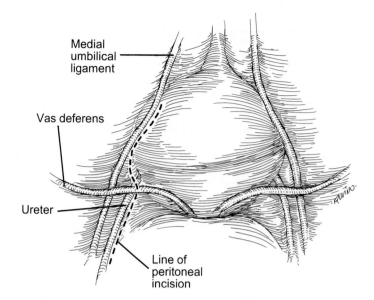

Figure 17. Position of the distal left ureter in relationship to the vas deferens and medial umbilical ligament. The *dotted line* indicates the line of incision.

midureter with a 5-mm atraumatic grasping forceps aids in dissecting the distal ureter. When the ureterovesical junction and a surrounding 1- to 2-cm margin of bladder are clearly visible, the ureteral catheter is deflated and removed along with the guidewire. Next, the laparoscopic tissue GIA 30 stapler is passed through the lower midline port and fired across the bladder cuff just distal to the ureterovesical junction. Using the Foley catheter, indigo carmine-stained saline is instilled to rule out leakage from the staple line. Now, the ureter is dissected proximally as far as possible.

There are two other methods for completing the ureterectomy portion of the procedure. According to the technique of Rassweiler, the ureteral tunnel is resected transurethrally up to and through the ureterovesical junction, thereby effectively detaching the ureter from the bladder. Now, the ureterectomy can be completed during the nephrectomy portion by simply tugging on the midureter in order to pull the distal ureter away from the bladder. In contrast, Breda begins his laparoscopic nephroureterectomy by passing a ureteral stone basket retrograde up the ureter. Then, after completing the laparoscopic nephrectomy portion of the procedure, a 9-mm clip is placed on the proximal ureter, and the ureter is incised. The remaining patent ureteral stump is longitudinally cut in continuity into four approximately 2-cm long strips. The stone basket is opened, and the ureteral flaps are passed through the opened wings of the basket. The basket is closed and slowly pulled retrograde. The sides of the ureter are grasped distal to

Table 3. *Laparoscopic*

Author (Ref.)	Attempted	Completed	Age (y)	OR time (h)
Rassweiler (19)	4 (36)[a]	—	—	3–4
Gershman (18)	4	4	—	1–3
Clayman	11	11	63 (5–83)	8.1 (5.5–10.6)
Total:	19	100%	—	Average: 6.0

[a] Number in parentheses indicates total number of laparoscopic procedures in the series and includes both nephrectomies and nephroureterectomies. Values in table are tabulated for *all* patients in the series.

See Table 1 for abbreviations.

the basket to facilitate intussusception of the proximal ureter into the midureter. With continued retrograde traction, the entire ureter is pulled inside out at the level of the ureteral tunnel. The renal specimen can now be entrapped and delivered as previously described, and the port sites can be closed. The patient is then placed into the dorsal lithotomy position and the intussuscepted ureter can be transurethrally incised and delivered. Alternatively, if the ureteral orifice is circumferentially incised at the time of placing the stone basket, then when the ureter is delivered through the urethra, the surgeon can continue to exert traction on the ureter and thereby avulse it at the point where the orifice was circumscribed. This variation precludes the need for repositioning the patient.

Following the distal ureteral dissection, the patient is turned to the lateral decubitus position. Two 5-mm ports are placed along the anterior axillary line: subcostal and opposite the umbilicus (Fig. 16B). The cephalad portion of the lateral colonic-peritoneal reflection (line of Toldt) is incised. Alternatively, a combined approach with retroperitoneal assistance using the modified Gaur balloon as described previously can be used initially to help develop the retroperitoneal space. In either case, Gerota's fascia is left intact along the midportion and lower pole of kidney; however, Gerota's fascia is incised over the upper pole of the kidney thereby allowing displacement of the adrenal gland superiorly. The hilar vessels are individually secured and divided as described previously, using five 9-mm clips for the renal artery or its branches and a vascular GIA stapler for the renal vein. The kidney, ureter and bladder cuff are manipulated away from the renal bed. The intraabdominal pressure is lowered to 5 mmHg, and the abdomen is inspected for any bleeding.

An impermeable 5 × 8-in. entrapment sack is delivered via the uppermost 12-mm port; the specimen is maneuvered into the sack and the entire specimen is removed intact with the sack by extending the 12-mm suprapubic port in the midline, to 5–7 cm. (If the specimen is too large to maneuver into the entrapment sack, then the incision is enlarged to 12–15 cm, and the kidney is delivered manually.) Intraabdominal pressure is again lowered to 5 mmHg in order to inspect for hemostasis. The ports are removed under direct vision, and the port sites are closed as previously described for performing a nephrectomy. The Foley catheter is removed on the second postoperative day. If the technique of Rassweiler or Breda has been used, then the Foley catheter is left in place for 5 days; a cystogram is performed before the catheter is removed.

Clinical Results

The first laparoscopic nephroureterectomy was performed at Washington University in St. Louis, Missouri in May 1991. Since this initial report, other investigators have likewise reported a sanguine, although limited, experience with laparoscopic nephroureterectomy (Table 3).

nephroureterectomy

EBL (ml)	Analgesics (MS) (mg)	Oral intake (days)	Hospital (days)	Compli- cations	Bladder cuff
—	—	—	—	—	0
—	—	—	1–2	0	?
211 (50–400)	16 (0–48)	0.76	4.6 (2–8)	1	11
211	16	<1	3.8	7%	—

Since 1991 we have performed 11 laparoscopic nephroureterectomies at Barnes Hospital: 10 were for transitional cell carcinoma of the upper tract and one was for recurrent pyelonephritis in a refluxing nonfunctioning kidney in a 5-year-old girl. Because of the size of the specimen, a transperitoneal approach is recommended; use of the dilating balloon in the retroperitoneum facilitates the procedure. The average age of patients was 63 years (range: 5–83). Operative time averaged 8.1 hours (range: 5.5–10.6 hours), including the time spent to unroof the ureter. Specimen size varied from 229 to 730 g. Blood loss averaged 211 ml (range: 50–400 ml). On average, the patients' analgesic requirements were low: 22 mg of morphine sulfate. In general, patients were eating within 24 hours of their procedure and were discharged from the hospital on the fifth day. The ensuing 2.8 weeks were spent in convalescence. In this group there has been only one, albeit major, complication. A 73-year-old, high-risk (ASA IV) cardiac patient suffered a significant postoperative hemorrhage that required open exploration and electrocoagulation of a small branch of the adrenal vein. After recovering from postoperative adult respiratory distress syndrome, the patient had a fatal cardiac arrythmia on postoperative day 67.

Kerbl compared our laparoscopic experience with upper tract transitional cell carcinoma to eight consecutive patients undergoing standard open nephroureterectomy at our teaching hospital. The operative time for the laparoscopic approach was more than twice that for the open procedure (7.29 vs 3.37 hours); however, operative blood loss was less with the laparoscopic approach (180 vs 340 ml). Moreover, the open surgical patients did not resume oral intake for 4.3 days as opposed to 1 day in the laparoscopic patients. Narcotic analgesic use in the open surgical group was 149 mg, sixfold greater than in the laparoscopic patients. Length of hospital stay was half as long (4.6 vs 9.25 days) in the laparoscopic series. No complications occurred in the surgical group vs the aforementioned major complication in the laparoscopic group. Lastly, patients resumed normal activity in only 2.8 weeks vs 6 weeks following the open procedure. The obvious advantage of laparoscopic surgery lies in the rapid convalescence of the patient, minimal narcotic requirements, and decreased hospital stay. While the patients' well-being and productivity are significantly promoted by the laparoscopic approach, any cost savings due to shortened hospital stay are counterbalanced by the longer operative times and the expense of the laparoscopic equipment.

▲ COMPLICATIONS

Fluid overload, particularly in older patients, is likely to occur if the anesthesiologist erroneously depends on urine output as a guide to assess fluid status. A number of investigators have noted that during lengthy laparoscopic procedures urine output is dramatically reduced, despite adequate cardiac filling pressures. This is likely due to a shift in blood flow from the renal cortex to the medulla during laparoscopy at 15 cm H_2O intraperitoneal pressure. For patients with cardiopulmonary compromise, left heart monitoring is the most reliable way to assess fluid status and avoid overaggressive fluid resuscitation; a central venous line is of little value. The surgeon should be reassured that after release of the pneumoperitoneum, urine output and renal function normalize in 1–2 hours.

Nerve palsy or compartment syndrome occurs during lengthy procedures with the patient in a lateral decubitus position. Muscular patients are especially prone to develop a compartment syndrome in the dependent lower extremity. Generous foam padding between the legs, such that the superior leg is parallel and on a level with the flank prevents undue stretch on the hip and excessive weight on the dependent leg. The dependent leg should be flexed to about 20 degrees. A carefully placed axillary roll and padding between the superior and dependent arms protects the brachial plexus. All dependent bony pressure points (e.g., ankles, knees, hips, elbows, wrists) are heavily padded with foam. Patient restraints are also padded with a foam or egg-crate pad.

Incisional hernias occur most commonly with inadequate fascial closure of 10- to 12-mm ports and occur with greater frequency in obese patients in whom exposure of the anterior abdominal fascia is limited. Closure of the fascia *and* peritoneum of ≥10-mm ports should be done under continuous endoscopic monitoring. A variety of port closure devices and techniques have recently been described that facilitate secure fascial closure; however, our experience favors the Carter-Thomason device, as a broad secure closure of the fascia is assured regardless of patient size.

Xanthogranulomatous pyelonephritis (XGP) and pyonephrosis are associated with severe perirenal adhesions that jeopardize safe laparoscopic dissection of the kidney. Failed laparoscopic nephrectomy has been associated with XGP in a number of series in addition to our own. For the less experienced laparoscopist, these kidneys are better approached through an open incision, as there is a substantial risk of bleeding or injury to adjacent structures. The surgeon approaching this type of problem laparoscopically can anticipate a 50% conversion rate to an open laparotomy.

Significant bleeding from the renal hilar vessels or the adrenal vein requiring immediate conversion to open nephrectomy, or delayed bleeding requiring transfusion or exploration, have been reported sporadically; with increased experience, this complication is rare. Securing the renal vein with the 3-cm endoGIA stapler (vascular load) reduces the risk of bleeding from a renal vein that is too broad for the standard 9-mm titanium occlusive clips. In addition, on the left side, particular attention should be directed at securing all branches of the renal vein (the adrenal vein, the gonadal vein, and the ascending lumbar veins) before securing the main renal vein. Clips placed on these venous branches should be at least 1–2 cm away from the main renal vein in order to facilitate subsequent placement of the endoGIA stapler across the left renal vein.

✓ CONCLUSIONS

Laparoscopic nephectomy for *benign* disease has become an accepted alternative to open surgery in many centers worldwide. While operative times are admittedly longer for the laparoscopic approach, the shorter hospital stay, less postoperative discomfort, and shorter convalescence make the procedure very appealing to patients. Also, as our instrumentation and skill improve, the time for the laparoscopic surgery should further decrease and eventually become similar to current open surgical operative time.

Presently, we have extended the indications for a laparoscopic approach to include malignant disease, whether of a parenchymal or urothelial nature. As with nephrectomy for benign disease, procedural times are lengthy; however, patient discomfort and recovery are minimal. Preliminary data support the contention that the laparoscopic approach is equivalent to the open approach in achieving a satisfactory cancer operation. However, longer follow-up is needed to properly test this most important hypothesis.

RECOMMENDED READING

1. Weinberg JJ, Smith AD. Percutaneous resection of the kidney: preliminary report. *J Endourol* 1988;2:355.
2. Ikari O, Netto R Jr, Palma PCR, D'Ancona CAL. Percutaneous nephrectomy in nonfunctioning kidneys: a preliminary report. *J Urol* 1990;144:966.
3. Clayman RV, Kavoussi LR, Long SR, Dierks SM, Meretyk S, Soper NJ. Laparoscopic nephrectomy: initial report of pelviscopic organ ablation in the pig. *J Endourol* 1990;4:247.

Positioning the entrapment sack and subsequent kidney entrapment may turn an otherwise routine procedure into a daunting experience. The sack is introduced through the *medial* upper port; the grasper securing the ureter enters by way of the *lateral* upper port. The sack is *pulled* into the abdominal cavity using grasping forceps passed through a lower port. The laparoscope is then shifted to the upper medial port. Traumatic locking graspers, passed through the three widely spaced *lower* ports are used to triangulate open the mouth of the sack. The lower edge of the sack is then pulled downward and cephalad such that its lower lip lies just beneath the inferior edge of the liver or spleen. Meanwhile, the kidney, held by the ureteral stump, should be manipulated until it rests on the body of the liver or spleen. The sack can then be triangulated open by pulling the three grasping forceps in different directions; the sack is further expanded by passing the laparoscope into the sack and moving it in ever widening circles. Upon withdrawing the laparoscope, the sack should be wide open; the kidney can then be rolled off of the surface of the liver or spleen onto the leading lower lip of the sack. The kidney is pushed deeper into the sack via the grasper on the ureter; this grasper hugs the superior anterior sack wall. As this is being done, the grasper on the inferior tab of the sack can be slowly raised upward thereby pushing the trailing pole of the kidney into the sack.

When dealing with the renal hilum of a large kidney (i.e., ≥400 g), the surgeon should perform a meticulous anterior dissection of the renal vein. The kidney is then rolled anteriorly to put the renal hilum on stretch. The renal artery will now be encountered

vessels, although, rarely, surgical clips may be employed. Irrigation of the area with suction may be necessary due to blood or lymphatic tissue obscuring vision. Once the nodal packet is freed, it should be held only by a few attachments at the iliac bifurcation. Again using blunt and sharp dissection the packet is completely freed from the pelvis (Fig. 12). Care must be taken not to injure the ureter at this point.

The nodal packet is removed by passing the tissue through an 11-mm port under direct vision (Fig. 13). Occasionally the packet is so large that it must be divided to effect removal. One must be careful not to drop the packet and lose it in the abdomen. An alternative is to place the packet in a laparoscopic bag prior to removal, although we have not found this necessary. If immediate prostatec-

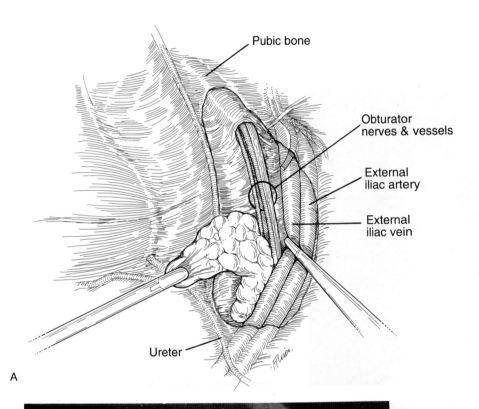

A

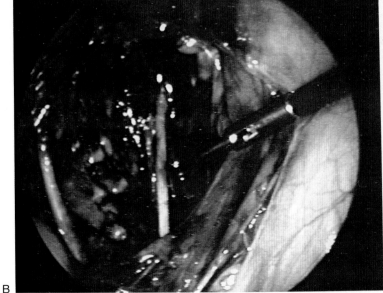

B

Figure 12. Utilizing blunt and sharp dissection the lymphatic packet is freed from all surrounding tissues. **A:** Diagram. **B:** Intraoperative appearance.

tomy is planned, the nodal packet is sent for frozen section. After the dissection is complete, and if there is no gross hemorrhage, the patient is tilted in the opposite direction and the opposite side node dissection is performed.

Once the nodal specimens are removed, the obturator fossa is irrigated using heparinized saline (5,000 U/l). Adequate hemostasis is obtained. If hemostasis is difficult to obtain using coagulation current or clips, one alternative is to place a small swatch of Surgicel into the obturator fossa under direct vision (Fig. 14). The peritoneum is left open to prevent lymphocele formation. The pneumoperitoneum pressure should be lowered to 5 to 7 mmHg to detect any venous bleeding that may have been tamponaded by the pneumoperitoneum. The abdominal cavity is inspected and all trocars removed under direct vision. All carbon dioxide should be allowed to escape from the abdomen. Fascial defects are closed with 2-0 Vicryl suture. The skin is closed with subcuticular suture and Steri-strips applied.

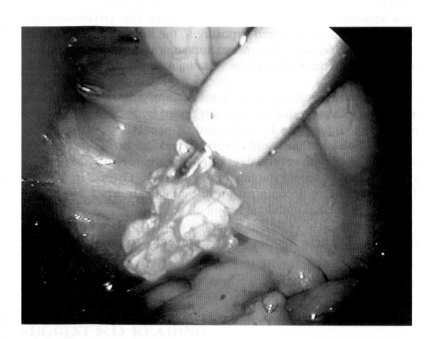

Figure 13. Nodal packet is removed by passing tissue through an 11-mm port under direction vision.

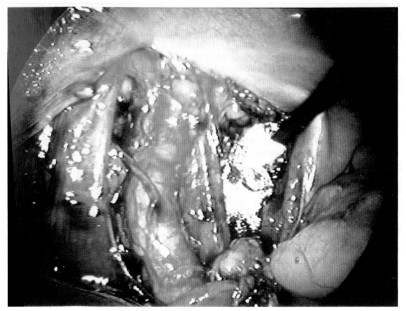

Figure 14. Use of a swatch of Surgicel, which is placed in the obdurator fossa under direct vision to assist in hemostasis.

the liver superiorly and medially. As the peritoneum is freed from the loose retroperitoneal aerolar tissues, it is displaced medially as well.

At this point, the scope is moved to the most dorsal port to allow a better view of the lateral and posterior aspects of the adrenal bed. The adrenal is first dissected laterally and superiorly. Then the inferior margin is freed (Fig. 27). Hemoclips are used before transection of small capillaries and veins. The gland is displaced medially, permitting further posterior dissection (Fig. 28).

Once again, the scope is moved to its original position in the subcostal port to allow a better view of the medial aspect of the adrenal gland and vena cava. Finally, the most difficult medial dissection is performed (Fig. 29). The central vein-vena cava junction must be carefully approached, because injury here is difficult to control. The vein is doubly clipped medially, singly clipped distally, and divided. The gland is then placed into a sterile plastic bag for removal through the initial port site. The wounds are closed in standard fashion.

Avoiding Pitfalls

As with the other approaches described here, port introduction and instrument manipulation must be performed meticulously. Parenchymal injury to the liver,

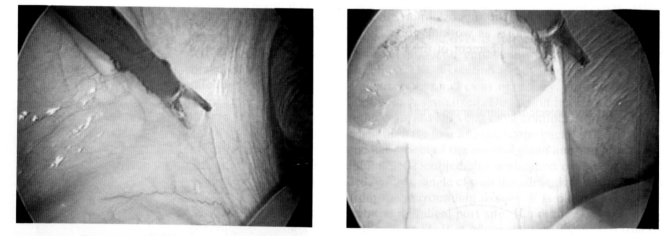

Figure 26. Incision of the peritoneum lateral to the liver, kidney, and right adrenal gland.

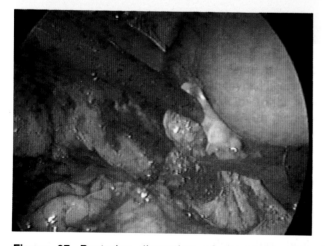

Figure 27. Posterior dissection of the right adrenal gland. The lateral and superior margins are approached first. Then the inferior aspect of the gland is approached.

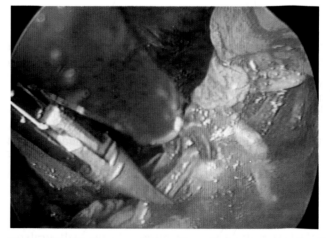

Figure 28. Further posterior dissection approaches the medial border of the adrenal.

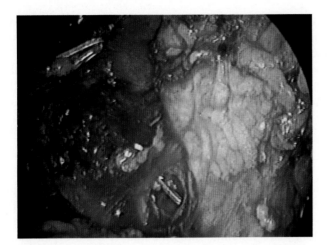

Figure 29. Access to the right central vein may be obtained from its posterior aspect (with the telescope in the dorsal port as shown here), or may be achieved anteriorly (with the scope in the more anterior subcostal port).

although not usually life-threatening, can result in significant loss of visual field because of blood accumulating in the retroperitoneal space.

Accessing and maintaining the best viewpoint of the anatomy requires not only a skilled camera controller, but also an alert surgeon who realizes when it is best to move the scope from one port site to another. This point cannot be overemphasized.

The other critical matter in the lateral approach to the right adrenal gland involves meticulous attention to detail as the medial dissection is performed. This should not be rushed. It is important for the surgeon to realize that, because this is one of the final steps in a procedure that may have been taxing and time-consuming, fatigue may become a factor and may influence decision-making as well as technical finesse. So extra caution should be exercised during the dissection of the medial aspect of the gland from the vena cava. Finally, a well-formulated and rehearsed plan for immediate conversion to open laparotomy in the case of caval hemorrhage should be in place.

▲ COMPLICATIONS

Hemorrhage

The most feared complication of any operation, especially in the retroperitoneum, is uncontrolled hemorrhage. The proximity of the adrenal glands to the great vessels, and their location high in the abdomen provides limited access for vascular control. These facts require the surgeon to use extreme caution when dissecting in this area. Hemostasis must be maintained as concurrently as possible; otherwise, the clarity of the field decreases sharply. This means that even small, and seemingly inconsequential, ''oozing'' vessels should be controlled before proceeding with any further dissection.

If more significant bleeding occurs, such as from a larger adrenal artery or the central vein, initial temporary control with pressure from a forceps is often essential to adequately assess the magnitude of the problem. Occasionally, a large-mouthed forceps may be used for temporary vascular control, if it can be applied safely and without injury to surrounding structures. After temporary control of the hemorrhage is obtained, the field should be irrigated and the excess blood aspirated away from the area. Definitive control with clips, sutures, or ligatures should then be accomplished. It may be necessary to place another port for access if a working port was used for insertion of an instrument which is maintaining temporary hemostasis.

If massive uncontrollable hemorrhage occurs, the surgeon should not hesitate to convert to open laparotomy. During the conversion, however, there may be benefit to maintaining some "pressure" control with a laparoscopic instrument if it truly appears to decrease the rate of bleeding.

Visceral Injury

On the left side, the spleen and pancreas are the most easily injured organs, although the splenic flexure of the colon, the stomach, and the left kidney are also at risk. On the right side, the liver, hepatic flexure of the colon, duodenum, and the right kidney are potential sites for injury. Solid organ injury generally occurs during retraction or dissection. Most commonly it involves puncture or laceration of the parenchyma by a retractor or dissecting instrument. If the resultant bleeding is not controllable with cautery or suture, conversion to open laparotomy may be necessary. In the case of injury to the liver or pancreas, it may be wise to leave a drain in place in the early postoperative period.

Hormonal Consequences

The most common intraoperative hormonal effects are cardiovascular. These occur especially with adrenalectomy for pheochromocytoma, although they may occur with other hormonally active tumors as well. It is vitally important that the patient undergo adequate preoperative preparation as previously described in this chapter. Close communication with the anesthesia team is also essential so that swings in blood pressure or changes in cardiac function may be addressed in a timely fashion.

Equally important is the conduct of the dissection. Great care must be taken to minimize the amount of manipulation of the tumor, especially in the case of pheochromocytoma. As previously mentioned, this may be easier to accomplish laparoscopically than in open surgery because of the ability of the scope to generate a better view of the anatomy than is generally obtained by direct vision at laparotomy. In this regard, it is important for the surgeon to recognize when it is best to move the scope to a different port site.

Pneumothorax

Although pneumothorax has not been reported to date, it is important to realize that accidental injury to the diaphragm could occur when dissection is so near to it. Puncture or laceration of the diaphragm with sharp dissecting instruments or those connected to unipolar cautery can occur. The resultant transmission of intraabdominal pressure to the chest produces tension pneumothorax. Immediate release of intraabdominal pressure is the first step in treatment. Repair of the diaphragm, with or without placement of a thoracostomy tube, is usually definitive treatment.

Wound Dehiscence

Although wound dehiscence is much less common than in open adrenalectomy, it may still occur. It is important for the surgeon to close all fascial wounds 10 mm or greater in size. The choice of suture material depends on the preference of the surgeon. Skin closure is much less potentially troublesome and may be accomplished with any number of methods, again depending on the surgeon's preference.

✓ CONCLUSIONS

Inherent Requirements for Adrenalectomy and Their Achievement in Laparoscopy

The location of the adrenal glands, their friable parenchyma, and the proximity of the great vessels pose significant demands on the surgeon, whether he approaches the gland laparoscopically or "open." First, the amount of space in which to work is limited. This requires long, narrow instruments. Laparoscopic instruments are especially suited to this task. Second, the viewing area is limited, and the amount of light needed to illuminate the area is crucial. Again, the laparoscope with the camera and the halogen light sources available today seem to meet these challenges particularly well. Not only can the scope negotiate places that the surgeon's head cannot, but it provides much-needed magnification and illumination, not possible in conventional surgery. Third, it is necessary to minimize manipulation of the gland. This, again, is more easily accomplished laparoscopically than in open surgery owing to the ability to move the scope to alternate sites for different views of the anatomy that would otherwise require significant retraction of the gland in an "open" approach.

In all, purely from an intraoperative viewpoint, and notwithstanding the postoperative benefits of decreased pain, fewer pulmonary complications, and better cosmesis, it appears that a laparoscopic approach should be preferred over an "open" approach to adrenalectomy for most cases.

The space around the adrenal glands is filled with fatty and loose areolar tissue that lends itself well to judicious use of blunt dissection, which may be accomplished with scissors, a blunt-tipped instrument, or the suction-irrigator. Surgical judgment is the key concept here. Assess the tissues with palpation (using an instrument) and if they appear amenable to blunt, atraumatic, hemostatic dissection, then use it. The small peripheral aterial blood vessels and the central vein should be readily identified with the magnification afforded by the scope, and can be secured with clips or cautery as appropriate. This is a great technique if it is not overused.

Preparation of the Surgeon

The single most important consideration in successful performance of laparoscopic adrenalectomy is that of surgeon preparation. The degree of difficulty, and the consequences of intraoperative mishap are so significant that only those surgeons who are accomplished advanced laparoscopists should consider attempting laparoscopic adrenalectomy. The surgeon must have mastered skills such as suturing, knot-tying, tissue manipulation, and control of hemorrhage before proceeding with this operation. He should have an inherent appreciation of even the most subtle nuances of laparoscopic surgery, from an understanding of the support equipment such as insufflators, cameras, and monitors, to the intricate details of how to obtain the best exposure or obtain hemostasis in any situation. If these fundamentals are present, the surgeon should consider himself ready to perform laparoscopic adrenalectomy, and should reasonably expect an excellent outcome.

RECOMMENDED READING

1. Bruining HA, Lamberts SWJ, Ong EGL, van Seyen AJ. Results of adrenalectomy with various surgical approaches in the treatment of different diseases of the adrenal glands. *Surg Gynecol Obstet* 1984;158:367–369.
2. Brunt LM, Molmenti EP, Kerbl K, et al. Retroperitoneal endoscopic adrenalectomy: an experimental study. *Surg Laparosc Endosc* 1993;3:300–306.
3. Constantino GN, Mukalian GG, Vincent GJ, Kliefoth WL Jr. Laparoscopic adrenalectomy. *J Laparoendosc Surg* 1993;3:309–311.
4. Fernandez-Cruz L, Benarroch G, Torres E, et al. Laparoscopic approach to the adrenal tumors. *J Laparoendosc Surg* 1993;6:541–546.
5. Gagner M, Lacroix A, Bolte E. Laparoscopic adrenalectomy in Cushing's syndrome and pheochromocytoma [Letter]. *N Engl J Med* 1992;327:1033.

6. Gagner M, Lacroix A, Bolte E, Pomp A. Laparoscopic adrenalectomy: the importance of a flank approach in the lateral decubitus position. *J Laparoendosc Surg* 1994;8:135–138.
7. Go H. Laparoscopic adrenalectomy. *Nippon Hinyokika Gakkai Zasshi* 1993;84:1675–1680.
8. Guazzoni G, et al. Surrenalectomia laparoscopica: case report. *Arch Ital Urol* 1993;65:265–267.
9. Higashihara E, et al. A case report of laparoscopic adrenalectomy. *Nippon Hinyokika Gakkai Zasshi* 1992;83:1130–1133.
10. Higashihara E, et al. Laparoscopic adrenalectomy: the initial 3 cases. *J Urol* 1993;149:973–976.
11. Petelin J. Laparoscopic adrenalectomy. Paper presented at the *Third World Congress of Endoscopic Surgery. Bordeaux, France. June 1992.*
12. Petelin J. Laparoscopic adrenalectomy. Video presented at the *International Symposium of Laparoscopic Surgery, Saskatoon, Saskatchewan, Canada, August 1992.*
13. Petelin J. Laparoscopic adrenalectomy. Paper presented at *Minimally Invasive Surgery and New Technology Congress. Luxembourg, September 1992.*
14. Petelin J. Retroperitoneal endoscopic surgery: adrenalectomy. Paper presented at *SAGES* (Society of American Gastrointestinal Endoscopic Surgeons) *Scientific Session. Phoenix, Arizona, 1993.*
15. Rassweiler JJ, Henkel TO, Potempa DM, Coptcoat M, Alken P. The technique of transperitoneal laparoscopic nephrectomy, adrenalectomy and nephroureterectomy. *Eur Urol* 1993;23:425–430.
16. Rassweiler JJ, et al. Laparoskopisches training in der Urologie. *Urol A.* 1993;32:393–402.
17. Salky BA, Bauer JJ, Gelernt IM, Kreel I. The use of laparoscopy in retroperitoneal pathology. *GastroIntest Endosc* 1988;34:227–230.
18. Sardi A, McKinnon WMP. Laparoscopic adrenalectomy for primary aldosteronism. *JAMA* 1993; 269:989–990.
19. Sardi A, McKinnon WMP. Laparoscopic adrenalectomy for primary aldosteronism. *Surg Laparosc, Endosc* 1994;4:86–91.
20. Suzuki K, et al. Laparoscopic adrenalectomy: clinical experience with 12 cases. *J Urol* 1993;150: 1099–1102.

STOMACH

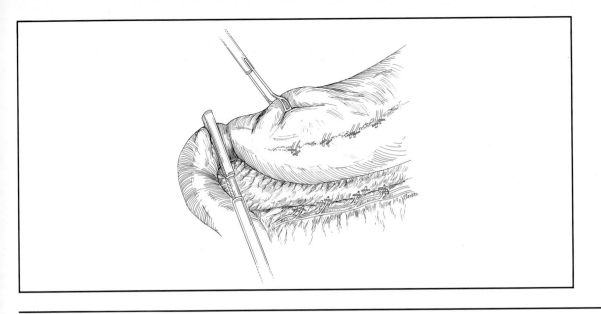

30

Gastrectomy

Peter M. Y. Goh and Cheng K. Kum
Department of Surgery
National University Hospital
Singapore 0511
Malaysia

Operative Laparoscopy and Thoracoscopy, edited by
B. V. MacFadyen, Jr. and
J. L. Ponsky. Lippincott-Raven
Publishers, Philadelphia © 1996.

The first laparoscopic Billroth II gastrectomy was performed by a team of surgeons in Singapore on February 10, 1992. This description is a modification of the original technique using the improved instrumentation now available. The technique described is suitable for a gastrectomy for benign gastric ulcer at the incisura of the stomach.

◉ ANATOMY

The vascular arcade of the greater curve of the stomach is important in the initial mobilization of the greater curve, which is the first part of the dissection. The proximal limit of the dissection is the first short gastric vessel that comes from the spleen. The distal dissection extends into the first part of the duodenum. In a patient with fatty omentum, the best strategy is to keep dissection as close to the stomach as possible. In a thinner individual, it is possible to choose the most avascular plane, that is, the one requiring the least dissection and clipping of omental vessels, and which curves toward the stomach wall only at the point of proximal transection.

The level of the pylorus externally can be identified by the vein of Mayo. If this is obscure, gastroscopic localization should be done to determine the exact level of the pylorus. The first part of the duodenum must be mobilized sufficiently to apply the EndoGIA stapler. The vascular supply to the duodenum comes from three directions: superior, inferior, and posterior. These vascular attachments are very fragile and must be carefully dissected, clipped, and transected. The position of the supraduodenal bile duct should be ascertained to prevent accidental stapling. The origin of the right gastroepiploic vessel is inferior to the duodenum and can usually be avoided. Occasionally it is in the way and has to be clipped and transected or stapled. The duodenum is attached to the pancreas inferiorly by fine vessels. These can give rise to troublesome bleeding and must be individually coagulated before transection. Vessels larger than 1 mm should be clipped.

Branches of the left and right gastric artery and their accompanying veins run along the lesser curve of the stomach (Fig. 1). There is an avascular area in the lesser omentum above this vascular arch that facilitates the dissection. It is not advisable to dissect between the arcade and the stomach. The gastric ulcer is usually located at the incisura and may be difficult to localize externally. If the ulcer is chronic, there is usually a patch of inflammatory tissue in the lesser omentum just adjacent to the ulcer.

The left gastric pedicle is located about two-thirds up along the lesser curve. It is seldom necessary to dissect out this vessel unless operating for cancer or in a high lesser curve ulcer. A large vein usually accompanies the left gastric pedicle, with several smaller vessels around it.

The identification of the duodenal jejunal junction is important for selecting a loop of small bowel for anastomosis. It is best found by sweeping the transverse colon cephalad. A loop of small bowel is selected in the upper left quadrant and followed proximally to the junction.

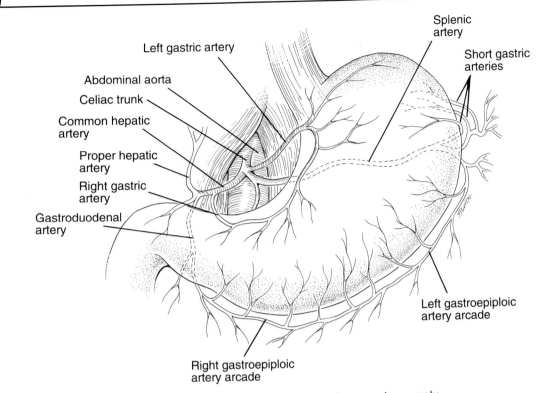

Figure 1. Anatomy of the stomach and its vascular supply.

▶ PREOPERATIVE PLANNING

Laparoscopic Billroth II gastrectomy is mainly performed for benign chronic gastric ulcer. The indications for surgery are as follows:

1. Resistant or recurrent ulcer disease after a suitable course of medical treatment (at least 3 months)
2. Bleeding gastric ulcer that is resistant to or recurs after endoscopic hemostasis
3. Perforated ulcer with minimal soilage

The patient must be fit for general anesthesia. Age itself is not a contraindication, but the operation should not be considered in patients with concomitant medical problems who are over 75. Previous upper abdominal surgery is not an absolute contraindication as the operation is still possible, for instance, after a previous cholecystectomy or repair of a perforated duodenal ulcer. The presence of adhesions does make the operation more difficult and is a contraindication if there are other concomitant medical problems.

The only absolute contraindication is a patient who is unfit for general anesthesia. Cancer of the stomach should not be operated on if there is a chance for cure or benefit from extensive lymph node dissection. At present, a meticulous lymph node dissection is still unreliable by the laparoscopic route. The operation should only be considered for very early gastric cancer or for cancer with metastasis where the gastrectomy is done for palliation of bleeding or obstruction.

The patient should have upper gastrointestinal endoscopy and the ulcer should be biopsied and proven to be benign. Standard preoperative workup—hematology, electrolytes, coagulation profile, electrocardiogram, and chest radiograph—are all that is required. Other investigations are ordered only if there are concomitant medical problems. Blood should be matched and available. The stomach should be washed out if pyloric stenosis is present.

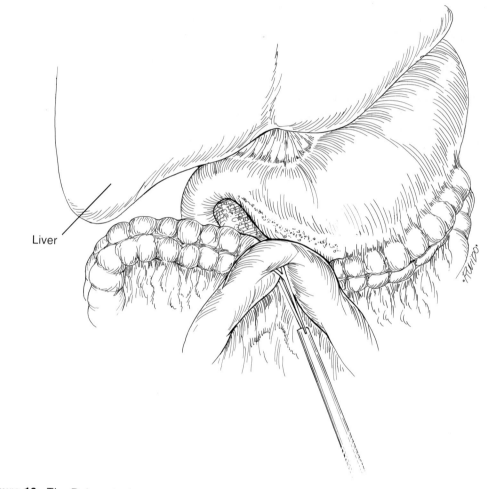

Figure 10. The Babcock clamp is inserted through the lower left trocar, grasps the jejunum, and pulls an antecolic loop up to the dependent portion of the stomach.

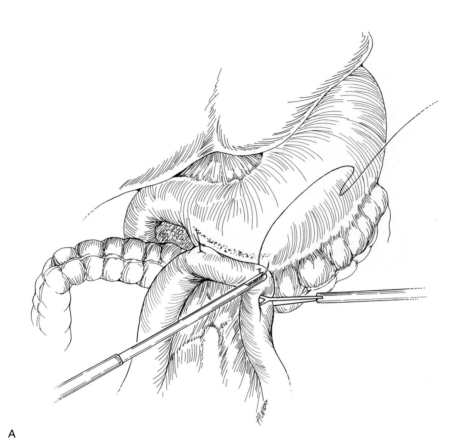

A

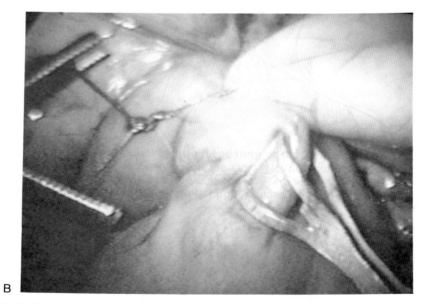

B

Figure 11. A: Babcock clamps hold the jejunum in place to the dependent antrum while a needle-holder is used to place stay sutures 6–8 cm apart through both jejunum and stomach. **B:** An extracorporeal knotter sets one of the knots.

Table 2. *Preoperative evaluation*

History
Physical examination
Laboratory studies (± serum gastrin)
Endoscopy (± upper gastrointestinal contrast study)
Acid secretion studies
Gastric emptying scan

Preoperative Evaluation

The preoperative evaluation is very similar to that for patients being considered for conventional ulcer surgery (Table 2). All patients are subjected to a routine history, physical examination, and laboratory evaluation. Patients with atypical presentations of ulcer diathesis should also undergo a workup to exclude gastrinoma. All patients should undergo upper gastrointestinal endoscopy as well as contrast studies to determine the extent and severity of disease. In addition, to evaluate the effectiveness of this procedure, patients should have determinations of their acid secretion (basal and pentagastrin-stimulated) and gastric emptying capacity. Repeat studies are performed between 1 and 6 months after surgery to confirm the effectiveness of the procedure. A thorough assessment of the patient's operative risk should also be made, similar to that for any major abdominal operation.

▼ INTRAOPERATIVE MANAGEMENT/SURGICAL TECHNIQUE

Patient Positioning

The patient should be positioned in the modified lithotomy position, which will allow the surgeon to stand between the patient's legs, in excellent position to perform the operative dissection of the distal esophagus and stomach (Fig. 4). When placing the patient in the lithotomy position, the proper precautions must be taken to prevent neurovascular compromise of the lower extremities. "Booted" stirrups should be used to elevate the lower extremities and appropriate padding placed to protect the calf. An alternative to the lithotomy position is to use a "split-leg" orthopedic table. This will allow the patient's legs to remain flat, but apart, to allow easy access for the surgeon between the patient's legs.

It is important to insert a nasogastric (or orogastric) tube and a urinary catheter as soon as possible to decompress the stomach and bladder. The gastric tube may subsequently be replaced with a large esophageal tube (Maloney dilator) or a flexible gastroscope to distend the distal esophagus and facilitate its identification during the early stages of the operative dissection. However, due to the inherent limitations of laparoscopic surgery, care must be taken to ensure proper retraction of the stomach during the passage of any large esophageal tube. Careful coordination between the anesthesiologist and the surgeon during this process will avoid inadvertent perforation of the stomach or esophagus during insertion of a semirigid esophageal dilator.

Trocar Placement

A total of five primary laparoscopic cannulas are employed in most cases (Fig. 5). The ports should be placed as evenly as possible across the abdominal wall. If the ports are located too close together they tend to interfere with each other.

clamp
junctic
or gasi
the esc
contro
should
the esc
"pool"
this rej

Th(
aspect
esopha
dissect
(Fig. 1
quite j

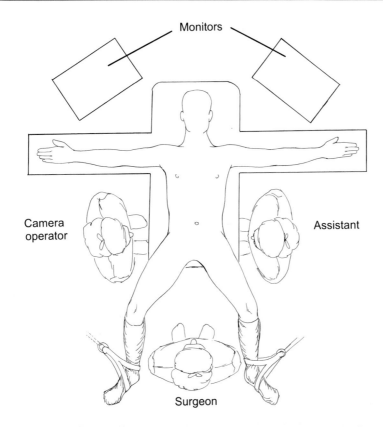

Figure 4. The modified lithotomy position is employed during laparoscopic vagotomy. It allows the surgeon to stand in an optimal position during the operative dissection.

Figure
esopha
phragm

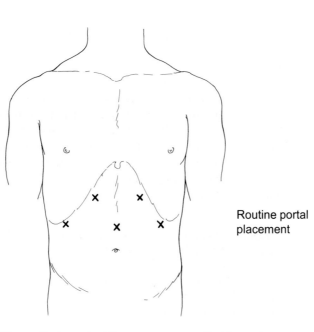

Figure 5. A total of five trocars, usually 10 mm in diameter, are routinely used during laparoscopic vagotomy.

Figure
from th
ment o
histolo(

the posterior aspect of the stomach can also be exposed by making an opening through the gastrocolic omentum (Fig. 24). Additional dissection of the epiploic vessels is at the discretion of the surgeon but should be strongly considered.

Having completed the highly selective vagotomy (Fig. 25), the operative field is copiously irrigated with saline and carefully inspected to ensure adequate hemostasis. The stomach wall along the lesser curve and the distal esophagus should be inspected for signs of ischemia or perforation. Care must be taken not to accidentally dislodge any of the previously placed clips during this final inspection process.

Specific Operative Techniques

Most of the laparoscopic procedures share many technical aspects; however, all laparoscopic antiulcer procedures have their own specific considerations, some of which are discussed below.

Posterior Truncal Vagotomy and Anterior Seromyotomy

An operation to treat patients with intractable ulcer disease, which has been popular in Europe for the past two decades, is a posterior truncal vagotomy combined with anterior seromyotomy. This procedure has been popularized by the work of Taylor and colleagues in the United Kingdom. The small gastric branches of the anterior vagus nerve course obliquely through the seromuscular layer of the stomach before reaching the acid-secreting mucosal layer. Dividing the seromuscular layer interrupts these small branches, thereby accomplishing a highly selective vagotomy of the anterior aspect of the stomach (Fig. 26). Ongoing clinical investigation by Taylor and others have shown that posterior truncal vagotomy and anterior seromyotomy does not significantly alter gastric motility or emptying, and therefore a gastric emptying procedure is not necessary.

The seromyotomy may be performed using either an electrocautery (hook-spatula) probe, laser, or with sharp dissection. Care must be taken not to penetrate the mucosa or to cause extensive thermal damage with the electrocautery or laser modalities. It appears that small perforations of the mucosa are not uncommon with this technique, but they can be easily repaired under laparoscopic guidance. To avoid a "missed" gastric perforation, the seromyotomy is completed by adding

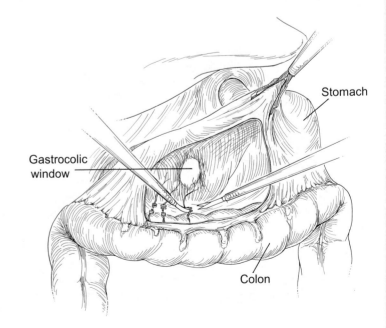

Figure 24. Retrogastric approach to stomach through gastrocolic omentum.

a running, "overlapping" suture that approximates the edges and closes any small perforations. The important factor is to ensure that such perforations do not go unrecognized at the time of surgery. The stomach should be distended with a methylene blue/saline solution at the end of the case to exclude the presence of a gastric leak.

Posterior Truncal Vagotomy and Anterior Linear Gastrectomy

Recently, a group of surgeons in Mobile, Alabama developed a modification of the anterior seromyotomy that utilizes a laparoscopic stapling instrument. In this procedure, Hannon and colleagues perform a posterior truncal vagotomy but complete an anterior highly selective denervation by dividing the fundic branches of the anterior vagus nerve with a laparoscopic stapling device.

Following ligation and division of the posterior vagus nerve the remainder of the distal esophagus is carefully dissected to ensure completeness of the vagotomy. The course of the anterior vagus is then identified to avoid subsequent injury with the stapler. A stapled division (and simultaneous reanastomosis) of the anterior wall of the stomach is then accomplished by firing a 3-cm laparoscopic GIA (Fig. 27). A long strip of gastric wall, approximately 1.5 cm from the lesser curvature,

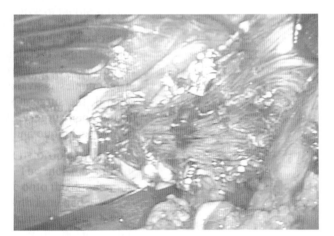

Figure 25. Completed view of standard (anterior and posterior) highly selective vagotomy.

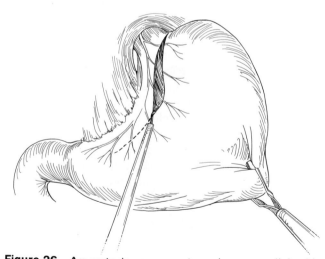

Figure 26. An anterior seromyotomy is accomplished by incising the gastric wall along the lesser curve, approximately 1.5 cm away from the anterior vagal trunk. The incision is carried down to the level of the gastric mucosa, thereby interrupting the small vagal fibers to the anterior portion of the stomach.

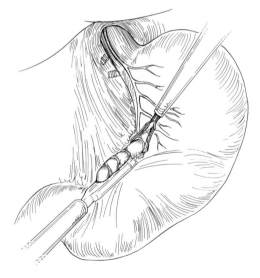

Figure 27. An anterior linear gastrectomy may be performed to achieve a highly selective vagotomy of the anterior stomach. A 3-cm laparoscopic stapling device is used to perform this technique.

of the perforation and the individual's clinical status. Laparoscopic management appears most appropriate for those patients with signs of progressive chemical peritonitis who are seen within 12 hours following ulcer perforation. In patients who present 48 hours or more after ulcer perforation and who remain stable with minimal peritoneal findings, the opening may have already been sealed. In these individuals, continued medical management and another gastric tube suctioning and antibiotic administration and acid reducing medication may be the most appropriate therapy. In contrast, patients presenting with a rigid abdomen and septic shock are not candidates for laparoscopic intervention. These individuals require immediate fluid resuscitation, stabilization of their vital signs and, when appropriate, exploratory open laparotomy.

▼ INTRAOPERATIVE MANAGEMENT/SURGICAL TECHNIQUE

Gastric Outlet Obstruction

Two types of procedures are used for gastric outlet obstruction: laparoscopic total vagotomy and gastrojejunostomy. A second procedure, laparoscopic antrectomy with total truncal vagotomy (V and A) is discussed in the section below on management of recurrences after vagotomy.

Laparoscopic Total Vagotomy

The patient is placed in a supine position with legs spread apart. The operating surgeon stands between the patient's legs in the so-called "French" position. The normal peritoneum is created by insufflation carbon dioxide at a pressure of 14 mmHg electronically controlled. Five trocars are introduced in the upper part of the abdomen; one for the video laparoscope, one for the operating instruments, two lateral trocars for the grasping forceps, and one subxyphoid port for the retractor or the irrigator (Fig. 2).

The abdominal cavity is explored as soon as the video laparoscope is inserted to ensure that the planned operation is feasible, particularly that the liver can be retracted. Other associated lesions amenable to laparoscopic surgery are noted

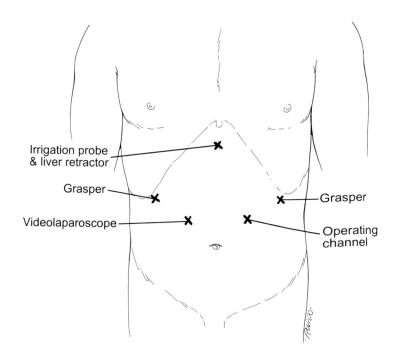

Figure 2. Trocar position for vagotomy.

and, for us, cirrhosis is the usual contraindication for advanced laparoscopic procedures.

Posterior Truncal Vagotomy

The left lobe of the liver is retracted using xiphoid palpation probe and the vascular part of the lesser sac is opened with electrical scissors above the hepatic branch of the vagus nerve and the dissection is continued to the level of the right crus of the diaphragm.

The two landmarks for a posterior truncal vagotomy are the caudate lobe and the right crus of the diaphragm (Fig. 3). The right crus is ceased with the right grasping forceps and retracted to the right to expose the esophageal peritoneum, which is incised along the length of the border of the right crus. This allows the separation of the abdominal esophagus outward and permitting access to its posterior wall. Within the depths of this angle, the right cord of the posterior vagus is localized and recognized by its pearly aspects. The nerve is transected between two clips and a 1-cm section is removed for histologic confirmation (Fig. 4).

Anterior Truncal Vagotomy

Several trunks of the anterior vagus are sectioned. Transection of these fibers is easy because of their position on the muscular fibers of the esophagus. The only difficulty occurs on the left edge of the esophagus where there is the possibility of overlooking some branches, even large ones (criminal branch of Grassi); with the use of the traction forceps the esophagus can be rolled to the right to expose its left edge to control those criminal nerves.

Laparoscopic Gastrojejunostomy

The same ports can be used, but one lateral one should be enlarged to allow the introduction of the endolinear cutter 60 (Ethicon Inc., Cincinnati, Ohio). The first loop of the jejunum is grasped approximated to the greater curvature. It is

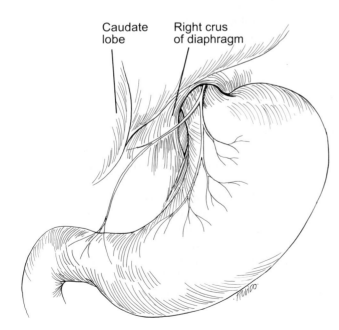

Figure 3. Lateral approach to the hiatus.

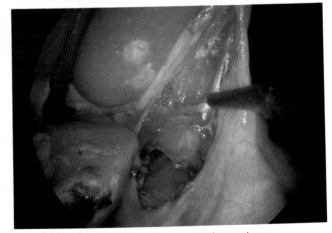

Figure 4. Posterior truncal vagotomy.

3, and 4. The commonest form is the simple sliding hiatal hernia in which the lower esophageal sphincter moves into the chest dragging the stomach behind it. A less common type is the co-called "mixed" hiatal hernia in which there is a sliding component together with a rolling component with the upper stomach moving up alongside the lower esophageal sphincter. The least common variant is the true paraesophageal hiatal hernia in which the lower esophageal sphincter remains in its normal position and the fundus of the stomach moves up into the chest alongside the esophagus. In some of these cases there is no evidence of gastroesophageal reflux with all of the symptoms due to the herniated stomach in the chest. Paraesophageal hernias may have gastritis or even ulceration present in the herniated stomach, which can lead to significant bleeding. Endoscopic examination will give a good impression of which of the three types of hernia is present. Endoscopy of the gastric mucosa may reveal the presence of gastritis, which should alert the endoscopist to the possibility of *Helicobacter pylori* or alkaline reflux. The presence of duodenal ulceration may suggest gastric acid hyposecretion as the underlying etiologic mechanism for both reflux disease and the ulcer.

Cinefluoroscopy

Cinefluoroscopy is frequently an ancillary test to endoscopy. Further information on diverticula, ulcers, and strictures can be obtained. The exact size and position of a hiatal hernia and the nature of paraesophageal hernias can be deter-

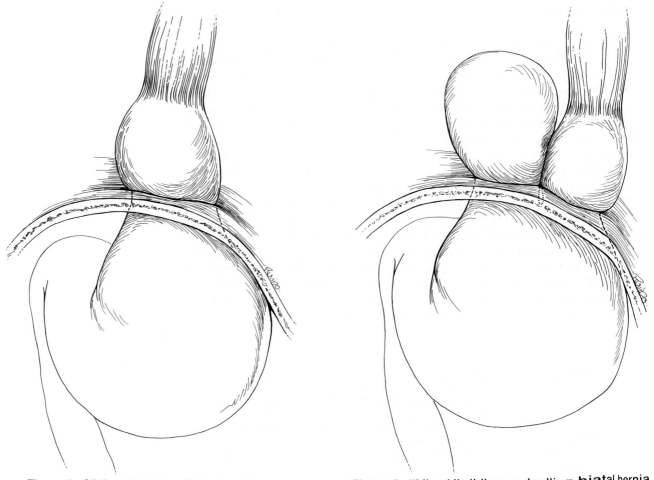

Figure 2. Sliding hiatal hernia. Lateral view.

Figure 3. "Mixed," sliding, and rolling hiatal hernia. Lateral view.

mined. The rate of passage of barium through the esophagus can give information on its motor power. Spasm or esophageal dilation can be identified. Free reflux of barium into the esophagus is not diagnostic for gastroesophageal reflux disease.

Esophageal Manometry

Esophageal manometry is available in many centers and offers excellent information on the motor characteristics of the lower esophageal sphincter, esophageal body, and upper esophageal sphincter. The test is easily performed by passing a manometric catheter through the nose into the stomach. Five water-filled perfusion ports spaced 5 cm apart are usually used. These are progressively withdrawn through the lower esophageal sphincter allowing for exact measurement of its total length, intraabdominal length, and mean resting pressure. The catheter is then placed in the esophageal body and the peristaltic response to swallows tested. It is also possible to measure relaxation of the lower esophageal sphincter with swallowing. Abnormalities such as scleroderma in which there is absent lower esophageal motility, diffuse esophageal spasm, the nutcracker esophagus with pressure waves over 180 mmHg, and nonspecific motor disorders may be identified. These frequently masquerade as gastroesophageal reflux disease, and each requires its own specific therapy. In achalasia there is inappropriate relaxation of the lower esophageal sphincter with swallowing, usually associated with poor or absent esophageal body motility and increased lower esophageal sphincter resting

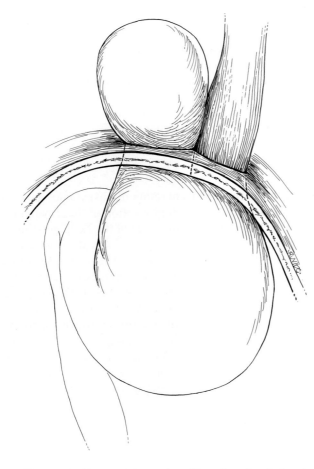

Figure 4. Paraesophageal rolling hernia. Lateral view.

The Hill procedure is an operation that essentially relies on fixation of the cardia to the preaortic fascia by several sutures. There is also a lesser curvature gastric plication (Fig. 7). This presumably produces elongation of the intraabdominal segment of the lower esophageal sphincter and results in posterior angulation at the esophagogastric junction. These anatomic alterations give the procedure its antireflux properties. This procedure was popularized by Dr. Lucius Hill, who obtained excellent results, particularly when he carries out intraoperative manometry to gauge the tightness and number of stitches placed at the hiatus. Others have found this to be a technically challenging procedure and fail to be able to identify the preaortic fascia with confidence. The procedure can be carried out laparoscopically, but is more difficult to do than the Nissen fundoplication.

Laparoscopic Nissen Fundoplication

The laparoscopic Nissen is our standard operation for gastroesophageal reflux disease. The procedure is performed regardless of previous abdominal operations or the weight of the patient.

The patient is placed in lithotomy and a steep reverse Trendelenburg position. The surgeon stands between the legs of the patient and the assistants are positioned on the patient's right and left sides. An incision is made above the umbilicus in the midline for establishment of the pneumoperitoneum. This can either be created by blind puncture using a Veress needle or by the open Hassan technique. A 10-mm port is placed through this wound. It is important to place this port for the camera superior to the umbilicus as the distance from the umbilicus to the hiatus is often too long for adequate visualization of this area. Further 10-mm ports are

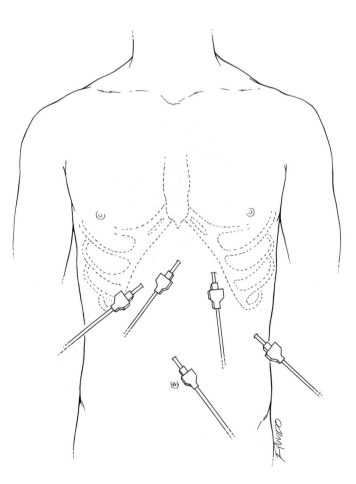

Figure 8. Placement of ports for laparoscopic fundoplication.

placed in the upper midline, right subcostal area and two in the left subcostal area (Fig. 8). The trocars are placed far enough apart to avoid instruments interfering with each other. Only 10-mm ports are used to provide more flexibility in introducing instruments into the peritoneal cavity. The left lobe of the liver is retracted using a liver retractor inserted through the right subcostal port. The triangular ligament is not divided as it holds the left lobe of the liver off the esophagus. The gastrohepatic omentum is divided without cutting vagal branches to the liver. Accidental damage to these branches results in an increased risk of gallstones and delayed gastric emptying. It is important to identify an aberrant left hepatic artery in the gastrohepatic omentum. This can be damaged and may cause troublesome bleeding. This is a branch of the left gastric artery and should be preserved intact if possible. The vessel is seen in approximately 23% of patients. The right crus of the diaphragm is then easily identified to the left of the caudate lobe of the liver. The anterior edge of the right crus is incised allowing access to connective tissue and fat behind it. The dissection may be carried superiorly along this edge to the point where the right and left crura meet anterior to the esophagus. The esophagus and anterior vagus nerve are not in danger of being damaged if the dissection is kept close to the edge of the crus (Fig. 9). The peritoneum can easily be identified and dissected off the inferior edge of the left crus. It is important to retract the gastric fundus to the right for exposure of the posterior part of the left crus. This gives access to the mediastinum on the anterior and left of the esophagus. The left crus of the diaphragm curves behind the esophagus and should be separated from the esophagus as far posteriorly as possible to prepare for creation of the window behind the esophagus. There is no need to dissect the anterior vagus nerve, as this often lies intimately attached to the anterior wall of the esophagus. This nerve will remain within the fundoplication. The esophagus is then retracted to the left side for access to the connective tissue behind the esophagus and the posterior vagus nerve (Fig. 10). This usually lies separate from the esophagus and is easily identified and dissected off the posterior wall of the esophagus. The fundus will eventually be brought through posterior to the esophagus and anterior to the posterior vagus nerve. This placement will help secure the fundopli-

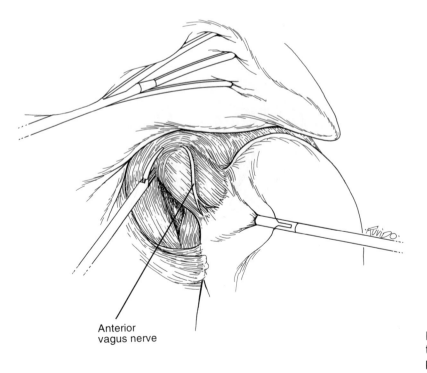

Anterior
vagus nerve

Figure 9. Laparoscopic Nissen fundoplication. Dissection of right crus of the diaphragm.

35

Gastric and Small Bowel Access for Enteral Feeding

Stephen W. Unger
Department of Surgery
Mt. Sinai Medical Center of Greater Miami
Miami Beach, Florida 33140-2893

David S. Edelman
The Gallbladder and Laparoscopic Surgery Center of Miami
Miami, Florida 33176

Operative Laparoscopy and Thoracoscopy, edited by
B. V. MacFadyen, Jr. and
J. L. Ponsky. Lippincott-Raven
Publishers, Philadelphia © 1996.

the insertion site, and if not mobile enough at the conclusion of the procedure and the reach seems a little bit tight, the pneumoperitoneum may be released, thus bringing the abdominal wall downward and shortening the distance between the viscus and the abdominal wall.

☑ CONCLUSIONS

Overall, as experience and technique become standardized, the laparoscopic placement of enteral feeding tubes should be equal to or better than the results of open operative or endoscopically placed tubes, since the procedure is inherently identical to the former without an incision and avoids the endoscopic morbidity of the latter. In fact, for these patients that cannot be endoscoped, a laparoscopically placed tube will become the primary procedure of choice.

REFERENCES

1. Russell TR, Brotman M, Norris F. Percutaneous gastrostomy, a new simplified and cost effective technique. *Am J Surg* 1984;148:132.
2. Edelman DS, Unger SW. Laparoscopic gastrostomy. *Surg Gynecol Obstet* 1991;173:401.
3. Edelman DS, Unger SW, Russin DJ. Laparoscopic gastrostomy. *Surg Laparosc Endosc* 1991;1: 251–253.
4. Duh QY, Way LW. Laparoscopic gastrostomy using T-fasteners as retractors and anchors. *Surg Endosc* 1993;7:60–63.
5. Duh QY, Way LW. Laparoscopic jejunostomy using T-fasteners as retractors and anchors. *Arch Surg* 1993;128:105–108.
6. Murphy C, Rosemurgy AS, Albrink MH, Carey LC. A simple technique for laparoscopic gastrostomy. *Surg Gynecol Obstet* 1992;174:424–425.
7. Reimer DS, Leitman IM, Ward RJ. Laparoscopic Stamm gastrostomy with gastropexy. *Surg Laparosc Endosc* 1991;1:189–192.
8. Sangster W, Swanstrom L. Laparoscopic guided feeding jejunostomy. *Surg Endosc* 1993;7: 308–310.
9. Reed DN. Percutaneous peritoneoscopic jejunostomy. *Surg Gynecol Obstet* 1992;174:527–529.
10. Albrink MH, Foster J, Rosemurgy AS, Carey LC. Laparoscopic feeding jejunostomy: also a simple technique. *Surg Endosc* 1992;6:259–260.

COLON AND SMALL BOWEL

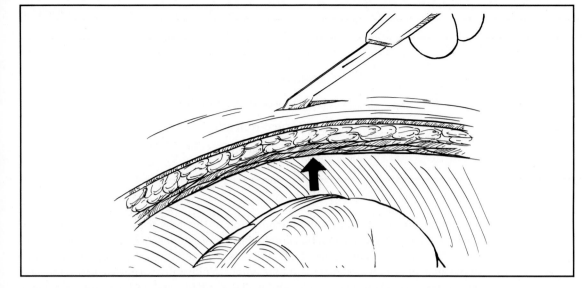

36

Left and Right Colon Resection

Jose M. Ramos
Department of Surgery
University of the Witwatersrand
Johannesburg, South Africa

Robert W. Beart
Department of Surgery
University of Southern California
Los Angeles, California 91103

Operative Laparoscopy and Thoracoscopy, edited by
B. V. MacFadyen, Jr. and
J. L. Ponsky. Lippincott-Raven
Publishers, Philadelphia © 1996.

KEY WORDS

Colectomy

Colon resection

Descending colon

Endoloop

Extracorporeal resection

Peritoneal reflection

Sigmoid resection

It is important to stress that the introduction of this new technique does not alter the underlying surgical principles applicable to colonic resection. Traditional surgical judgment is perhaps even more important in this operation and attention to detail and uncompromising technique vital. While intracorporeal resection and anastomosis is certainly possible, and well described, current techniques are cumbersome, costly, lengthen the procedure, and require leaving the bowel open in the abdomen for a lengthy period of time. Therefore, with the existing technology, we feel that colonic resections should be laparoscopic-assisted rather than totally intracorporeal. The technique described herein consists of laparoscopic mobilization of the relevant segment of colon, and isolation and division of the main mesenteric vessels supplying that segment. The mobilized bowel is then exteriorized through a small abdominal incision where further mesenteric division, bowel resection, and anastomosis are performed.

▣ ANATOMY

Individual variations influenced by build, body length, mesenteric length and attachments, and the presence or absence of adhesions, make the disposition of the colon within the peritoneal cavity inconsistant. Under normal conditions, the surgical anatomy is similar in most patients. The presence of teniae coli, haustrations, and appendices epiploicae distinguish the colon from the small bowel (Fig. 1). On the right side, the cecum and ascending colon are usually retroperito-

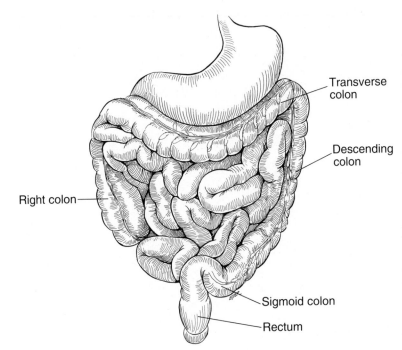

Figure 1. Abdominal colon anatomy.

neal structures, bound to the posterior abdominal wall by the overlying peritoneum. The lateral peritoneal reflection is marked by the line of Toldt. In up to 10% of individuals, the cecum and ascending colon are very mobile with a long mesentery. Lying between the hepatic flexure and the more superiorly situated splenic flexure, the transverse colon is freely mobile, usually hanging down into the lower abdomen, and is distinguished by its attachment along its superior border to the stomach by the gastrocolic omentum. Posteriorly, the transverse mesocolon tethers the transverse colon to the retroperitoneum. The splenic flexure and descending colon are firmly bound to the posterior abdominal wall by the overlying peritoneum. The lateral reflection is again marked by the line of Toldt. At the pelvic brim the colon acquires a mesentery and becomes variably mobile, this change marking the junction between the descending and sigmoid colon. The length, fixity, and position of the sigmoid is somewhat variable and the apex of the loop may be tethered to the anterior rectum, other pelvic structures, or the lateral abdominal wall by adhesions. At the level of the sacral promontory, the taeniae become confluent marking the rectosigmoid junction. In its upper third, the rectum is invested anteriorly and laterally by peritoneum, lower down only the anterior aspect being covered. At this level, the rectum loses its posteriorly situated mesentery, the blood supply and lymphatic drainage being situated laterally.

As in open surgery, the relations of the various parts of the colon are important to note when contemplating laparoscopic colon resection. On the right, the ureter lies posteromedial to the cecum and ascending colon and is exposed by dividing the peritoneal reflection laterally and mobilizing the colon medially (Fig. 2). The ureter descends on the psoas and crosses anterior to the bifurcation of the common iliac artery to enter the pelvis. The gonadal vessels and, more laterally, the right kidney, are other posterior relations of the right colon. The second and third parts of the duodenum lie posteromedial to the ascending colon and part of the hepatic flexure. This flexure is related anterosuperiorly to the undersurface of the right lobe of the liver and may be attached to the gallbladder. On the left side, the colon is similarly related posteriorly to the left ureter, gonadal vessels, and left kidney.

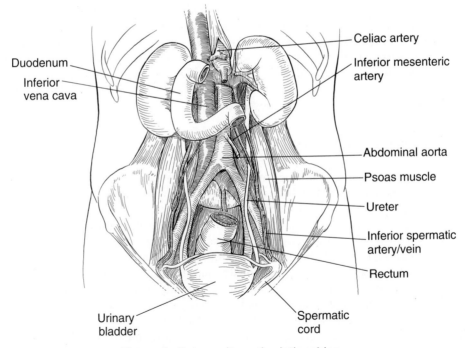

Figure 2. Retroperitoneal relationships.

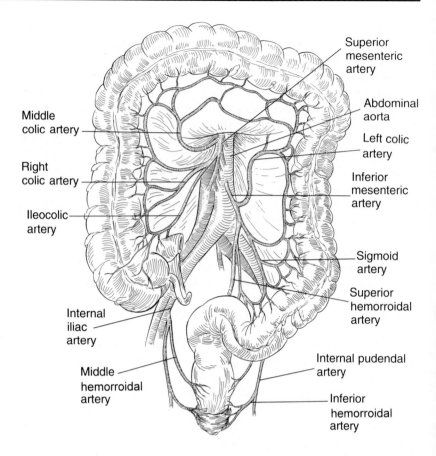

Figure 3. Colonic blood vessel anatomy.

The ureter, coursing down on the left psoas, is exposed by dividing the lateral peritoneal reflection of the descending and sigmoid colon and reflecting these medially.

The right colon is supplied by the superior mesenteric artery via its ileocolic, right, and middle colic branches, the anatomy and distribution of which are fairly constant (Fig. 3). The transverse colon is supplied by left and right branches of the middle colic artery. The left colon is supplied by the inferior mesenteric artery via the left colic and various sigmoidal branches, the inferior mesenteric artery terminating as the superior hemorrhoidal artery and supplying the proximal rectum. The marginal artery of Riolan provides a variable link between the superior and inferior mesenteric territories, forming an arcade along the inner border of the colon. Recognition of this anatomy and ligation of the vessels at their origin simplifies the laparoscopic colon resection.

▶ PREOPERATIVE PLANNING

The workup planned for a laparoscopic colon resection should include evaluation of factors relevant to the disease (such as cardiac, pulmonary, and coagulation assessments) and the patient's ability to undergo general anesthesia. Diagnostic accuracy is vital as the ability to assess intraluminal pathology with the laparoscope is limited. Thus preoperative colonoscopy and/or contrast enema is necessary to accurately locate the disease-containing segment. Colonoscopic localization of colonic pathology is notoriously unreliable, therefore the site of the pathology must be marked by endoscopic tattooing using a permanent marker such as India ink. Other markers, such as methylene blue, are rapidly absorbed and tend to disappear within a short time. While it is possible to perform the colonoscopy intraoperatively, it is preferable to perform it earlier, with the advantages of saving anesthetic time and limiting the degree of gaseous colonic distension. The ability to detect lymphatic and hepatic metastases laparoscopically is limited, thus accurate preoperative imaging with computed tomography (CT) scans or magnetic resonance imaging (MRI) may be important. While patient factors such as obesity may make the procedure more difficult, this would not constitute an absolute contraindication to laparoscopic colon resection. Adhesions from previous surgery or intraabdominal infections can usually be dealt with laparoscopically, although a history of dense adhesions documented at a previous operation would probably make the patient unsuitable for this procedure. The position of previous abdominal incisions may necessitate slight changes to port placement.

Laparoscopic colon resections should probably be limited to the right colon, left colon, sigmoid, and rectum. While it is possible to mobilize the transverse colon laparoscopically, the proximity of the vessels in the transverse mesocolon to the root of the small bowel mesentery, with the risks involved in dissecting in this confined area, and the degree of dissection necessary, make this a more hazardous and usually lengthy procedure.

The indications for laparoscopic colectomy include obstruction, bleeding, perforation, tumors, fistula, diverticulitis, and widespread polyp disease, although lesions in the transverse colon are probably better dealt with at open surgery. Active lower gastrointestinal bleeding requiring emergency surgical intervention should also be dealt with by traditional open methods. Intestinal obstruction, either small or large bowel, sigmoidovesical fistula, and dense adhesions are considered to be contraindications to the laparoscopic approach. There is some disagreement as to the role of laparoscopic resection in cancer of the colon. We believe that, provided traditional surgical oncologic principles are upheld, cancer does not preclude a laparoscopic approach. It is certainly possible to do a standard cancer operation using this technique. It is, however, important to exercise surgical judgment as those patients with large or locally complicated lesions should probably have an open procedure.

The patient should be made fully aware of the surgical strategy before the operation, and it must be stressed that the procedure will be converted to a standard open procedure should the need arise. This occurrence should not be misconstrued as a surgical failure but rather as the use of a more appropriate surgical technique in that particular instance.

In order to prepare the bowel, the patient is given 90 g of Fleet's Phospho-soda orally at 6:00 P.M. and is encouraged to drink water or juice liberally. Three hours later a further 45 or 90 g of Phospho-soda is taken, the amount varying according to the nature and consistency of the stool passed. A Fleet enema is administered on the evening prior to surgery and again early on the day of surgery. Antibiotic prophylaxis consists of Neomycin 2 g and Flagyl 2 g given orally at 6 P.M. and again at 11 P.M. on the day prior to surgery. Intravenous antibiotics are not routinely used.

Deep venous thrombosis prophylaxis may be provided by the use of elastic stockings or sequential compression devices.

▼ INTRAOPERATIVE MANAGEMENT/SURGICAL TECHNIQUE

General anesthesia is recommended both for patient comfort and to allow speedy conversion to an open procedure should the need arise. The use of a nasogastric tube and urethral catheter is optional but may be useful if the procedure is expected to be prolonged. In addition to standard anesthetic monitoring, the regular measurement of arterial blood gases is recommended in order to limit the likelihood of complications arising from acidosis, particularly in prolonged procedures.

The patient is placed in the supine position for both left and right colon resections, with both arms placed alongside the patient so as not to interfere with the operating team. Secure straps are applied to make it possible to tilt and rotate the table without the patient moving. Whenever possible, placement of an evacuable beanbag under the patient, on the ipsilateral side, helps to minimize movement. The camera operator is always in the left upper quadrant and the nurse in the right lower quadrant. Two monitors are placed at the feet and all members of the operating team must have an unrestricted view of these throughout the procedure (Fig. 4). The patient is placed in steep Trendelenburg position and is rotated away from the side being resected; this maneuver displaces the small bowel from the operative field.

In most cases, four ports are adequate for this procedure, two 10- to 11-mm and two 5-mm cannulae being used (Fig. 5). The camera must be placed in a position which allows for clear visualization of both lower quadrants and colonic flexures, and the left upper quadrant is ideally suited to this. A small skin incision is made in the left upper quadrant (Fig. 6) and the dissection carried out to the posterior rectus sheath which is incised (Fig. 7). Fascial sutures are placed and a Hasson introducer is inserted into the peritoneal cavity under direct vision and fixed with the fascial sutures. A pneumoperitoneum is induced via this port and the camera inserted. Insufflation pressures should be kept to 10–12 mmHg to avoid extensive retroperitoneal and subcutaneous emphysema. The 0-degree laparoscope is used routinely and provides adequate visualization in most instances.

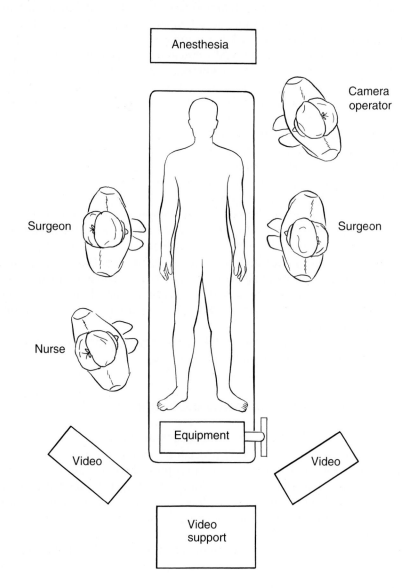

Figure 4. Theater layout for both right and left colon resection, the surgeon standing opposite the side being resected.

Another 10- to 11-mm cannula is placed suprapubically in the midline and two 5-mm cannulae are placed at the edges of the rectus sheath on either side at or just below the level of the umbilicus, these being referred to later as the midabdominal ports (Fig. 8). It is advisable to avoid placing ports in or adjacent to the umbilicus, as this tends to interfere with the mesenteric dissection, the vessels being close to the midline at that level.

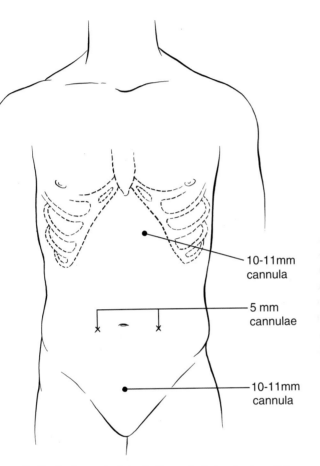

10-11mm
cannula

5 mm
cannulae

10-11mm
cannula

Figure 5. Port placement and sites of abdominal wall incision.

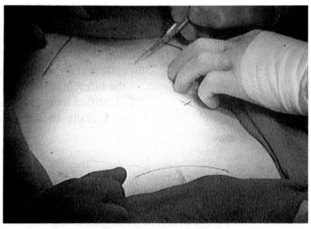

Figure 6. Sites for port placement indicated. Incision being made in left upper quadrant.

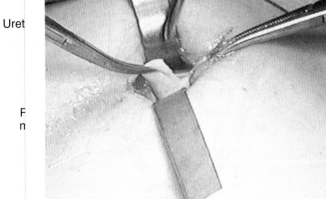

Figure 7. Peritoneum exposed and opened using the Hasson technique.

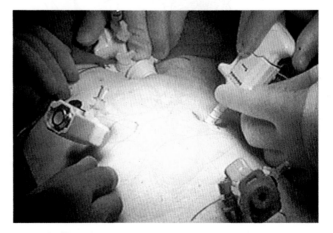

Figure 8. Port placement completed.

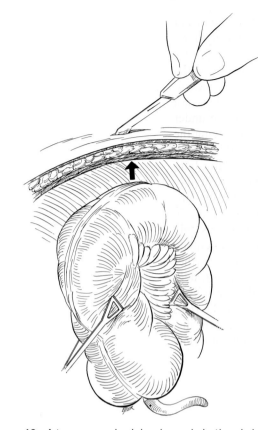

Figure 13. A transverse incision is made in the abdominal wall from the lateral border of the rectus abdominus muscle.

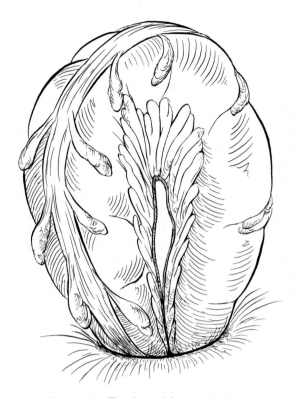

Figure 14. The bowel is exteriorized.

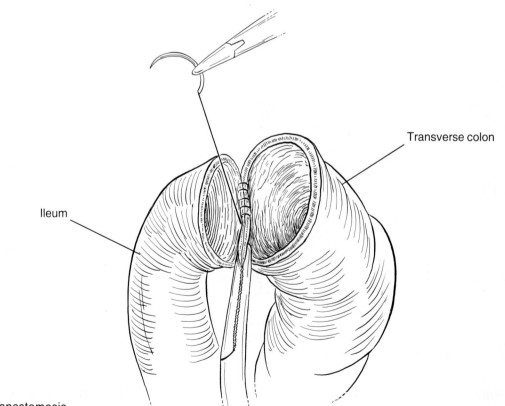

Transverse colon

Ileum

Figure 15. Extracorporeal anastomosis.

to ensure a thorough cancer operation, but also to minimize the need for dissection and clipping of multiple vascular branches. Although the mesentery can be divided using a vascular linear stapler, unless the head can be angled it is difficult to place the staple line perpendicular to the structures being divided, particularly in cases requiring high ligation. Furthermore, the extra costs of using staplers may be difficult to justify.

Once the major vascular pedicle has been divided, the colon should be fully mobile and prepared for exteriorization. The optimal site for placement of the transverse abdominal incision through which the bowel is exteriorized can be determined by elevating the bowel towards the anterior abdominal wall. The colon to be resected is then grasped with a Babcock forceps and held. A transverse incision is made in the abdominal wall, adjacent to the right midabdominal port, proceeding laterally from the lateral border of the rectus abdominous muscle (Fig. 13). The mobilized colon is exteriorized and further mesenteric division is performed as necessary under direct vision (Fig. 14). Division of the transverse mesocolon and greater omentum is performed readily at this stage. Following resection of the colon, an extracorporeal anastomosis is performed using a two-layer handsewn technique, any other standard technique being suitable (Fig. 15). The mesenteric defect is then closed and the bowel returned to the abdominal cavity (Fig. 16). The abdominal incision is closed in two layers using absorbable monofilament sutures, and the pneumoperitoneum reestablished in order to examine the opera-

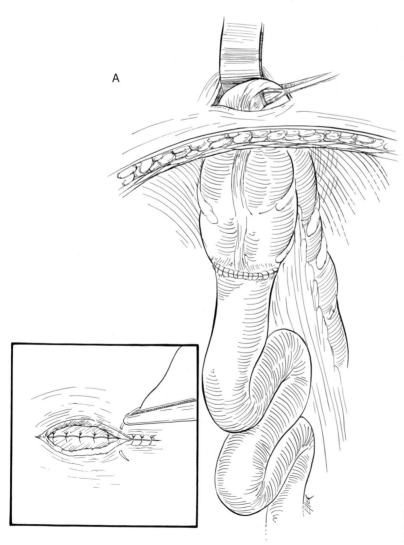

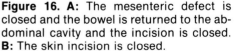

Figure 16. A: The mesenteric defect is closed and the bowel is returned to the abdominal cavity and the incision is closed. **B:** The skin incision is closed.

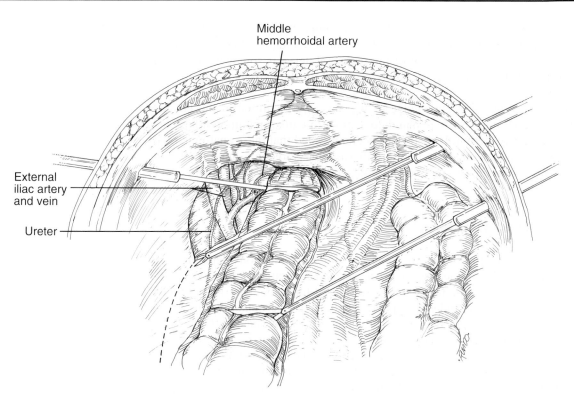

Figure 2. Anatomic landmarks in the early low anterior resection. Colon displaced medially.

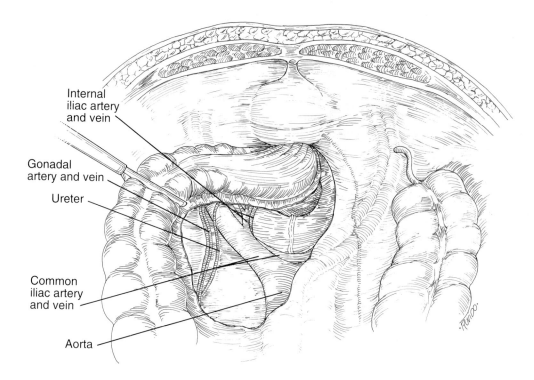

Figure 3. Anatomic landmarks in the early low anterior resection. Colon displaced laterally.

resection into the area of the rectum, and resultant dissection needed for completion of the procedure.

The workup for a patient being considered for a laparoscopic low anterior resection is virtually the same as that for a patient being considered for an open procedure. However, we believe several tests are mandatory, especially (a) colonoscopy, to identify the exact location and extent of the lesion and to clear the remainder of the colon of polyps, and (b) rigid proctoscopy to more accurately access the location of the tumor, so that one can determine exactly how low the resection must be. A barium enema is almost always added to the workup to evaluate colon redundancy and anatomy. We frequently add a CT scan to the workup to rule out ureteral obstruction as well as potentially discover the presence of metastatic disease in the pelvic and periaortic lymph nodes or in the liver. A very specific history and physical examination with particular regard to cardiac status and prior abdominal surgery should be obtained. The clinical presentation is usually for obstruction, bleeding, tenesmus or a palpable rectal mass by digital examination. Usually this operation should be performed electively with an adequate bowel preparation. However, as one gains experience with this procedure, it can be performed safely in acute situations where a Hartmann's pouch and/or diverting colostomy are performed.

Patient Selection

Although early in our series we had a great number of exclusionary factors, over the past $2\frac{1}{2}$ years we have practiced no specific patient selection other than attention to the presence of other disease processes that might interfere with a laparoscopic colon resection. In particular, we have considered large tortuous aorta, large aortic and/or iliac aneurysms, extensive malignant disease, and the potential for multiple adhesions secondary to prior inflammatory processes or prior operations to be relative contraindications, which to some extent, influenced patient selection. Ideally, the patient who has an increased chance of bleeding secondary to preexisting liver disease and portal hypertension should not be considered for laparoscopic low anterior resections. The ideal patient, of course, is the thin patient with benign disease, no prior operations, and no contraindications for general anesthesia. At the present time, however, the only patients we exclude from laparoscopic low anterior resection are those in whom general anesthesia is considered to be an exorbitant risk, although, with the current high level of anesthesia, this number is continually dwindling.

Indications

Currently, we feel all colonic pathology, especially benign disease, including adenomatous polyps, diverticular disease, prior diverticulitis (complicated and uncomplicated), and closure of ostomies requiring additional resection of the lower portion of the colon, are candidates for laparoscopic low anterior resections.

Procedures regarding carcinoma are controversial. Our current recommendations are as follows: The patient should be fully informed of the procedure under consideration and the lack of a randomized, prospective study; individual hospital and institutional review board approval, including the department of surgery, should be obtained before undertaking laparoscopic low anterior resections for carcinoma; meticulous records must be kept, including the patient's presentation, hospital course, and progress, as well as the results of procedures performed and the outcome, and this information should be placed in one of the ongoing nationwide studies or a local study which will be published.

All patients with colonic pathology of any type are currently included as candidates for laparoscopic low anterior resections for benign and malignant disease;

the indications for this procedure are the same as those for open low anterior colon resections.

Contraindications

Contraindications can be divided into two distinct groups: absolute and relative. We believe there are no absolute contraindications to laparoscopic low anterior resections at this time. Disease processes considered as relative contraindications are severe liver disease with portal hypertension or massive hepatosplenomegaly and/or bleeding dyscrasias (Fig. 4). These disease processes tend to cause increased bleeding that may be difficult to control and/or make the operation dangerously long and tedious. The presence of a large abdominal aortic aneurysm and/or biiliac aneurysms can also make the resection extremely difficult. Patients with an inability to tolerate general anesthesia and/or a change in position, such as in cases of severe advanced pulmonary disease and massive preexistent edema of the head and face, should be strongly considered for a different type of therapy. Relative contraindications also include multiple severe adhesions such as seen in patients with multiple prior operations, severe inflammatory processes in the past, and prior abscesses, particularly in the pelvis. While we seriously consider these relative contraindications, it is our feeling that the patient could be evaluated laparoscopically, and if the adhesions are so severe that no progress can be made after a preset period of time, then conversion to an open procedure can be undertaken. Advanced carcinoma with adjacent organ involvement, such as the bladder and/or multiple loops of bowel, should also be considered a relative contraindication to laparoscopic low anterior resection, and these patients would be candidates for alternative therapy. A frozen pelvis, particularly with carcinoma is another relative contraindication. Prior radiation therapy, although not a complete contraindication, should alert the would-be laparoscopic surgeon to the possibility of bleeding and/or adhesions, which may be so massive as to necessitate conversion to an open procedure.

Inflammatory bowel disease, especially in the acute phase, presents a situation that can be evaluated laparoscopically, but only if there is a very low tolerance for conversion to an open procedure, as a thinned wall can rupture quite easily

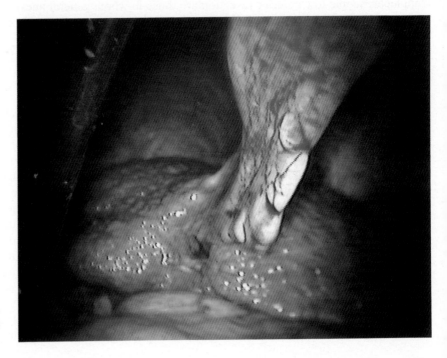

Figure 4. Cirrhosis of the liver, a relative contraindication to laparoscopic colon resection.

and extremely thickened bowel and mesentery are difficult situations to handle laparoscopically.

An additional area of relative contraindication would be a patient's or surgeon's unwillingness to enter the patient into an ongoing study. This is a philosophical point; however, it is my strong contention that any patient undergoing laparoscopic surgery should be entered into a local or a nationwide study in order to share the experience and aid in delineation of indications and contraindications as well as outcome in this new approach to lower colonic pathology.

Also very high on the list of relative contraindications is the surgeon's experience. The novice would-be laparoscopic colonic resectionist would be well advised to avoid an extremely difficult low anterior resection, as these particular procedures are indeed more difficult than perhaps some simpler procedures such as a right hemicolectomy, or even a laparoscopically assisted sigmoid colon resection.

▼ INTRAOPERATIVE MANAGEMENT/SURGICAL TECHNIQUE

Patient Positioning

It is imperative to have an acceptable patient, to very carefully plan a laparoscopic low anterior resection, and to position the patient properly. There must undoubtedly be anal access, and the position we have found to be most advantageous is with the patient's buttocks at the edge of the operating table with the end flap completely retracted or removed. The legs can be extended by Allen or Lloyd-Davis stirrups, depending on the preference of the individual surgeon. It

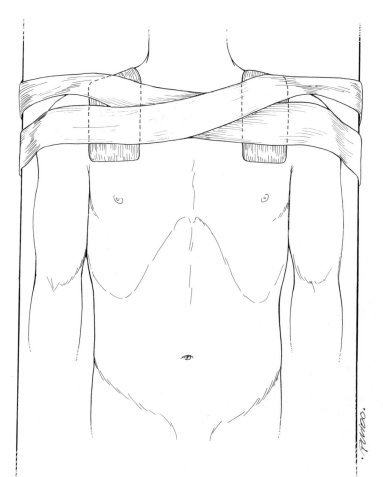

Figure 5. Taping of the shoulders.

of laparoscopic instruments were interchanged and CO_2 use was high. Anesthesia considerations are of prime interest in that these patients accumulate CO_2 when the retroperitoneal space is opened and CO_2 absorption is increased through the tissues in this area at a greater rate than the intact peritoneum alone. Therefore, the anesthesiologist should be aware of this potential problem and begin hyperventilation with a more rapid removal of CO_2 at an earlier point in the surgery rather than waiting for secondary evidence of hypercapnia to develop, by which time it may be too late to correct the situation.

Irrigation fluid utilized is primarily that of genitourinary (1,000 ml of normal saline to which is added 100,000 U of polymyxin B, 1 g of neomycin), irrigant to which is added 7,500 U/l of heparin.

All our procedures are performed totally intracorporeally with intraoperative colonoscopy to check margins and ensure cleanliness of the colon as well as adequacy of the bowel preparation. We irrigate with Betadine solution intraluminally routinely and check the integrity of the anastomosis. Our primary variation with other authors is that of a completely intracorporeal technique with mobilization, vascular control, resection, and anastomosis, all done on the inside as well as transanal removal of the specimen in approximately 75% to 85% of the cases. Additionally, we now bag virtually 100% of the specimens on a routine basis regardless of the disease process (i.e., benign or malignant).

We use a dedicated camera holder, and cannula placement is essentially as illustrated in Figure 8. The cannula placement is variable from patient to patient,

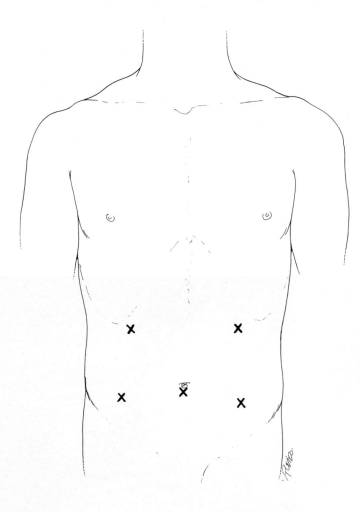

Figure 8. Cannula placement.   **X** 10 mm

depending on the body habitus as well as the location of the disease process. Generally speaking, we like to use five ports, all of which are the 10-mm type ports. These ports are placed at the umbilicus; if the patient has had prior surgery an alternative site is used initially until adhesions can be cleaned from the subumbilical area. Additional ports are placed approximately lateral to the umbilicus on the right and left, and approximately at McBurney's point on the abdominal wall, again depending on the habitus of the patient. If the patient is very tall, the ports are moved caudally. If the patient is very small, the ports are moved cephalad in order to accommodate the instrumentation and avoid clashing of instruments during the procedure. A general rule of thumb is to keep the port sites approximately one handbreath apart, which aids greatly in avoiding outside instrument clashing. Instruments should be laid alongside the proposed site to the anticipated lower edge of the dissection in order to ensure adequate length of the instruments with a given proposed port site to perform the procedure.

Preparation of the patient for surgery is perhaps as demanding as the actual surgery itself. This includes proper positioning of the patient on the table to allow adequate anal access, proper padding of all exposed areas to prevent nerve damage due to prolonged procedures, proper draping to avoid finger and exposed surfaces contact with the metal table. Arms should be strapped at the patient's side to allow freedom of movement around the shoulders. Additionally, it is important to exercise temperature maintenance mechanisms such as a plastic bag on exposed extremities, which we have found will result in conservation of at least 1 degree of body temperature loss over a 2-hour procedure compared with not bagging the extremities. We routinely use sequential compression devices on the lower extremities and have completely avoided thrombophlebitis with this maneuver. We have found that a gynecologic drape, which allows anal access with a flap mechanism, is also advantageous compared with routine open draping. The operative opening of the drape over the abdominal cavity is usually expanded to allow access to the anterior abdominal wall. Care must be taken in placing camera lines, light source lines, and insufflator lines, to allow adequate movement of the foot portion of the table as the patient is placed in steep Trendelenburg position and turned side to side. Longer light cords are advisable. Monitors must be placed relatively close to the patient's feet on each side, but leaving adequate room for movement of the patient or the table. We have found very distinct advantages to using two separate monitors, one for the surgeon and one for the assistant surgeon.

After satisfactory general endotracheal anesthesia has been administered, central lines are placed as needed, arterial lines placed as needed, and temperature monitoring devices as well as capneograph placed in 100% of the patients. Insufflation of the abdominal cavity can be carried out in a number of ways, but we have preferred the Veress-type needle insertion, and have been extremely successful without injury to underlying organs by following a few simple rules. If a patient has had no prior surgery, the umbilicus is used for the initial needle insertion site. If the patient has had prior surgery of any kind, an alternative site is used, preferably in the left upper quadrant or the right upper quadrant, well away from any prior surgery sites. While this method is not foolproof, we feel the degree of safety afforded with this method, particularly with judicious placement of the Veress needle, and gaining a sense of feel of the needle as it passes through the layers of the abdominal wall is a superior method to that of the Hasson technique. When placing the Veress needle, however, the liver or spleen must be carefully palpated to avoid injury with the initial insertion of the Veress needle. Immediately after insufflation is accomplished, the cannulae are placed as previously outlined (Fig. 8). We have routinely used Marcaine injections before placement of incisions for cannulae as this seems to diminish postoperative pain. Often the initial step in the procedure, particularly in low anterior resection for carcinoma is to ascertain the presence of metastasis in the liver. We have found that the CT scan, while helpful in many conditions, frequently will fail to detect smaller lesions on the surface of

Fig. 3). Dissecting the anterior peritoneum as the final portion of the low rectal dissection has had a distinct advantage in avoiding drip and rundown from this area, which would cloud the remainder of the dissection. Additionally, the dissection is much easier when the dissection planes have already been developed posteriorly. Thus, we incise the peritoneum and perform the anterior dissection after the entire posterior and lateral dissection has been completed. After completion of the pelvic portion of the dissection and establishment of an adequate distal margin, our next maneuver is to clean the colon distally, at the predetermined lower margin of the resection circumferentially, starting from the posterior and working anteriorly. Almost invariably the superior sacral artery is identified and should be doubly clipped, proximally and distally, and then divided. We have found that partial division of any vessel initially is much better than complete transection with the first incision, as additional branches may be present, and it is much easier to secure this vessel partially transected rather than completely divided. The superior hemorrhoidal vein is also readily identified in this area, is dissected free from surrounding posterial rectal fat, and divided as well.

Care must be taken to clean the colon circumferentially in order to allow placement of a linear stapling device such as an Endo-GIA 60. After completion of this portion of the dissection, usually the common iliac arteries can be readily identified and can be traced proximally to the bifurcation of the aorta by careful blunt dissection. Immediately above the bifurcation of the aorta the inferior mesenteric artery can be identified in most patients. We generally perform slow, meticulous blunt dissection in this area, using blunt unopened instruments and/or 10-mm scissors with virtually no cutting but only spreading maneuvers. The inferior mesenteric artery can then be encircled and either clipped or divided with an Endo-GIA stapler or ligated. We prefer ligation of this vessel, similar to what we have usually accomplished with open procedures. We use an extracorporeal tie for this procedure in the following manner: The inferior mesenteric artery is separated from the surrounding tissue; we have found that a curved dissector is most advantageous for this (Fig. 15). A suture of 40 in. or more is then brought through the superior cephalad trocar, looped around the vessel and an extracorporeal knot (Westin knot, developed in conjunction with our laboratories) is then constructed and

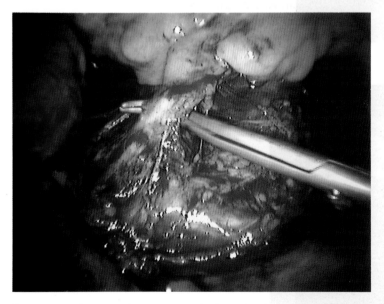

Figure 15. Curved dissector encircling the inferior mesenteric artery.

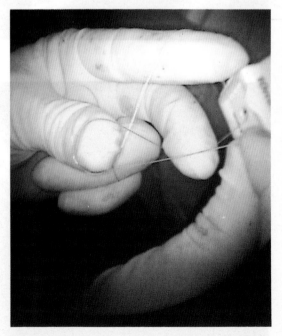

Figure 16. Extracorporeal tie for ligation of large artery.

tightened around the vessel (Figs. 16 and 17). A second intracorporeal throw is added for additional security.

A second technique utilizes a new device—laparoscopic Bulldog clamps (Fig. 18)—and entails dissecting the vessel free, placing Bulldog clamps proximally and distally, dividing the vessel, then placing a pretied loop over the vessel. While this seems a bit clumsy at first, with minimal practice this becomes quite easy, taking less than 2 minutes to complete.

After division of the inferior mesenteric artery and complete control of the bleeding, dissection is then carried out adjacent to the artery until the inferior mesenteric vein has been identified (Fig. 19). Care should be taken here to avoid injury to the left ureter which is immediately adjacent to vessels laterally. When dealing with cancer, the inferior mesenteric vein is then dissected free until it is found to disappear under the ligament of Treitz. Here a ligation is carried out, usually with multiple clips, with a minimum of two being applied on the proximal side and frequently a pretied loop applied over a Glassman clamp or clips on the

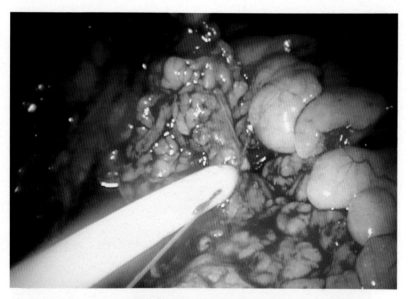

Figure 17. Knot tightened.

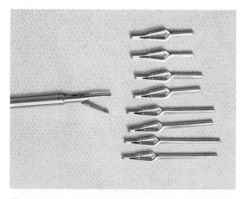

Figure 18. Laparoscopic bulldog clamps.

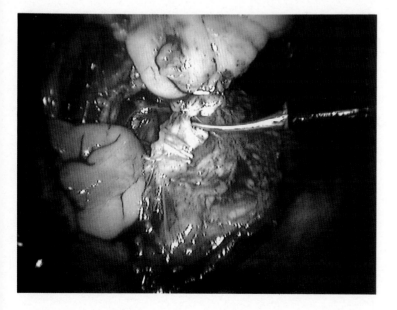

Figure 19. Division of inferior mesenteric artery.

distal portion of the vessel (Fig. 20). The proximal line of colonic dissection should have been ascertained by colonoscopic examination and is now directly visualized. The colon is held distally with the left hand of the assistant, proximally with the right hand of the assistant, and holding the colon much like an open book, dissection is now carried out up to this point through the mesentery. Blunt dissection is preferred over sharply incising this area, as sharp division results in bleeding that is frequently very difficult to control. The marginal artery of Drummond will be divided and is extremely variable in location, often near the inferior mesenteric artery, often quite lateral, virtually next to the colon itself (Fig. 21). Careful dissection should be carried out in this area until the colon is reached, then a segment of at least 2 cm of colon should be circumferentially cleaned in order to facilitate the division of the colon and the subsequent anastomosis (Fig. 22).

After completion of the proximal portion of dissection, we have found it advantageous to place this portion of the colon into the pelvis to be sure adequate length is present. If adequate length is not present, this is the point where splenic flexure mobilization should be accomplished, and we feel it is better to complete this

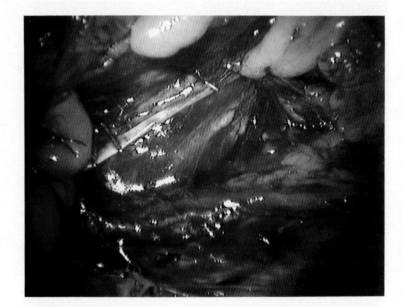

Figure 20. Inferior mesenteric artery ligated at ligament of Treitz.

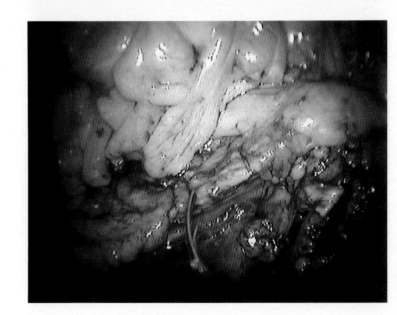

Figure 21. Marginal artery of Drummond clipped.

dissection now, before division of the colon. (It has been our routine to place the proximal line of resection deep into the pelvis to ensure adequate length without undue tension before division of the colon.)

If intraoperative colonoscopy has not been performed, this is a good opportunity to do so. The colonscope can be introduced after the colon has been occluded at least 6 cm above the proposed site of proximal division. The colonoscope is used to clearly define the margins of resection as well as to ensure cleanliness (Fig. 23). Intraluminal irrigation with Betadine solution is also routinely performed at this point unless the patient has a near-occluding carcinoma. Again, it must be emphasized that it is better to mobilize the colon first then perform colonoscopy rather than to do this in the reverse order.

Division of the colon can be accomplished in a variety of methods. I have preferentially chosen to use the KTP laser because of the resultant relatively blood-free field and a minimum of lateral tissue injury compared with standard cautery techniques. It is my understanding that newer cautery techniques, particularly with needle tips, will alleviate the extensive lateral injury, and perhaps this

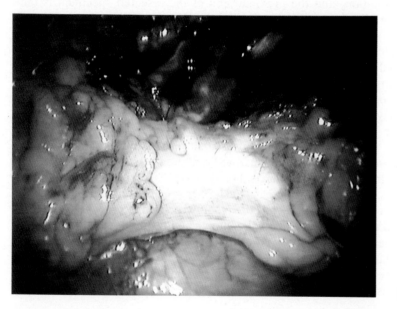

Figure 22. Proximal line of dissection cleaned.

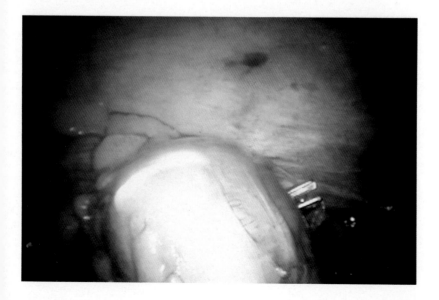

Figure 23. Colonoscopic examination of colon prior to division.

will indeed replace the laser (Fig. 24). Scissors can be used; however, this frequently results in a very bloody field, and it takes little to lose one's sense of direction and to perform an oblique transection—perhaps venturing into dangerous territory—rather than a straight transverse transection. Endo-GIA staplers can be used for division of the colon if the surgeon is willing to take down the line of staples and/or to do a laparoscopically assisted procedure where the proximal end of the colon is brought out and the anvil placed externally. Additional techniques for placement of the anvil can be used if a device is available for placing the anvil above the proposed line of resection with a suture being left attached, which then allows freeing the pointed end of the anvil through the side wall of the colon. A variety of techniques can be used for securing the proximal portion of the colon, and/or division of the same, and each laparoscopic surgeon will determine the best technique for his own use. We have performed intracorporeal anastomosis on all of our patients and feel this is a very acceptable way of completing this technique. The laparoscopic Bulldog Glassman clamp is left in place during the division of the colon to prevent proximal rundown of uncontrolled intracolonic material (Figs. 11A and 18). The cut edges of the colon are irrigated thoroughly with Betadine solution, and the proximal end of the resected specimen is then closed with a pretied loop in order to alleviate the possibility of tumor/bowel spillage. Attention is then turned to the distal line of resection where a division is made in much the same manner after adequate proximal tension on the colon has been applied. Again the laser is used in this area and has been used as low as 4 to 5 cm. Angulation is a problem much below this point unless a laser tip is used that can be turned 70 to 90 degrees. After very low division of the colon, CO_2 leakage may occur through the rectum, although if a rectal stump has been left that is 5 cm or longer, this will collapse and prevent further loss. Ongoing CO_2 loss can be prevented by having an assistant place a moistened laparotomy pad at the rectum, virtually in the anus, and holding pressure in this area. The distal aspect of the resected specimen is then ligated with a pretied loop to prevent tumor spillage as well. A specimen bag is placed in the abdominal cavity, and the specimen is placed in the bag, which is then tightly secured to prevent inadvertent or unrecognized spillage of intraluminal contents and/or tumor cells. A judgment must then be made as to the most efficacious manner for removal of the tumor specimen. We have found that if the lower line of resection is below the pelvic brim and into the larger part of the rectum, approximately 75% of specimens can be removed transanally by slowly dilating the anus to at least 2 to 3 fingerbreaths

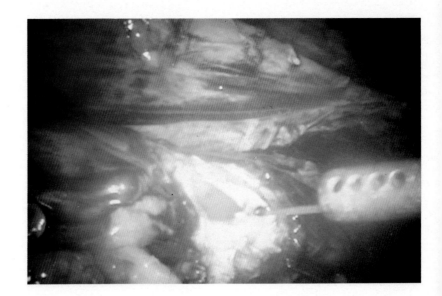

Figure 24. KTP laser division of colon: note blood-free field.

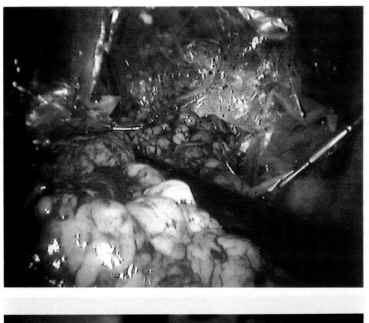

A

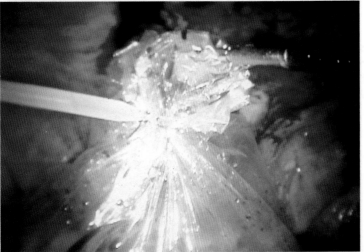

B

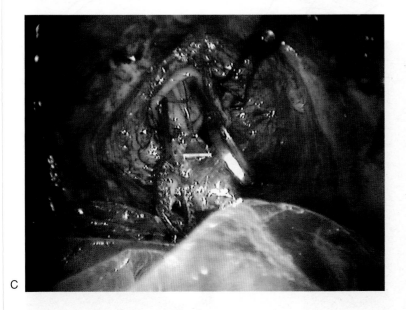

C

Figure 25. A: Bag open to receive specimen. **B:** Specimen bagged and Endo-loop applied. **C:** Bag being removed through rectum.

using 3-0 Vicryl or Polysorb suture or other suitable suturing materials (Fig. 32). The laparoscopic Bulldog Glassman clamp is left in place and serves to occlude the proximal colon to prevent its irretrievable distention. The entire area is then checked for bleeding, preferably with intraperitoneal pressure decreased, and a 10-mm Jackson-Pratt drain is placed in the pelvis, usually being brought out through the McBurney's Point port on the left side, and sutured into place. If the specimen has not been removed transanally, it is now removed through an old incision site, or from the infraumbilical incision as previously described. The specimen is removed much like that described for the transanal extraction procedure, and the fascia is then closed. The abdomen is reinsufflated, the entire dissected area is rechecked for additional bleeding, the area is irrigated thoroughly with 10% Betadine solution, followed by a saline solution to completely clear the area.

All port sites should now be irrigated with dilute Betadine solution or distilled water to remove debris as well as lessen the chance of tumor implantation in trocar sites, which has been reported but has not occurred in our series with proper techniques and precautions.

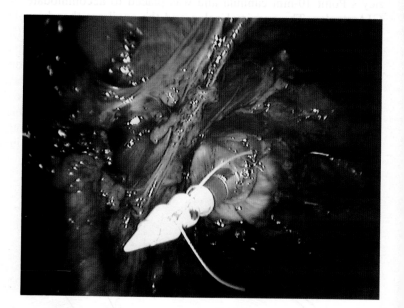

Figure 29. Spike through closed rectum.

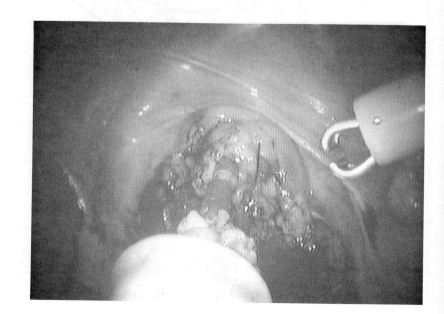

Figure 30. Anvil and head of stapler joined.

The individual ports should then be closed very meticulously to prevent postoperative Richter-type hernias. We have recently described a method of closing the ports wherein a Truecut needle is used to introduce a suture on one side of the port with the suture being left inside. The Truecut needle is then directed toward the opposite side of the cannula, and the suture is grasped and brought back out to the surface of the skin as a large U stitch (Fig. 33). All sutures are placed before removal of the cannula, then each cannula is removed under direct vision to check for bleeding, and the suture is tightened under direct vision except the last suture, which is tightened as the scope is withdrawn and the pneumoperitoneum has been evacuated. Using this technique we have completely avoided Richter's hernia in any case where 10-mm ports have been made. We feel very strongly that ports that are 10 mm or greater in diameter or any port in the midline of the linea alba should have a fascial closure.

It is our strong feeling that very low anterior anastomoses are best completed with at least a partial intracorporeal anastomosis because mobilization of an adequate amount of colon much below 12 cm to an anterior incision is virtually impos-

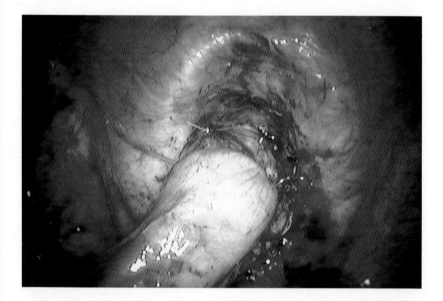

Figure 31. Completed anastomosis.

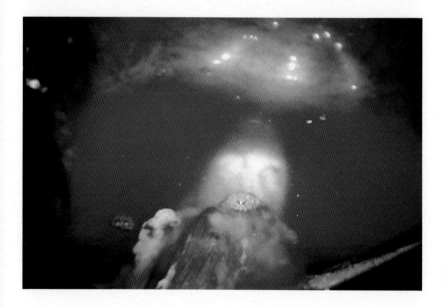

Figure 32. Colonoscopic testing of anastomosis.

Figure 33. Closure of cannula sites: **A:** Suture introduced. **B:** Fascial suture completed. **C:** Port site closed.

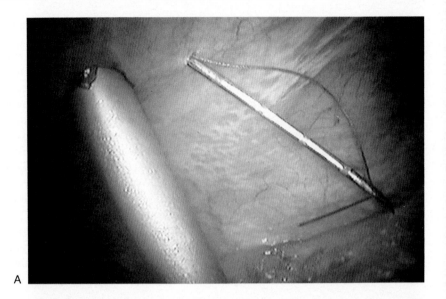

A

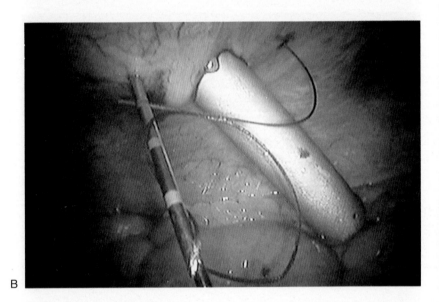

B

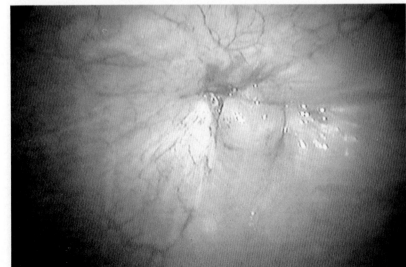

C

sible for a hand-sewn or stapled anastomosis performed extracorporeally. In this case, a totally intracorporeal technique can be used instead, or a laparoscopically assisted technique can also be used, as described above with the totally intracorporeal anastomosis.

▲ COMPLICATIONS

As with any type of surgery that entails removing tissues, taking tissues apart, and, most importantly, putting tissues back together, with the intent of healing, myriad complications can occur. The top five complications for laparoscopic low anterior resections are bleeding, hypothermia, small bowel injuries recognized and unrecognized, disorientation accompanied by ureteral injury, and anastomotic leaks.

Bleeding is most commonly caused by the following: inflammatory process, nonrecognition of vessels, poor control of vessels in the dissecting process, rough or excessive sharp dissection, and tearing of tissue by excessive force. Control of bleeding can best be accomplished by slow, meticulous dissection and control of each bleeding vessel at the time it begins to bleed. If one allows even capillary bleeding to proceed without complete control, as frequently occurs with small vessels in the open operative situation, laparoscopically this can snowball. Pooling of blood can obscure the field, and since clots are difficult to remove, this bleeding should not be allowed to proceed, but each individual vessel should be controlled with cautery, clips, or ligation as it appears. It is very important to identify the major vessels in the pelvis, as discussed earlier, and it is imperative to know the anatomy impeccably, and to avoid cutting a vessel unless it is totally controlled. We also advise very strongly not to divide vessels totally despite apparent good proximal and distal control, as retraction of the vessel will result in a very difficult situation in finding the cut ends of the vessel and controlling them on a second occasion should bleeding occur. We feel that excessive cautery should be avoided, particularly on unidentified vessels, as this can result in a partial tear of the vessel and in bleeding that would appear to be controlled at the time of surgery, only to open up and bleed at a later point when pressure is reduced. The argon beam coagulator can be used for diffuse oozing as frequently seen in the posterior pelvis and at the peritoneal incision sites, especially with a very large vascular pool in that area. However, care must be emphasized in identification of the ureter and avoiding use of the argon beam coagulator on top of the ureter. We feel it is important to ligate larger vessels and we use extracorporeal ties to accomplish this. We also use clips on smaller vessels (2–5 mm) and cautery on much smaller vessels (less than 2 mm). We consider the Endo-GIA stapler to be an excellent device for control of vessels, but cost seems prohibitive at the current time for its routine use on all mesentery vessels.

The second major complication is hypothermia, which very frequently occurs in prolonged laparoscopic procedures regardless of the type of procedure performed. The primary factor contributing to hypothermia in a patient undergoing a laparoscopic procedure is heat loss of the extremities. The extremity heat loss is best controlled by tucking the arms at the side of the patient and maintaining covering as much as possible with a Bair Hugger or heating device over the shoulders and head, and by covering the exposed extremities. The lower extremities are the most vulnerable to heat loss, and this can be controlled with plastic bags after sequential compression devices have been applied. Another source of heat loss is irrigation with unheated fluids, and we strongly advise preheating the fluids or running them through a heating solution such as a blood warmer. Heat loss can also be caused by cold insufflation gases of anesthesia, and this can be completely averted by using a warming device for these gases. One of the more obscure sources of heat loss is that of infusion of cold CO_2, into the abdominal cavity.

tions, than conventional open surgery; however, the well-being of the patient, the much smoother postoperative course with more rapid discharge from the hospital, and, for the most part, avoidance of complications, certainly make the slightly increased cost of the surgical procedure itself more than worthwhile. Extensive studies have been performed that show that—even with the higher cost of equipment at the time of surgery on the front end of the hospitalization—the diminished stay on the back end of hospitalization and the lack of complications in the hands of competent surgeons result in overall tremendous savings. Additionally, the diminution in pain and suffering by patients undergoing laparoscopic procedures and the faster return to full function are rarely factored into standard cost equations but is worth an incalculable amount to most patients.

The exact role of low anterior resection in the care of patients with carcinoma is yet to be determined, although preliminary studies seem to show that a comparable procedure is being performed and, in some instances, particularly with very low anterior resections where direct visualization of all anatomic plains and structures is possible, perhaps a better procedure is being performed laparoscopically.

RECOMMENDED READING

1. Franklin ME, Rosenthal D, Ramos R. Laparoscopic colectomy: utopia or reality. *Gastrointest Endosc Clin North Am* 1993;3:353–365.
2. Franklin ME, Ramos R, Rosenthal D, Schessler W. Laparoscopic colonic procedures. *World J Surg* 1993;17:51–56.
3. Phillips EM, Franklin ME, Carroll BJ, et al. Laparoscopic colectomy. *Am Surg* 1992;216:703–707.
4. Voyles CR, Tucker RD. Electric conductivity. Equipment design: equipment failure, equipment safety. Intraoperative complications. *Am J Surg* 1992;164(1):57–62.
5. Jacobs M, Verdeja JC, Goldstein HS. Minimally invasive colon resection (laparoscopic colectomy). *Surg Laparosc Endosc* 1991;1:144–150.

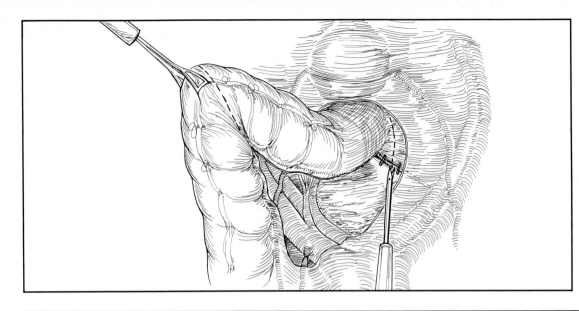

38

Abdominoperineal Resection

Bruce V. MacFadyen, Jr.
Arlene E. Ricardo
Department of Surgery
The University of Texas Medical School
Houston, Texas 77030

Barry A. Salky
Department of Surgery
Mt. Sinai Medical Center
New York, New York 10029

Operative Laparoscopy and Thoracoscopy, edited by
B. V. MacFadyen, Jr. and
J. L. Ponsky. Lippincott-Raven
Publishers, Philadelphia © 1996.

KEY WORDS

Anal Verge   Perineum

Colonoscopy   Rectum

Inferior Mesenteric Artery

Abdominoperineal resection, although becoming more and more infrequent because of the increasing technical abilities to perform low anterior anastomosis, is probably the best operation to perform laparoscopically because there are no abdominal incisions except the colostomy. As is true with any cancer operation, operative cancer principles must be maintained and the bowel and lymph node dissection must be equivalent to an open procedure. The belief that such dissection cannot be performed laparoscopically has led to much scepticism regarding this procedure for cancer. Before attempting resection in primary cancers, experience has been obtained in laparoscopic colectomies for benign disease and in palliative resections for cancer with unresectable metastases. During this time, efficient techniques for laparoscopic colectomy have been developed that are compatible with oncologic mesenteric resection. Preliminary results in regards to morbidity, mortality, local tumor recurrence, and survival are indicating similar outcomes with the laparoscopic technique when compared to the open procedure.

⬤ ANATOMY

The primary blood supply of the colon includes the ileocolic, the right colic, the middle colic, and the inferior mesenteric artery (Fig. 1). The middle colic artery divides into a right and left branch, which connects to the right colic and

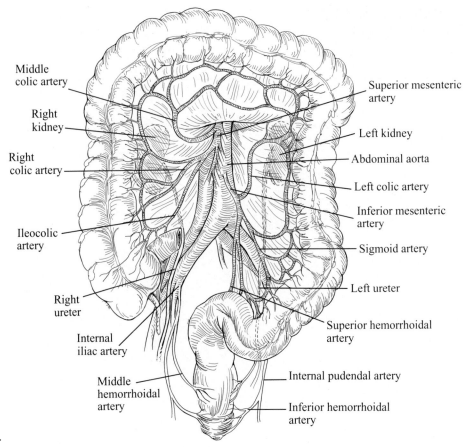

Figure 1. Blood supply to colon.

left colic arteries, respectively, via the marginal artery of Drummond. The inferior mesenteric artery bifurcates into the left colic artery, three to four sigmoid branches, and the superior hemorrhoidal artery, which supplies the upper rectum (Fig. 2). The middle and inferior hemorrhoidal arteries supply the middle and distal rectum and originate from the internal iliac arteries bilaterally, whereas the middle sacral artery from the distal aorta supplies the anterior surface of the rectum. The venous drainage corresponds to the arterial blood supply, and the lymphatic drainage parallels the blood vessels (Fig. 3). The number of lymph nodes resected

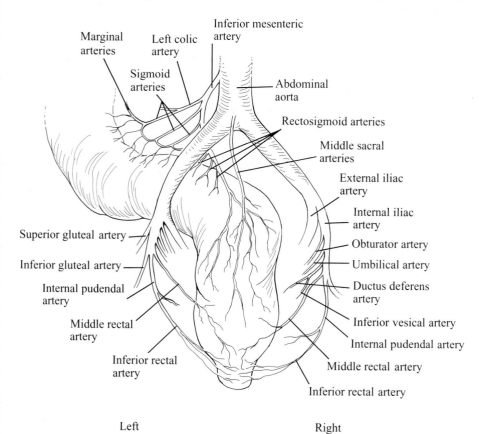

Left   Right

Posterior view

Figure 2. Blood supply to rectum

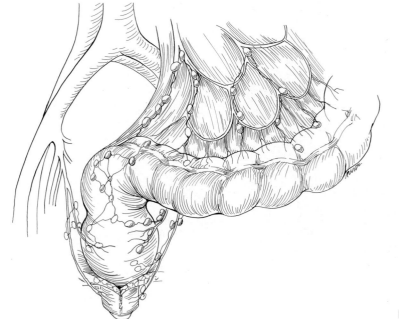

Figure 3. Colon lymphatics.

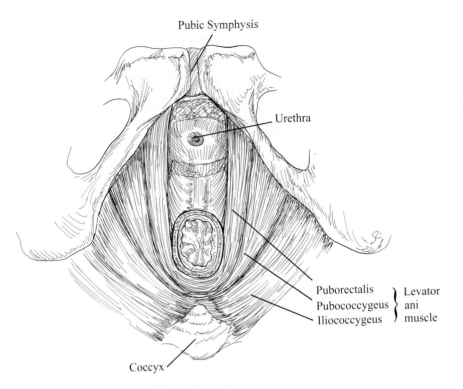

Figure 4. Rectum through levator.

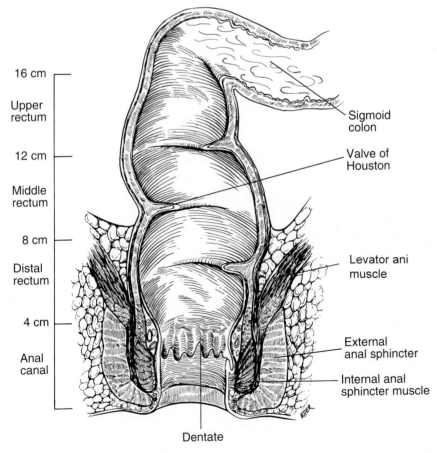

Figure 5. Dentate line.

in an abdominoperineal procedure is less than in other colon operations, and therefore resection of the rectum and surrounding tissue to the lateral pelvic side walls is important in order to ensure an adequate cancer operation.

The rectum penetrates the muscles of the levator ani approximately 5 cm from the anal verge at the level of the anorectal ring (Fig. 4). The rectal mucosa is composed of columnar cells which transitions to squamous mucosa at the dentate line approximately 2.5 cm from the anal verge (Fig. 5). The entire rectum is 15 to 17 cm long and has three valves within its lumen. The superior rectal valve is located at 11 to 13 cm from the anal verge, middle rectal valve is 8 to 9 cm from the anal verge, and the inferior rectal valve is at 5 to 6 cm from the anal verge (Fig. 5). The sphincteric muscle mechanism around the distal rectum is illustrated in Fig. 5 and is not important in this procedure, whereas preserving these sphincter muscles is important when a low anterior rectal resection is performed.

In the posterior dissection of the rectum, the surgeon must stay in the plane of the presacral space. The dissection below the presacral fascia can result in

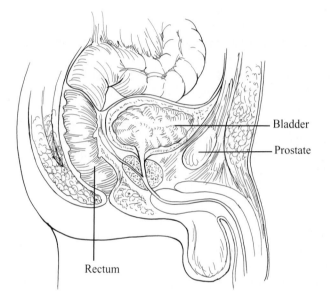

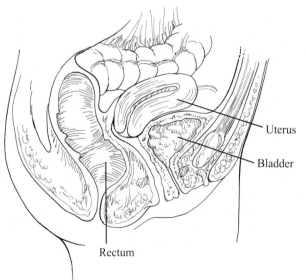

Figure 6. Anterior anatomy.

significant hemorrhage from the plexus of small veins and arteries in this region. The anatomic course of the ureter in the pelvis is illustrated in Figure 1. The ureters consistently cross the bifurcation of the common iliac arteries and descend into the pelvis along the lateral pelvic side walls and then enter the bladder in the posterior lateral and inferior section. Bilateral identification of the ureters is essential during the abdominoperineal resection.

The surgeon should also be familiar with the anatomy anterior to the rectum to avoid injury to the bladder in males and the uterus in females (Fig. 6). Since the sigmoid colostomy should be placed in the lower left rectus muscle, knowledge of the anatomy of this region and the inferior epigastric vessels is important.

▶ PREOPERATIVE PLANNING

Abdominoperineal resection is usually reserved for patients with cancers located less than 5 cm from the anal verge. Lesions which are above this region can usually be removed by a laparoscopic low anterior resection and colorectal or colo-anal anastomosis. However, when anal incontinence occurs as a result of the necessary cancer operation, abdominoperineal resection is the procedure of choice rather than a low anterior resection.

A relative contraindication may include those patients with dense pelvic adhesions due to previous colonic surgery in the area of the rectosigmoid colon. In addition, previous pelvic radiation therapy may also lead to dense adhesions and friable tissue which will increase the likelihood of conversion to open surgery. Another relative contraindication is liver cirrhosis with portal hypertension since portocaval shunting, especially in the area of the rectum, will be significantly increased thus potentially causing excessive bleeding. Morbid obesity may also make pelvic dissection more difficult. Standard diagnostic evaluations include computed tomography (CT) scans of the abdomen and pelvis, chest radiograph, serum CEA and C-125 levels, along with standard hematologic and chemistry studies. An intravenous pyelogram may be considered if there is any question regarding the normal position of the ureters.

Colonoscopy should be performed to more accurately assess tumor size and location as well as make the pathologic diagnosis. In addition, colonoscopy can be used to rule out other intrinsic colon lesions. If colon polyps are observed, they should be removed and evaluated preoperatively. If other tumors are noted, tissue diagnosis should be obtained, as their result may alter the chosen procedure. If the colon cannot be completely evaluated with colonoscopy, a barium enema can be used secondarily to assess anatomy and other lesions.

Since most patients undergoing this procedure are being treated for cancer, an extensive evaluation is important to rule out the possibility of preoperative metastatic disease. If the rectal tumor is large, preoperative radiation therapy and chemotherapy may be beneficial. These modalities may decrease tumor size and make a potentially inoperative patient into an operative candidate, and may also decrease the likelihood of local recurrence after the abdominoperineal resection. In addition, some patients may also become amenable to low anterior resection and thus avoid the sigmoid colostomy associated with abdominoperineal resection.

The bacterial content of the bowel can be greatly minimized by placing the patient on a clear liquid diet for 24 hours prior to surgery. In addition, a full bowel preparation should be administered utilizing 4 L of ethylene glycol and standard oral antibiotics. A bisacodyl suppository and 2 bisacodyl tablets after the colonic cleansing help to evacuate the small and large bowel so that there is very little small or large bowel gas. Preoperative colostomy site selection and teaching are important, and the site should be marked with indelible ink the night before surgery.

▼ INTRAOPERATIVE MANAGEMENT/SURGICAL TECHNIQUE

The patient is placed in a modified lithotomy position with the thighs slightly flexed. It is important to keep the thighs in a more parallel position, so movement of the laparoscopic instruments is not impaired (Fig. 7). The perineum is placed just off the end of the operating room table to provide access for the resection. A Foley catheter and Venodyne boots are placed routinely as is an orogastric tube. Nitrous oxide is not utilized by the anesthesiologist to minimize bowel distention. While I prefer operating from the left side of the table with the assistant on the right, the reverse is just as comfortable.

Access to the abdominal cavity is begun at the infraumbilical fold using a Veress needle approach. Open Hassan insertion is another option depending on the routine of the surgeon. I prefer the use of a 45-degree telescope, but less angled scopes are adequate. A 0-degree laparoscope does not provide the proper perspective of the anatomy, because the important anatomic landmarks (ureter, iliac vessels) are seen in a parallel fashion, and therefore, its use is not recommended. Figure 8 demonstrates the size and location of the other trocar sites in the performance of an abdominoperineal resection. The 18-mm trocar should be placed in the midrectus muscle as this is where the colostomy will be matured.

The view of the pelvic anatomy as seen through the 45-degree laparoscope is superior (Fig. 9). A thorough exploration of the abdominal cavity is commenced before any dissection. Retraction sutures are placed extracorporelly on both sides of the anterior pelvic peritoneum to aid in the exposure of the pelvic structures (Fig. 10). With the assistant elevating the sigmoid colon, the superior hemorrhoidal vessels are identified at their base. Using the two-handed technique, the peritoneum over the blood vessels is divided, and the vessels are dissected until a large

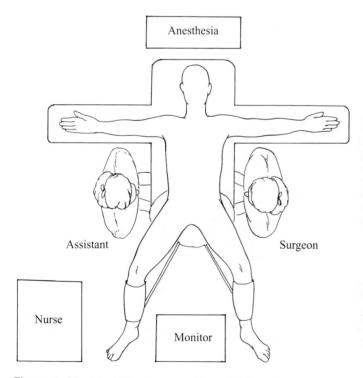

Figure 7. Modified lithotomy position with legs in a more parallel position and operating room setup.

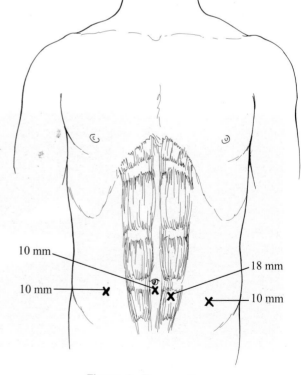

Figure 8. Trocar sites.

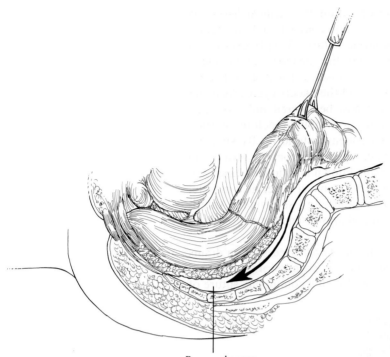

Figure 20. Posterior dissection in the presacral space.

Presacral space

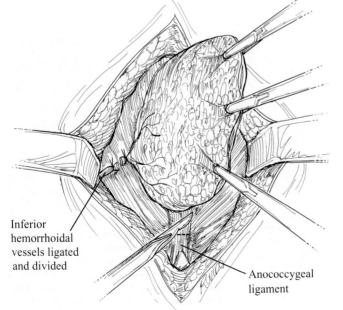

Inferior hemorrhoidal vessels ligated and divided

Anococcygeal ligament

Figure 21. The inferior hemorrhoidal vessels are ligated and divided, and the anococcygeal ligament is divided.

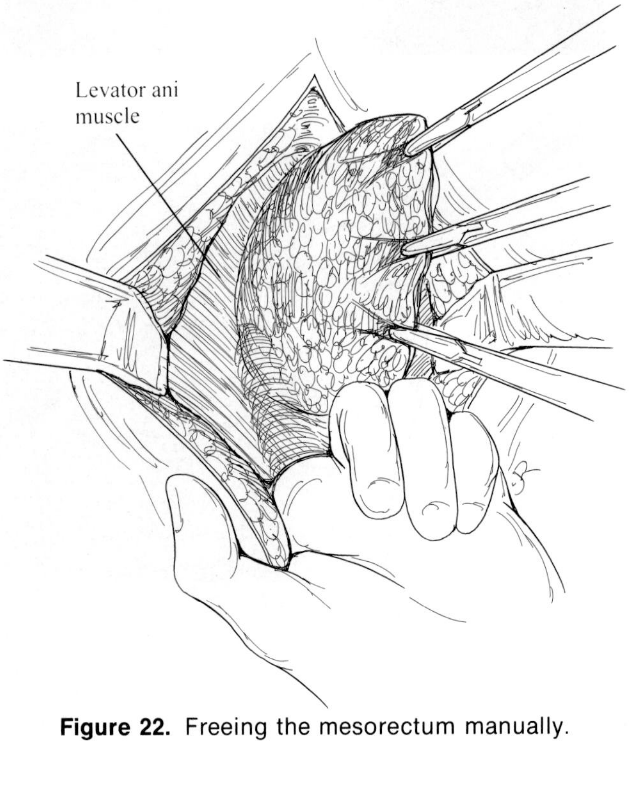

Levator ani muscle

Figure 22. Freeing the mesorectum manually.

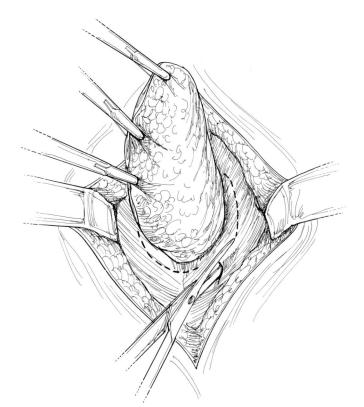

Figure 23. Dividing the levator ani muscles.

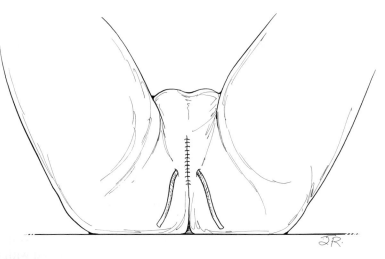

Figure 24. Closure of the peineum.

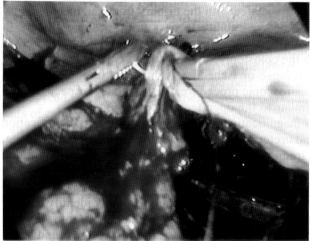

Figure 25. The pelvic peritoneum is closed with a running suture of 2-0 Vicryl. All ties are placed intracorporeally. A closed suction drain is seen in the rectal space which is passed for the perineum.

2. Decanini C, Milsom JW, Bohm B, Fazio VW. Laparoscopic oncologic abdominoperineal resection. *Dis Colon Rectum* 1994;37:552–558.
3. Chindasub S, Charntaracharmnong C, Nimitvanit C, Akkaranurukul P, Santitarmmanon B. Laparoscopic abdominoperineal resection. *J Laparoendosc Surg* 1994;4:17–21.
4. Larach SW, Salomon MC, Williamson PR, Goldstein E. Laparoscopic assisted abdominoperineal resection. *Surg Laparosc Endosc* 1993;3:115–118.
5. Sackier JM, Berci G, Hiatt JR, Hartunian S. Laparoscopic abdominoperineal resection of the rectum. *Br J Surg* 1992;79:1207–1208.
6. Pollard AO, Nivatvongs S, Rojanasakul A, Ilstrup DM. Carcinoma of the rectum: profiles of intraoperative and early postoperative complications. *Dis Colon Rectum* 1994;37:866–874.
7. Petrelli NJ, Nagel S, Rodriquez-Bigas M, Piedmonte M, Herrera L. Morbidity and mortality following abdominoperineal resection for rectal adenocarcinoma. *Am Surg* 1993;59:400–404.

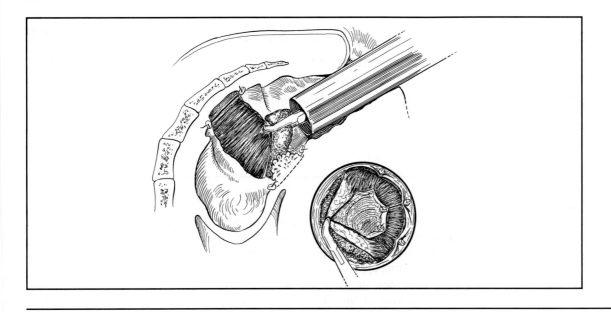

39

Endoluminal Rectal Surgery

Lee E. Smith
Department of Surgery
George Washington University
Washington, DC 20037

Operative Laparoscopy and Thoracoscopy, edited by
B. V. MacFadyen, Jr. and
J. L. Ponsky. Lippincott-Raven
Publishers, Philadelphia © 1996.

A special gas insufflation machine, similar to that used in laparoscopic surgery, is employed (Fig. 4), which insufflates carbon dioxide up to 6 l/min. Hence exposure can be maintained even in the upper rectum. Usually the pressure is maintained at the 15 mmHg. The pressure is constantly monitored and is increased or decreased depending on the desired pressure. A special suction device is used in concert with the insufflation machine so that its suction power is less than that of the insufflation pressure; hence suction can occur without completely depleting the carbon dioxide atmosphere holding the exposure. An electrocautery and light source are other essential parts of the system.

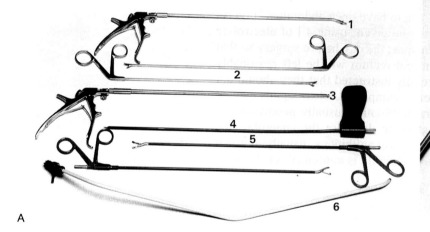

A

C

Figure 3. A: Transanal endoscopic microsurgery (TEM) instruments: *1*, needle holder; *2*, right- and left-angled scissors; **3,** clip applier; *4*, electric knife; *5*, angled forceps; *6*, suction-irrigation probe. **B:** The tips of the TEM instruments: *1*, electric knife; *2*, right- and left-angled forceps; *3*, suction-irrigation probe tip; *4*, left- and right-angled scissors; *5*, needle holder; *6*, clip applier. **C:** Electrified instruments: *1*, forceps; *2*, suction-irrigation probe; *3*, electrified knife.

muscle rel
attached to
6B). The w
tin arm) ca
can be cla
the procto

A

B

Anesthesia

General or regional anesthesia may be administered. The position of the patient needs to be decided in advance so that the anesthesiologist may modify the type of anesthesia depending on whether or not it is deemed safer to be under general anesthesia.

Patient Position at Surgery

The patient is positioned such that the center of the tumor is directly down toward the operating table. The patient may be placed in the prone jackknife, left lateral, right lateral, or lithotomy positions. The hips must be acutely flexed regardless of positions. The most difficult position to work in is in the knee-chest position because the hips must be flexed to right angles and the legs spread so that the operator can sit closely up toward the buttocks where the operating procto-scope projects and lean over the proctoscope to use the operating microscope. For large lesions the surgeon must be prepared to make frequent changes in the scope orientation to allow better access to the tumor. The portion of the tumor that is being operated on should be placed in the middle of the field. Achieving the optimal position may require a combination of shifting the scope, turning the patient, or shifting the surgeon. When the scope or patient cannot be turned adequately to keep the working field centered under the microscope, sometimes it is necessary to remove the face plate and to perform a portion of the procedure under direct vision.

Operative Techniques

The circulating nurse and the scrub nurse should be introduced to the equip-ment ahead of time so that the surgeon does not have to explain their jobs during the surgery.

The back table is prepared as if to have an abdominal operation. The abdominal operative field is draped over, and the anus is left uncovered because the anal area is the site of proposed surgery; the rectum is inspected with a sigmoidoscope for cleanliness; it is usually washed out with dilute povidone-iodine solution. A

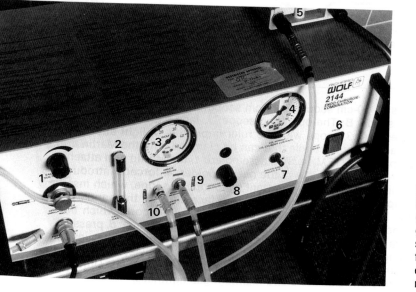

Figure 4. The insufflation-suction-irriga-tion machine: *1,* irrigation regulator; *2,* gas flow indicator; *3,* gauge for pressure generated; *4,* tank volume indicator; *5,* suction pump; *6,* power switch; *7,* gas flow switch; *8,* gas flow rate knob; *9,* gas outflow port; *10,* port for gas pressure monitoring.

D

bands, together with the so-called haustra or sacculation coli and epiploic appendages, allow the surgeon to easily distinguish the large and small bowel.

The large bowel begins with the cecum at the ileocecal junction and transitions to the ascending colon. The ascending colon, as well as the descending colon, are usually retroperitoneal structures as a result of the embryologic posterior attachment of the mesentery with the formation of the peritoneal lateral reflection called the white line of Toldt. When mobilization of the colon is performed, the incision of this peritoneal reflection allows access to an avascular plane, which often results in bloodless dissection.

The transverse colon is a bridge between the ascending and descending colons, lies freely in the abdominal cavity because it is completely intraperitoneal, and is attached to the stomach by the gastrocolic ligament. The greater omentum is connected to the transverse colon and drops over the loops of small bowel.

The sigmoid colon is also completely intraperitoneal and mobile and runs from the base of the descending colon to the right and then inferiorly toward the sacrum where the rectum begins at the level of the sacral promontory. The upper portion of the rectum is intraperitoneal, whereas the distal end is completely extraperitoneal.

From a surgical point of view, it is important to define the relationship between the left and right colons and the respective ureters (Fig. 3). The ureter descends retroperitoneally on the psoas muscle and is crossed anteriorly by the gonadal vessels at the level of the aortic bifurcation. As it descends into the pelvis, the ureter crosses the bifurcation of the common iliac vessels as it divides into the external and internal iliac arteries. It then descends on the pelvic side wall reaching the bladder posteriorly and laterally.

The blood supply to the large bowel is comprised of both the superior and inferior mesenteric arteries (Fig. 2). The first major branch of the superior mesenteric artery is the middle colic artery, followed by the right colic artery, the ileocolic artery, and then the jejunal and ileal vascular arcades. These supply the proximal one-half to two-thirds of the transverse colon, ascending colon, cecum,

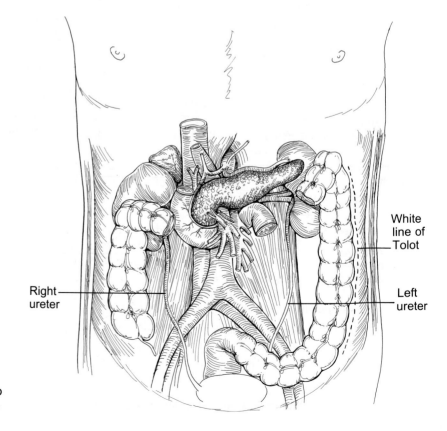

White
line of
Tolot

Right
ureter

Left
ureter

Figure 3. Course of ureter with relation to colon. Course of inferior mesenteric vein.

and small intestine, respectively. The inferior mesenteric artery gives rise to the left colic artery, sigmoid artery and branches, and the superior hemorrhoidal artery. These supply the distal one-half to two-thirds of the transverse colon, descending colon, sigmoid colon, and upper rectum. The anastomosis between the branches of all these arteries forms an arterial arcade in the mesentery close to the bowel wall and is known as the marginal artery of Drummond. The anastomosis between the left branch of the middle colic artery and the ascending branch of the left colic artery, known independently as the arc of Riolan, is absent in approximately 50% of the population, making the most distal portion of the transverse colon and the splenic fixture vulnerable to ischemia.

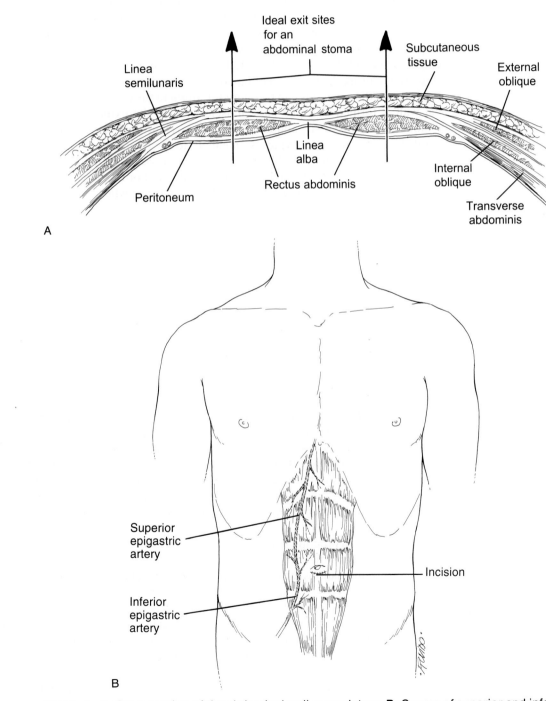

Figure 4. **A**: Cross section of the abdominal wall musculature. **B**: Course of superior and inferior epigastric arteries.

fashion. The pelvis is irrigated, hemostasis is obtained, and the perineum is closed. Next, the abdomen is reinsufflated and the stapled end of the sigmoid colon is grasped with a Babcock clamp inserted through the trocar in the lower left quadrant (Fig. 13). A 3- to 4-cm circular incision of skin around the trocar is performed. The trocar is removed and a 3- to 4-cm cruciate incision is made in the rectus sheath and muscle. The Babcock clamp is withdrawn from the abdomen pulling the sigmoid colon to the skin surface (Fig. 14). The colon serosa is secured to the rectus sheath, and the mucosa is then sutured to the skin. Careful visualization with the camera ensures the sigmoid colon is untwisted and tension-free.

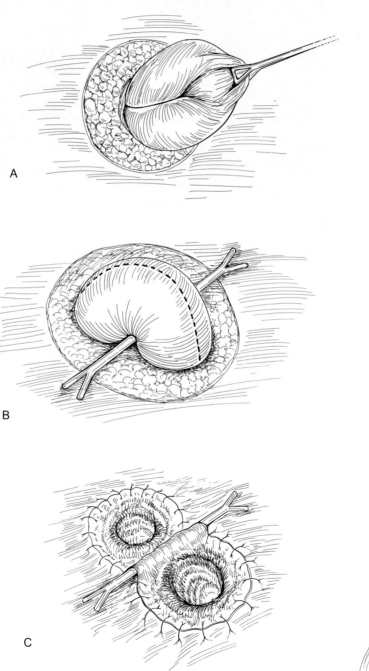

A

B

C

Figure 12. A: Loop ileostomy through the cruciate incision. **B**: Longitudinal incision. **C**: Sutured to skin anchored by bridge.

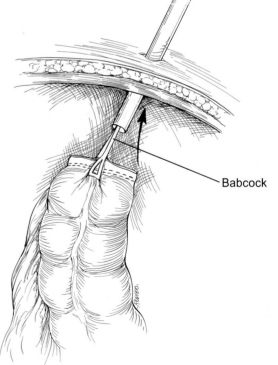

Babcock

Figure 13. Babcock grasping end sigmoid.

Loop Colostomy

The most common loop colostomies performed are in the transverse and sigmoid colons.

In preparing for a sigmoid loop colostomy, the patient is placed in the Trendelenburg position with the left side up, and the camera is inserted through a 10-mm periumbilical trocar. One 5-mm trocar is placed in the left upper quadrant, and possibly another 5-mm trocar is inserted in the right lower quadrant. A 10- to 12-mm trocar is inserted in the preselected stomal site in the left lower quadrant through the midportion of the rectus muscle (Figs. 8D and 15). Through the left lower quadrant port, the sigmoid colon is grasped with a Babcock clamp and elevated toward the anterior abdominal wall (Fig. 16). The left colon is mobilized as necessary along the white line of Toldt. A 3- to 5-cm circular piece of skin is excised around the left lower quadrant trocar and a 3- to 5-cm cruciate incision is made in the rectus fascia around the stomal port. The trocar and Babcock clamp are withdrawn from the abdomen, and the colon is exteriorized and secured with a plastic bridge between it and the skin, a longitudinal colotomy is made in the taenia coli and the colostomy is matured (Fig. 17). Reinsufflation allows for careful visualization with the camera to ensure that the colon is tension-free and untwisted. Following this procedure, the trocars are removed and the wounds are closed in a standard fashion.

For a laparoscopic transverse loop colostomy, a right upper quadrant 5-mm trocar is inserted with a 10- to 12-mm trocar at the preselected stomal site in the midportion of the left or right upper rectus abdominus muscle. A 10-mm periumbilical trocar is used for the camera (Fig. 8E). Through the right upper quadrant

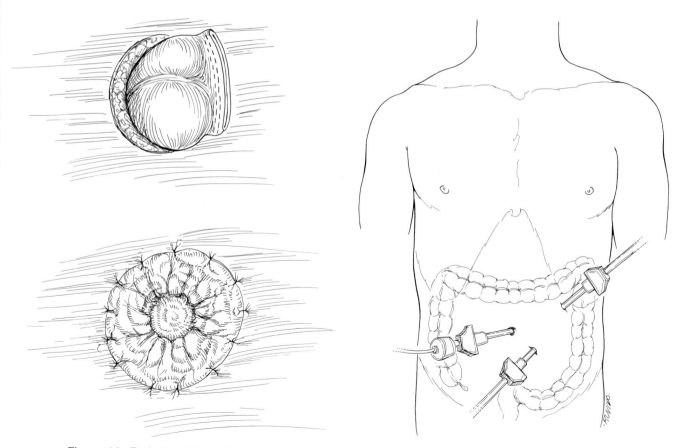

Figure 14. End sigmoid at skin surface.   **Figure 15.** Trocar site for loop sigmoid colostomy.

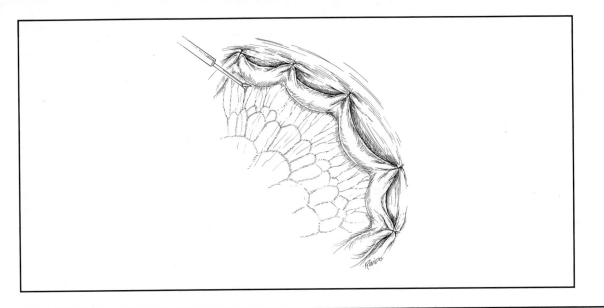

41

Small Intestinal Resection

David M. Ota
Department of Surgery
University of Missouri Ellis Fischel Cancer Center
Columbia, Missouri 65203

Timothy King
Department of Surgical Oncology
The University of Texas
M.D. Anderson Cancer Center
Houston, Texas 77030

Charles A. Staley
Department of Surgical Oncology
Emory University School of Medicine
Atlanta, Georgia 30322

Michael J. Miller
Department of Plastic Surgery
The University of Texas
M.D. Anderson Cancer Center
Houston, Texas 77030

Operative Laparoscopy and Thoracoscopy, edited by
B. V. MacFadyen, Jr. and
J. L. Ponsky. Lippincott-Raven
Publishers, Philadelphia © 1996.

KEY WORDS

Autologous jejunal transplantation   Small bowel tumors

Laparoscopic small bowel resection   Small intestine congenital defects

In 1959 Seidenberg and colleagues (1) introduced the concept that an autologous jejunal segment could be harvested with an intact vascular pedicle and transplanted to the neck for reconstruction of the cervical esophagus. Considerable advances in microsurgical vascular techniques led to successful revascularization of the transplanted jejunum and in a high flap survival rate (2–4). At the University of Texas M. D. Anderson Cancer Center this procedure was performed in 50 patients who had a cervical esophagectomy for neoplastic disease. There was a 95% success rate with this procedure, making it a viable option to reconstruct the cervical esophagus. The advantages of a jejunal interposition graft are (i) similar luminal diameter to the esophagus, (ii) tolerance to postoperative radiation therapy, and (iii) intestinal motility for swallowing. Because an exploratory laparotomy is needed to harvest the jejunum and place a gastrostomy tube, a laparoscopic approach could reduce the postoperative morbidity and hospitalization time in a jejunal resection for autologous transplantation after cervical esophagectomy for malignant disease. The requirements of this laparoscopic intracorporeal procedure are (i) identification of the proximal jejunum, (ii) meticulous dissection of the nutrient artery, vein, and mesentery, (iii) transection of the proximal and distal bowel and reanastomosis, and (iv) an intact vascular pedicle.

● ANATOMY

The blood supply to the human proximal jejunum is fairly consistent. As shown in Fig. 1 the superior mesenteric artery and vein supply segments of the small intestine. Major branches come off the mesenteric vessels and bifurcate into minor vessels that form an arcade. The terminal branches emanate off this arcade perpendicularly to the bowel wall. Thus, these 20- to 30-cm segments of the small bowel are fed by an adjoining nutrient artery and vein, and there is extensive collateral circulation to the small intestine. The objective of the laparoscopic dissection is to carefully isolate the arcade and nutrient vessels from the mesenteric fat. Another feature of the mesenteric blood supply should be noted. The laparoscopic surgeon should take advantage of the avascular windows within the mesentery. As shown in Fig. 1, there are avascular areas between the terminal branches and the laparoscopic technique makes use of these windows to travel down the mesentery to the arcade without concern for hemostasis. Because laparoscopic surgery has taken away our tactile sensation, it is imperative that the vascular anatomy is understood before embarking on this procedure.

▶ PREOPERATIVE PLANNING

The jejunal resection for autologous transplantation requires no special tests. Obviously, previous abdominal surgery can lead to adhesions that may make it difficult to identify the ligament of Treitz. If extensive adhesions do not permit adequate visualization, the procedure should be abandoned.

Small bowel pathology such as Meckel's bleeding diverticulum may require a preoperative technetium scan. Intussusception and small bowel tumors may require preoperative barium studies to document and locate the site of pathology. Small bowel tumors such as metastatic melanoma or partially obstructing lymphoma can be removed laparoscopically (see Fig. 2). Small bowel carcinoid tumors can metastasize to regional lymph nodes and should not be resected laparoscopically unless the surgeon feels that an adequate node dissection can be done or if the procedure is done to palliate obstructing symptoms in the face of stable hepatic metastasis.

▼ INTRAOPERATIVE MANAGEMENT/SURGICAL TECHNIQUE

Patients who require resection of the cervical esophagus often require a jejunal interposition for reconstruction. A preoperative intravenous broad-spectrum antibiotic is given on the morning of surgery. In the operating room the patient is

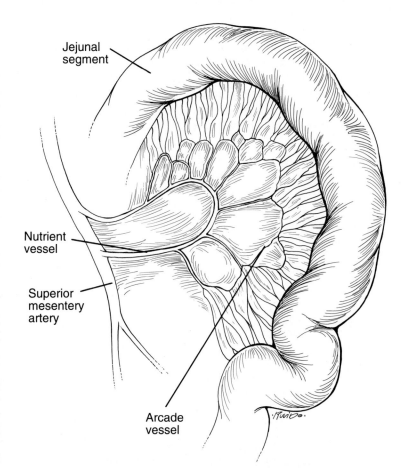

Jejunal
segment

Nutrient
vessel

Superior
mesentery
artery

Arcade
vessel

Figure 1. The jejunal segment and its vascular supply are shown in this diagram. In an individual with mesenteric fat, the nutrient vessel must be identified by transillumination. Once the vessel location has been mapped out, the avascular windows can be used to facilitate blunt dissection.

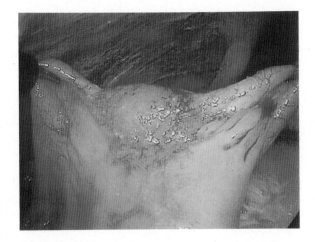

Figure 2. This is an intraoperative video print of a partially obstructing recurrent intestinal lymphoma. The lesion was found by running the small bowel from the ligament of Treitz to the ileocecal valve. This segment was resected laparoscopically and retrieved in a plastic bag. The two ends were reanastomosed intracorporeally, and the patient made an uneventful postoperative recovery. The patient was discharged 48 hours after operation.

placed in a supine position with both arms down to the side. The neck, chest, and abdomen are prepped and draped. After the neck procedure including esophagectomy is completed, the operating room is set up for the laparoscopic procedure.

Figure 3 shows the positions of the video monitors and the surgeons. The operating surgeon stands to the right of the patient and the assistant is to the left. The port sites are also shown in Fig. 3. The camera port accommodates the 0-degree laparoscope and is placed in the left lower quadrant through an open technique and utilizes a Hasson cannula. Two 10-mm ports are placed on the right side of the abdomen and they become the working ports for the surgeon. A fourth port (10 mm) is placed in the left upper quadrant and is used for instruments and the transilluminating light source.

The patient is then placed in a Trendelenburg position. Using either graspers or laparoscopic Babcock clamps the surgeon and assistant gently lift the greater omentum cephalad over the transverse colon. The transverse colon is gently lifted up and the underside of the transverse mesocolon is exposed. The ligament of Treitz is identified at the base of the mesentery and the jejunum is traced distally to about 40 cm. This is done by the surgeon and assistant working together to grasp and exchange the bowel as they move distally. The surgeon then holds up the jejunum with the mesentery facing the viewing laparoscope. A 30-degree laparoscope is then inserted in the left upper port and the light source cable is

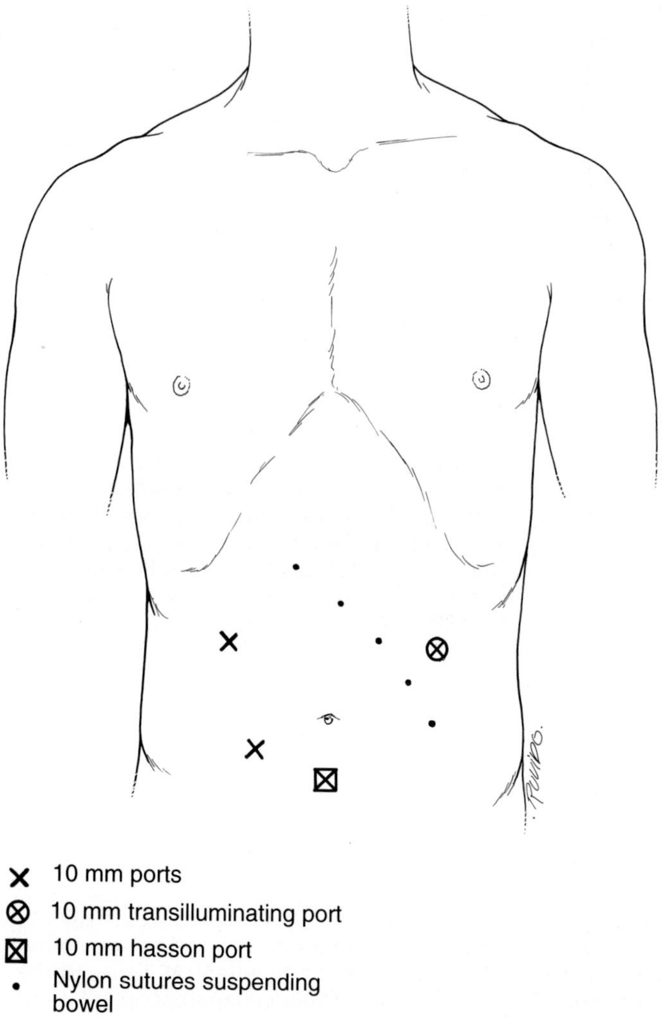

X   10 mm ports
⊗   10 mm transilluminating port
⊠   10 mm hasson port
·   Nylon sutures suspending bowel

A

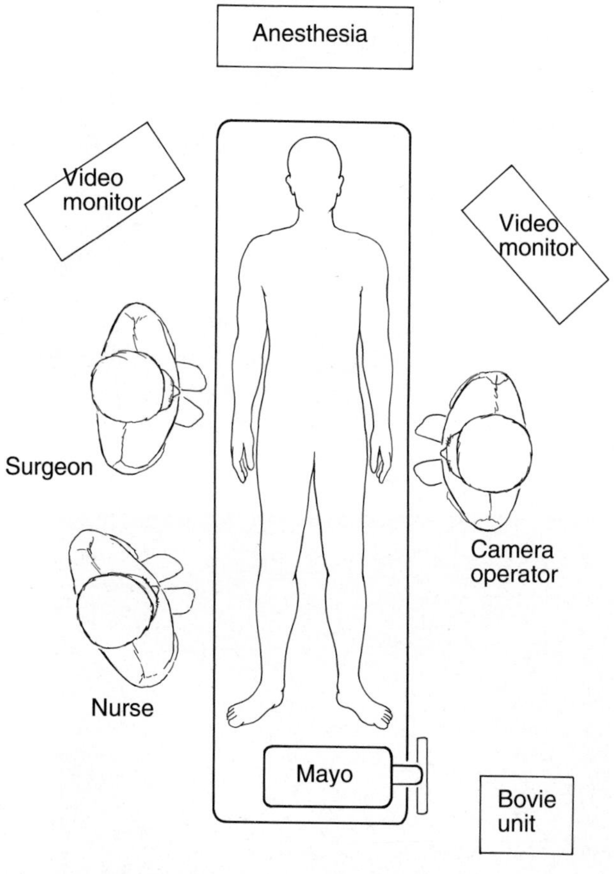

B

Figure 3. A, B: The port locations and video monitor placements are shown. The Hasson cannula is placed in the left upper quadrant. Because of the length of the 60-mm stapler, the right and left ports should be placed far from each other in order to perform the intracorporeal anastomosis.

transferred to it. By illuminating the backside of the mesentery the camera operator can scan the mesentery for the nutrient vessel. During transillumination the surgeon and operator can also see the arcade and thus map out the area to be resected.

Next a series of four to six 3-0 nylon sutures on a Keith needle are passed through the abdominal wall into the peritoneal cavity (see Fig. 3 for location of sutures). These sutures are placed into the abdomen in order to suspend the jejunum from the anterior abdominal wall. The first needle is placed in the right upper quadrant by the assistant and passed into the peritoneal cavity. Intracorporeally, the surgeon then passes the needle through the proximal part of the bowel that is to be resected. The needle should be placed near the bowel-mesentery interface closest to the surgeon in order to achieve maximum retraction of the mesentery. The Keith needle is passed out of the abdomen at the point of insertion and the suture is clamped on the surface of the abdomen. The next sutures are placed and tied along the anterior abdominal wall in order to suspend and position the jejunum and mesentery in view of the surgeon and the 0-degree laparoscope (see Fig. 4). The last distal suture is clamped on the surface of the abdomen. The left upper quadrant port is behind the bowel in order to transilluminate when necessary.

Using transillumination the surgeon can see the nutrient vessels, arcade terminal branches, and the proximal and distal avascular windows (Fig. 5). Just distal to the proximal abdominal suture the surgeon scores the peritoneum over the proximal window with a spatula cautery and creates an opening in the mesentery using a dissector (see Fig. 6). The location of the proximal window is important. By placing it just distal to the nylon suture the stitch can be used for traction during the bowel transection and for identifying the proximal end after the jejunal segment is removed. A dissector and a spatula are placed in the opening and gently spread. This maneuver opens the mesentery to a point of resistance which is the arcade vessels (see Fig. 7). With a dissector and grasper the surgeon exposes the arcade vessels. ML clips are placed proximally and distally and the vessels are cut. The dissection continues further along the mesentery until the nutrient vessels are identified (see Fig. 8).

The distal mesenteric window is identified just proximal to the distal abdominal suture. Approximately 30 cm of jejunum should be resected. As before, the distal nylon suture will remain on the distal end after the laparoscopic stapler is fired. The window is opened to the arcade vessel, which is then taken. The mesentery is taken down to the nutrient vessels. The artery and vein are carefully dissected out, avoiding injury to the vessel walls (see Fig. 9). Sufficient length of artery and vein are cleared so that the microvascular surgeon can complete the microvascular anastomosis with an adequate lumen. The vein and artery are doubly clipped and

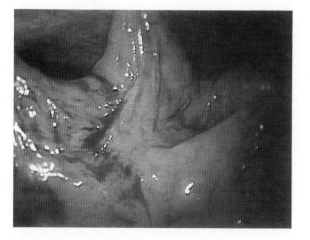

Figure 4. The jejunal segment is fixed to the anterior abdominal wall using nylon sutures on a Keith needle. This suspension technique stabilizes and exposes the small bowel mesentery for dissection.

transected. The inner abdominal wall sutures suspending the small bowel are cut and removed. The proximal and distal nylon sutures are loosened. The laparoscopic intestinal stapler is introduced through the left upper quadrant port. Instruments through the right ports are used to feed and position the proximal jejunum into the jaws of the stapler (see Fig. 10). The intestinal stapler is fired and then reloaded. The distal jejunal segment is likewise transected. While feeding the bowel into the jaws of the stapler, the surgeon should use the nylon suture for traction and should be left intact after the stapler is fired. This will allow the operator to find the proximal and distal ends.

The resected jejunum is brought out through the Hasson port site and given to the microvascular surgeon who prepares the graft for interposition. The Hasson port is replaced and the proximal and distal jejunal limbs are identified with their nylon sutures. A 0.5-cm enterostomy is made at the proximal and distal ends on the antimesenteric borders. After reloading the laparoscopic stapler, is placed through the left upper port and opened in the abdominal cavity. The proximal enterostomy is fed into the long fork of the stapler using a grasper and Babcock clamp through the right ports. The nylon suture is then removed. The distal enterostomy is fed onto the short fork and the nylon suture is removed. The stapler is fired and then withdrawn, reloaded, and reinserted. The common enterostomy is then placed into the stapler, which is fired and removed along with the residual tissue. The anastomosis is then examined for an intact staple line. Through an enlarged left upper port the stomach is exteriorized and a Witzel 12 French Foley gastrostomy tube is placed (5). The stomach is attached to the anterior peritoneum and the fascia is closed. The jejunum distal to the anastomosis is brought out through the left lower port and a Witzel feeding tube is placed. The port sites are closed at the fascia and skin. Postoperatively, the gastrostomy tube is placed to straight drainage and jejunal feedings are started 24 hours later.

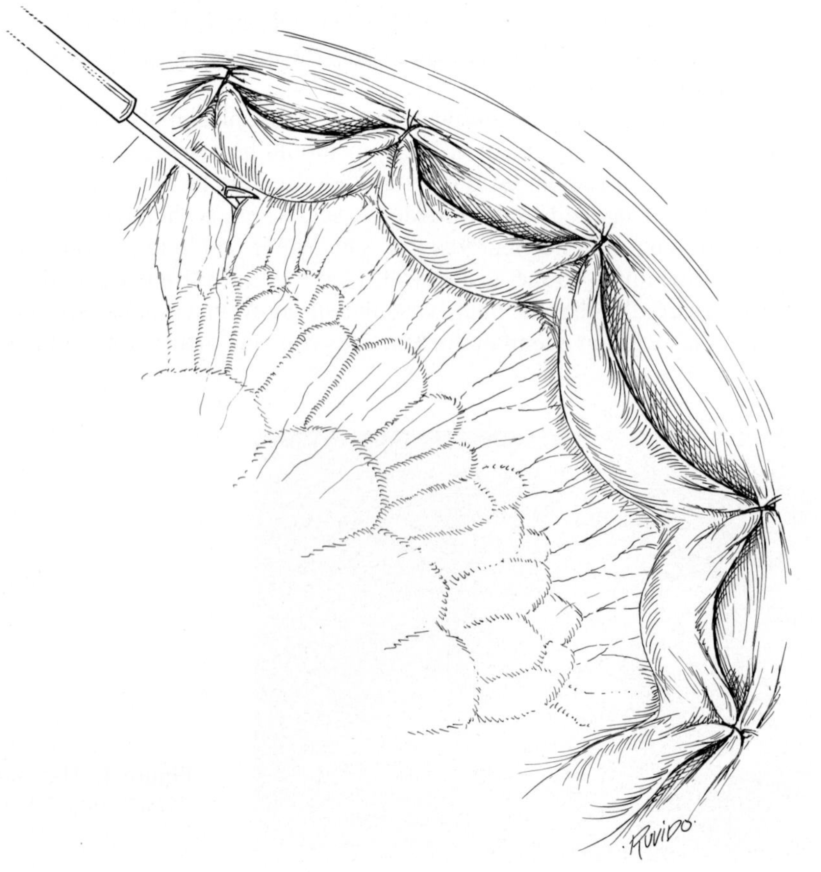

Figure 5. After the jejunal segment is temporarily anchored to the abdominal wall, the surgeon can immobilize and expose the mesentery to dissect the nutrient vessels. Approximately 30 cm of jejunum should be resected.

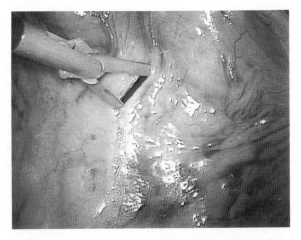

Figure 6. An avascular window at the proximal end is identified and the peritoneum is incised. The window is opened with blunt dissection.

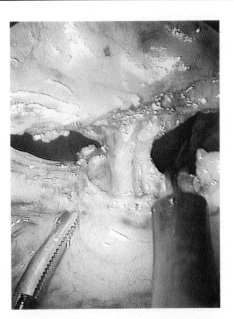

Figure 7. The arcade vessel is dissected from the surrounding tissue. These vessels are clipped and cut.

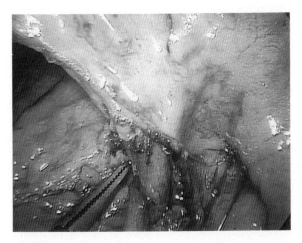

Figure 8. The dissection continues to the base of the mesentery. The nutrient artery is carefully dissected from the surrounding fat. The vein is then exposed.

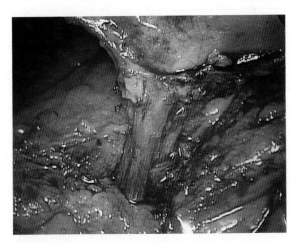

Figure 9. After the distal mesentery has been dissected to the nutrient vessels, the artery and vein are clipped and cut. The abdominal nylon sutures are cut.

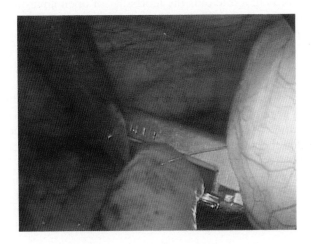

Figure 10. A 60-mm intestinal stapler is placed through the LUQ port and the proximal jejunum is fed into the jaws of the stapler. The bowel is fired and reloaded. The distal segment is similarly transected. The resected specimen is placed in a specimen and carefully removed through the LUQ port. The two ends are fed into the stapler, which is fixed and reloaded. The common enterostomy is closed with another staple load.

Suspension of the jejunum from the anterior abdominal wall with transabdominal sutures.

Transillumination of the mesentery is important for dissection. The light source is placed on a laparoscope behind the mesentery while another laparoscope and camera are positioned in front of the mesentery.

Do not use the cautery or a laser near the nutrient or arcade vessels.

There must be sufficient distance between the ports in the right upper and lower quadrants, left upper quadrant, and the suspended jejunum in order to maximize instrument utilization and visualization.

▲ COMPLICATIONS

When the proximal jejunum is harvested for autologous transplantation, injury to the intima or adventitia of either the nutrient artery or vein can result in thrombosis and graft failure. For this reason the nutrient vessels cannot be dissected out blindly. Also, inadequate length of the nutrient vessels can make the revascularization procedure difficult.

In performing the anastomosis we found that there must be adequate distance between the parts to facilitate movement of the grasping instruments and the 60-mm laparoscopic intestinal stapler. The port placement shown in Fig. 3 was ideal for accommodating the 60-mm stapler and laparoscopic Babcock clamps.

Other potential, but fortunately rare, complications include intestinal anastomotic disruption, bowel ischemia, anastomotic stricture, or bleeding. Such complications should be rare and are avoidable by observing the general principles of bowel anastomosis. If there is any difficulty with the laparoscopic anastomosis, the bowel can be exteriorized through the extraction site to connect or complete the anastomosis.

☑ CONCLUSIONS

The important maneuver of this procedure is suspending the jejunum from the anterior abdominal wall. This does several things. First, fewer port sites are needed because the assistant does not have hold the bowel. Second, the suture suspension fixes the intestinal segment so that, as the surgeon dissects the mesentery, the tissue is not constantly moving. This is essential if the nutrient vessels are to be isolated without intimal injury or adventitial hematomas. The success of the revascularization procedure greatly depends on taking these vessels with the least amount of trauma. Third, this technique provides maximum traction and exposure to the base of the mesentery in order to dissect the nutrient vessels. Fourth, the use of sutures to suspend the bowel is less traumatic to the bowel and mesentery compared with instruments.

Another important step was transillumination of the mesentery. This assisted in identifying the location of the mesenteric vessels. If the mesentery is so thick that transillumination is inconclusive, then open laparotomy should be done. The last technical comment is to avoid using the cautery near the nutrient vessels. The heat from cauterization can injure the vessel wall, resulting in thrombosis after revascularization.

There have been two patients who have undergone a successful laparoscopic jejunal resection for autologous transplantation. Both patients made a successful postoperative recovery and have excellent swallowing capability. The advantage of the laparoscopic procedure is that it avoids the morbidity of open laparotomy. The bowel suspension technique allows excellent exposure of the mesentery and minimizes the number of port sites, laparoscopic instruments, and assistants to complete the procedure. Because this is a combined neck and abdominal procedure, laparoscopy also reduces the postoperative stress. Another potential advantage of laparoscopy is a lower incidence of adhesion formation.

This procedure to harvest a segment of jejunum may have broad implications for reconstructive surgery. The jejunal segment provides a well-vascularized tissue that is flat and could be used to cover flat surface defects. The bowel wall could be opened longitudinally, and the mucosa could be stripped from the submucosa. A skin graft could then be placed over the flap after revascularization.

There are several reports of laparoscopic small bowel resection. Darzi and coworkers (6) reported that a bleeding Meckel's diverticulum was resected laparoscopically. Saw and coworkers (7) presented a case of intussuscepted Meckel's diverticulum which was resected by laparoscopic assistance. Eltringham and colleagues (8) described a full thickness intestinal biopsy technique. Scoggin and associates (9) reported a laparoscopic resection for a perforated jejunal diverticulum. It is conceivable that small bowel tumors and inflammatory bowel disease could be resected laparoscopically.

While the concept of jejunal harvest for autologous transplantation is not new, the application of laparoscopic technology to this procedure is unique. The use of bowel wall suspension during the laparoscopic procedure allows full exposure of the mesentery. This technique has proven to be satisfactory and can be used for resecting small bowel for congenital, neoplastic, or inflammatory diseases or reconstructive purposes.

ACKNOWLEDGMENTS

This work was supported in part by Ethicon Endo-Surgery. We thank Dr. Michael Clem and Mrs. Karen Geren for their assistance.

REFERENCES

1. Seidenberg B, Rosenak SS, Hurwitt ES, et al. Immediate reconstruction of the cervical esophagus by a revascularized isolated jejunal segment. *Ann Surg* 1959;149:162–171.
2. Sasaki TM, Baker H, McConnel D, Vetto R. Free jejunal flap reconstruction after extensive head and neck surgery. *Am J Surg* 1980;139:650–653.
3. Fischer S, Cole T, Meyers W, Seigler H. Pharyngoesophageal reconstruction using free jejunal interposition flaps. *Arch Otolaryngol* 1985;111:747–752.
4. Coleman J, Searles J, Hester R, et al. Ten years experience with the free jejunal autograft. *Am J Surg* 1987;154:394–398.
5. Ellis LM, Evans DB, Martin D, Ota DM. Laparoscopic feeding jejunostomy tube in oncology patients. *Surg Oncol* 1992;1:245–249.
6. Darzi A, Menziesgow N, Bartram C, Silk D. Laparoscopic excision of a bleeding Meckel's diverticulum. *Minim Invasive Ther* 1993;2:85–87.
7. Saw EC, Ramchandra S. Laparoscopically assisted resection of intussuscepted Meckel's diverticulum. *Surg Laparosc Endosc* 1993;3:149–152.
8. Eltringham WK, Roe AM, Galloway SW, Mountford RA, Espiner HJ. A laparoscopic technique for full thickness intestinal biopsy and feeding jejunostomy. *Gut* 1993;34:122–124.
9. Scoggin SD, Frazee RC, Snyder SK, Hendricks JC, Roberts JW, Symmonds RE, Smith RW. Laparoscopic-assisted bowel surgery. *Dis Colon Rectum* 1993;36:747–750.

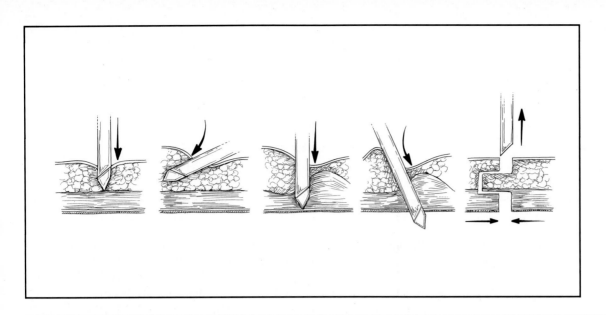

42

Appendectomy

Kurt K. S. Semm

Department of Obstetrics and Gynecology
Michaelis-School of Midwifery
Christian-Albrechts University
24105 Kiel, Germany

Operative Laparoscopy and Thoracoscopy, edited by
B. V. MacFadyen, Jr. and
J. L. Ponsky. Lippincott-Raven
Publishers, Philadelphia © 1996.

KEY WORDS

Abscess

Appendiceal stump

Cooled CO_2 gas

Endostapler

Endosuture

Laser

Roeder knot

The appendix was described first in 1521 by the anatomist Giacomo Berengario a Capri (1470–1530) as a "malicious wurmilike appendix of the caecal" and later in 1542 by Charles Estienne (1504–1564) (2). The illness "appendicities" was first described by Heister (9) in 1711 and the first appendectomy was performed by chance during the resection of a prolapsed hernia in 1735 by Claudius Amyand (1681–1740) (1,2). McBurney (14) and Sprengel (15) best described the appendectomy technique used today.

From 1985 to 1992, during gynecologic pelviscopy, I observed that 33% of my patients had had an appendectomy, and the smaller the skin scar, the more severe the intraabdominal adhesions (37). In fact, 10% to 15% of my patients had infertility

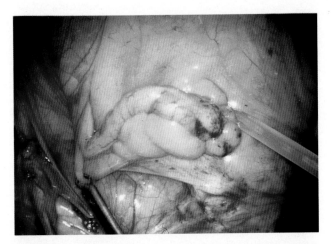

Figure 1. Endometriosis of the appendix with multiple periappendicular peritoneal endometriosis implants: setting the guide loop.

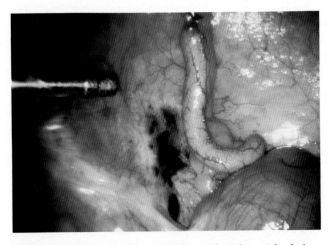

Figure 2. Periappendicular peritoneal endometriosis implant demonstrated with the point coagulator heated to 100°C = thermocolor test (hemosiderin effect). When untreated, these implants result in chronic pain in the area of the appendix without coexisting appendicitis.

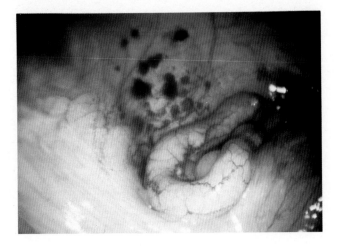

Figure 3. Chronic appendicitis with periappendicular peritoneal endometriosis implants.

problems as a direct result of these adhesions and another 10% to 15% remained infertile. I also observed that appendectomy was often performed on patients who did not appear to have the periappendicitis that occurs as a result of endometriosis (Figs. 1, 2, and 3) on and around the appendix. These patients were treated for appendicitis, and the endometriosis was never properly treated. I performed the first laparoscopic appendectomy in 1980, following the classic operation described by McBurney in 1889.

Götz (6,7) introduced the operation to general surgeons but changed the technique by cauterizing the appendicular artery with high-frequency current for hemostasis and by resecting the appendix with high-frequency current coagulation. However, high-frequency cautery causes elastin and the Warburg respiratory enzymes to become thermolabile, and these enzymes are destroyed at 54°C and 57°C, respectively. This maneuver results in the cell death of the grasped tissue and the surrounding tissue as well, which may lead to bowel and bladder injury and increased pain. Today, most surgeons use the classic technique laparoscopically, as described in this chapter.

● ANATOMY

The location of the appendix on the anterior abdominal wall at McBurney's point. This area is positioned on a line at the junction of the middle and distal thirds is usually between the umbilicus and the anterior superior iliac spine.

The appendix is located inside the abdomen at the apex of the cecum at the confluence of the three taenia coli of the colon. Its length is usually 6–10 cm, and its diameter is 0.5–1 cm (Fig. 4). The blood supply to the appendix is the appendiceal artery, which arises from the ileocolic artery, whose origin is at the superior mesenteric artery. The appendiceal artery lies close to and parallel to the base of the appendix and can be inadvertently injured, causing troublesome bleeding, during dissection. The position of the appendix usually lies behind the cecum (60–65%), but it can also be found lying in the pelvis, medial to the cecum and anteriorly (Fig. 5). Knowledge of these anatomic variations are important during

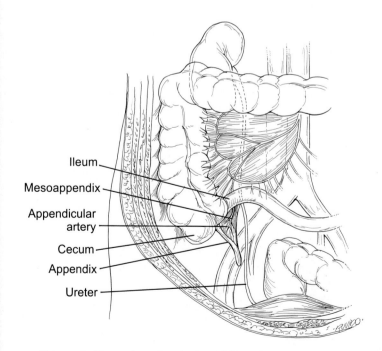

Ileum
Mesoappendix
Appendicular artery
Cecum
Appendix
Ureter

Figure 4. Normal anatomical position of the appendix.

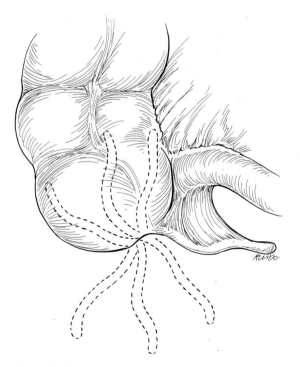

Figure 5. Anatomical variations of the appendix.

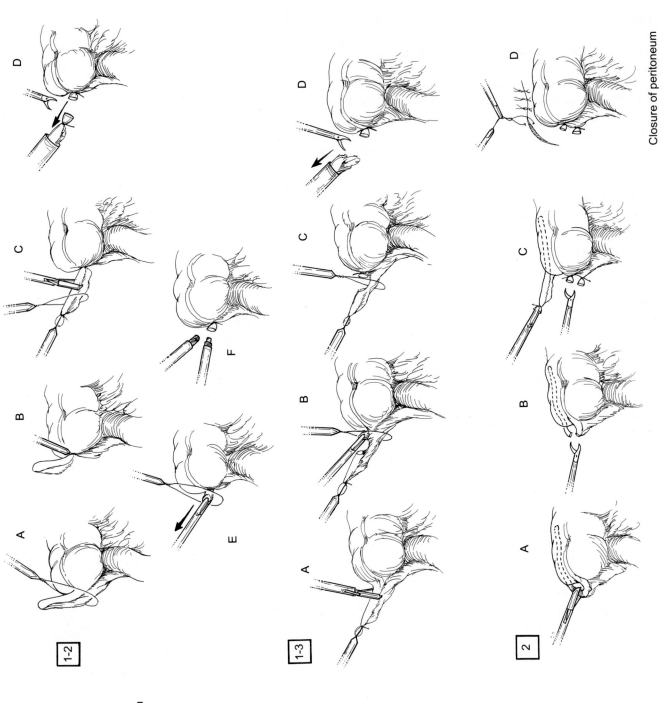

1-2

D   C   B   A

F   E

"Only" loop ligation

1-3

D   C   B   A

Endocoagulation
and loop ligation

2

D   C   B   A

Closure of peritoneum

Retrograde

appendectomy, since different surgical techniques may be necessary to remove the inflamed organ.

▶ PREOPERATIVE MANAGEMENT

In the preoperative assessment of the patient with right lower quadrant and pelvic pain, the history and physical examination are extremely important. Laboratory tests should include a complete blood count, coagulation studies, and serum chemistry studies. The classic patient with acute appendicitis has an increased white blood cell count (10,000–15,000/ml) and rebound tenderness in the right lower quadrant. A pelvic ultrasound scan may help to differentiate pelvic disease from acute appendicitis, but even with positive physical findings and an elevated white blood cell count, the accuracy of diagnosing acute appendicitis will range from 80% to 85% positive. However, a delay in diagnosis may lead to a perforated appendix with attendant morbidity and mortality of 10% compared to a mortality of 0.1% in nonperforated appendicitis.

The most common indications for laparoscopic appendectomy include acute appendicitis, appendicular adhesions, diseases affecting the right adnexa, appendicular endometriosis, periappendicular peritoneal endometriosis, and chronic lower back pain. The advantages of endoscopic appendectomy include direct visual diagnosis, visualization and evaluation of periappendicular peritoneal endometriosis, which may not be detected when the open right quadrant gridiron incision is used. In addition, immediate postoperative mobilization of the patient may ensure a short hospital stay. Postoperative adhesions are significantly reduced, thereby lowering the incidence of postoperative iatrogenic female sterility, and the decreased postoperative pain may reduce recuperative time. These patients return to work between 10 and 20 days postoperatively compared to 25 to 30 days after the open operation. Additional advantages include differentiating acute appendicitis from adnexal infection or ectopic pregnancy.

▼ INTRAOPERATIVE MANAGEMENT/SURGICAL TECHNIQUE

There are several factors that are important when performing endoscopic appendectomy. The Quadro-Test can control the establishment and maintenance of the pneumoperitoneum. Direct visual control of insertion of the trocar and the Z-track incision of the abdominal wall minimizes the risk of postoperative hernias, bowel and omentum prolapse, and adhesion formation at the trocar sites. The classic laparoscopic techniques are described in Fig. 6.

Suture and Ligation Technique

The proper placement of the trocars is depicted in Fig. 7. With practice, two trocars are sufficient to ligate, resect, and remove the appendix. The instruments are shown in Fig. 8, and the surgeon's ability to suture and knot-tie intracorporeally is very important. Other equipment includes a CO_2 gas insufflator with electronic pneutherm with the Quadro-Test system (Fig. 9), CO_2 aquapurator, which allows for heated water irrigation to aid in dissection and irrigation, and a 0- and 30-degree 10-mm endoscope. In addition to the 10-mm trocar for the endoscope, two 5 mm trocars are used and inserted as seen in Figure 7. Initial inspection

Figure 6. Laparoscopic appendectomy with needle, suture material, and loop ligation following the classic abdominal rules according to McBurney and Sprengel with pursestring and Z suture techniques.

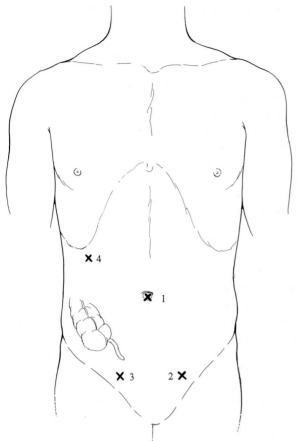

Figure 7. Trocar insertion points 1, 2, and 3 for orthograde appendectomy. No. 4 is for retrograde appendectomy.

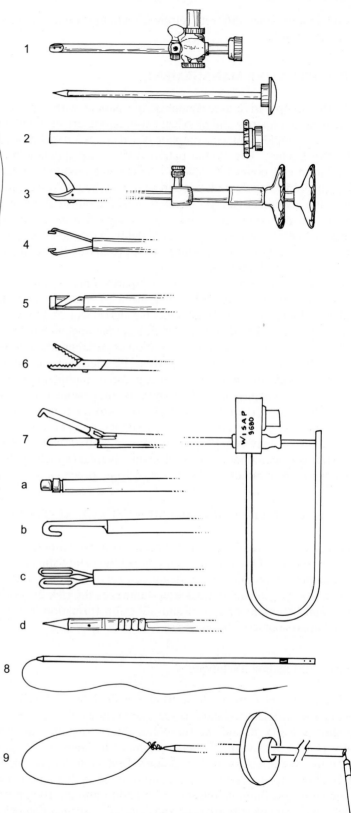

Figure 8. Classic instruments for appendectomy: *1,* trocars; *2,* appendix extractor; *3,* hook scissors; *4,* bowel grasper; *5,* needle blocker; *6,* needle-holder; *7,* crocodile forceps for the endocoagulator: *a,* point coagulator; *b,* melting hook; *c,* biopolar forceps; *d,* laser-tool; *8,* endosuture for extracorporeal knotting technique; *9,* loop ligature.

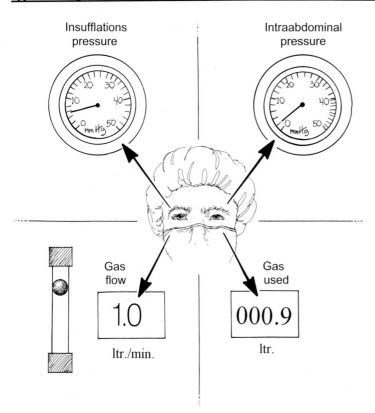

Insufflations pressure

Intraabdominal pressure

Gas flow

1.0

ltr./min.

Gas used

000.9

ltr.

Figure 9. Quadro-Test for the insufflation apparatus gives safe insufflation even in cases of prelaparotomized patients. Note the gauges for immediate visual control of insufflation pressure, intraabdominal pressure, gas-flow, and volume of gas used.

of the abdominal cavity can be performed with a 5-mm pelviscope placed in the right lower quadrant or intrabilically. The diagnosis is determined, and the appendectomy is started.

First, the appendix is isolated and a guide suture is set at the tip of the appendix using a Roeder loop. At this point, the mesoappendix is viewed. Next, the appendicular artery is ligated with an endosuture, using the extracorporeal knotting technique. The needle is grasped with a needle-blocker (Fig. 8), and a second needle-holder is introduced through trocars 2 and 3 (Fig. 7) and the appendicular mesentery is suture-ligated (Fig. 10). In cases where adhesions are present, an atraumatic bowel grasper allows the surgeon to grasp the bowels without risk. After the first suture is tied, the appendicular artery is ligated and partial skeletonization of the appendicular mesentery occurs.

A Roeder loop (Fig. 11) is then set around the entire appendix approximately 0.5 cm away from the cecum. The fecal contents are expressed from the appendix

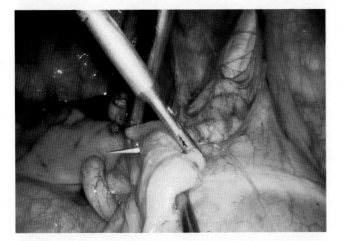

Figure 10. Suture ligature of the appendicular artery with a needle using the extracorporeal knotting technique.

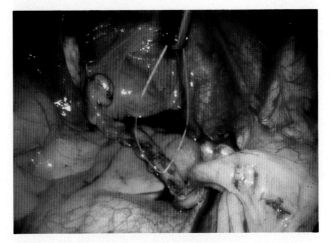

Figure 11. Introduction of the loop over the appendix, which has been completely skeletonized.

with a crocodile forceps (Fig. 12) heated to 100°C so that disinfection of the resection area occurs. Transection of the appendix (Fig. 13) within the coagulated area follows, using the hooked scissors. The appendix is then removed through the appendix extractor, or an intracorporeal bag is used to prevent contamination.

A second ligature is then set around the stump for security, and the stump is disinfected (Fig. 14) by using a small iodine swab. This is followed by coagulation of the stump using the point coagulator attachment of the endocoagulator set at 110°C.

As a final step, the appendix stump is inverted by using the classic purse-string technique with 2-0 silk suture, and a Z-suture technique is used to complete the operation. For the past eight years, we have omitted this step in our technique as it appears to be unnecessary.

The pneumoperitoneum is then deflated after the Z-track puncture canal is checked for bleeding while simultaneously removing the 10-mm trocar and pelviscope. The umbilical wound is closed using skin clips. Because of the Z-track puncture technique, the wound closes itself in different layers and suture closing techniques are therefore not necessary.

Similarly, an endo-GIA stapler (2.5-mm staples) can be used to divide the appendiceal stump. The mesentery can be similarly divided with a stapler. However, bleeding at the staple line can be noted and should be sutured or clipped. Staples significantly increase the cost of the operation.

The only other variation of the suture and ligation technique is to omit the pursestring Z-suture on the appendiceal stump. However, these variations do not appear to significantly alter the leakage rate from the appendiceal stump, abscess formation, or wound infection.

Single Ligation Technique

The single ligation technique simplifies appendectomy, is safe, and can be used by surgeons who are beginners in laparoscopic appendectomy. As described in Fig. 6, top the appendix is fixed on a Roeder loop (Fig. 6 top, A) but can be grasped with a forceps except in highly infectious cases where the thickened mesentery and appendix may be lacerated and may increase contamination with the contents of the appendix.

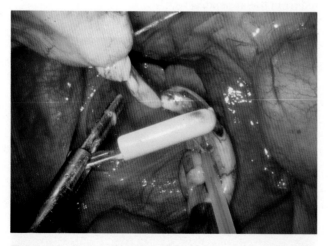

Figure 12. Removal of the crocodile forceps set at 90°C, followed by double ligation of the intended area of resection.

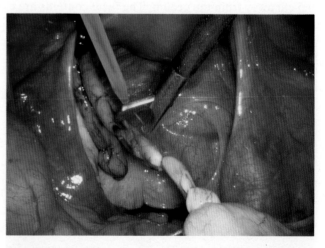

Figure 13. Cutting of the second ligature thread after expressing the feces and thermosterilization of the intended area of resection.

If the mesentery of the appendix is adherent to the abdominal wall, it can be dissected free without significant blood loss. If any bleeding occurs, a Roeder loop ligation controls it immediately. If the appendix is mobile, a Roeder chrome catgut loop is set 0.5 cm above the cecal pole (Fig. 6 top, A and B) which ligates the appendix, appendicular artery, and appendicular mesentery. If the proper placement of the Roeder loop proves to be difficult, an atraumatic forceps is helpful, and the crocodile forceps of Semm's endocoagulator can be used simultaneously (Fig 6 top, C) heated to 100°C to sterilize this part of the appendix, since *Escherichia coli* is especially thermolabile. Then a second Roeder loop is positioned directly beside the forceps on the distal side (Fig 6 top, C and D). Next, the guide ligature pulls the appendix into the appendix extractor, and hooked scissors transect the appendix between the two ligatures (Fig. 6 top, D). Finally, the remaining stump is grasped with biopsy forceps that have been put through a Roeder loop (Fig. 6 top, E), and the appendix is ligated for a second time. The stump is sterilized with the endocoagulator set at 100°C and with an iodine swab (for example) (Fig. 6 top, F).

At the end of the procedure, the appendix stump is pushed backward if possible, and the appendectomy is finished. Figure 15 shows the actual healing process 48 hours postappendectomy with no scarring and no adhesions.

In summary, the single ligation technique is the simplest and most efficient method and is associated with the fewest complications.

Endocoagulation Technique

Endocoagulation is a simple technique that only omits the suturing and extracorporeal knotting techniques. It is based on the technique of Götz, who uses the high-frequency technique (see the next section) and is based on the amputation procedure usually employed for the removal of the retrograde appendix.

The appendix is first located and isolated using trocars 2 and 3 (Fig. 6) and then coagulated (Fig. 16) for 20 seconds using the crocodile forceps set at 110°C and 1 cm distal to the cecal pole. Amputation of the appendix (Fig. 17) is performed without blood loss and without contamination using the hook scissors by butting within the endocoagulated area.

The appendicular mesentery is then inspected by using two bowel forceps, thereby ensuring proper separation of the cut edges. The remaining appendicular

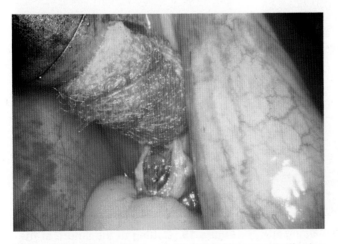

Figure 14. Disinfection of the ligated appendicular stump with iodine. *Left:* periappendicular peritoneal endometriosis implants.

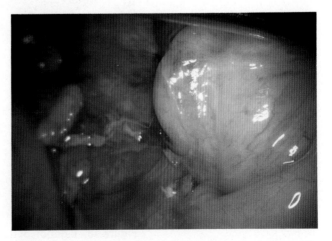

Figure 15. Appendix stump 48 hours after surgery. No scar is visible despite the once severely adherent appendix.

stump is ligated 0.5 cm distal to the cecum (Figs. 18 and 19) using a Roeder loop (when possible with chromic catgut or polydioxanone). The loop is introduced through trocar 3, and the biopsy forceps pulls the tissue into position through trocar 2. The entire appendicular mesentery and appendicular artery are ligated in toto by a second Roeder loop (Fig. 6 middle, C and 20).

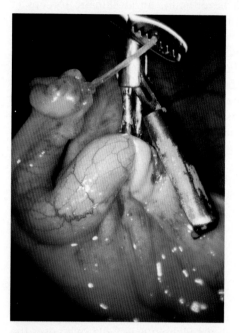

Figure 16. Removal of the crocodile forceps. The area of hemostasis is clearly visible. The thread of the loop fixing the tip of the appendix is visible behind the periappendicular peritoneal endometriosis implants.

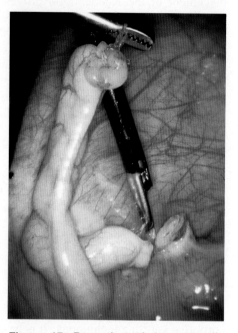

Figure 17. Resection of the appendix without blood loss at the midpoint of the endocoagulated area.

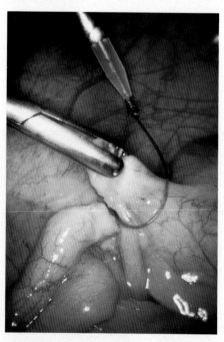

Figure 18. Ligation of the remaining appendicular stump at the cecal pole with a chromic catgut Roeder loop.

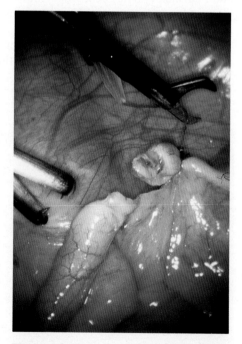

Figure 19. Cutting of the suture of the stump ligature and grasping the appendix before total ligation of the appendicular artery and the mesentery.

The mesentery and the attached appendix are resected, using the hook scissors introduced through trocar 3. The tissue bundle is then removed through a trocar that is either 10 or 15 mm in diameter, depending on the size of the specimen. A second ligature is set around the appendicular stump for security. The wound pedicle is sterilized, using the point coagulator set at 110°C, and disinfected, using an iodine swab (Fig. 6 top, F). An additional pursestring and Z-suture are not necessary; the appendiceal region 3 years postappendectomy is shown in Figure 21.

High-Frequency Current Technique

The difficulties associated with endoscopic intraabdominal suturing and ligating have caused some authors (6,7) to substitute the suture and ligature technique with various coagulation methods.

In this operation, coagulation of the appendicular artery is first performed with the bipolar instrument. The appendicular mesentery is then dissected and the appendix coagulated with the bipolar forceps 1 cm away from the cecal pole. Sharp dissection of the appendix follows using the hook scissors. In case of infection, a second loop is applied to the free end of the appendix, which prevents the contamination of intestinal contents from the resected appendix. The appendicular mesentery is pulled together with the appendix into the appendix extractor. If necessary, the mesentery is partially resected, using the hook scissors.

Laparoscopic Laser Appendectomy

Coagulation of the appendicular artery and transection of the appendix itself may also be performed with an Nd:YAG Laser beam. The CO_2 laser is not suitable for this surgery unless the surgeon is adept at using a backstop. The Nd:YAG or Argon laser are practicable when the amount of money at your disposal is unlimited.

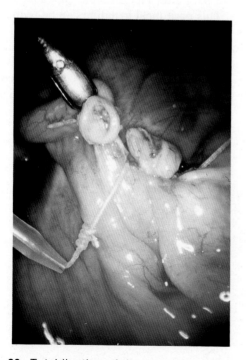

Figure 20. Total ligation of the appendicular mesentery and the appendicular artery.

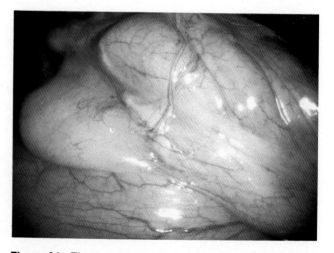

Figure 21. Three years status postappendectomy: No visible scarring.

Retrograde, Laparoscopic Appendix Amputation

As at laparotomy, difficulties may arise in locating and dissecting the appendicular artery when the appendix lies in the retrograde position and extends superiorly—sometimes as far up as the liver. This is particularly true when the appendix is in a very acute state, thickened, and adherent to the lateral pelvic wall.

In these cases, it is important to immediately ensure a proper view of the operative field by first performing adhesiolysis. Water dissection may be employed when necessary. The base of the appendix is exposed in Fig. 6 bottom, A. Coagulation and resection of the appendix is performed as described in Fig. 6 bottom, A and B.

Two Roeder loops are then set around the two pedicles for security thus freeing the appendicular mesentery from adhesions and the whole appendix can be mobilized (Fig. 6 bottom, C). Any gaping peritoneal wounds should be closed using endosuture with the intra- or extracorporeal knotting technique (Figs. 6 bottom, D and 22).

Postoperative Care

Due to minimally invasive intraabdominal surgery, it is possible to offer patients clear liquids when they have recovered from the general anesthetic. Often a regular diet can be given 8 to 12 hours postoperatively, and the patient can be discharged shortly thereafter. Postoperative therapy is determined by the degree of infection. In cases of severe infection, a closed silicone drain may be used (Fig. 23A, B). This drain can be introduced into the abdominal wall through one of the 5-mm trocars.

Until now, cooled CO_2 gas has been used to insufflate and maintain a pneumoperitoneum at all laparoscopic surgery. After 3 years of clinical research at the University Women's Clinic in Kiel, we have shown that this reduces body temperature sometimes to as low as 28°C. This produces in turn peritoneal irritation, which causes the patient severe postoperative pain. Many surgeons have reported that patients have more postoperative pain after laparoscopic appendectomy as compared to the classical procedure. This peritoneal irritation can be reduced by using warmed CO_2 gas, which has an isothermic effect. The Flow-Therme with its heating cable can be adapted to all types of CO_2 gas insufflators. In clinical studies, patients who have undergone laparoscopic surgery with warmed CO_2 gas have required 34% less analgesia postoperatively as compared to the control group, and have 47% less shoulder pain. In addition, the initial tachycardia at the

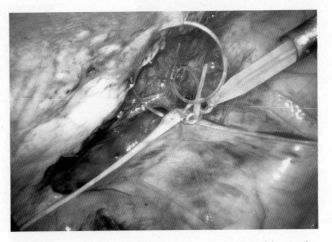

Figure 22. Closing a gaping peritoneal wound by endosuture or clips.

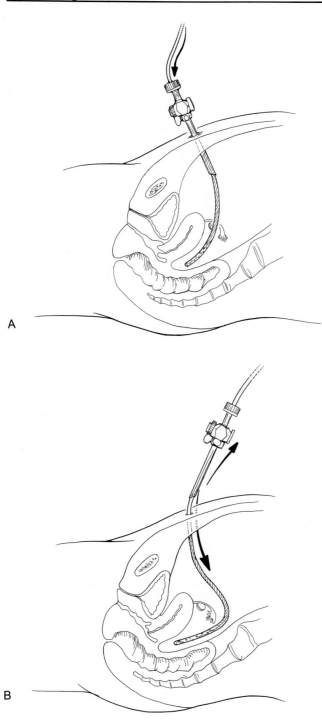

A

B

Figure 23. Insertion of a silicon drain through a 5 mm trocar after ruptured appendix **(A)** and trocar extraction after proper positioning of the drain **(B)**.

beginning of laparoscopy is totally absent. The use of warm CO_2 gas is now imperative in laparoscopic surgery.

▲ COMPLICATIONS

Difficulties at Endoscopic Appendectomy

Only in cases with advanced degrees of infection or with perforation and abscess formation is the endoscopic appendectomy rendered more difficult. A thick appendix, such as in the case of the myxedematous appendix, may also be problematic. For the easy extraction of such tissue, appendix extractors, 15 or 20 mm in diameter, are available; an atraumatic dilation set enlarges the smaller trocar sites so as to accommodate these instruments.

Trocars should never be inserted straight! If all trocars are pushed through the abdominal wall in a Z-track technique (Figs. 24 and 25), hernias and other complications are avoided. This is also true if 10- to 20-mm trocars are used. The different layers of the abdominal wall are closed in an overlapping manner. Only conical trocars should be used in the Z-track technique. The blades of the sharp trocars can cut vessels and muscle fibers (8,19,20).

High-frequency current is uncontrollable, and serious injuries to the cecum, small intestine, and ureter have been reported. These complications have caused many surgeons to doubt the applicability and acceptance of pelviscopy/laparoscopy in general.

Surgeons should note that each cell has thermostable and thermolabile enzymes that are important for the proper functioning of a cell. For example, elastase is destroyed at 53°C and the Warburg respiratory enzymes at 57°C. If such high temperatures are applied in the area of the cecal stump, enzymes are destroyed and two sequelae may result:

1. If the initial temperature damage is tolerated by the cecal tissue, it may repair itself, but sharp abdominal pain may result between the 2nd and 10th day postoperatively.
2. If the temperature damage cannot be repaired by the cecal tissue, a cecal fistula will develop after a few days.

Complications resulting from laparoscopic appendectomy are seen only when high-frequency and laser techniques are used. If only the suture techniques are used, the postoperative complications of laparoscopic appendectomy are comparable to those seen at classic laparotomy.

Appendicular Abscess

The experience gathered by gynecologists in the endoscopic treatment of falloppian tuboovarian abscess has shown that opening of the ovary or tube allowing the pus to escape has not led to the grave consequences that occur when these structures are opened at laparotomy. It is important that the abscess be emptied before appendix transection and generously irrigated with the CO_2 aquapurator. When required, sutures and ligatures should be used to minimize contamination and possible abscess formation.

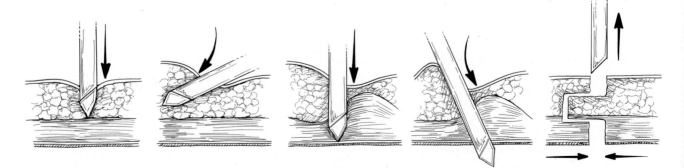

Figure 24. Demonstration of the effectiveness of the Z-track puncture performed with the conical trocar (see also Figure 25). After removing the trocar sheath, the wound in the abdominal wall is closed immediately by overlapping of the various layers.

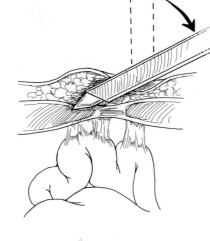
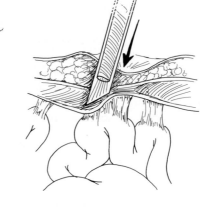
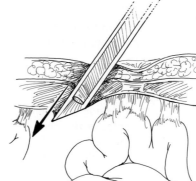
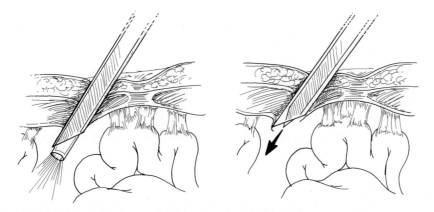

Figure 25. Z-track incision to avoid hernias and to allow perforation of the parietal peritoneum under endoscopic visual control. **1:** The elliptically shaped tip of the 5-mm-diameter trocar sheath is fitted with a conical trocar and is inserted down to the muscle layer following the Z-puncture technique. **2:** After the conical trocar has been replaced by the 5-mm-diameter pelviscope, the trocar sheath is advanced through the abdominal musculature under visual control down to the level of the peritoneum. **3:** In cases of the peritoneal adhesions to omentum or bowel, a white surface will be visible due to the total reflection of the light. **4:** Through lateral movement of the elliptical trocar on the rectus fascia and the peritoneum, a translucent peritoneum will be seen, demonstrating the vessels very clearly. **5:** By means of blunt pressure, the parietal peritoneum is perforated under visual control allowing a free view into the adhesion-filled abdominal cavity. **6:** In cases where the procedure described in number 5 cannot be performed, e.g., due to a thick fascia, perforation of the peritoneum is performed in the classical way after exchange of the optics system for the conical trocar.

A mandatory prerequisite for optimal treatment is an experienced surgeon who has a complete understanding of the endoscopic suture and ligature techniques. Tissue trauma is exaggerated only when methods of thermal necrosis are employed.

When pus is encountered, it should be sent to the laboratory for culture, sensitivity tests, and Gram stain, thereby ensuring a specifically targeted postoperative antibiotic therapy. The abdominal cavity and pelvis should be irrigated intraoperatively with 4 to 5 L of physiologic saline, and the intraabdominal instillation of antibiotics can sometimes be of value in grossly contaminated cases, since systemic antibiotics require a lot of time and a high concentration to be effective in abscess cavities.

Thick Appendix

In cases of severe infection, increase in appendiceal diameter can occur and the appendix may be too thick to be removed through the 10-mm trocar, a dilutation to a 15 mm or 20 mm trocar inserted by means of a Z-track puncture should be used for removal of the appendix. Only occasionally is it necessary to remove the appendix piece by piece with a large claw forceps or an open operation. However, postoperative abscess and wound infection rates may increase.

Acute Intraoperative Hemorrhage

During coagulation or ligation, an unexpected hemorrhage may occur, for example, in the case of an aberrant appendicular artery, which can be arrested in either procedure by a Roeder loop. If after ligation or coagulation the appendicular artery slips away into the retroperitoneal area and provokes a retroperitoneal hematoma the abdomen should be opened immediately. However, in most cases, careful dissection of the retroperitoneal area usually reveals the bleeding artery, which is grasped with biopsy forceps previously pushed through a Roeder loop, thereby facilitating immediate ligation. Because of magnification with the laparoscope, a bleeding vessel is often easier to find than at laparotomy. However, massive hemorrhage may obscure the field and may necessitate an open operation to complete the surgery.

When using the classic gridiron open incision, one cannot avoid contaminating the lymphatic vessels with infecting toxins and bacteria. This is prevented at endoscopic appendectomy, as the area of infection is not allowed to infect the abdominal wall. In cases of severe and advanced infection, appropriate antibiotics may be given intraabdominally and at the end of the endoscopic procedure.

☑ CONCLUSION

When compared to the classic operative therapy of appendicitis the advantages of the endoscopic therapy are evident. The operative steps have been simplified over the past 10 years of development. The operation time is short and does not exceed the time required to perform the same procedure by laparotomy. Postoperative therapy is dependent on the severity of appendiceal inflammation. Reduction in the length of hospital stay is often decreased to 1 till 4 days. Convalescence at home often requires only 7 to 10 days as opposed to 3 to 4 weeks after the open operation. The laparoscopic approach can significantly reduce adhesions; this is particularly important, as these adhesions can cause sterility, especially if periappendiceal endometriosis develops.

Contraindications to endoscopic appendectomy are few, although advanced gangrenous appendicitis may be very difficult to manage laparoscopically. However, with careful technique and attention to detail, laparoscopic appendectomy can be safely performed in 95% to 98% with minimal complications.

SURGICAL PEARLS

Initially, use very little dissection at the base of the appendix to avoid injury to the appendiceal artery.

The base of the appendix should be dissected 1 cm above the cecum and the suture or staples pulled down the cecum.

If bleeding occurs at the suture or staple line, an enodoclip or suture will rapidly control bleeding.

The use of warmed CO_2-intraoperatively will decrease postoperative pain.

Massaging the appendix so as to empty the appendix of fecal contents prior to transection is important to decrease the possibility of spreading infection.

SUGGESTED READING

1. Amyand C. Of an inguinal rupture, with a pin in the appendix coeci, incrusted with stone, and some observations on wounds in the guts. *Philos Trans Soc Lond* 1736;39:329–342.
2. Bishop W. *The Early History of Surgery*. London: Oldbourne Science Library, 1955.
3. Creese PG. The first appendectomy. *Surg Gynecol Obstet* 1953;97:645–652.
4. Doll D. Zur Geschichte der Appendizitis. *Münch Med Wochenschr* 1908;21:2143–2145.
5. Ebstein E. Sektionsbefund Lorenz Heister über eine akute brandige Blinddarmentzündung aus dem Jahre 1711. *Virchows Arch* 1919;226:96–100.
6. Götz F. Pier A, Bacher C. Modified laparoscopic appendectomy in surgery: a report on 388 operations. *Surg Endosc* 1990;4:6–9.
7. Götz F, Pier A, Bacher C. Laparoscopic appendectomy: indications, technique and results in 653 patients. *Chirurg* 1991;62:253–256.
8. Haarmann W. Experience with complicated appendicitis. *Chirurg Gastroenterol* 1993;9:237–239.
9. Heister L. *Medizinische, chirurgische und anatomische Wahrnehmungen*. Vol. 1. Rostock: Kern Verlag, 1753.
10. Hufschmidt M, Raguse T, Adamenk L. Intraoperative antibiotic prophylaxis in appendicitis. *Chirurg Gastroenterol* 1993;9:245–249.
11. Hurry JB. *Imhotep, the vizier and physician of King Zoser and afterwards the Egyptian god of medicine*. 2nd Ed. Chicago: University of Chicago Press, 1928.
12. Koch C, Häring R. *Senile Appendicitis. Chirurg Gastroenterol* 1993;9:250–252.
13. Lyons AS, Petrucelli RJ. *Geschichte der Medizin im Spiegel der Kunst*. Köln: Dumont, 1980.
14. McBurney C. Experience with the early interference in cases of appendicitis, with a description of a new method operating. *Ann Surg* 1889;20:38–49.
15. McBurney C, Sprengel O. Appendektomie. In: Grewe H-G, Kremer K, eds. *Chirurgische Operationen*. Vol. 2. Stuttgart: Thieme, 1977.
16. Pier A. Die laparoskopisch/endoskopische Appendektomie nach Semm in der Modifikation nach Götz, eine Untersuchung von 255 Fällen. *Diss Vorber Linnich* 1990.
17. Pier A, Götz F, Bacher C. Laser-assisted laparoscopic appendectomy. *Z Gastroenterol* 1991;29: 77–78.
18. Pier A, Götz F, Thevissen P. Laparoskopische Versorgung einer indirekten Inguinalhernie (Fallbeschreibung). *Endosk Heute* 1991;4:5–16.
19. Raguse T, Hufschmidt M. Complications in endoscopic appendectomy. *Chirurg Gastroenterol* 1993;9:229–232.
20. Reding R. Complicated appendicitis. *Chirurg Gastroenterol* 1993;9:233–236.
21. Reith HB. Zur Geschichte der der Appendizitis. In: Reith HB, ed. *Chirurgie 1990: Aktueller Stand und Perspektiven*. Hamelin: TM-Verlag, 1990.
22. Reith HB. Appendicitis and perityphlitis: a historical review. *Chirurg Gastroenterol* 1993;9: 184–197.
23. Semm K. Das Pneumoperitoneum mit CO_2. *Endosk Method Ergeb Vis* 1967;6:167–169.
24. Semm K. Pelviskopische Chirurgie in der Gynäkologie. *Geburtsh Frauenheilk* 1977;37:909–920.
25. Semm K. *Operative Pelviskopie–Laparoskopie–Endoskopische Ligaturen mit Hilfe der Schlingen-Unterbindung*. Hamburg: Ethikon/Norderstedt, No. 32, 1978.
26. Semm K. Die Automatisierung des Pneumoperitoneums für die endoskopische Abdominalchirurgie. *Arch Gynäkol* 1980;232:738–741.
27. Semm K. Advances in pelviscopic surgery (appendectomy). *Curr Probl Obstet Gynecol* 1982;10: 1–54.
28. Semm K. Die endoskopische intraabdominale Naht. *Geburtsh Frauenheilk* 1982;42:56–57.
29. Semm K. Endoscopic appendectomy. *Endoscopy* 1983;15:59–64.
30. Semm K. Die endoskopische Appendektomie. *Gynäkol Prax* 1983;7:131–140.
31. Semm K. Die pelviskopische Appendektomie. *Dtsch Med Wochenschr* 1988;113:3–5.
32. Semm K. Operative pelviscopy: an alternative to laparotomy. *Women Wellness* 1988;2:1–8.
33. Semm K. *Operationslehre für endoskopische Abdominal Chirurgie*. Stuttgart: Schattauer, 1984.
34. Semm K. Technische Operationsschritte der endoskopischen Appendektomie. *Langenbecks Arch Chir* 1991;376:121–126.
35. Semm K. Operative Pelviskopie: ein Leitfaden. 3rd Ed. Kiel: Universitäts-Frauenklinik, 1991.
36. Semm K. Das Pneumoperitoneum, Fehler und Gefahren. *Laparo Endosk Chir* 1992;1:1–20.
37. Semm K. 25 years of laparoscopic surgery: personal reflections: problems in laparoscopy in the past and present. *Dev Surg Surg Res* 1993;2:27–35.
38. Shepard JA. Acute appendicitis: a historical survey. *Lancet* 1954;11:299–302.
39. Siemer P, Lorenz D, Thriene W. Gentamicin-collagen combination for the prophylaxis postoperative wound healing disorders in phlegmonous gangrenous appendicitis: a prospective, randomized multicenter phase IV study. *Chirurg Gastroenterol* 1993;9:240–244.
40. Smith DC. A historical overview of the recognition of appendicitis. Part I. *State J Med* 1986;86: 571–583.
41. Smith DC. A historical overview of the recognition of appendicitis. Part II. *State J Med* 1986;86: 639–647.
42. Sprengel O. Zur Frühoperation bei akuter Appendizitis. *Verh Dtsch Ges Chir* 1901;30:601.

SECTION X

HERNIA

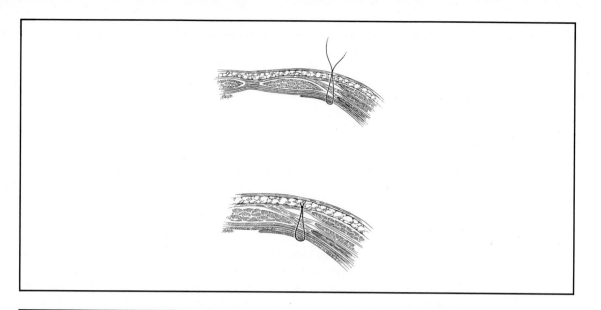

Intraperitoneal Inguinal Hernioplasty

Frederick K. Toy and Roy T. Smoot, Jr.
Department of Surgery
University of Maryland School of Medicine
Baltimore, Maryland 21201; and
Nanticoke Memorial Hospital
Seaford, Delaware 19973

Stephen D. Carey
Department of Surgery
F. Edward Hibent School of Medicine
Bethesda, Maryland 20892

Operative Laparoscopy and Thoracoscopy, edited by
B. V. MacFadyen, Jr. and
J. L. Ponsky. Lippincott-Raven
Publishers, Philadelphia © 1996.

KEY WORDS

Cooper's ligament   Iliopubic tract

ePTFE   Onlay patch

Endo-suture passer

● ANATOMY

When viewed through the laparoscope introduced via the umbilicus, the posterior surface of the anterior abdominal wall is divided into several fossae. In the midline, between the pubic bone and umbilicus, is a fibrous band that comprises the remains of the urachus. The fold of the peritoneum over the urachal remnant is the *median umbilical ligament.* At 3 to 4 cm lateral to the median umbilical ligament is another fibrous cord covered with peritoneum. This cord, which extends from the sides of the urinary bladder to the umbilicus, is the *medial umbilical ligament* and is the fibrous remnant of the obliterated umbilical arteries. This is an important landmark because it lies directly over the pubic tubercle. At 3 or 4 cm lateral to the medial umbilical ligaments are the *lateral umbilical ligaments,* which are a slight protrusion of the inferior epigastric vessels and the interfoveolar ligament. Occasionally, there are transverse folds in the contracted bladder that extend laterally from the fundus to the pelvic side walls. These folds constitute a false ligament known as the *transverse vesical folds.*

The ductus deferens is covered only by peritoneum. It is usually identified easily as it exits the pelvic cavity over the pelvic brim and crosses ventral to the external iliac vein and artery obliquely. It then curves around the lateral side of the inferior epigastric vessels, where it joins the spermatic vessels (Fig. 1, left inguinal region).

At the level of Cooper's ligament, the ductus deferens lies directly over the external iliac vein and acts as a landmark for the lateral extent of exposure of Cooper's ligament.

The spermatic vessels are made up of the testicular artery and vein. The testicular artery is a branch of the aorta. The two testicular veins at the level of the internal inguinal ring unite to form a single vein that drains on the right side into the inferior vena cava and on the left side into the left renal vein. The spermatic vessels are covered only by the peritoneum and run along the pelvic wall over the anterior psoas muscle.

The spermatic vessels merge with the ductus deferens, forming the spermatic cord, which enters the internal ring and traverses the inguinal canal. The junction of the ductus deferens and the spermatic vessels forms the apex of an imaginary triangle—''triangle of doom.'' Within the triangle are the external iliac artery and vein, covered by the peritoneum and the transversalis fascia. It is essential to identify this triangle because it is paramount not to staple or suture within this area (Fig. 2).

The *transversalis fascia,* also known as the *endoabdominal fascia,* is the internal investing layer of deep fascia that lines the entire abdominal cavity. This layer is now generally called the transversalis fascia, although formerly this name was applied only to the deep fascia covering the internal surface of the transversus abdominis muscle. Various subdivisions of the transversalis fascia are still referred to by their more specific regions, such as the iliac, psoas, or obturator fascia. The transversalis fascia is a complex layer, sometimes covering bones, muscles, aponeurosis, and ligaments in different areas. It may be very thin and adherent in one place or thickened and independent in another. In some areas, it gives rise

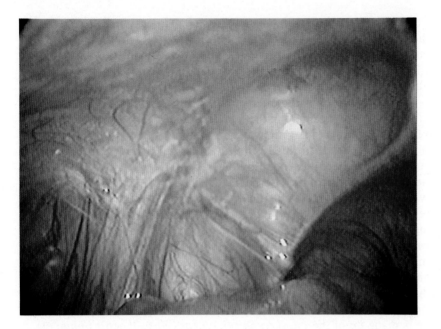

Figure 1. Intraoperative view of the left inguinal area showing the spermatic vessels and ductus deferens going into the internal ring, forming a triangle with the iliac artery and iliac vein within this triangle.

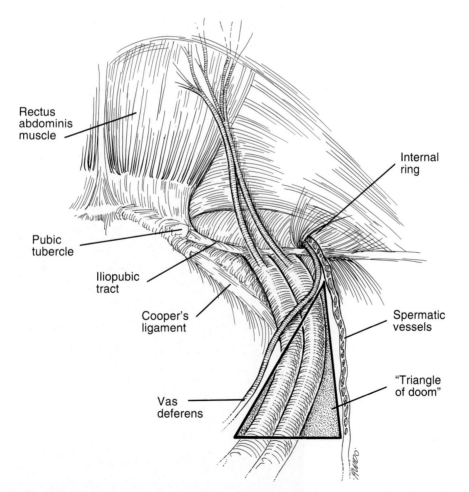

Figure 2. The left inguinal area, showing the spermatic vessels and the ductus deferens going into the internal ring with the triangle of doom in which the iliac artery and vein are identified. Cooper's ligament runs across the superior edge of the superior ramus, the iliopubic tract, the transversus abdominis arch, and the inferior epigastric vessels.

to specialized structures, such as thickened strong bands or tubular investments. Between the transversalis fascia and the peritoneum lies a layer of *subserous fascia,* commonly known as the preperitoneal space. This is the fibroareolar connective tissue supporting the peritoneum. It commonly contains varying thicknesses of adipose tissue.

The *internal inguinal ring* is the interruption in the transversalis fascia where the spermatic cord (round ligament in the female) penetrates the anterior abdominal wall. It is an oval form and lies midway between the anterosuperior iliac spine and the pubic symphysis. It normally fits rather closely about the penetrating structures unless it has been distended by the sac of an *indirect inguinal hernia* (Fig. 3). The superior border of the internal inguinal ring is the *transversus abdominis arch,* which is the inferior edge of the transverse abdominis muscle aponeurosis and inserts medially to the pubic tubercle. The inferior border of the internal inguinal ring is the *iliopubic tract,* an extension of the transversalis fascia that extends from its lateral attachment the anterosuperior iliac spine, medially to the superior pubic ramus. At about midway through its course, the iliopubic tract forms the inferior boundary of the internal inguinal ring and the transition of the transversalis fascia to the anterior femoral sheath. The iliopubic tract is distinct from the inguinal ligament, which lies superficial to it. The medial border of the internal ring is made up of the *interfoveolar ligament (Hesselbach's ligament),* a crescentic band of fibers that fan out medially along the inferior epigastric vessels as they ascend to the rectus muscle from the external iliac vessels and the transversalis fascial sling. The interfoveolar ligament is felt to be the most important structure making up the medial border of the internal ring.

A second structure in this area, first described by Franz K. Hesselbach, a German surgeon, is *Hesselbach's triangle.* The boundaries of this triangle are the lateral border of the rectus muscle medially, the inferior epigastric vessels laterally, and the inguinal ligament inferiorly (the iliopubic tract from the laparoscopic perspective). This is the site of *direct inguinal hernias* (Fig. 4).

When viewed laparoscopically, the femoral canal is triangular in shape and measures about 1.25 cm in length. Its boundaries are the external iliac vein laterally, the iliopubic tract superiorly, and Cooper's ligament inferiorly along the upper edge of the superior pubic ramus. This is the location of the *femoral hernia.*

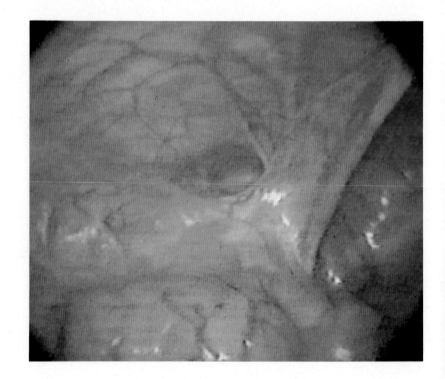

Figure 3. Intraoperative view of a left indirect hernia. The hernia defect is just lateral to the inferior epigastric vessels. The medial umbilical ligament is also seen.

Cooper's ligament (pectineal ligament) is a strong, narrow, tendinous ridge densely adherent to the pectineal line along the superior edge of the superior pubic ramus. It was first described by Sir Astley Cooper, an English anatomist and surgeon. Cooper's ligament is covered by peritoneum and subserous fascia and, when dissected, is a white, glistening, easily identified ligament (Fig. 5). When performing laparoscopic inguinal hernioplasty, it is paramount to dissect the peritoneum and fatty areolar tissue off Cooper's ligament from the pubic tubercle to the external iliac vein to ensure adequate fixation of the prosthetic patch. Although this dissection is usually uneventful, there are two structures one needs to be aware of.

The inferior epigastric artery gives off a small branch at its origin called the *pubic branch*. This tiny artery runs medially on the iliopubic tract and then courses inferiorly along the medial border of the femoral canal. It crosses Cooper's ligament and gives off a tiny branch (arteria corona mortis), which continues medially on the surface of Cooper's ligament. The pubic branch continues inferiorly and joins the obturator artery. This tiny artery is often accompanied by several slightly

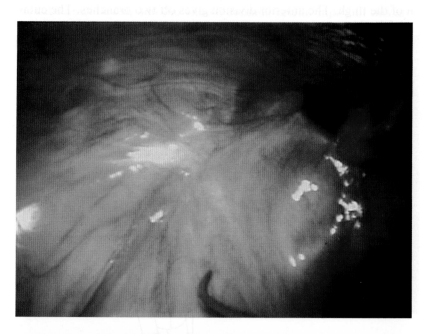

Figure 4. Intraoperative view of a left direct hernia. The spermatic vessels and the ductus deferens can be seen going into the internal ring. The inferior epigastric vessels with the defect medial to them are easily identified.

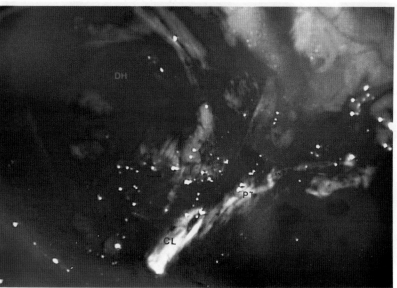

Figure 5. A large direct hernia with the peritoneum and subserous fascia covering Cooper's ligament and the pubic tubercle dissected away exposing the white glistening ligament.

component of the femoral nerve comprises largely the cutaneous branches, and the major muscular branches lie in the deep posterior division of the femoral nerve.

The genitofemoral nerve arises from the first and second lumbar nerves. It passes down through the psoas major muscles and emerges on its ventral surface at the level of the third or fourth lumbar vertebra. It is covered by the endoabdominal fascia (psoas fascia) and peritoneum. On the surface of the muscle, or occasionally within the substance of the muscle, the nerve divides into a genital and a femoral branch.

The genital branch continues caudally on the surface of the psoas muscle. It then pierces the endoabdominal fascia at the internal inguinal ring and converges with the testicular vessels, the ductus deferens, to form the spermatic cord. It lies against the dorsal aspect of the cord, supplying the cremaster muscle and the skin of the scrotum. In the female, it accompanies the round ligament of the uterus.

The femoral branch continues caudally on the surface of the psoas, lateral to the genital branch, and passes under the inguinal ligament with the external iliac artery within the femoral sheath. It lies anterior and lateral to the artery and then pierces the sheath and fascia lata to supply the skin to the proximal part of the anterior surface of the thigh for approximately 7.5 cm.

The genital and femoral branches may be injured when dissecting flaps and the hernia sac from the spermatic cord structures at the internal ring. Both of these branches lie beneath the spermatic vessels as they travel caudally on the anterior surface of the psoas muscle. The femoral branch, however, is more lateral and may be injured if stapling is done just lateral to the spermatic vessels. Injury to these nerves would result in a sensory deficit and/or pain to the dermatomes in the scrotum and a small area on the anterior thigh, just below the inguinal ligament.

The lateral femoral cutaneous nerve arises from the second and third lumbar nerves. It emerges midway down the psoas muscle from its lateral edge and runs across the iliacus muscle obliquely toward the anterosuperior iliac spine. It passes under the inguinal ligament at its lateral end and enters the thigh, where it divides into anterior and posterior branches, which supply the skin of the lateral aspect of the thigh and knee. It also supplies the skin of the lower lateral quadrant of the buttocks. This nerve can be injured when dissecting large peritoneal flaps laterally near the anterior superior iliac spine and inferior to the iliopubic tract. This would result in a sensory deficit and/or pain in the dermatome in the anterolateral thigh.

▶ PREOPERATIVE PLANNING

The surgeon has various options to repair an inguinal hernia whether it be direct, indirect, or femoral. Surgical repair is the only option and one of the common complications of inguinal hernia is that of incarceration of the bowel or ovary with possible strangulation. General anesthesia is required in the laparoscopic technique and in those patients who have comorbid diseases such as chronic obstructive pulmonary disease, coronary artery disease, and congestive heart failure, may best be treated by local anesthesia using an anterior approach with mesh. In addition, pediatric patients under the age of 16 should most likely be treated by the anterior approach rather than laparoscopically. However, the laparoscopy is especially suited for recurrent and bilateral inguinal hernias.

In the laparoscopic technique there are three methods of repair: (i) an onlay patch using a Gore-Tex peritoneal onlay patch, (ii) a transabdominal preperitoneal placement of mesh, and (iii) the total extraperitoneal approach using mesh. The preferred method in our practice is with the use of an onlay patch of Gore-Tex because of its decreased ability to form adhesions with intraperitoneal tissue. On the other hand, polypropylene mesh is associated with a significant number of adhesions and the postoperative complication of bowel obstruction is a real concern. As has been shown with mesh used in the anterior technique, mesh infection is not a major concern in laparoscopy.

The Gore-Tex peritoneal onlay laparoscopic hernioplasty has undergone several modifications throughout its evolution.

The procedure is performed under general anesthesia. The patient is given antibiotic prophylaxis, and the bladder is decompressed with a Foley catheter; the stomach is decompressed with a nasogastric tube. The patient is supine in the Trendelenburg position. The television monitors are positioned at the patient's feet. A skin incision is made at the superior edge of the umbilicus, and a Veress needle is used to insufflate the abdomen with carbon dioxide for visualization of the peritoneal cavity. A 10/11-mm trocar is inserted into the peritoneal cavity via the umbilical incision, through which a 0-degree laparoscope is introduced. The abdominal cavity is then explored and the hernia defect confirmed. Two additional 10/11-mm trocars are inserted under direct vision. These are placed at the level of the umbilicus along the anterior axillary lines (Fig. 9). The contents of the sac, if present, are reduced into the peritoneal cavity. This is usually quite easy; however, it can be the most difficult part of the procedure, especially on large, direct hernias. These may be sliding hernias and have colon (usually sigmoid on the left and cecum on the right) making up the inferior portion of the sac and/or bladder making up the medial portion of the sac. The bowel or bladder fat is grasped with an atraumatic babcock and retracted cephalad. The peritoneal reflection between bowel and hernia sac is easily identified and incised with endoshears, delivering the bowel back into the peritoneal cavity. The demarcation between the bladder and the hernia sac is not so obvious. Early in our experience, while performing this portion of the dissection, we entered the bladder. This required an open repair of the bladder rent and a Lichtenstein hernioplasty. To avoid this complication, on large, direct hernia defects, dissection is started on the anterior abdominal wall component of the medial umbilical ligament and carried inferiorly, incising only the peritoneum and teasing bluntly all bladder and perivesicle fat from the medial portion of the hernia sac. Dissection can also be started lateral to the defect at the level where the ductus deferens crosses Cooper's ligament. The peritoneum is incised and the fatty areolar tissue is bluntly teased away, exposing Cooper's ligament. This blunt dissection is carried medially up to the

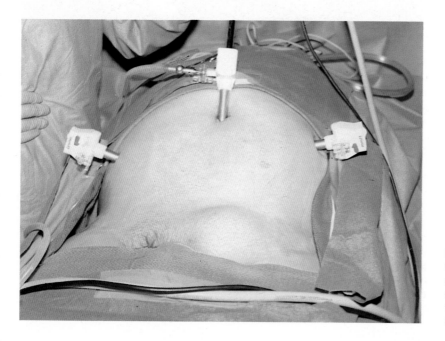

Figure 9. The scope is introduced via the umbilical trocar. The two additional trocars are placed at the anterior axillary line at the level of the umbilicus under direct vision. The bulge of the left inguinal hernia can be seen.

pubic tubercle. These two maneuvers safely reduce the bladder into the peritoneal cavity and clears the medial edge of the hernia defect for patch fixation. The sac is left in situ with no ligation of the internal ring. When there is no sliding component on the medial edge of the defect, the medial umbilical ligament is incised laterally and reflected medially with endoscopic scissors. Dissection inferiorly and laterally exposes the pubic tubercle and Cooper's ligament (Fig. 10). The dissection is carried laterally along Cooper's ligament up to the ductus deferens, which courses over the external iliac vein at this level. Any redundant, floppy, medial umbilical ligament is stapled medially to the anterior abdominal wall to prevent it from obstructing the surgeon's view.

An expanded polytetrafluoroethylene (ePTFE) dualmesh biomaterial, 1-mm thick (W.L. Gore & Associates, Inc., Flagstaff, Arizona), is cut to 8.0 × 12 cm in size and tailored inferiorly to conform with the oblique Cooper's ligament and iliopubic tract (Fig. 11).

After a thorough review of the experimental and clinical data on biomaterials, ePTFE was felt to be the best biomaterial in the intraperitoneal position. When compared to all the other biomaterials available, ePTFE is the strongest, has the best fixation-retention, has the best durability, is the most inert, has the least

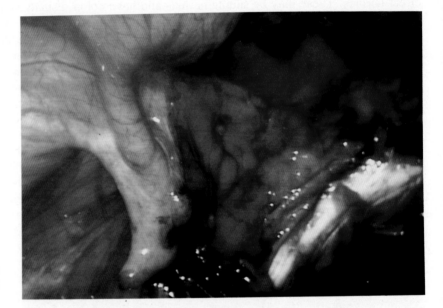

Figure 10. An intraoperative dissection of Cooper's ligament up to the tubercle; a large indirect hernia is to the left.

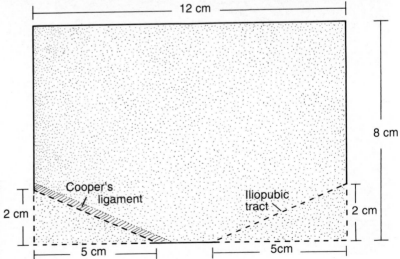

Figure 11. A template for the cutting of the Gore-Tex dualmesh biomaterial. The Cooper's ligament side is marked with a sterile marking pencil for easy identification intraabdominally.

acute inflammatory response, has the least infectability, has the least foreign-body response, and is the softest, most pliable, and least abrasive. Experimental studies and clinical experience with full-thickness abdominal wall defect repairs have shown a lower incidence and grade of visceral adhesion formation and/or adhesion-related complications with ePTFE when compared to the polypropylene and polyester mesh materials. The cardinal determining factor for the choice of prosthetic material in the peritoneal position is erosion of abdominal viscera resulting in obstruction, abscess, and fistula formation. Experimental studies and clinical experience with polypropylene and polyester meshes are replete with complications of erosions and fistulization. ePTFE in the peritoneal position has never had a reported case of erosion and fistulization. The edge to be stapled to Cooper's ligament is highlighted with a sterile marker for easy orientation. CV-2 Gore-Tex sutures are attached to all four corners, leaving approximately 6-in. strands. The patch is then attached to a 2-pronged Endo-Patch Spreader (Fig. 12) with 2-0 Ethibond sutures. The medial (pubic tubercle) corner of the patch is attached to the short prong (Fig. 13). This greatly facilitates introduction of the patch into the peritoneal cavity and the spreading and positioning of the inferomedial edge of the patch over the pubic tubercle and Cooper's ligament. The Endo-Patch Spreader is inserted through the contralateral 11-mm trocar. Through the ipsilateral 11-mm

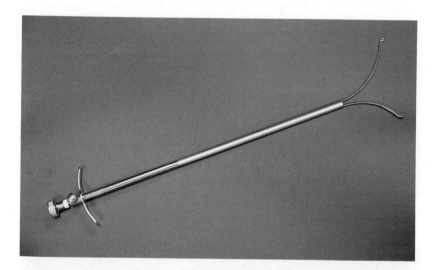

Figure 12. The two-pronged patch spreader is used to introduce and spread the Gore-Tex soft tissue patch. This greatly facilitates introduction and positioning of the patch.

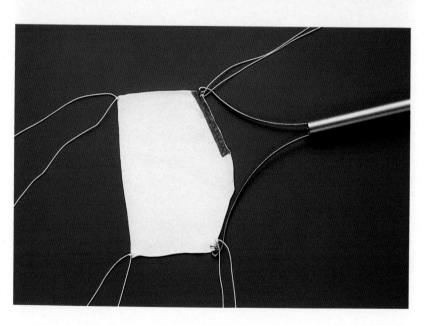

Figure 13. The patch cut with Cooper's ligament highlighted with a marking pencil and attached to the two-pronged patch spreader. Note that the shorter limb of the patch spreader is attached at the pubic tubercle on the Cooper's ligament side for easier positioning. Sutures are placed at all four corners. The strands are left about 6 in. long for suture fixation.

trocar, the Endopath EMS hernia stapler (Ethicon, Inc., Cincinnati, Ohio) (Fig. 14) is inserted. It is paramount to use a stapler that has a sturdy straight-drive mechanism and a box staple. This is necessary to drive the staple out through the 1-mm Gore-Tex dualmesh biomaterial and deep into the fascia. The staple then closes into a box, fixing the patch securely to the fascia. The only commercially available stapler that meets these criteria is the Endopath EMS hernia stapler. Articulating staplers are *not* adequate. Several staples are placed, securing the Gore-Tex patch to the pubic tubercle and Cooper's ligament up to the external iliac vein (Fig. 15). The sutures attaching the patch to the spreader are then cut, and the Endo-Patch Spreader is removed. The inferior lateral corner is grasped and positioned over the iliopubic tract and fixed with staples. The iliopubic tract is easy to identify without any dissection. It lies parallel and deep to the inguinal ligament (Poupart's ligament). Anterior abdominal wall countertraction is applied just above the inguinal ligament; this countertraction can be seen laparoscopically and palpated with the stapler head. The stapler head is then rolled inferiorly, just below the palpable fingers. This is the iliopubic tract from the laparoscopic perspective. It is paramount not to staple inferior to the iliopubic tract, so as to avoid injury to the femoral, genitofemoral, and/or lateral femoral cutaneous nerves. The Endo-Suture Passer (Fig. 16) secures previously placed sutures at each corner. The location of the corners is identified on the skin surface with

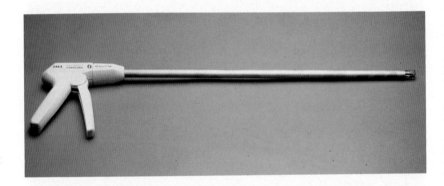

Figure 14. The endo-path EMS straight multifire stapler.

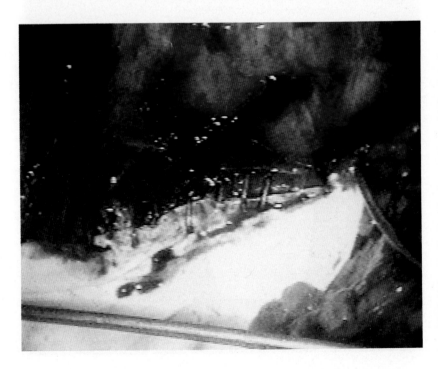

Figure 15. The two-pronged patch spreader holding the patch in place over Cooper's ligament and the pubic tubercle with multiple staples placed fixing the Gore-Tex soft tissue patch to Cooper's ligament.

bimanual palpation and/or passing a spinal needle for localization. A 2-mm nick is made in the skin with an 11-blade. The Endo-Suture Passer is passed through the abdominal wall, opened, and the sutures placed in the Endo-Suture Passer with a smooth grasper (a 5-mm needle holder works well) from the opposite trocar. The suture is then grasped and pulled out through the skin (Fig. 17). After retrieving both strands, the suture is tied down to the fascia easily, pushing through the subcutaneous fat (Fig. 18). This is done at all four corners. The EMS stapler is introduced via the contralateral trocar, and the patch is stapled anteriorly to the transversalis fascia and laterally to the endoabdominal fascia. Good fascial fixation of the staples anteriorly and laterally is facilitated by anterior abdominal wall countertraction. This provides secure and reliable fixation of the patch to the fascial structures, covering the indirect, direct, and femoral hernia spaces (Fig. 19).

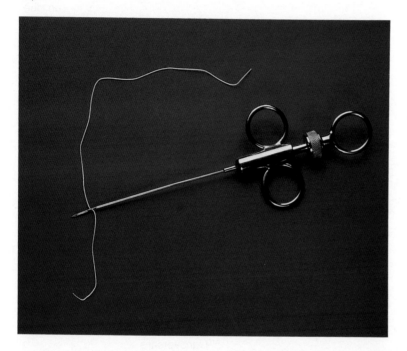

Figure 16. The Endo-Suture Passer with a suture in its grasp.

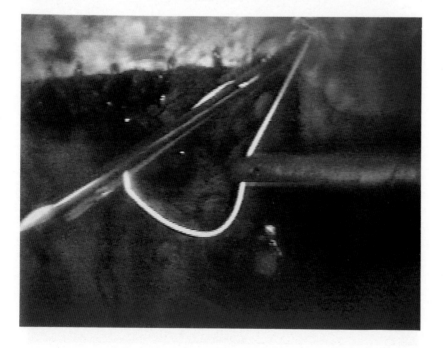

Figure 17. An intraabdominal view of the Endo-Suture Passer, which has been passed through the abdominal myofascial layers and Gore-Tex patch. The Endo-Suture Passer is opened, and the suture is being loaded into it using a blunt-tip needle driver.

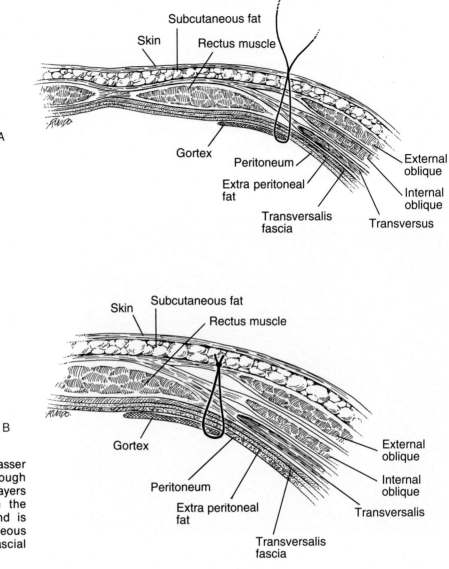

Figure 18. How the Endo-Suture Passer works. **A:** The suture is passed through the same skin incision and various layers of myofascial tissue and through the Gore-Tex. **B:** The knot is tied, and is pushed down through the subcutaneous tissue and secured to the anterior fascial layers.

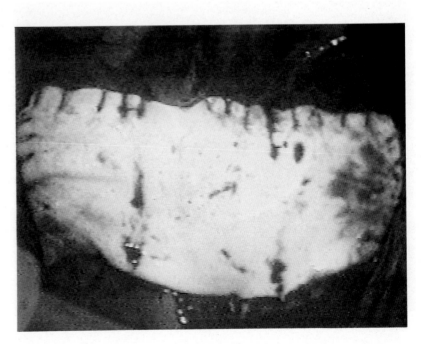

Figure 19. A complete repair demonstrating the Gore-Tex soft tissue patch in position over a left inguinal hernia.

Additional sutures are placed wherever it is felt necessary, depending on the size and the type of hernia. For the additional sutures, the location is identified and a skin nick made, the 2-0 nonabsorbable suture is grasped with the Endo-Suture Passer and passed through the abdominal wall and Gore-Tex patch. The suture is released and grasped with a smooth grasper. The Endo-Suture Passer is then passed through the same skin incision, but at a slightly different angle. The suture is then passed to the Endo-Suture Passer, grasped, and pulled out through the skin. By changing the angle slightly, the suture passes through the fascia, muscle, and/or Gore-Tex patch at a slightly different location. When this is tied down to the fascia, it is with a mattress stitch, which incorporates the Gore-Tex patch and all of the myofascial layers of the abdominal wall.

We have seen one small bowel obstruction from a Richter's hernia via a trocar site (Fig. 20). This was 4 days postoperatively. The patient was relapaorscoped,

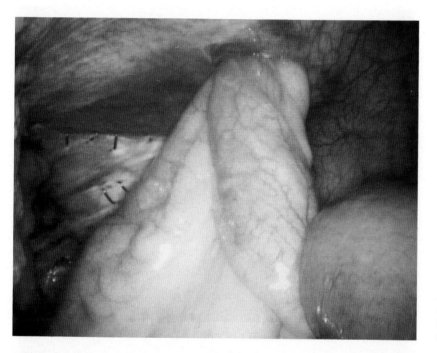

Figure 20. Richter's hernia. The bowel is up in the trocar site. The hernia repair is in the background. This is 4 days postoperative.

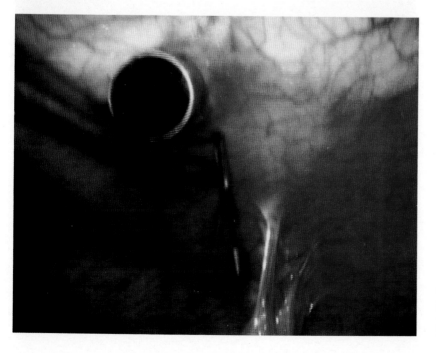

Figure 21. An Endo-Suture Passer with a 2-0 Ethibond suture mounted in it is passed through the skin incision of the trocar site adjacent to the trocar.

and the bowel was reduced and viable. The trocar site was then closed using the Endo-Suture Passer. We now close all our trocar sites to prevent this complication. While the abdomen is still insufflated and all the trocars are in place, a suture is grasped in the Endo-Suture Passer and passed through the same skin incision adjacent to the trocar. Intraabdominally, it is released and grasped with a blunt grasper (Fig. 21). The Endo-Suture Passer is removed and passed adjacent to the trocar on the opposite side, the suture is passed to the Endo-Suture Passer, grasped (Fig. 22), and pulled out through the skin (Fig. 23). All of the sutures are passed for each trocar under direct vision, leaving the strands long enough to tie later. The pneumoperitoneum is released, and the trocars are removed; the sutures are tied, closing the trocar sites. The skin is closed with 4-0 Vicryl, subcuticular sutures, and Steri-Strips. The patient is discharged to home when fully recovered.

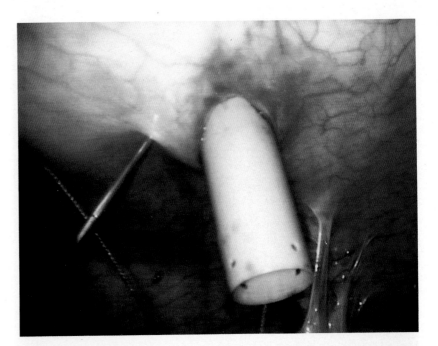

Figure 22. The suture is grasped by the Endo-Suture Passer, which is passed on the opposite side adjacent to the trocar. This is then pulled out, forming a Halsted mattress-type suture.

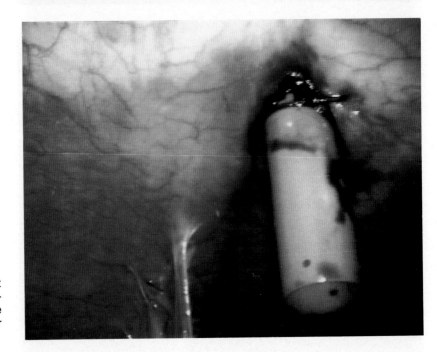

Figure 23. The sutures are pulled out with the trocar still in place. At completion, the trocars are all removed and the sutures are all tied, closing the trocar sites.

▲ COMPLICATIONS

The complication of the Gore-Tex peritoneal onlay laparoscopic hernioplasty can be divided into minor and major. The minor complications have been such things as urinary retention and abdominal wall hematomas, all of which resolved spontaneously. We had one pubic ostitis, which resolved after injection of the area with Depo-Medrol. We have had three major complications, all of which have been discussed in this chapter. The bladder injury early in our experience has been alleviated by always starting dissection of Cooper's ligament laterally and dissecting toward the pubic tubercle, teasing all the fatty areolar tissue from the defect bluntly in all direct hernias. The anterior thigh pain, which resulted from injuries to the femoral, lateral femoral cutaneous, or femoral branch of the gentiofemoral nerves, resolved spontaneously over a 3-month period. This complication has been eliminated with the tailoring of the patch's inferior edge and all fixation of the patch's inferior lateral edge to the iliopubic tract. We have seen one Richter's hernia, resulting in a small bowel obstruction 4 days postoperatively. This is an easily preventable complication with routine closure of all trocar sites greater than 10 mm. We have had five recurrences out of a total of 223 hernioplasties over the past 33 months; this is a recurrence rate of 2.2%. These recurrences were all early in the evolution of the procedure, prior to exposing Cooper's ligament, increasing the patch size from 5 × 7 cm to 8 × 12 cm, and the addition of the suture technique.

> *SURGICAL PEARLS*
> Always expose Cooper's ligament to ensure adequate staple fixation.
> Always dissect lateral to medial with direct hernias to avoid bladder injury.
> Never staple or suture below the iliopubic tract laterally.
> Close all trocar sites larger than 10 mm.

RECOMMENDED READING

1. Spaw AT, Ennis BW, Spaw LP. Laparoscopic hernia repair: the anatomic basis. *J Laparoendosc Surg* 1991;1:269–277.
2. Toy FK, Smoot RT. Laparoscopic hernioplasty update. *J Laparosc Surg* 1992;2:197–205.
3. Brown GL, Richardson DJ, Malangoni MA, Tobin GR, Ackermaan D, Polk HC Jr. Comparison of prosthetic material for abdominal wall reconstruction in the presence of contamination and infection. *Ann Surg* 1985;201:705–711.
4. Law NH, Ellis H. Adhesion formation and peritoneal healing on prosthetic materials. *Clin Mater* 1988;3:95–101.
5. Bauer JJ, Salky BA, Gelernt IM, Kreel I. Repair of large abdominal wall defects with expanded polytetrafluoroethylene (PTFE). *Ann Surg* 1987;206:765–769.
6. Law NW. A comparison of Polypropylene mesh, expanded polytetrafluoroethylene patch, and polyglycolic acid mesh for the repair of experimental abdominal wall defects. *Acta Chir Scand* 1990;156:759–762.
7. Kaufman Z, Engelberg M, Zager M. Fecal fistula: a late complication of Marlex mesh repair. *Dis Colon Rectum* 1981;24:543–544.
8. Voyles CR, Richardson JD, Bland KI, et al. Emergency abdominal wall reconstruction with polypropylene mesh: short-term benefits versus long-term complications. *Ann Surg* 1981;194:219–223.

44

Transabdominal Retroperitoneal Inguinal Herniorrhaphy

Maurice E. Arregui
Department of Surgery
St. Vincent Hospital and Health Care Center
Indianapolis, Indiana 46260

Operative Laparoscopy and Thoracoscopy, edited by B. V. MacFadyen, Jr. and J. L. Ponsky. Lippincott-Raven Publishers, Philadelphia © 1996.

KEY WORDS

Blunt dissection   Onlay mesh

CO_2 Preperitoneal space

Direct, indirect hernias   TAPP (transabdominal preperitoneal approach)

Because of the remarkable success associated with laparoscopic cholecystectomy, it seems logical to extend the principles of minimally invasive surgery to the second most common general surgical procedure performed. Approximately 700,000 hernias are repaired annually in the United States, of which 500,000 are inguinal hernias.

Traditional herniorrhaphy without mesh under general anesthesia is the most commonly used technique throughout the United States and internationally. There is considerable pain associated with this procedure and a convalescence of approximately 6 weeks before patients are allowed unrestricted activity. The potential improvement in the pain, cosmesis, and convalescence has served as the impetus for developing laparoscopic hernia repairs. Moreover, the high recurrence rate associated with traditional techniques and the associated costs and discomfort of repairing recurrent hernias serves as an added incentive. At a recent symposium on inguinal hernia repair in Indianapolis, an estimated 15% of these repairs were for recurrences. This would add up to approximately $15,000,000 in the United States alone (500,000 × 0.15 × $2,000). The unseen costs of a prolonged convalescence have not even been considered. They could be substantial.

Preliminary studies have shown that laparoscopic hernia repairs can be performed with reasonably low complication rates and very few recurrences even during the learning curve. Numerous techniques are being performed, but currently the most commonly used is the transabdominal preperitoneal approach (TAPP).

● ANATOMY

Peritoneal Landmarks

More than with any other laparoscopic procedures, the anatomy and perspective of inguinal hernia repair is quite different and less familiar to the surgeon. Upon entering the peritoneal cavity, one is particularly struck by the multiple folds and fossae, which are exaggerated by the pressurized intraperitoneal cavity. The median umbilical fold represents the obliterated urachus extending from the bladder to the umbilicus. This is often not clearly seen. The next fold is the medial umbilical fold, which represents the obliterated umbilical arteries. This extends from its origin at the internal iliac vessels to its termination at the umbilicus. Medial to this fold lies the bladder. A good rule of thumb is to avoid cutting the peritoneum and preperitoneal tissues medial to this to lessen the chances of a bladder injury. The next landmark is the lateral umbilical fold, which represents the inferior epigastric vessels. Between the medial and lateral folds is the site of occurrence of direct groin hernias. Lateral to the epigastric vessels lies the orifice of the internal ring, which is the site of indirect inguinal hernias (Fig. 1).

Periperitoneal Anatomy

Critical to a safe preperitoneal dissection is an understanding of the preperitoneal fascias. The bladder, umbilical ligaments, and preperitoneal fatty layer surrounding these structures are contained between the peritoneum and the umbilical prevesicular fascia or preperitoneal fascia. This discrete layer also surrounds the cord structures and, when present, the indirect hernia sac as they enter the internal inguinal ring. In fact, it is this preperitoneal fascia rather than the transversalis fascia that continues into the inguinal canal to form the internal spermatic fascia (Fig. 2). The blood supply to the structures contained by the preperitoneal fascia is derived from the internal iliac vessels and branches to the bladder as well as the spermatic artery. Dissection within the preperitoneal fascia medial to the medial

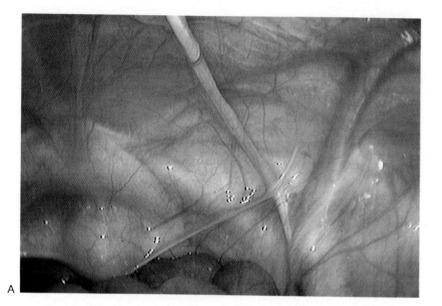

A

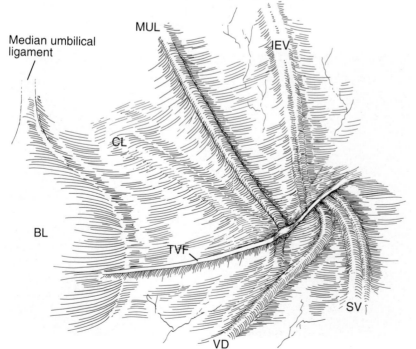

B

Figure 1. A: Laparoscopic photo of a thin elderly female undergoing laparoscopic cholecystectomy demonstrates the inguinal anatomy quite well. (From Arregui et al., ref. 5, with permission.) **B:** The peritoneal landmarks in a male: BL, bladder; MUL, medial umbilical ligament; IEV, inferior epigastric vessels; TVF, transverse vesicular fold; VD, vas deferens; SV, spermatic vessels; CL, Cooper's ligament.

umbilical ligament could result in a bladder injury. The correct space of dissection is superficial to the umbilical prevesicular fascia and the posterior lamina of the transversalis fascia. This latter structure represents an attenuated continuation of the posterior rectus sheath. The blood supply to this and the anterior abdominal wall is derived from the inferior epigastric vessels. The preperitoneal space extends inferiorly to the space of Retzius and laterally and posteriorly to the retroperitoneal space (Fig. 3).

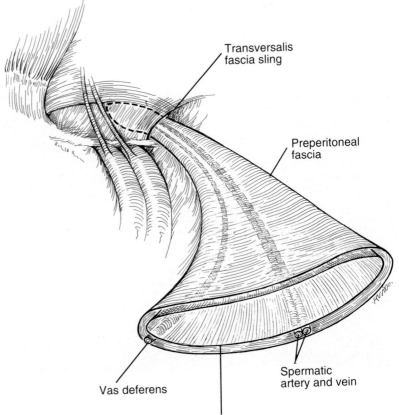

Transversalis fascia sling

Preperitoneal fascia

Vas deferens

Peritoneum

Spermatic artery and vein

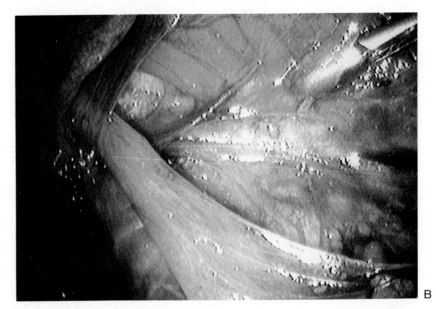

B

Figure 2. A: Preperitoneal fascia at right internal ring. **B:** Extraperitoneal dissection showing the preperitoneal fascia surrounding the cord structures at the right internal ring.

Anatomy of the Nerves and Vessels

Early reports of nerve injuries due to laparoscopic hernia repairs attest to the fact that surgeons' understanding of this area has been lacking. To avoid these injuries, a clear knowledge of the relationship of these structures is essential. Contained within the triangle formed by the spermatic cord and the spermatic vessels are the external iliac vessels and femoral nerve. Also contained within and following the cord structures into the canal is the genital branch of the genitofemoral nerve. Lateral to the spermatic vessels and inferior to the lateral iliopubic

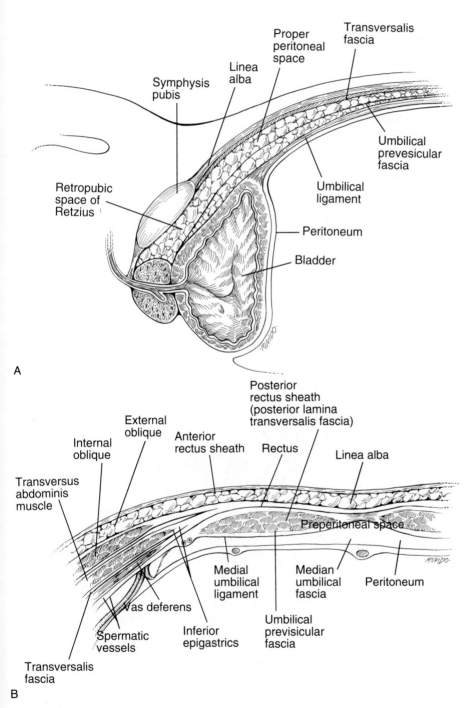

Figure 3. A: Longitudinal midline view of the preperitoneal space, which is continuous with the space of Retzius. **B:** Transverse view of the preperitoneal space and fascias at the level of the internal inguinal ring.

tract is located the femoral branch of the genitofemoral nerve and further laterally is the lateral femoral cutaneous nerve (Fig. 4).

Myopectineal Orifice of Fruchaud

The basic concept of the transabdominal preperitoneal placement of a large prosthesis is to cover the myopectineal orifice of Fruchaud, which represents the areas of potential weakness in the groin. The myopectineal orifice is bounded inferiorly by the superior ramus of the pubis or Cooper's ligament, inferior laterally by the iliopectineal fascia covering the iliopsoas muscle, anteriorly and laterally by the transversus abdominis muscle, superiorly by the aponeurosis of the transversus abdominis muscle, and medially by the rectus abdominis (Fig. 5).

▶ PREOPERATIVE PLANNING

Preoperative assessment requires careful evaluation of the hernia type, previous surgery, age, and risk factors. Patients must be thoroughly informed of the risks of laparoscopic versus open hernia repairs. They must also be informed of the uncertainty of the long-term results of this evolving technique.

Physical Examination

Physical examination confirms the presence of a groin hernia and can often determine the hernia type. Symptoms compatible with groin hernias without a

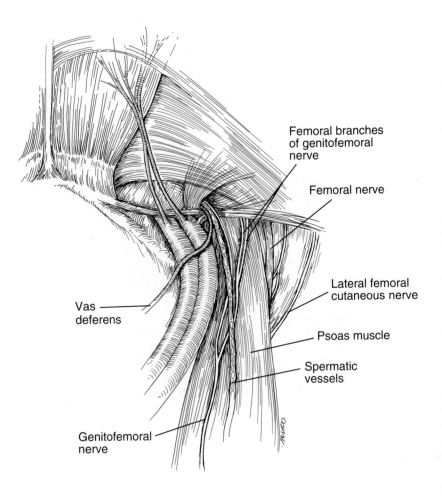

Figure 4. Anatomy of the nerves and vessels of the preperitoneal and retroperitoneal inguinal space.

palpable bulge could represent an occult hernia. Herniography is used by some to determine the presence of an occult hernia. Ultrasonography can be useful to find nonpalpable femoral hernias but is not useful in our experience to identify other types of occult groin hernias. It is useful in differentiating hernias from other groin masses such as enlarged lymph nodes, abscesses, and lipomas. We have also found ultrasound useful to distinguish direct from indirect hernia.

Type of Hernia

To properly prepare for surgery, one must know the type of hernia. Several classifications are used. L. M. Nyhus has developed a simple classification scheme, which has become widely accepted by most surgeons and serves well for open as well as laparoscopic inguinal hernia repair. By maintaining consistency in classification, we can better assess his results as well as to plan the best surgical approach. Small congenital or indirect hernias are classified as type I hernias. Most would agree that these require simple high ligation, which can be performed laparoscopically or open. Direct hernias, large or complex hernias, recurrent, and bilateral hernias suggest a weakness in the myopectineal orifice due to a collagen deficiency and are best repaired with a mesh reinforcement.

Previous Surgery

Previous surgery in the lower abdomen may make laparoscopic hernia repair more difficult and risky. A midline incision may pose access problems. Lower quadrant incisions may make dissection of the peritoneum and preperitoneal tissues much more difficult. If extensive lower abdominal surgery has been performed, consideration should be given to an anterior approach. We have not found previous lower abdominal surgery an absolute contraindication.

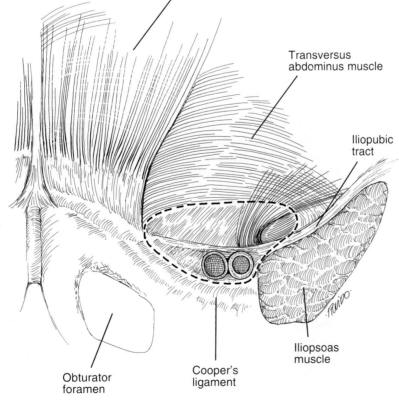

Figure 5. Myopectineal orifice of Fruchaud—posterior view right side.

portion left in place (see Fig. 10). Because of increased intraabdominal pressure any oozing or seroma formation will collect in the hernia sac, and this may result in a postoperative hematoma or seroma. This problem will not be eliminated even if the sac is dissected out, since the space remains. A large indirect sac cannot be inverted as can a direct sac.

Selecting the Mesh and Anchoring

The mesh is usually soaked in an antibiotic solution of 500 mg of cephalothin mixed in 500 ml of normal saline. The selected mesh is trimmed to size, folded in half, then rolled. The end to be inserted is grasped with a grasping forceps and introduced directly into the 11-mm umbilical port into the peritoneal cavity. The mesh is unrolled and positioned in the preperitoneal space.

Initially we used a 3 × 5 in. Prolene mesh (Ethicon, Inc., New Brunswick, NJ) but have gradually increased the size to 4 × 6 in. This larger size allows complete coverage of the myopectineal orifice of Fruchaud with good overlap. Prior to the development of stapling devices, we used suturing technique to anchor the mesh. This worked quite well but was cumbersome. Stapling devices were soon substituted but were not always reliable nor that easy to use. Moreover, by any technique the risk of injury to nerves was pervasive (Fig. 12). We no longer anchor the mesh.

Closing the Peritoneum

Once the mesh is in place laying over the direct, indirect, and femoral space and overlying the cord structures, the peritoneum must be closed. Most use staples for closure but we prefer to close with absorbable Vicryl suture using the purse-string technique. Meticulous closure is necessary to avoid exposure of mesh and preperitoneal fat and fascia, which can predispose to adhesion formation. The peritoneal defect should closely resemble the minimal puckering seen with a high ligation during open surgery (Fig. 13).

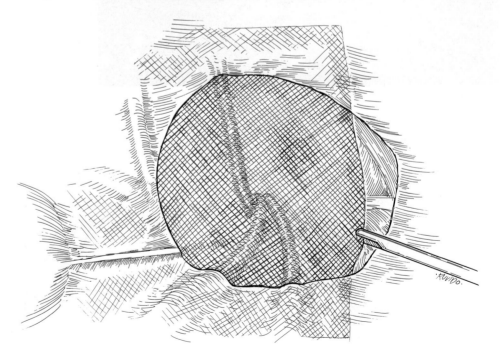

Figure 12. Positioning of the mesh in the preperitoneal space.

Final peritoneal inspection is carried out to look for any peritoneal defects that must be repaired. The CO_2 in the extraperitoneal space is aspirated out to check the final position of the mesh. It is very important to be certain that the mesh is lying flat without curling of the edges (Fig. 14). Marcaine 0.5% is introduced into the preperitoneal space prior to removal of the trocars.

Any trocar site 10 mm or greater is closed with absorbable 2-0 Vicryl. The umbilical trocar site is also closed with 2-0 Vicryl. Subcutaneous sutures of 3-0 Vicryl are used to close the skin incisions.

Postoperative Care

The patient is kept in the recovery room for approximately 1 hour before transfer to the third-stage recovery area where observation for an additional 2 to 3 hours is carried out prior to discharge. A prescription for 15 tablets of 7.5 mg hydrocodone bitartrate (Lortabs 7.5 mg, Whitby Pharmaceuticals, Richmond, VA) with one refill is given.

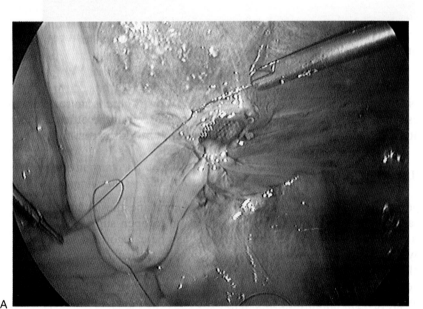

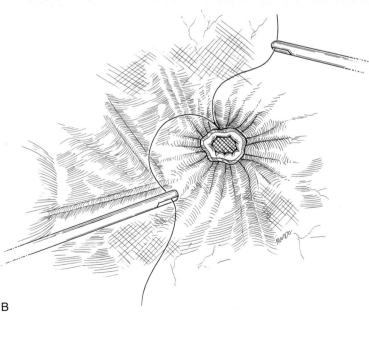

Figure 13. A: Purse-string closure of the peritoneal defect. **B:** Purse-string closure of the peritoneum. **C:** Inspection of the mesh. (From Arregui, ref. 4, with permission.)

lems should be mostly eliminated. It is important, however, to be aware of the potential pitfalls. Currently, the laparoscopic approach is a more invasive technique than that of open repair and is more costly. Careful consideration should be given to individual patients and their individual needs. We have not yet demonstrated that the laparoscopic approach has any advantage over open anterior repair using mesh, which can be performed with local anesthesia. For simple unilateral primary hernias, this is an excellent technique. Those who perform this operation routinely report minimal pain with a rapid return to full activity. Prospective studies are being performed to compare these techniques. Currently, the optimal indication for laparoscopic repair of inguinal hernia with a large prosthesis is on patients with recurrent, bilateral, or complicated hernias.

RECOMMENDED READING

1. Arregui ME, Nagan RF, eds. *Inguinal hernia: advances or controversies*. Oxford, UK: Radcliffe, 1994.
2. Arregui ME, Navarrete J, Davis CJ, et al. Laparoscopic inguinal herniorrhaphy: techniques and controversies. *Surg Clin North Am* 1993;73:513–527.
3. Arregui ME, Navarrette JL. Laparoscopic preperitoneal repair of inguinal hernias with mesh. In: *Minimal access general surgery*. Oxford, UK: Radcliffe, 1993.
4. Arregui ME. Laparoscopic hernia repair. In: *Laparoscopy in focus*. Vol. 1. McMahon Group, 1992.
5. Arregui ME, Castro D, Nagan RF. Anatomy of the peritoneum, preperitoneal fascia and posterior of lamina of the transversalis fascia in the inguinal area. In: *Inguinal hernia: advances or controversies?* Oxford, UK: Radcliffe, 1993.
6. Lichtenstein IL. Herniorrhaphy: a personal experience with 6,321 cases. *Am J Surg* 1987;153:553–559.
7. MacFadyen BV, Arregui ME, Corbitt J Jr, et al. Complications of laparoscopic herniorrhaphy. *Surg Endosc* 1993;7:155–158.
8. Nyhus LM. The preperitoneal approach and iliopubic tract repair of inguinal hernia. In: Nyhus LM, Condon RE, ed. *Hernia*. Philadelphia: JB Lippincott; 1989:154–177.
9. Rutkow IM, Robbins AW. Demographic, classificatory, and socioeconomic aspects of hernia repair in the United States. *Surg Clin North Am* 1993;73:413–426.
10. Stoppa RE, Warlaumont CR. The preperitoneal approach and prosthetic repair of groin hernia. In: Nyhus LM, Condon RE, eds. *Hernia*. Philadelphia: JB Lippincott; 1989:199–255.
11. Wantz GE. *Atlas of hernia surgery*. New York: Raven Press, 1991.

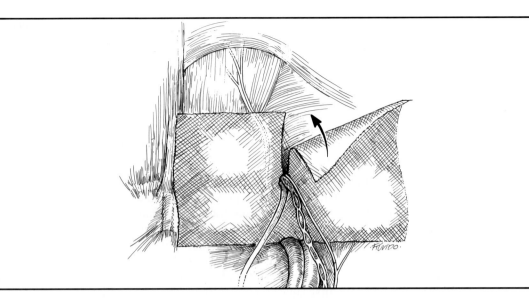

45

Extraperitoneal Inguinal Herniorrhaphy

J. Barry McKernan
Department of Surgery
Emory University School of Medicine
Atlanta, Georgia 30322; and
Medical College of Georgia
Augusta, Georgia 30912-4000

Operative Laparoscopy and Thoracoscopy, edited by
B. V. MacFadyen, Jr. and
J. L. Ponsky. Lippincott-Raven
Publishers, Philadelphia © 1996.

inguinal hernias. Furthermore, we consider this laparoscopic extraperitoneal procedure for active, postpubertal patients with primary inguinal defects because of the increased speed of recovery and diminished pain associated with this and other laparoscopic procedures. The only absolute contraindication is an inability to tolerate general anesthesia.

RECOMMENDED READING

1. Nyhus LM, Condon RE, Harkins HN. Clinical experiences with preperitoneal hernial repair for all types of hernia of the groin with particular emphasis to the importance of transversalis fascia analogues. *Am J Surg* 1960;100:234.
2. Stoppa R, Petit J, Henry X. Unsutured Dacron prosthesis in groin hernias. *Int Surg* 1975;60:411.
3. Stoppa RE, Warlaumont CR. The preperitoneal approach and prosthetic repair of groin hernia. In: Nyhus LM, Condon RE, eds. *Hernia,* 3rd ed. Philadelphia: JB Lippincott; 1989:199.

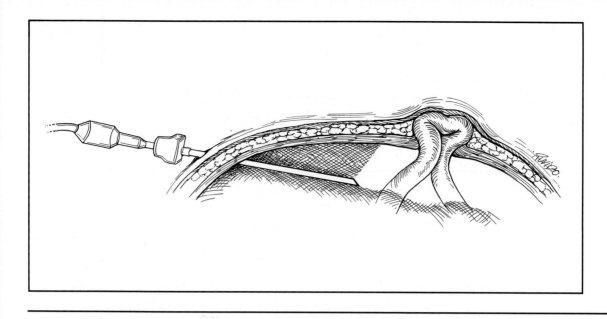

46

Ventral Hernia Repair

Robert W. Sewell
350 Westpark Way, #205
Euless, Texas 76034

Operative Laparoscopy and Thoracoscopy, edited by
B. V. MacFadyen, Jr. and
J. L. Ponsky. Lippincott-Raven
Publishers, Philadelphia © 1996.

KEY WORDS

ePTFE prosthesis   Spigelian hernia

Herniaplasty   Tension-free prosthesis

Polypropylene mesh   Transversalis fascia

By entering the abdominal cavity to perform a diagnostic or therapeutic procedure, the surgeon knowingly creates the potential for a ventral hernia. While some types of ventral hernias occur naturally, the majority are iatrogenic and therefore more accurately classified as incisional hernias. Many factors influence whether or not a particular patient will develop an incisional hernia, the most notable of which are wound infection, underlying malignancy, obesity, malnutrition, chronic cough, prostatism, and other chronic illnesses. In addition, the specific technique used to close the original abdominal incision may also play a significant part in the development of incisional hernias.

Incisional hernias are far from uniform in size or location, and frequently they may occur as multiple defects within a single incision. This wide variability has led to the development of many different techniques for their repair, which have in turn yielded variable results. This chapter deals with the feasibility and applicability of laparoscopic techniques in the repair of ventral hernias. I have used this procedure to successfully repair a variety of defects, both large and small. The technique, known as laparoscopic ventral herniaplasty, involves the placement of a tension-free prosthetic bridge across the musculofascial defect rather than attempting to approximate the fascial edges, as in a more traditional herniorrhaphy (Fig. 1).

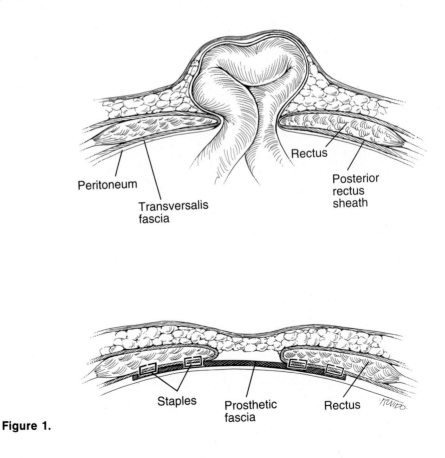

Figure 1.

● ANATOMY

The gross anatomy of the abdominal wall, as viewed from the exterior, is well known to all abdominal surgeons. However, when the abdominal wall is viewed from the interior, as it is during laparoscopy, its appearance is less familiar. Before attempting to repair a ventral hernia laparoscopically, the surgeon must first have a clear understanding of the interior of the anterior abdominal wall, from the inside out (Fig. 2).

The parietal peritoneum covers the interior of the entire abdominal wall, with the majority of its surface having no distinguishing characteristics. However, there are four specific peritoneal folds radiating out from the umbilicus. These elevations in the topography provide important landmarks for the laparoscopic surgeon. The most obvious of these landmarks is the falciform ligament, which drapes over the obliterated umbilical vein, also known as the ligamentum teres. This obliterated vessel passes cephalad from the umbilical annulus, beneath the dense umbilical fascia for several centimeters before emerging as an obvious peritoneal fold. It courses slightly to the right of the midline toward its eventual entrance into the substance of the liver. The curtainlike falciform ligament contains a variable amount of adipose tissue, and this structure may occasionally interfere with laparoscopic visualization of the upper abdomen. If necessary, this structure may be divided, but the ligamentum teres will frequently bleed if not adequately ligated.

Extending caudad from the umbilicus are three additional peritoneal folds, the median umbilical fold in the midline, and a pair of medial umbilical folds. The median umbilical fold is the remnant of the urachus, extending from the umbilicus to the dome of the urinary bladder. Usually it is very indistinct and difficult to identify, particularly in those patients with considerable amounts of preperitoneal

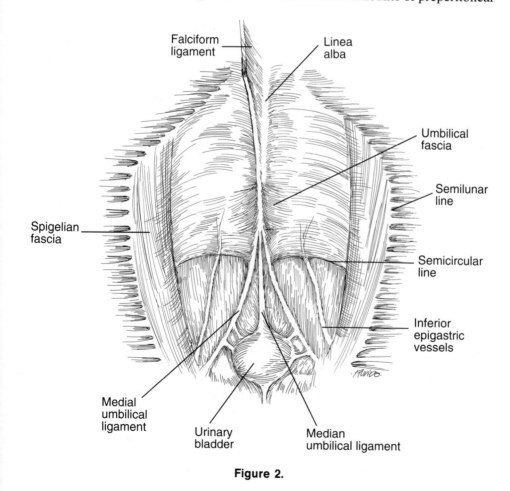

Figure 2.

fat. Although the urachus is normally obliterated, the possibility of patency should be considered anytime a procedure is performed in this area.

The medial umbilical folds are reflections of the peritoneum over the obliterated umbilical arteries. Each of these folds extends from the umbilicus to the rim of the true pelvis, just lateral to the urinary bladder. They too can occasionally be difficult to identify, but usually are very obvious. Like the falciform ligament, a variable amount of adipose tissue is found within these folds. The umbilical artery may be patent and should therefore be ligated whenever this peritoneal fold is divided.

The lateral umbilical folds are a pair of peritoneal elevations found lateral to each of the medial umbilical folds. These more subtle prominences are due to the underlying inferior epigastric vessels as they course cephalad from the inguinal region, along the posterior aspect of the rectus muscles. These vessels generally penetrate into the substance of the muscle within 6 to 8 cm of their origin, thus the lateral umbilical folds are quite short and often indistinct. The surgeon should attempt to identify each of these landmarks during laparoscopic procedures to ensure proper orientation. Unfortunately, any of these folds can be displaced by a ventral hernia, making their identification more difficult. But, generally, at least one of these structures can be found and used as an important frame of reference.

The parietal peritoneum is extremely well vascularized by a network of small vessels that can be seen running along its surface. Because of this superb blood supply, the peritoneum can be incised in virtually any direction, even to the point of creating large flaps, without significant risk of devascularization. This layer also has extraordinary regenerative capabilities, resulting in eventual complete reperitonealization of exposed surfaces.

Immediately anterior to the peritoneum is a layer of adipose tissue. This preperitoneal fatty layer is far from uniform, and may be totally absent in some areas. Typically, the largest deposits of fat are found below the semicircular line and along the lower midline up to the periumbilical region. Sizable deposits of preperitoneal fat may also be found in the flanks, as well as in the various peritoneal folds.

Anterior to the preperitoneal space is the transversalis fascia, a thin layer of dense connective tissue, which is continuous throughout the entire abdominal wall. Since this is the only truly continuous fascial layer, it may actually be the most important anatomic barrier to hernia formation. If this layer could be maintained intact, and unattenuated, there would not be a hernia, regardless of the status of the other structural elements of the abdominal wall. Unfortunately, when this layer is not supported by additional musculaponeurotic layers, it often lacks sufficient strength to prevent herniation. The placement and reinforcement of defective areas in the transversalis fascia, using a sheet of prosthetic material, is the fundamental principle of laparoscopic herniaplasty. Anterior to the transversalis fascia, the rectus abdominis muscles occupy most of the central portion of the abdominal wall. The upper two-thirds of these muscles is covered posteriorly by a dense fascial layer, the posterior rectus sheath. This sheath is absent below the semicircular line, leaving the transversalis fascia as the only connective tissue layer posterior to the rectus muscle. The linea alba, extending along the midline from the xiphoid to the pubis, between the rectus abdominis muscles, is well defined above the semicircular line, being formed by the decussation of fibers from both the anterior and posterior rectus sheaths. Below the semicircular line, it is less obvious when viewed from the inside because its fibers come exclusively from the anterior rectus sheath. The urinary bladder rises into the preperitoneal space above the pubis, and lies adjacent to the insertion of the rectus abdominis muscles. Just lateral to the rectus muscle is the transversus abdominis aponeurosis, also known as the spigelian fascia. Further lateral, beyond the semilunar line, this layer becomes muscular. Further anterior lie the remaining flat musculoaponeurotic layers, the internal and external obliques.

▶ PREOPERATIVE PLANNING

The diagnosis of ventral hernia is generally obvious when a palpable defect is present in the abdominal wall. Such defects frequently cause pain or disturbances in bowel function, prompting the patient to seek medical care. Even in those cases where a defect is not easily palpable, patients will typically point to an area in the abdominal wall where they have consistent pain or a sensation of weakness. In these situations, computed tomographic examination or ultrasonic scanning may confirm the diagnosis of herniation, but other radiographic studies are usually not helpful. On those occasions when a hernia is strongly suspected but cannot be confirmed, it may be appropriate to perform a diagnostic laparoscopy. Defects in the abdominal wall are easily identified from the inside when the peritoneal cavity is distended by a pneumoperitoneum (Fig. 3). If a hernia should be found during diagnostic laparoscopy, it can be repaired using a laparoscopic technique. Even if no hernia is found, the patient's symptoms are often substantially improved or eliminated by the simple lysis of any adhesions between the viscera and the abdominal wall.

In the absence of specific contraindication, ventral hernias should be treated with surgical repair. This is not only the best treatment for relieving symptoms, but also helps avoid the well-known complications of incarceration and bowel obstruction. Obviously this repair can be performed with any of a variety of techniques, including the laparoscopic approach.

For some patients, any surgical treatment may be inappropriate. In particular, very elderly patients with asymptomatic defects, and those with concomitant serious medical conditions, may be better managed with observation alone. Trusses or abdominal binders will provide symptomatic relief for some, but these constricting devices can impair respiratory effort, and may be contraindicated in patients with existing respiratory compromise.

In selecting patients for this procedure, the surgeon should consider the size of the defect, the size of the patient, the nature of the symptoms, as well as his or her own level of laparoscopic experience. Occasionally these procedures can be technically difficult, taxing the skills of even the most experienced laparoscopist. While this approach can be used to repair most types of ventral hernias, some defects are more easily managed laparoscopically than are others.

The location of the defect is generally not a significant limitation, since the entire anterior abdominal wall can be accessed laparoscopically. The size of the defect, on the other hand, may be a more limiting factor. Extremely large defects are poorer candidates for this repair, because these major defects may actually require musculofascial approximation to reestablish a functional abdominal wall.

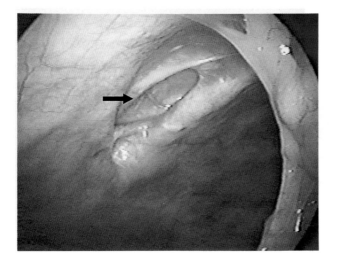

Figure 3. Occult hernia in a transverse right upper quadrant scar, identified laparoscopically.

level of the umbilicus. The spigelian aponeurosis is actually the continuation of the transversus abdominis and internal oblique muscles. When a defect exists in this layer, either congenital or acquired, it is not generally associated with any defect in the external oblique aponeurosis. Because this strong superficial layer is intact, the underlying hernia remains concealed, making the diagnosis difficult (Fig. 24).

Spigelian hernias are often associated with intermittent, nonspecific abdominal pain, occasionally accompanied by nausea and vomiting or changes in bowel habits. The duration of symptoms is usually brief and followed by periods of total resolution. Physical examination is typically unremarkable, but the examiner may be able to illicit point tenderness over the defect. This single finding is obviously inadequate to establish a diagnosis. The nonspecific nature of the symptoms and negative examination, frequently leads to an exhaustive evaluation, including various barium studies, esophagogastroduodenoscopy, colonoscopy, abdominal computed tomography scan, and occasionally even psychiatric evaluation. Despite these efforts, the diagnosis often remains elusive. However, if the surgeon is fortunate enough to examine the patient during an attack of pain, a palpable fullness in the abdominal wall is usually present, corresponding to the underlying defect. By applying gentle pressure, the hernia can be reduced, resolving both the abdominal wall mass and the symptoms. When spigelian hernia is suspected, laparoscopic examination of the abdominal wall provides an ideal means of confirmation. Using an initial periumbilical cannula, a 30- or 45-degree telescope can be used to inspect the abdominal wall thoroughly. The defect will be seen as a small opening in the peritoneum along the lateral margin of the rectus abdominis muscle (Fig. 25). If a spigelian hernia is found, it can readily be repaired using the same basic laparoscopic technique described for ventral hernia.

Additional cannulas are placed, on either side of the telescope port, and the dissection is initiated with a peritoneal incision, superior and medial to the defect. The hernia sac and preperitoneal fat are reduced out of the fascial defect using constant gentle traction. Then surrounding fascia is exposed, using the blunt irrigation technique previously described (Fig. 26). Care should be exercised when dissecting medially, since the inferior epigastric vessels can potentially be injured along the posterior aspect of the rectus muscle.

For repairing a spigelian hernia, a sheet of polypropylene mesh is cut, large enough to overlap several centimeters onto the normal fascia. It is placed in the abdomen, and stapled to the fascia, in the same manner described for other ventral hernias (Fig. 27). Sufficient peritoneum should always be available to cover the mesh, if the surgeon has taken the time to dissect out the sac (Fig. 28).

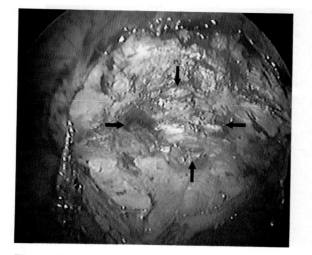

Figure 22. Multiple fascial defects are well defined after peritoneum has been removed.

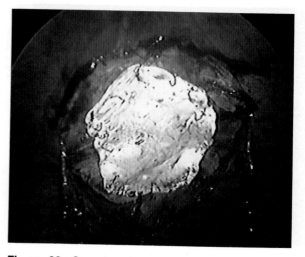

Figure 23. Completed repair with ePTFE. The peritoneum is always inadequate to cover the repair in this region.

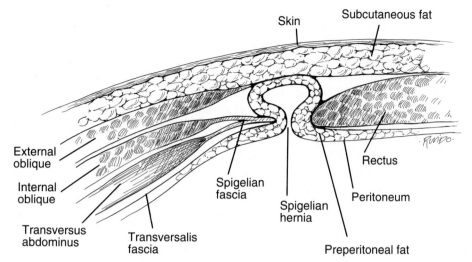

Figure 24.

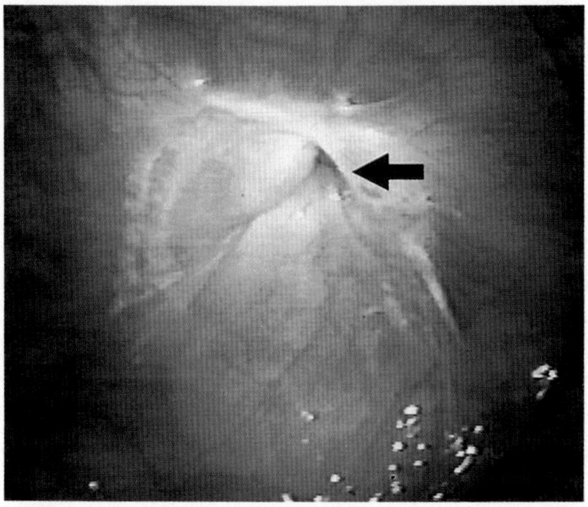

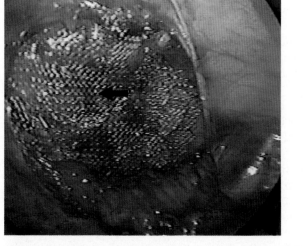

Figure 25. Laparoscopic appearance of left spigelian hernia.

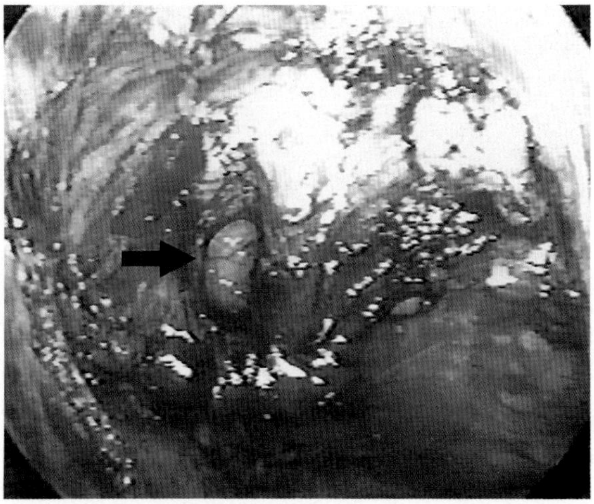

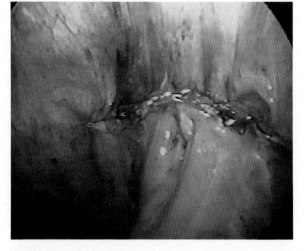

Figure 26. Spigelian defect after peritoneum has been reflected off the fascia.

Figure 27. Mesh repair of spigelian hernia. *Arrow* indicates location of fascia defect.

Figure 28. Completed peritoneal closure, completely covering the mesh repair.

▲ COMPLICATIONS

There are a few obvious risks associated with laparoscopic ventral herniaplasty. These include recurrence of the hernia, bowel injury, bleeding, infection, postoperative intestinal obstruction and fistula formation. Each of these possibilities must be considered prior to recommending this procedure. Fortunately, I have not yet observed any of these specific complications in conjunction with this technique. Those complications observed have thus far been relatively minor.

The problem of postoperative seroma in the hernia sac has occurred, but in each instance has resolved spontaneously within a few weeks. The avoidance of this problem, by placing a suction drain anterior to the prosthesis, has previously been discussed. Another patient experienced persistent pain in the abdominal wall, presumed secondary to an inflammatory reaction to either the mesh or staples. This symptom resolved completely following 6 weeks treatment with oral nonsteroidal antiinflammatory medication.

The long-term stability of this repair is unknown, and will require additional study. However, once the mesh has become firmly incorporated into the surrounding normal fascia, recurrence would seem unlikely. Early experience, with this laparoscopic technique, appears to offer hope for improving on the relatively high recurrence rates of many conventional repairs. Injuries to the bowel and other viscera may occur when manipulating tissues during herniaplasty. The surgeon must exercise great care during the placement of trocars, and in the dissection of adhesions. This is particularly true if there is any element of obstruction, since distended bowel is more prone to injury. Also, by using atraumatic instruments to handle the bowel, and by avoiding the indiscriminate use of energy sources, the risk of such injuries should remain very low. Major bleeding during laparoscopic ventral herniaplasty is unlikely, except in patients with portal hypertension. Large, collateral vessels are frequently encountered in these patients, especially around the umbilicus. This area, known as the caput medusa, can be as dangerous as the name implies, and laparoscopy should be avoided in these patients.

Troublesome bleeding can occur in any patient, during the preperitoneal dissection, if the proper avascular plane is not followed. This is especially true in the lower one-third of the abdominal wall, where aggressive dissection may injure the inferior epigastric vessels. Electrocoagulation is totally ineffective for controlling significant bleeding. To control these vessels, they should be ligated, both above and below the site of bleeding. If not addressed quickly, brisk hemorrhage from the inferior epigastrics creates an almost immediate problem with laparoscopic visibility, and may even necessitate laparotomy.

Another potential source of bleeding is along the anterior wall of the urinary bladder. If a hernia exists in this region, the fascia is more difficult to identify, and the bladder may actually extend out into the defect. Any significant bleeding encountered during a suprapubic dissection should be assumed to be coming from the bladder wall, as this is the most highly vascularized structure in the area. Proceeding in the face of uncontrolled bleeding is treacherous, inviting a disastrous bladder injury.

Wound infections have not been seen with this procedure, and logically they should be less common than with conventional approaches. During open procedures, tissues of the abdominal wall are exposed to potential airborne and cutaneous bacterial contamination for the duration of the operation. In addition, open procedures involve dissection through poorly vascularized scar tissue, which offers less resistance to infection. The laparoscopic procedure on the other hand, takes place within the sterile confines of the peritoneal cavity. The only contact with the patient's skin occurs during the initial placement of the cannulas. There is virtually no opportunity for contamination of instruments or prosthetic materials, provided good sterile technique is followed. In short, unless the peritoneal cavity is actually contaminated before the procedure, or the bowel or bladder is entered, the chances of suffering a postoperative infection are minimal. Nevertheless, to provide prophylaxis against this risk, a single intravenous dose of a broad-spectrum antibiotic is routinely administered 1 to 2 hours before the procedure.

Perhaps the complication most widely feared following laparoscopic herniaplasty is small bowel obstruction. On two occasions, I have encountered early postoperative small bowel obstruction following laparoscopic inguinal rather than ventral hernia repairs. The etiologies of these two obstructions were such that they could easily have followed the ventral herniaplasty technique, and therefore are included in this discussion. One patient developed a bowel herniation through a stapled peritoneal closure. This problem has already been discussed, and suffice it to say, can be avoided by careful closure of the peritoneum. The other obstruction was due to herniation through a lateral cannula insertion site in the lower abdomen. Despite a specific effort to insert the cannula obliquely through the abdominal wall, a loop of ileum still managed to become incarcerated in this small fascial opening. This problem can and should be avoided by employing some commonsense techniques. The practice of removing the telescope first, then opening all cannulas to evacuate the pneumoperitoneum, should not be done. A loop of bowel can be partially drawn into a cannula due to the negative pressure that is created by the rapidly escaping gas. Then, as the cannula is removed, the bowel may actually be pulled through the fascial opening. In at least one case, this resulted in an immediate incarceration. To prevent this complication, each cannula should be removed under direct laparoscopic observation, the same way it was inserted. Additionally, all cannula sites greater than 5 mm in diameter, should have their fascial openings sutured closed. This requires at least one suture per site, and ideally should approximate the deep fascial layer. In some patients, especially those with a thick layer of subcutaneous fat, it may be necessary to enlarge the skin incision slightly to accomplish this closure. A slightly larger skin incision does not cause any increase in postoperative pain, and may help to ensure against a trocar site hernia. Following the closure of the lateral cannula sites, reinsufflating the abdomen through the midline cannula can be a very useful technique for assessing the completeness of these closures.

The problems of enteric fistualization due to prosthetic materials have been well documented. Although this situation has not been seen following this technique, the risk clearly exists. Without question, polypropylene mesh offers a greater potential for fistula formation than ePTFE, but this risk is minimal unless the bowel and mesh are in direct contact. Whenever possible, the patient's own peritoneum provides the best means of isolating the preperitoneal prosthesis from the internal viscera. In the event there is not enough peritoneum available, the mesh repair can be covered by either the omentum or a sheet of ePTFE. If an enteric fistula occurs, surgical intervention would be required to repair the bowel and remove the prosthesis.

☑ CONCLUSIONS

By employing modern laparoscopic techniques, it is possible for the surgeon to repair hernias of the anterior abdominal wall with a minimum of pain and inconvenience to the patient. While these are welcome advantages, the most promising aspect of this procedure rests in the early evidence that it may provide a lower incidence of recurrence. Many open, or so-called conventional techniques, are associated with high recurrence rates due to excessive tension on the approximated fascial edges. The laparoscopic repair is a tension-free herniaplasty, which relies on permanent prosthetic materials to replace the weakened or absent native fascia. While this technique can be used to repair most ventral hernias, it is particularly well suited for recurrent defects, including recurrent umbilical hernias. Laparoscopic ventral herniaplasty provides both surgeon and patient an excellent alternative to conventional, open hernia repairs.

SURGICAL PEARLS

Since the interior of the inflated abdomen is spherical, the optimum angle for dissecting instruments is obtained by placing all ports as far away from the operative field as possible. The length of the instruments is the main limiting factor.

When reflecting the peritoneum back toward the telescope it is difficult to assess the depth and quality of this dissection. Here it can be very helpful to temporarily move the telescope to one of the lateral ports, to improve the view of this area.

Orienting polypropylene mesh within the abdomen can frequently be quite difficult. This problem can be solved by marking the mesh at the 12 o'clock position, with a sterile marker or tied suture. Positioning will be much quicker, and it will mark the point for the first staple placement.

During the closure of the peritoneum, lowering the intraabdominal pressure to 6 to 8 mmHg greatly facilitates the reapproximation of this layer by reducing the tension. This can also be useful when stapling the mesh, but during the enterolysis and preperitoneal dissections, keeping the pressure at 12 to 14 mmHg improves visualization.

RECOMMENDED READING

1. Lanzafame RJ. Techniques for the simultaneous management of incarcerated ventral herniae and cholelithiasis via laparoscopy. *J Laparoendosc Surg* 1993;3:193–201.
2. Wantz GE. Incisional hernioplasty with mersilene. *Surg Gynecol Obstet* 1991;172:129–137.
3. Deysine M. Hernia repair with expanded polytetrafluoroethylene. *Am J Surg* 1992;163:422–424.
4. Read RC, Yoder G. Recent trends in the management of incisional hernia. *Arch Surg* 1989;124: 485–488.
5. Spanger L. Spigelian hernia. *Surg Clin North Am* 1984;64:351–366.

THORACOSCOPY

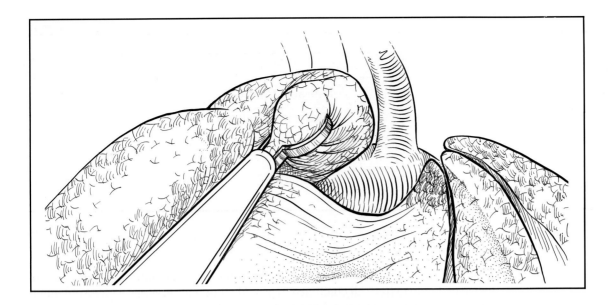

47

Exploratory Thoracoscopy

Joe B. Putnam, Jr.
Department of Thoracic and Cardiovascular Surgery
The University of Texas
M.D. Anderson Cancer Center
Houston, Texas 77030

Operative Laparoscopy and Thoracoscopy, edited by
B. V. MacFadyen, Jr. and
J. L. Ponsky. Lippincott-Raven
Publishers, Philadelphia © 1996.

Chamberlain procedure or an anterior parasternal mediastinotomy. Paratracheal lymph nodes and subcarinal lymph nodes are difficult to visualize thoracoscopically from the left side.

▶ PREOPERATIVE PLANNING

Patient Selection

Patient selection as well as indications for exploratory thoracoscopy remain in flux as advantages and disadvantages for video assisted thoracic surgery (VATS) techniques continue to be defined. Patients undergoing exploratory thoracoscopy rarely will undergo exploration alone. The purpose of exploratory thoracoscopy is to accomplish the following:

1. Establish a diagnosis or evaluate the extent of the thoracic disease process
2. Provide appropriate staging information for the oncology patient
3. Assist in the treatment or management of the patient's disease

Exploratory thoracotomy may yield findings or cause complications that require immediate and accurate correction. Surgeons attempting VATS techniques or exploratory thoracotomy should be intimately familiar with thoracic anatomy and physiology. As open thoracic procedures are frequently required after exploratory thoracoscopy, thoracoscopic procedures should be performed by thoracic surgeons.

Indications/Contraindications

Exploratory thoracoscopy may be performed for many different thoracic diseases (Table 1). Its usefulness depends on the surgeon's ability to incorporate information obtained from thoracoscopy with the patient's treatment. If VATS exploration will yield no additional information, or information that is superfluous, then this procedure should not be performed. VATS should be performed only when it is "value added" to the patient's care by minimizing or avoiding larger thoracic incisions or the morbidity of open exploration. VATS exploration may be performed before a planned open procedure for diagnosis, staging, or possible treatment. For example, VATS exploration may be used for diagnosis of a solitary indeterminant pulmonary nodule, staging and treatment of a stage 1 (T1N0) lung carcinoma in a patient with poor pulmonary function, initial or subsequent management of spontaneous or acquire pneumothorax, or drainage of pleural effusion and talc pleurodesis.

Table 1. *Thoracic diseases amenable to exploratory thoracoscopy with or without additional procedures*

Wedge resection of lung	Pleural diseases
Metastasis, solitary	Symptomatic pleural effusion
Indeterminate pulmonary nodule	Pleural biopsy
Benign/other/pneumothorax/excision of blebs	Mediastinal diseases
Occult metastases	Esophageal tumors
Lymphoma	Thymectomy/thymus biopsy
Staging	Pericardial window
Lung cancer	Other
Pulmonary metastases	Diaphragm nodule/repair
Esophageal cancer	Thoracic sympathectomy
Mesothelioma	
Lymphoma involving the lung or mediastinum	

Relative contraindications for exploratory thoracoscopy are as follows:

1. Morbidly obese patients may have a chest wall thickness that impairs instrument placement and subsequent manipulations.
2. Chronic obstructive pulmonary disease, inability to tolerate one-lung anesthesia, or prior surgery within the ipsilateral hemithorax may make VATS difficult.
3. An elevated hemidiaphragm or an enlarged heart that obscures visualization of the thoracic abnormality, active hemorrhage, or a hemodynamic unstability may suggest that an open procedure may be more prudent than exploratory thoracoscopy.

Physiologic Criteria

The selection of patients for VATS should include those tests that would be required for an open thoracotomy. Patients with solitary nodules and good pulmonary function may only need a chest radiograph before resection. Those patients with a smoking history or those with other underlying medical or cardiopulmonary dysfunction may require further investigations. Extended testing could include studies such as chest radiograph, computed tomographic (CT) scan of the chest and abdomen (to look for metastases), CT scan of the brain (for symptoms), and bone scan (for symptoms). Pulmonary function studies with and without bronchodilators, D_{LCO}, xenon ventilation perfusion lung scan, and oxygen consumption ($\dot{V}o_2$) may be required, particularly for patients with a history of poor pulmonary function or marginal cardiopulmonary reserve.

Even though VATS only is planned, the patient should be prepared physically and mentally for an open thoracotomy should that be needed. The conversion from a closed thoracic procedure to an open procedure is rare, but it does occur. Proper evaluation of the patient and planning of both the VATS portion of the operation as well as the potential open portion of the operation are critical and enhance the potential for a stable and predictable postoperative recovery. Patients are not permitted to smoke for a minimum of 2 weeks prior to surgery. Bronchorrhea, from smoking, coupled with any thoracic procedure often leads to prolonged intubation, increased secretions, atelectasis, poor pulmonary function, and pneumonia. Increased mucus production within the first few days following cessation of cigarette smoking compounds the problem of adequate pulmonary hygiene with thick secretions. Reintubation may be required. Incentive spirometry begun before surgery and continued throughout the perioperative course minimizes atelectasis.

Physically active patients with a normal electrocardiogram (EKG) may not require further evaluation of cardiac function before surgery. Advanced age (60 or above), known heart disease, or abnormal EKGs will require further evaluation.

Even with VATS as a clean or clean-contaminated procedure, routine perioperative antibiotics such as a second-generation cephalosporin are recommended. Trauma to the skin from trocar sites and manipulation of instruments may increase risk of wound infections.

All patients need deep-vein thrombosis/pulmonary embolus prophylaxis. Subcutaneous heparin (5,000 units every 8–12 hours) is inexpensive and well tolerated. Elastic hose or intermittent compression stockings may also be effective.

▼ INTRAOPERATIVE MANAGEMENT/SURGICAL TECHNIQUE

In the operating room all appropriate radiographic studies are displayed prominently. A radial artery catheter, and two large-bore intravenous infusion units are

SURGICAL PEARLS

Always face the lesion you want to evaluate. In this manner, the right and left hands use the instruments naturally, and the operation may proceed similarly to the open procedure. If the lesion is ventral, stand at the patient's back; if the lesion is dorsal, stand at the patient's front.

Whenever possible, use trocars to protect the tissues of the chest wall as instruments traverse the thorax. In some instances, tumor seeding of the trocar tracts may occur. Also use bags when withdrawing specimens to protect the chest wall.

Never hesitate to open the chest. Progression of the operation from VATS/exploratory thoracoscopy to an open procedure is often natural and to be expected for even minor concerns of diagnosis, staging, or treatment.

The use of VATS/exploratory thoracoscopy is new, and indications and results are not well established. Keep accurate records of your procedures, complications, and follow-up data to best evaluate the value of exploratory thoracoscopy in your patient population.

the patient is discharged. In the operating room, as the lung is inflated, the staple line should be visualized for bleeding and for excessive air leak. If an excessive air leak exists, repeat stapling or suturing of the staple line may be required.

Intrathoracic Hemorrhage

With the excellent visualization afforded by VATS, intrathoracic hemorrhage is rare. In patients with dense adhesions or tumors involving the great vessels or the pulmonary hilum, VATS should be limited to needle biopsy or small tissue biopsy for diagnosis. These patients should be treated by open thoracotomy. Persistent biopsies in the hilum or along the great vessels are subject to sudden and catastrophic hemorrhage, which could be controlled only by rapid open thoracotomy. Hemorrhage from the chest wall trocar sites or pulmonary parenchymal biopsies are also rare. All trocar sites and biopsy sites should be inspected before reinflation of the lung. Trocar site bleeding may be readily controlled by electrocauterization under direct vision. Intraparenchymal hemorrhage may require open thoracotomy and lobectomy for control.

Tumor Recurrence

Late complications of exploratory thoracostomy are only recently being identified. Recurrence of chest wall tumors, or seeding from manipulation of tissue or retraction of contaminated instruments through the chest wall may only become evident months to years after the primary thoracoscopic procedure. To prevent such occurrences, all instruments should be protected by a trocar sheath to minimize contamination of the chest wall by instruments. In addition, all tissue biopsies from suspected neoplasms should be removed from the chest through the trocar sheath if small enough, or within a plastic bag to minimize chest wall contamination.

☑ CONCLUSION

Video assisted thoracic surgery techniques are readily and safely applied to the thorax for the diagnosis, staging, and treatment of thoracic diseases. The novelty of this technique demands careful attention to the need for this procedure in selected patients. Not every patient will benefit from exploratory thoracoscopy; the cost as well as the information expected to be obtained should be weighed carefully before the surgeon decides to use this procedure. Surgeons performing exploratory thoracoscopy should be well trained in the comparable open procedures. Prospective data collection will assist the practitioner in optimizing patient selection as well as refining the skills necessary for facile exploratory thoracoscopy.

RECOMMENDED READING

1. Kaiser LR. Video-assisted thoracic surgery: current state of the art. *Ann Surg* 1994;220:720–734.
2. Rusch VW. Thoracoscopy. Surgical technique supplement 2. In Wilmore DW, Brennan MF, Harken AH, Holcroft JW, Meakins JL, eds. *Care of the surgical patient.* New York: Scientific American; 1993:1–20.
3. Landreneau RJ, Mack MJ, Hazelrigg SR, Naunheim KS, Keenan RJ, Ferson PF. Video-assisted thoracic surgery: a minimally invasive approach to thoracic oncology. In: DeVita Jr VT, Hellman S, Rosenberg SA, eds. *Principles and practice of oncology,* Vol. 8, 4th ed. JB Lippincott; Philadelphia: 1994:1–14.
4. Allen MS, Deschamps C, Lee RE, Trastek VF, Daly RC, Pairolero PC. Video-assisted throacoscopic stapled wedge excision for indeterminate pulmonary nodules. *J Thorac Cardiovasc Surg* 1993;106:1048–1052.

48

Dorsal Sympathectomy

Harold C. Urschel, Jr.
Department of Thoracic and Cardiovascular Surgery
University of Texas Southwestern Medical School
Baylor University Medical Center
Dallas, Texas 75246

Operative Laparoscopy and Thoracoscopy, edited by B. V. MacFadyen, Jr. and J. L. Ponsky. Lippincott-Raven Publishers, Philadelphia © 1996.

Transaxillary Approach with a Transthoracic Sympathectomy

The patient is placed in the lateral thoracotomy position with an axillary roll under the downside arm. The upper arm is suspended at 90 degrees from the chest wall over a pulley system with a 1-lb weight (14). An arm-holder is employed to be certain that no hyperabduction or hyperextension of the shoulder occurs and that relaxation occurs every 3 minutes. Three ports are used between the second and fourth interspaces. The camera should be placed either anteriorly or in the midaxillary port (Fig. 4). A double-lumen endotracheal tube is used, and the upside lung is collapsed, ventilating only the downside lung (19). This shunts blood through the downside lung selectively, and excellent oxygenation usually results. The lung is retracted and the sympathectomy performed. The mediastinal pleura is cut open and the sympathetic chain identified on the vertebral body near the neck of the ribs (Fig. 5). Nerve hooks are employed to elevate the dorsal sympathetic chain, and the nerve connections, including the gray and white rami which are clipped before cutting or cauterization (Fig. 6). The stellate ganglion is divided at the junction of the lower third, where it looks like a "cat's paw." The lower third is cut, it is not photoablated or cauterized because Horner's syndrome may result from either the heat or light injury in the adjacent C8 ganglion. It is important to do a frozen section in the resected ganglia to verify it pathologically. The lower ganglia can be cauterized, photoablated with the laser, or cut. Hemostasis is

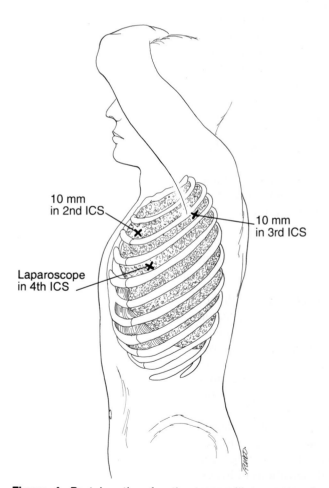

Figure 4. Port location for the transaxillary approach with a transthoracic sympathectomy. A 10-mm port is used in both second and third intercostal spaces and the thoracoscope inserted via the port in the fourth intercostal space.

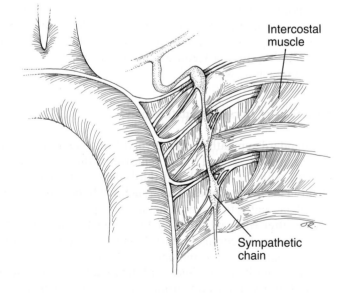

Left chest

Figure 5. Location of the sympathetic chain near the neck of the ribs.

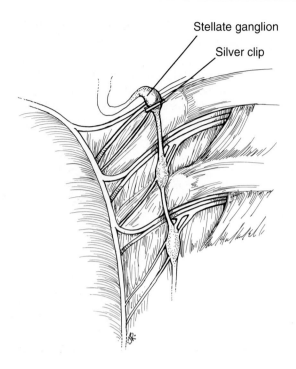

Stellate ganglion

Silver clip

Figure 6. Clip across the sympathetic chain.

Left chest

achieved with cautery. The pleura is left open and the chest tube placed through one of the ports to allow drainage. There is a curvature of the sympathetic chain so that in many cases the stellate ganglion lies transversely, rather than vertically, on the transverse process of the vertebral body. Special knowledge of the anatomy is important as well as the location of the thoracic duct, which can simulate the sympathetic chain and be injured if not appropriately identified. Similarly, these ganglia can be removed more easily from the right mediastinal area because the thoracic duct is not usually seen. However, the azygous vein and its branches are visible, and care must be taken to avoid injury to these structures (Fig. 7).

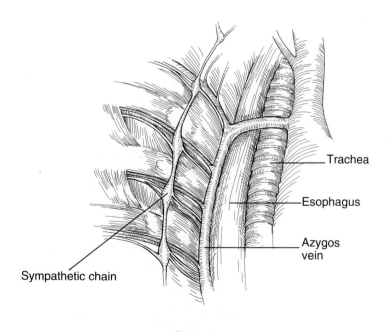

Trachea

Esophagus

Azygos vein

Sympathetic chain

Right chest

Figure 7. Relationship of the sympathetic chain and the azygous vein in the right mediastinum.

Transaxillary First Rib Resection for Thoracic Outlet Syndrome with Retraction of the Pleura and Sympathectomy

The transaxillary technique differs slightly from the usual video-assisted thoracoscopy in that an actual incision is made transversely below the axillary hairline between the pectoralis major muscle anteriorly and the latissimus dorsi muscle posteriorly (Fig. 8A,B). The axillary roll is placed beneath the opposite axilla with

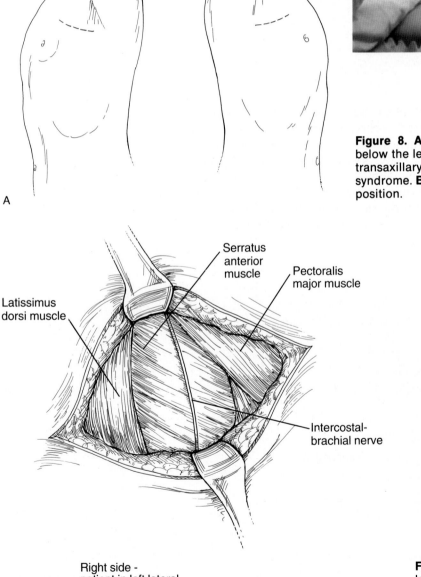

Figure 8. A: A transverse incision is made just below the left or the right axillary hairline during a transaxillary first rib resection for thoracic outlet syndrome. **B:** The patient is placed in a right lateral position.

Serratus anterior muscle

Pectoralis major muscle

Latissimus dorsi muscle

Intercostal-brachial nerve

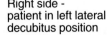

Right side - patient in left lateral decubitus position

Figure 9. Dissection through the subaxillary incision is performed to expose the intercostal-brachial nerve.

the patient in a lateral thoracotomy position. The arm is elevated to 90 degrees with a pulley system and a 1-lb weight. An arm-holder is used to be sure that hyperabduction and hyperextension of the shoulder does not occur and that the arm is relaxed every 3 minutes. The incision is carried down to the chest wall and up toward the axilla (Fig. 9). The intercostal-brachial nerve is retracted and not divided (Fig. 10). The first rib is identified and the scalenus-anticus muscle is divided (Fig. 11). The first rib is divided at its midportion, removing a triangular shape of bone with the vortex of the triangle at the scalene tubercle (Fig. 12). A right-angle breast retractor with a light is employed as one retractor. A Dever retractor is placed on the other side of the incision. The video camera is either a standard thoracoscope, a Wolf scope, or an Olympus flexible operating esophogastroscope. All of these provide magnification and have an excellent light source.

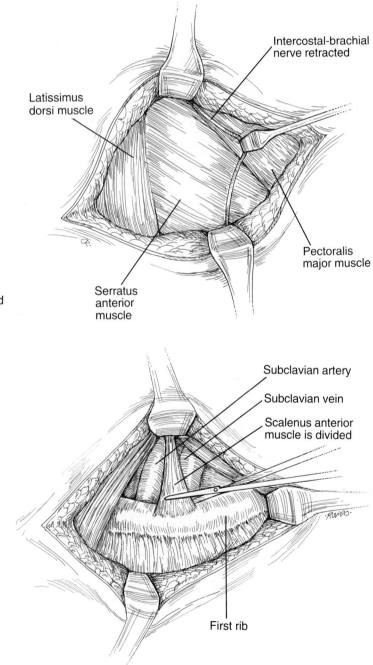

Figure 10. The intercostal-brachial nerve is spared by retracting, not dividing, it.

Figure 11. Identification of the first rib and division of the scalenus anterior muscle.

The anterior part of the rib is removed back to the sternal costal cartilage (Fig. 13). The costoclavicular ligament is divided, and the axillary-subclavian vein is decompressed. The posterior part of the rib is removed back to its articulation with the transverse process, and the axillary-subclavian artery is decompressed. The special Urschel-Lexall and pituitary ronguers are used to remove the head and the neck of the rib to avoid injuring T1 and C8 nerve roots, which lie on each side of the head and neck of the rib. Neurolysis of C7, C8, T1, and any part of the brachial plexus that appears to have scarring is carried out under video-assisted magnification. The lung is collapsed on the operated side during the rib resection.

The pleura is retracted inferiorly using a sponge stick, and the sympathetic chain is identified on the transverse process of the vertebral bodies (Fig. 14); it

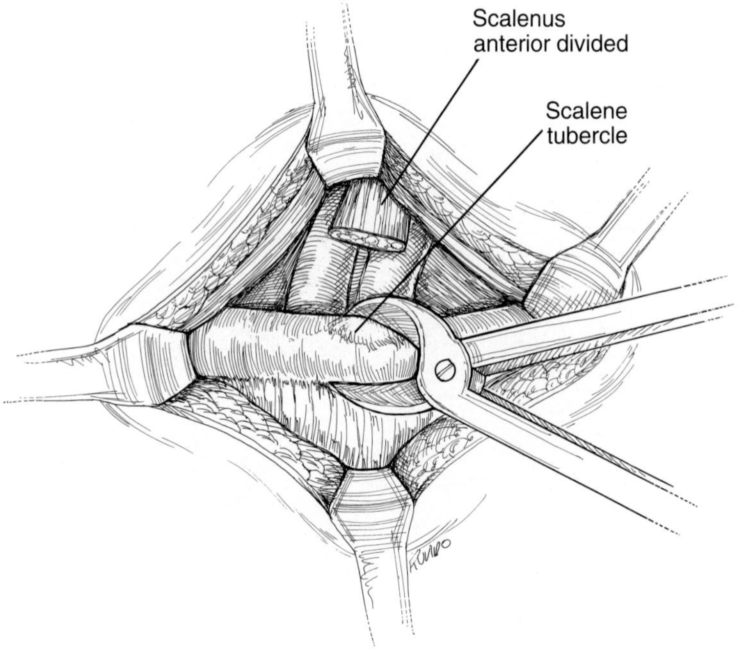

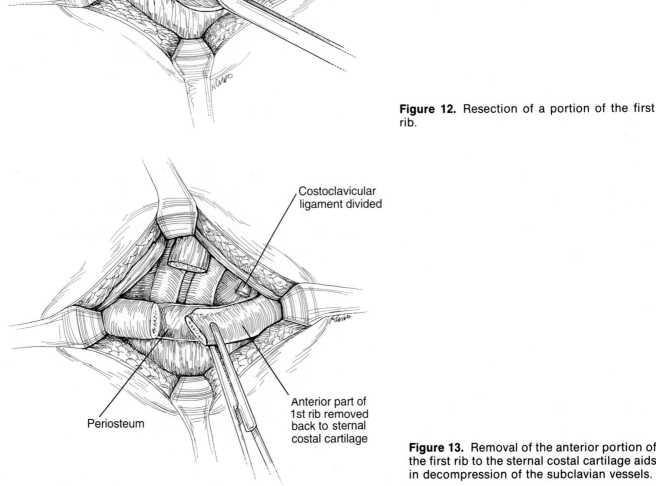

Figure 12. Resection of a portion of the first rib.

Figure 13. Removal of the anterior portion of the first rib to the sternal costal cartilage aids in decompression of the subclavian vessels.

is vertical between T2 and T3 ganglia. However, T1 is the lower part of the stellate ganglion, and it angles anteriorly and lies in almost a transverse position. Clips are placed on all the communicating rami of the sympathetic chain (Fig. 6). T2 and T3 ganglia are resected. The stellate ganglion is divided at the junction of its lower third, removing T1 (Fig. 15), with a sharp knife (Fig. 16). Cauterization or laser photoablation is not performed in the stellate ganglion. Cautery is used after the removal of the sympathetic chain to prevent sprouting and regeneration. Hemostasis is secured. A large round Jackson-Pratt drain is placed and DepoMedrol is injected over the nerve roots and plexus that have undergone neurolysis. The camera is removed and the wound closed in the usual fashion.

▲ COMPLICATIONS

Horner's Syndrome

If the fibers of C7 and C8 (the upper part of the stellate ganglion) are removed, Horner's syndrome results, which involves miosis, enophthalmos, drooping of the eyelid (ptosis), and flushing of that side of the face with loss of sweating in that area (20).

Postsympathetic Neuralgia

The complication of postsympathectomy neuralgia in the upper extremities is less common than in the lower extremities. The pain usually occurs in the shoulder and upper arm on the lateral aspect. Clinical history usually substantiates this diagnosis if the symptoms occur within the first 3 months. The confirmation may be obtained by a test involving skin resistance of pseudomotor activity detection. Characteristics of these tests reveal increased sympathetic activity, suggesting a rebound phenomenon from the nonsympathectomized adjacent dermatomes. Rebound may be a regeneration of nerve fibers on an increased response of peripheral nerves to catacholamines. Symptoms are usually resolved in 3 to 6 weeks with conservative management. Dilantin, Tegretol, and calcium channel blockers are used in the medical management of these symptoms (21).

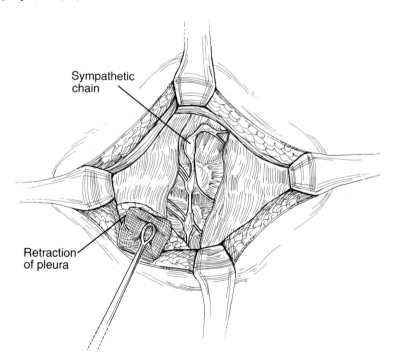

Figure 14. Retraction of the pleura allows identification of the sympathetic chain.

Wedge Resection for Diffuse Lung Disease

The operative technique is basically the same for lung biopsy for the diagnosis of diffuse lung disease as for lung nodules. If the disease process is present in both lungs we preferentially chose the right side, since tissue samples can be obtained from all three lobes. One advantage of the thoracoscopic technique compared to the traditional "open lung biopsy" is the ability to select by direct visualization pathologic tissue and therefore increase the chance of obtaining of a specific diagnostic result. It is important to include in the biopsy specimen a margin of adjacent "normal" lung tissue, since the most abnormal area often contains only fibrosis or necrosis without clues of the specific etiology. The inclusion of the margin or edge of the pathologic process may increase diagnostic yield. We also feel that lung biopsy with cup forceps yields an inadequate tissue sample compared with a stapled wedge resection.

Wedge Resection for Apical Blebs

For surgical intervention for suspected apical bleb disease, all trocars are placed more cephalad in order to more easily access the apex. The initial trocar is placed in the fifth intercostal space in the midaxillary line and the two remaining trocars placed anterior and posterior in the fourth interspace (Fig. 18). Optimal placement of the posterior trocar is medial to the scapula for placement of the endoscopic stapler across the apical bleb. Usually, placement of two staple firings

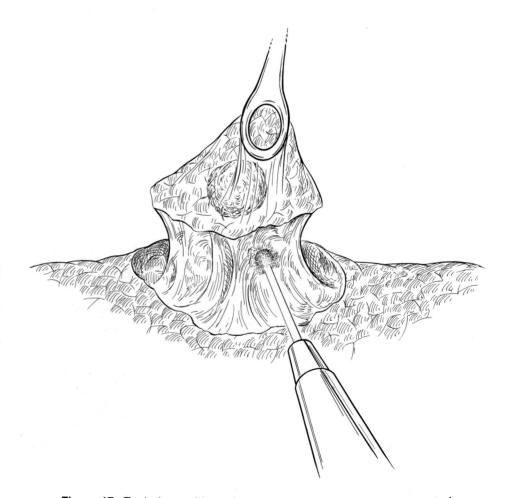

Figure 17. Technique of laser lung resection of a pulmonary nodule.

is necessary because of the angle necessary for application of the staples. The 3.5-mm staple is used as it is for most other lung resections. Of course, resection of the blebs is not necessary, and simple exclusion of the bleb from the remaining lung is sufficient. Therefore, use of an Endo-TA stapler or an EndoGIA stapler with the knife blade removed is an option.

If the bleb is small and a stapler is not available, or if concern exists regarding the expense of stapler usage there are alternative techniques available for blebectomy. An endoscopic surgical tie or loop can be used to ligate the base of the bleb. Two loops are used to assure secure ligation when the lung is reexpanded. Another simple technique for bleb ligation is with rubber bands traditionally used for hemorrhoid ligation. The same applier used for hemorrhoids can be introduced through a trocar site and the bleb snared and the base ligated with a rubber band. Very small blebs can also be coagulated with either an Nd:YAG laser or electrocautery.

At the conclusion of the bleb resection, a pleurodesis is performed. It is our practice to perform a mechanical abrasion of the parietal pleura using an endoscopic kittner or sponge introduced into the chest cavity. It is some surgeons' preference to perform an apical pleurectomy, which can also be easily accomplished by thoracoscopy. We do this only if a bleb has not been located in the lung, which occurs in 5% to 10% of cases.

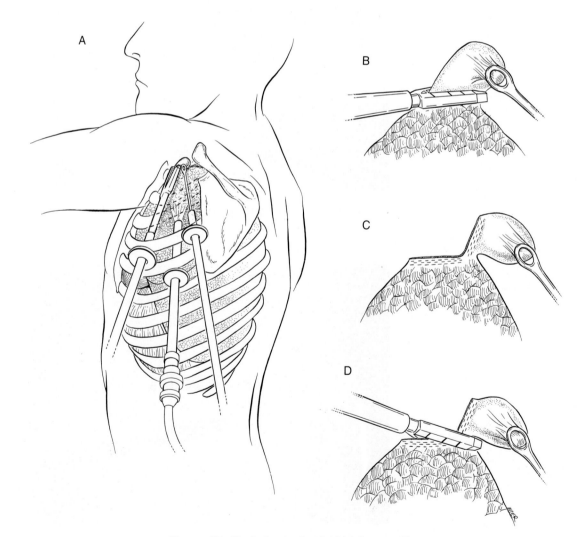

Figure 18. Technique of apical bleb resection.

Lung Resection for Bullous Lung Disease

Bullous lung disease represents an increasing application of thoracoscopy even though its benefit remains in doubt and the usage controversial. We presently feel that thoracoscopy is indicated only for large localized bullae with evidence of compressed adjacent lung and *not* for diffuse panacinar emphysema.

The technique usually involves initial shrinkage of the bullous with an Nd: YAG laser at low energy levels (8–10 W) (Fig. 19) and then application of the endoscopic stapler across the base of the shrunken bulla. If the bullous can be managed without perforation, it is optimal. If there is an air leak present or inadvertent perforation occurs, localization of the bronchial communication is performed, and it is oversewn by endoscopic suturing techniques. If a laser is not available, electrocautery or the argon beam coagulator can be used, but neither has the precision of the laser, and the coagulative necrosis formed on the shrunken bulla is not as satisfactory.

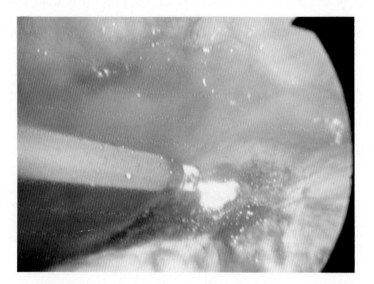

Figure 19. Laser coagulation of an emphysematous bulla.

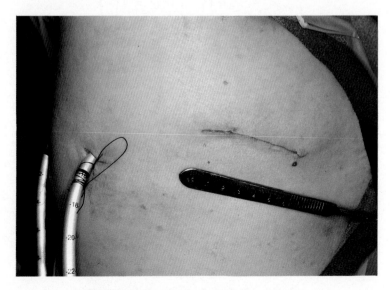

Figure 20. Incisions for VATS lobectomy.

VATS Lobectomy

Incisions

The surgical technique for video-assisted lobectomy involves two or three trocar sites and an additional 6-cm "accessory" or "utility" incision, which is necessary for removal of the specimen at the completion of the procedure (Fig. 20). Since this incision will ultimately be necessary for specimen retrieval, advantage is taken of condition, and the incision is made at the beginning of the procedure. Multiple standard instruments can then be placed through this site throughout the course of the procedure. The initial trocar is placed in the seventh intercostal space in the midaxillary line for exploratory thoracoscopy. An additional trocar is placed in the sixth intercostal space in the posterior axillary line. Chest tubes are placed through these trocar sites at the end of the procedure. The "accessory" or "utility" incision is made in the fifth intercostal space along the anterior axillary line. This corresponds to the major fissure and direct visualization is gained through this incision onto the interlobal pulmonary artery (Fig. 21). A standard, rigid, 10-mm 0-degree thoracoscope is used for the majority of the procedure, however, for upper lobectomy, it is helpful to use a 30-degree angled scope and to place an additional trocar more anteriorly, in the third intercostal space in the anterior axillary line. These two maneuvers give better visualization to the superior aspect of the hilum.

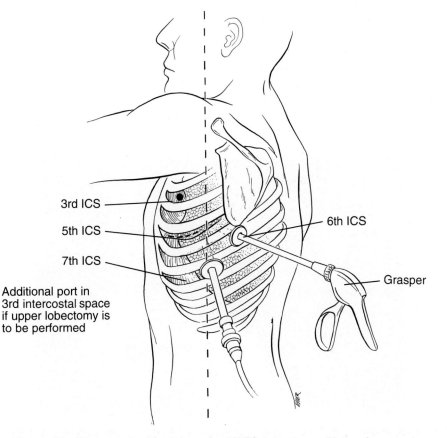

Figure 21. Placement of incisions for VATS lobectomy. Note placement of the "utility" incision over the fissure.

Initial Assessment

After the initial exploratory thoracoscopy is completed, and any evidence of pleural metastases is eliminated, attention is turned toward the hilum. Since dissection of the hilar vessels is the limiting step in the procedure, immediate assessment is made regarding the feasibility of the video-assisted technique. As mentioned under preoperative evaluation, extensive hilar lymphadenopathy and extension of the tumor toward the hilum make video-assisted technique more difficult. In addition, incomplete fissures, especially an incomplete minor fissure when contemplating a right upper or right middle lobectomy, make the video-assisted technique extremely difficult and serious consideration should be given to conversion to an open thoracotomy if this situation is present.

The mediastinum and hilum are also staged before proceeding with a lobectomy, since positive N2 nodes would mitigate toward preoperative adjuvant therapy before lobectomy. An assessment is made of the aortopulmonary window on the left side as well as the periesophageal and inferior pulmonary ligament lymph nodes. If the intraoperative staging is negative and the anatomic situation appears suitable for thoracoscopic lobectomy, the dissection is commenced. Standard thoracic surgical instruments are introduced either through the two trocarless incisions or through the utility incision (Fig. 22). We make frequent use of curved ringed forceps for retraction of the lung.

Pulmonary Vein

Dissection begins in the hilum at the interlobar artery. Exposure and control of this vessel is the most difficult aspect of the procedure and is often times helpful to perform this aspect first. By using a combination of sharp dissection with endoscopic scissors with blunt, curved blades and blunt dissection with endoscopic kittners as well as a suction apparatus, the interlobar artery can be exposed. Once it has been ascertained that the video-assisted technique will allow approach to the interlobar artery, we usually then turn our attention to the other hilar structures for both upper and lower lobectomies (as well as middle lobectomies). Better exposure of the hilum is next gained by sacrificing the pulmonary vein. If the inferior pulmonary vein is to be divided, the inferior pulmonary ligament is divided

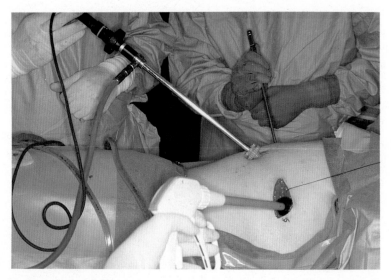

Figure 22. Placement of the endoscopic stapler through the utility incision for a VATS lobectomy.

first and the vein exposed from the inferior aspect. Using a standard right angle clamp, the pulmonary vein is encircled and a 0-silk tie placed around it. Extensive mobilization of tissue around the vein is performed so that the endoscopic stapler jaw can easily be placed around the vessel. Once the vein has been adequately freed from surrounding tissue, an endoscopic stapler with a 2.5-mm vascular staple is placed carefully around the pulmonary vein (Fig. 23). Care is taken to ensure that the jaws of the stapler will completely transect the vessel. An endoscopic grasping instrument is placed upon the proximal portion of the vessel in case stapler malfunction occurs. In our experience of over 25 lobectomies as well as hundreds of other endoscopic resections, we have not experienced staple malfunction; however, this remains a concern by some clinical investigators. If concern exists regarding this point, then the knife blade of the endoscopic stapler can be removed and six rows of staples alone applied ligating the vessel but not cutting it. Once the stapler is removed and an intact staple line ascertained to the surgeon's satisfaction, the endoscopic scissors can then be used to divide between the two sets of staple lines.

Pulmonary Artery

Next the pulmonary artery is approached. If a lower lobectomy is being performed, it is easiest to approach this vessel from the fissure (Fig. 24). If it is an upper lobe artery, this is best visualized by using a 30-degree angled scope placed through an anterior intercostal space. For the interlobal artery to the lower lobes, using an endoscopic kittner, the lung tissue is gently teased away from the pulmonary artery. The blunt endoscopic scissors can also be used to sharply dissect the artery free. Once it has been sufficiently mobilized, a standard right-angle clamp is placed carefully around the vessel and a 0-silk tie is used for traction. Once the artery has been freed sufficiently on the back side, an endoscopic stapler with a 2.5-mm vascular cartridge is placed across with the jaws completely encompassing the vessel. If the correct angle for placement of the stapler cannot be obtained, the utility incision as well as all different ports should be tried. Usually, there is an access site that gives the correct angle for placement of the stapler across the pulmonary artery. Once the jaws have been closed and secured, the stapler is fired. An endoscopic grasper is again used in case control of the pulmonary artery should be necessary. The stapler jaws are opened and an intact suture line is checked for.

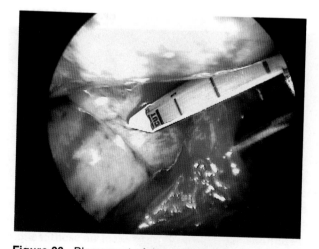

Figure 23. Placement of the endoscopic stapler with a vascular cartridge across the left inferior pulmonary vein.

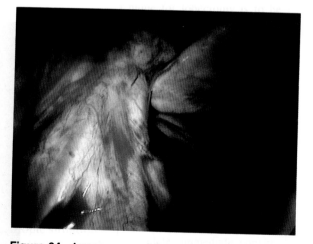

Figure 24. Appearance of the segmental pulmonary arteries to the left lower lobe in the fissure.

Video-assisted thoracic surgery (VATS) will undoubtedly have some role in the staging and treatment of esophageal cancer, but the current use of this new technique is limited. This chapter reviews the early experience with video surgery for the staging of esophageal cancer and presents an initial experience with Ivor Lewis esophagogastrectomy performed entirely with video surgery.

● ANATOMY

The key anatomic features for this operation relate to the blood supply of the stomach and all of the esophageal anatomy. The stomach has a very rich blood supply that allows its transposition into the chest. The vessels that supply the proximal stomach are transected in order to fully mobilize the stomach, including the short gastric arteries and the left gastric artery (Fig. 1). Up to five short gastric arteries feed the fundus. In the lesser sac, there is often a transverse pancreatic artery that goes approximately 3 cm from the pancreatic artery directly anteriorly to the posterior stomach. Additional arteries that need to be sacrificed include the branches of the left gastric, accessory left hepatic, left inferior phrenic, and, rarely, the right inferior phrenic that supply the abdominal portion of the esophagus.

The viability of the stomach then depends on the distal vessels to supply the entire stomach. The gastroepiploic arcade is found 1 to 2 cm lateral to the greater curvature, from the pylorus to the bare area near the spleen. Although the stomach is supplied by both the right gastroepiploic and splenic arteries, the collaterals are so extensive that the organ remains viable when the short gastric arteries are sacrificed. The right gastric artery on the lesser curve at the pylorus is the other major feeding artery for the transposed stomach.

The esophagus is 25 cm long in the adult (15 to 40 cm from the incisors). After traversing the thoracic inlet, the thoracic esophagus is posterior and slightly to the left of the trachea. At the tracheal bifurcation, the esophagus is dorsal to the left main stem bronchus. Inferior to the carina the esophagus is ventrally related

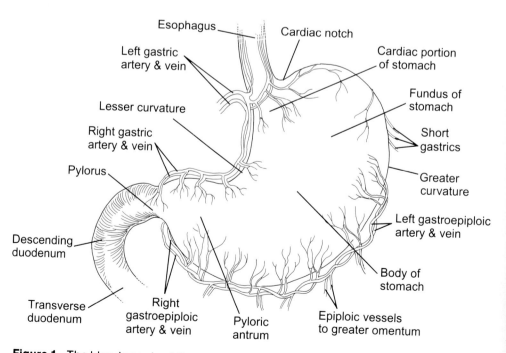

Figure 1. The blood supply of the stomach and its relation to the esophageal anatomy are important knowledge in order to perform this procedure.

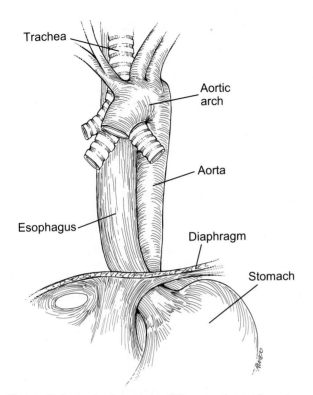

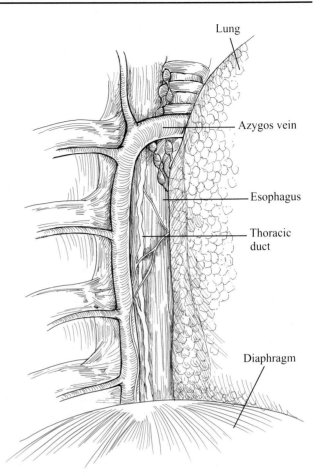

Figure 2. Important aspects of the esophageal anatomy: aortic arch, trachea, diaphragm, and stomach.

Figure 3. The lung is collapsed on the right side showing the esophagus, and it is visualized from the thoracic inlet to the diaphragm.

to the pericardium and the left atrium. At the level of the 9th thoracic vertebra, the esophagus passes through the diaphragm (Fig. 2).

The esophageal blood supply is segmental and without good collaterals, so it does not lend itself to segmental resection. The esophagus from the thoracic inlet to the carina receives its blood supply from bronchial arteries and directly from the aorta. Below the carina, the arterial supply is segmental without anastomotic connections between these vessels, which arise directly from the aorta.

The esophagus has a rich mucosal and submucosal lymphatic network that is independent of its blood supply. Injection studies have demonstrated that lymphatic drainage is longitudinal six times more often than it is transverse. The submucosal lymphatics may run a particularly long course, which leads to nodal metastases that may be quite distant to a tumor.

The thoracic duct begins in the abdomen at L1 or L2 as the cisterna chyli. It enters the thorax through the aortic hiatus on the right anterior surface of the aorta. During an esophagectomy, it should be identified and clipped in its normal location between the aorta and the azygos vein. As the duct courses superiorly through the chest, it passes from the right to the left at about the level of T5 (Fig. 3).

▶ PREOPERATIVE PLANNING

While screening has led to the early diagnosis of esophageal cancer in areas of very high incidence (e.g., Linxian Province in northern China), screening is

TABLE 1. *Incidence of abnormal bronchoscopic findings for thoracic esophageal cancer*

Location	Bronchoscopic finding (%)		
	Normal	Impingement	Invasion
Upper third	43	33	24
Middle third	63	18	19
Lower third	89	6	5

not practical in the United States, where virtually all patients are symptomatic at diagnosis. Dysphagia is present in 95% of patients and is a late symptom that indicates two-thirds of the circumference is involved. The mean time from onset of dysphagia to death is 4 months. Other symptoms include weight loss (46%), odynophagia (50%), retrosternal pain (20%), and respiratory symptoms (4%) (1).

Adenocarcinoma is now the most common type of esophageal cancer, occurring most often in Barrett's esophagus in white males in the fifth or sixth decade. Squamous cell carcinoma occurs in the sixth or seventh decade after a long history of alcohol and tobacco abuse. The male:female ratio is 5:1.

Surgery is indicated for patients who have potentially curable tumors and patients with a life expectancy long enough to justify a procedure to palliate their dysphagia and eventual problem with aspiration. Preoperative evaluation of resectability is difficult because noninvasive studies are not completely reliable.

Resection is contraindicated in cases with mediastinal invasion, extensive, fixed celiac nodal metastases, and hepatic metastases. The sensitivity of a computed tomography (CT) scan is only 56% for tracheobronchial invasion and 51% for aortic invasion. CT scans detect regional nodal metastases only when nodes are enlarged, so the sensitivity is only 27% and the accuracy is 57% for thoracic nodes. The CT scan evaluation of the celiac nodes is even worse. The accuracy for CT scan detection of visceral metastases is 96% (2).

Esophagectomy is not indicated in the presence of tracheobronchial invasion, so bronchoscopic examination of patients with cancers at or above the carina is mandatory. Table 1 shows the incidence of abnormal bronchoscopic findings for thoracic esophageal cancers (3). These findings do not correlate well with symptoms.

Surgical Staging of Esophageal Cancer

Dagnini and colleagues (4) performed laparoscopic evaluation of 369 patients with cancer of the esophagus (280) and of the cardia (89). They found no metastatic disease in 76%, but detected extension or metastases that precluded resection in 14%. Krasna and colleagues (5) performed right thoracoscopy to successfully evaluate the primary tumor and to biopsy mediastinal lymph nodes in 16 of 18 patients with thoracic esophageal cancer.

▼ INTRAOPERATIVE MANAGEMENT/SURGICAL TECHNIQUE

Current surgical approaches for esophagectomy range from the radical regional resection of Skinner to the transhiatal esophagectomy of Orringer. VATS provides a compromise between these two extremes.

Right thoracoscopy permits the esophagus to be mobilized with as much regional dissection as the surgeon desires, without the morbidity of the thoracotomy incision. A laparotomy and a cervical incision can then be used to complete the operation in the same fashion that transhiatal esophagectomy is performed. A cervical anastomosis is created.

Gosset and coworkers (6) were able to complete the operation in 11 of 14 patients with an average operating time of 125 minutes. In the remaining 3 cases, they were unable to collapse the lung or had difficulty in mobilizing the esophagus. Collard and associates (7) were also successful in 8 of 11 cases, but the operating time was quite long (ranging from 157 to 390 minutes).

Minimally Invasive Ivor Lewis Esophagogastrectomy

In 8 patients (6 were high-risk, elderly patients who were not good candidates for open procedures), we undertook an Ivor Lewis esophagogastrectomy with laparoscopy and thoracoscopy. Our goal was to perform video-assisted surgery following the same procedure as in an open operation—including gastric mobilization, pyloromyotomy, feeding jejunostomy, thoracic esophagectomy, and a high intrathoracic esophagogastrostomy.

Description of Procedure

The procedure is performed under general anesthesia with an arterial line and a double-lumen endotracheal tube. For the abdominal portion of the operation, five 12-mm trocars (Fig. 4) are used to allow maximal flexibility. During most of the procedure, the camera is placed through the umbilical trocar. The 0-degree lens is used primarily, but the 30-degree lens is helpful during dissection of the esophageal hiatus.

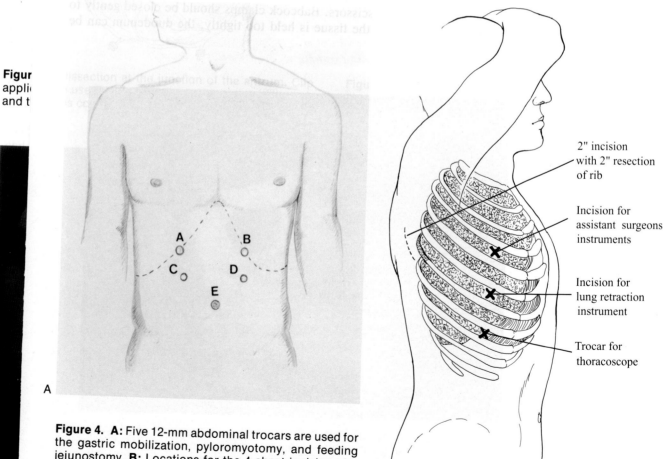

Figure 4. A: Five 12-mm abdominal trocars are used for the gastric mobilization, pyloromyotomy, and feeding jejunostomy. **B:** Locations for the 4 chest incisions for the thoracic part of the procedure.

2" incision with 2" resection of rib

Incision for assistant surgeons instruments

Incision for lung retraction instrument

Trocar for thoracoscope

A

B

KI

Ly

Pe

Pe

Figur
forme

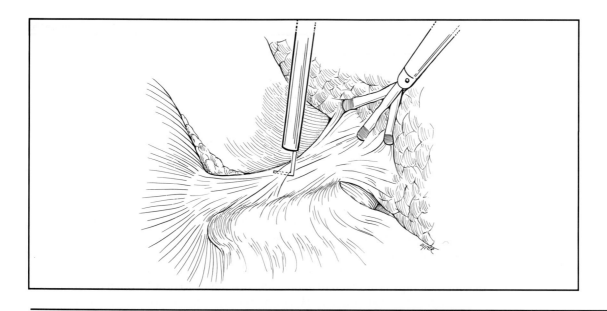

52

Cardiomyotomy for Achalasia

Carlos A. Pellegrini
Department of Surgery
University of Washington Medical Center
Seattle, Washington 98195

Operative Laparoscopy and Thoracoscopy, edited by B. V. MacFadyen, Jr. and J. L. Ponsky. Lippincott-Raven Publishers, Philadelphia © 1996.

the myotomy, one can use a bipolar instrument (which lessens the chance of thermal injury to the mucosa) or hook electrocautery. We prefer an electrocautery instrument that has suction and irrigation attached. This facilitates the procedure, as it is possible to clear the field immediately and proceed to further coagulation or with the myotomy. As the myotomy is carried downward, it is important to grasp the muscular wall on the assistant's side and use it to pull the esophagus upward. The surgeon may use the left hand to lower the diaphragm down as far as it is possible. This way the gastroesophageal junction is exposed and the myotomy can be carried down all the way through it. The lowest part of the myotomy represents the most delicate part of the procedure. It is, in fact, crucial to the outcome, and it is also the most difficult part of the operation because it is at this level that the muscle layers are less clearly identified and the mucosa is thinner, making the risk of perforation higher. The upper part of the myotomy is usually much simpler to perform and probably less important for the result on the average patient with achalasia. On the other hand, in patients with vigorous achalasia or with nutcracker esophagus, in whom the upper extent of the myotomy is important, one can pull the hilum of the lung with the lung anteriorly, open the pleura behind it, and carry out the myotomy all the way to the aortic arch.

At the completion of the myotomy, it is important to dissect the edges as far as possible, allowing the mucosa to protrude widely and exposing about 40% of its surface (Fig. 9). This way, early healing with stricture is avoided. This maneuver can be done in part by gentle insufflation of the esophagus, by movements of the esophagoscope laterally, and by a combination of blunt and sharp dissection.

Next, the lung is expanded, the chest tube is placed in position, and the thoracoports are removed. We close the entry sites with single sutures of reabsorbable material. This operation is usually accomplished in 2 to 3 hours, the blood loss is minimal, and the recovery rapid. The patient is extubated at the end of the procedure and taken to the recovery room.

Laparoscopic Approach

An esophageal myotomy can also be performed through a laparoscopic approach. In this case, the patient is positioned supine on the operating table, with

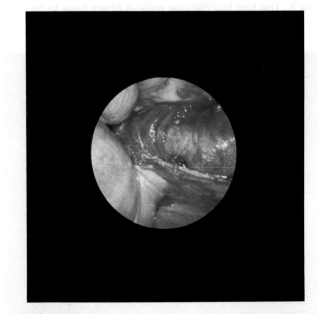

Figure 9. The esophagus and the site of myotomy (intraoperatively). Note the separation of the muscular edges and the bulging of the mucosa.

the legs extended on stirrups so that the surgeon can stand between them. We prefer to induce pneumoperitoneum by direct puncture over the right upper quadrant (as the umbilicus is not going to be used and the midline carries a risk of insufflation within the leaves of the falciform ligament). Trocar position is illustrated in Fig. 10. Usually the telescope port is placed about 1 to 2 in. above the umbilicus through the midline. There are four additional trocars required: two in the right upper quadrant and two in the left upper quadrant. These four trocars ought to be placed, in general, as close as possible to the costal margin. It is impossible to place a trocar too high for operations on the left upper quadrant. The two medial trocars are used for the left- and right-hand instruments of the surgeon (at each side of the telescope). The right lateral trocar is used for retraction of the liver. The left lateral trocar is used for most of the operation to introduce a Babcock clamp with which the gastroesophageal junction can be pulled down and the lower esophagus exposed.

With the left lobe of the liver pulled up (without dividing the falciform or triangular ligaments), using a fan retractor similar to that described for the thoracoscopic approach, and the surgeon using a grasper in the left hand and the scissors-electrocautery in the right hand, the hiatus is identified and the peritoneum overlying it is divided in a transverse fashion. We do not subscribe to the common procedure of opening the gastrohepatic ligament widely. Although this procedure facilitates exposure, it places both the branches of the left gastric artery and the branches of the nerve of Latarjet at risk. Furthermore, if a fundoplication is done, having divided the gastrohepatic ligament, the wrap may end over the stomach rather than the esophagus.

The next step is the identification of the esophagus (which again is aided greatly by having the endoscope in place) and the dissection of the esophagus from the diaphragmatic crus. At this point, it is important to identify (if not previously identified) and preserve the left (anterior) vagus at risk, particularly when performing the myotomy. Once the esophagus is exposed, the dissection is carried upward

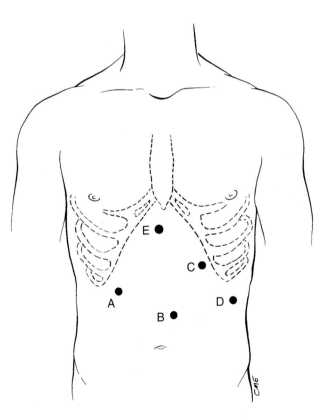

Figure 10. Trocar placement for laparoscopic myotomy. *A*, port used for the retraction of the left lobe of the liver; *B*, 2 in. above the umbilicus is used for the telescope, *C*, the instruments held with the surgeon's right hand; *D*, the Babcock clamp that will bring the esophagogastric junction down; *E*, the surgeon's left-handed instruments.

anteriorly and laterally, to expose sufficient length. The myotomy is otherwise carried out in a manner similar to that described above (Figs. 11, 12, and 13). When performing a laparoscopic approach the structures that support the antireflux mechanism are sacrificed. Thus, under those circumstances it may advisable to perform a partial wrap.

Postoperatively, the main source of complaint is the chest tube, which we remove in 24 hours, if possible. Oral feedings are usually started when the patient feels well enough to tolerate them. This usually occurs the evening of or the day after the operation. When done laparoscopically, the use of CO_2 may lead to some transient nausea. Since vomiting early after the operation may be deleterious, we try to prevent this by asking the patients how they feel before we start feedings, and we recommend that they be prudent in the type and amount of food they eat for the first few days. Patients can go home the second postoperative day and return to work within a week.

In our experience, patients are generally pain-free at the time of discharge from the hospital and able to resume regular activity within 1 week. Three patients complained of residual dysphagia postoperatively. Esophageal manometry revealed presence of a high-pressure zone of about 1 cm in length, indicating that the myotomy had not been extended enough distally. A laparoscopic myotomy was performed (all three had the first myotomy done through a thoracoscopic approach) with complete resolution of symptoms in two patients. In the third patient, dysphagia persisted despite the two myotomies, and, because he had a large, sigmoid esophagus, a total esophagectomy was performed. He can now swallow without difficulty. We subsequently learned how to gauge the extent of the myotomy, based on the endoscopic view from within the esophageal lumen, and this complication no longer occurs. Another patient developed a paraesophageal hernia, which required reoperation for repair 6 months after the Heller myotomy. At last follow-up, excellent (no dysphagia) or good (dysphagia less than once a week) results were obtained in 88% of patients (Table 1). It was found 90% of

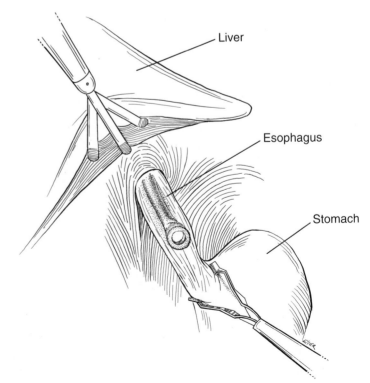

Figure 11. The left lobe of the liver is retracted upward, the esophagus is placed into view. The endoscope facilitates finding the esophagus and pulling its anterior wall forward.

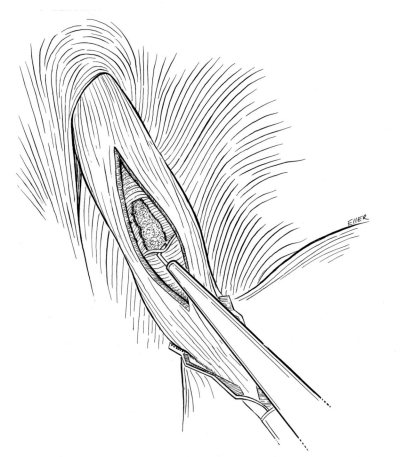

Figure 12. The myotomy from the laparoscopic approach.

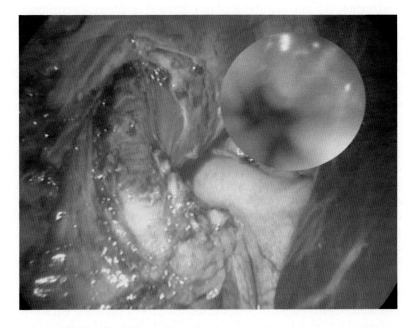

Figure 13. Intraoperative esophageal exposure during the course of a myotomy from the laparoscopic approach. The light on the end of the esophagoscope is clearly seen; the crura of the diaphragm have been separated from the esophagus.

Table 1. *Results of esophagomyotomy in 24 patients with achalasia*

Results	No. of patients	%
Excellent (no dysphagia)	17	71
Good (occasional dysphagia—less than once weekly)	4	17
Fair (occasional dysphagia—more than once weekly)	2	8
Poor (persistent dysphagia)	1	4

SURGICAL PEARLS

Use an endoscope. The use of the endoscope: *(a)* facilitates identification of the esophagus; *(b)* allows manipulation (lifting the wall, moving it, etc.); *(c)* determines when the obstruction has been completely relieved.

When dividing the circular muscle (inner layer) *lift each bundle far away from the mucosa* before activating the electrocautery unit. This way you will avoid thermal injury to the mucosa.

Beware of the lowermost part. When reaching the stomach, the fibers change in direction, and the mucosa thins out making it easier to enter the lumen. Go slow in this area, make certain you have lifted the muscle away from the mucosa and that the tip of the instrument is not engaging some of the mucosa distally.

Do a thorough functional workup of the patient beforehand. Only do this operation when the functional profile coincides with that of achalasia.

our patients have none or minimal dysphagia (excellent/none 71%; good/minimal dysphagia 18%).

▲ COMPLICATIONS

The most serious and most common complication that we have observed has been a laceration of the mucosa. This occurred in three of our patients and always in the lowermost site of the myotomy, at the level of the gastroesophageal junction. The perforation is immediately detected because the esophagus is distended with air during the operation. It is generally very small (1 or 2 mm). The hole can be closed with a single stitch (or two) of 4-0 absorbable suture. Since the stomach is close by, the closure may be reinforced with adjacent gastric wall tissue if needed. The first two times that this complication occurred, we chose to open the chest to repair the mucosa. It is surprising that the thoracostomy needed is small. The esophagus is mobilized, and the orifice is clearly visible. The hole can be closed using thoracoscopic suturing techniques.

Bleeding can occur on the entry sites—which is bothersome, particularly at the level of the telescope, since blood drips down slowly along the telescope and can obscure the vision substantially—and on the tissues adjacent to the esophagus. It is best to control bleeding as soon as it detected; in this area we usually induce coagulation. On the other hand, when bleeding points are close to the mucosa, we prefer to apply gentle pressure instead of coagulation and wait for the bleeding to stop. These bleeding points will usually stop without intervention, but coagulation in this area may be dangerous, as it could lead to thermal injury to the mucosa. An unrecognized burn to the mucosa may lead to a delayed esophageal perforation. Should this occur, the perforation should be handled as any other perforation of the esophagus.

Residual dysphagia is usually caused by the persistance of a narrowing in the lower part of the esophagus. In these cases, the myotomy has not been carried far enough. In our opinion, the endoscopic view of the obstruction allows adequate gauging of the extent needed. In fact, we continue our myotomy until it is clear that the obstruction has disappeared.

We have not added an antireflux procedure to the esophagomyotomy in these patients. It has been shown by others that extending the myotomy into the gastric wall for only 0.5 cm reduces the incidence of postoperative gastroesophageal reflux to around 3%. On the other hand, we were surprised by the finding that five of the eight patients, who received 24-hour pH monitoring postoperatively, showed evidence of abnormal reflux (all asymptomatic). However, in spite of the lack of peristalsis in the esophageal body, acid reflux was limited to the lower esophagus, suggesting that the volume of refluxate is very low. We think that a longer follow-up in a larger group of patients is necessary to determine if, in addition to the esophagomyotomy, an antireflux procedure is needed.

Postoperative manometry should be performed whenever possible to determine the level to which resistance has been decreased. In our patients, LES pressure decreased from 33.5 ± 7 to 14 ± 5 mmHg. The 24-hour pH monitoring is extremely important postoperatively, as asymptomatic reflux may occur.

Our experience shows that with minimally invasive techniques it is possible to perform an esophagomyotomy safely, achieving results that are similar to those obtained with open surgery. In addition, the hospital stay is short, the postoperative discomfort minimal, and the recovery is rapid with prompt return to work.

RECOMMENDED READING

1. Ferguson MK. Achalasia: current evaluation and therapy. *Ann Thorac Surg* 1991;42:336–342.
2. Csendes A, Braghetto I, Henriques A, Cortes C. Late results of a prospective randomized study comparing forceful dilatation and oesophagomyotomy in patients with achalasia. *Gut* 1989;30: 299–304.
3. Shimi S, Nathanson LK, Cushieri A. Laparoscopic cardiomyotomy for achalasia. *J R Coll Surg Edinb* 1991;36:152–154.
4. Pellegrini C, Wetter LA, Patti M, et al. Thoracoscopic esophagomyotomy: initial experience with a new approach for the treatment of achalasia. *Ann Surg* 1992;216:291–299.
5. Pellegrini CA, Leichter R, Patti M, Somberg K, Ostroff J, Way LW. Thoracoscopic esophageal myotomy in the treatment of achalasia. *Ann Thorac Cardiovasc Surg* 1993;56:680–682.

SECTION XII

FUTURE TECHNOLOGY

53

Future Directions

Richard M. Satava
Department of Surgery
Walter Reed Army Medical Center
Washington, D.C. 20307
Advanced Biomedical Technologies
Advanced Research Projects Agency (ARPA)
Arlington, Virginia 22203

Operative Laparoscopy and
Thoracoscopy, edited by
B. V. MacFadyen, Jr. and
J. L. Ponsky. Published by
Lippincott-Raven
Publishers, Philadelphia, 1996.

10. Satava RM. Robotics, telepresence and virtual reality: a critical analysis of the future of surgery. *Minimally Invasive Ther* 1992;1:357–363.
11. Satava RM. Speculation on future technology. In: Hunter JG, Sackier JE, eds. *High tech surgery: new approaches to old diseases*. New York: McGraw-Hill; 1993:339–347.
12. Satava RM. Surgery 2001: a technologic framework for the future. *Surg Endosc* 1993;7:111–113.
13. Satava RM. Virtual reality surgical simulator: the first steps. *Surg Endosc* 1993;7:203–205.
14. Sheridan TB: Telerobotics. *Automatica* 1989;25:487–507.
15. Sheridan TB. Defining our terms. *Presence* 1992;1:272–274.
16. Sheridan TB. Musings on telepresence and virtual presence. *Presence* 1992;1:120–125.
17. Timothy AG, Davies GL, Hibber RD, Wickham JEA. Use of robots in surgery: development of a frame for prostatectomy. *J Endourol* 1991;5:165–168.
18. Yeaple JA. Robot insects. *Pop Sci* 1991;3:52–56.

SUBJECT INDEX

ISBN 0-7817-0279-8